ESSENTIALS OF STRENGTH TRAINING AND CONDITIONING

National Strength and Conditioning Association

Thomas R. Baechle, EdD, CSCS
Creighton University, Omaha, Nebraska
Editor

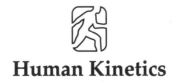

Human Kinetics

Library of Congress Cataloging-in-Publication Data

Essentials of strength training and conditioning / National Strength
    and Conditioning Association ; Thomas R. Baechle, editor.
        p.   cm.
    Includes index.
    ISBN 0-87322-694-1
    1. Physical education and training.   2. Muscle strength.
    3. Physical fitness--Physiological aspects.   I. Baechle, Thomas R.,
    1943-   .   II. National Strength & Conditioning Association (U.S.)
    GV711.5.E88   1994
    613.7'1--dc20   94-3915
                                                                            CIP

ISBN: 0-87322-694-1

Acquisitions Editor: Rick Frey, PhD
Developmental Editor: Christine Drews
Assistant Editor: Ed Giles
Copyeditor: Jay Thomas
Proofreaders: Kathy Bennett, Pam Johnson, Karin Leszczynski, Myla Smith, John Wentworth, Steve Wrone
Indexer: Theresa J. Schaefer
Production Director: Ernie Noa
Production Manager: Kris Slamans
Typesetters: Sandra Meier and Angela K. Snyder
Text Designer: Keith Blomberg
Layout Artist: Denise Lowry
Cover Designer: Jack Davis
Medical Illustrator: Katherine Galasyn-Wright
Artist for Line Drawings: Keith Blomberg
Artists for Computer-Generated Art: Thomas E. Janowski, Craig Ronto, Kathleen Boudreau-Fuoss, and Gretchen Walters
Printer: Braun-Brumfield

Printed in the United States of America   10 9 8 7 6 5 4

Human Kinetics
P.O. Box 5076, Champaign, IL 61825-5076
1-800-747-4457

Canada: Human Kinetics, Box 24040, Windsor, ON N8Y 4Y9
1-800-465-7301 (in Canada only)

Europe: Human Kinetics, P.O. Box IW14, Leeds LS16 6TR, United Kingdom
(44) 1132 781708

Australia: Human Kinetics, 2 Ingrid Street, Clapham 5062, South Australia
(08) 371 3755

New Zealand: Human Kinetics, P.O. Box 105-231, Auckland 1
(09) 523 3462

CONTENTS

CONTRIBUTORS

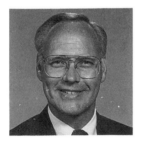

EDITOR

Thomas R. Baechle, EdD, CSCS, is the executive director of the Certified Strength and Conditioning Specialists (CSCS) Agency, the certifying body for the National Strength and Conditioning Association (NSCA). He has been a state and regional director of the organization, was president from 1983-1985, and served as its Director of Education from 1985-1990. He is an associate editor for NSCA's two periodicals—the *Journal of Strength and Conditioning Research* and *Strength and Conditioning*. In addition, he serves on NSCA's Tests and Measurements Committee, Research Committee, and Past President's Committee. Dr. Baechle has received various honors and awards from the NSCA, including the Outstanding Strength and Conditioning Professional of the Year in 1985. He is also a professor and chair of the Department of Exercise Sciences at Creighton University in Omaha, Nebraska.

For 16 years Dr. Baechle competed successfully in weightlifting and powerlifting, setting various Midwest records. For more than 20 years he has been involved in the strength training and conditioning of college athletes. Dr. Baechle is certified as a Level I weightlifting coach by the United States Weightlifting Federation, as a Certified Personal Trainer and Certified Strength and Conditioning Specialist by the CSCS Agency, and as an Exercise Test Technologist and Exercise Specialist by the American College of Sports Medicine (ACSM). He has written numerous articles and is the author of several popular texts on strength training. He has held various offices at the state and regional level in the American Alliance for Health, Physical Education, Recreation and Dance and is a member of NSCA, ACSM, National Association for Physical Education in Higher Education, and the National Organization for Competency Assurance.

CONTRIBUTORS

William B. Allerheiligen, MS, CSCS, earned his master's degree in physical education from the University of Wyoming in 1991 and is currently the NSCA's Director of Education. As a strength coach, Allerheiligen has held positions at the University of Nebraska, Kansas State University, Notre Dame University, and the University of Wyoming, as well as for the National Football League's Houston Oilers. He was also named National Strength Coach of the Year in 1988 by the NSCA. Allerheiligen has been a member of the board of directors for NSCA, co-chairman of the CSCS certification committee, and a lecturer at several NSCA national conferences.

Stephanie L. Armitage-Johnson, MS, CSCS, is currently an assistant strength coach at the University of

Washington. She earned her master's degree in physical education/coaching at Washington State University after completing research on female weightlifter training methods at the Hungarian Olympic Training Center for Weightlifting and Track and Field. Armitage-Johnson authored *Improved Work Performance and Injury Prevention for Firefighters*, and coauthored the NSCA Coaches Program clinic manual for volleyball conditioning for the National Volleyball Association.

Evan B. Brody, PhD, is owner and president of Performance Enhancement Consultants, Inc., a health and fitness consulting firm located in Silver Spring, Maryland. Brody has been a consultant to athletes in professional baseball and golf, an Olympic gold medalist, a Paralympic gold and bronze medal winner, and the NBA's Washington Bullets. He earned his master's degree in exercise physiology and his doctorate in kinesiology, with an emphasis in the psychology of sport and exercise, from the University of Maryland at College Park. Brody has 11 years of teaching experience at both the university and secondary-school levels, ranging from martial arts instruction to teaching courses on strength and conditioning, stress reduction, and sport psychology. He has published and presented nationally and internationally on topics including the psychophysiology of skilled athletic performance in marksmen and runners and the use of mental preparation strategies to enhance strength performance.

Michael S. Conley, MS, is a NASA pre-doctoral fellow in the Muscle Biology Lab at the University of Georgia and has presented at meetings of the NSCA, ACSM, and ASMA. Conley recently earned his master's degree in exercise science at Appalachian State University in Boone, North Carolina, where he was a research assistant in the Exercise Physiology Lab. Conley was also a sports science intern at the United States Olympic Training Center in Colorado Springs, Colorado.

Brian P. Conroy, MA, CSCS, is currently a medical student at the University of Nebraska Medical Center in Omaha. His research and publications cover the topics of bone mineral density adaptations to heavy resistance exercise, the interaction of parathyroid hormone treatment and mechanical loading on bone formation, and the biochemical analysis of Type II collagen defects in chondrodysplasia. Conroy earned his master's degree in exercise science from the University of Connecticut in Storrs.

Gary A. Dudley, PhD, CSCS, is currently on the faculty of the Department of Exercise Science at the University of Georgia. He is an applied muscle physiologist with more than 80 publications and reviews focusing on exercise and muscle. Dudley received his PhD in 1978 from the Ohio State University.

Roger W. Earle, MA, CSCS, earned his master's degree from the University of Nebraska at Omaha in 1991. He currently is the head strength and conditioning coach and is on the faculty of the Exercise Science Department at Creighton University in Omaha. He is also a member of the NSCA–Certified Personal Trainer certification examination committee and is the director of the Nebraska NSCA. Earle is coauthor of *Fitness Weight Training*, an upcoming book from Human Kinetics.

Karl E. Friedl, PhD, is a research physiologist and currently a Science & Technology Staff Officer at the headquarters of the U.S. Army Medical Research and Development Command, Fort Detrick, Maryland. Previously he was assigned to the Occupational Physiology Division at the U.S. Army Research Institute of Environmental Medicine in Natick, Massachusetts. Friedl received his doctorate in physiology from the University of California, Santa Barbara in 1984.

Everett Harman, PhD, CSCS, is a research physiologist and head of biomechanics research at the U.S. Army Research Institute of Environmental Medicine in Natick, Massachusetts. He was NSCA's vice-president for research from 1991 to 1994, and is associate editor for the *Journal of Strength and Conditioning Research* and the *National Strength and Conditioning Association Journal*. Harman earned his PhD from the University of Massachusetts in 1984.

Robert T. Harris, PhD, is a research assistant professor in the department of physiology at Marshall University in Huntington, West Virginia, where he is also a postdoctoral research associate in the division of health, physical education, and recreation. Harris received his doctorate in physiology from Ohio University in 1992. In a majority of his research, Harris has utilized high-level electrical stimulation of human skeletal muscle as a tool to investigate the influence of neural factors on the expression of muscular torque. He has also used magnetic resonance imaging and electromyograms to study patterns of muscle use during different types of muscle action.

Bradley D. Hatfield, PhD, is an associate professor of kinesiology with an emphasis in exercise and sport psychology at the University of Maryland at College Park. His research has focused on the mental states of elite athletes as well as the effects of aerobic exercise upon the aging of the brain. Subscribing to a biological psychology approach, Hatfield has published a number of papers on psychophysiological aspects of sport performance and exercise psychology. He has extensive speaking experience, nationally and internationally, and has consulted with a number of professional athletic teams on both physical and mental training.

Jean Barrett Holloway, MA, CSCS, is an instructor and advisory board member for UCLA Extension's Certificated Program in Fitness Instruction. She earned her master's degree in developmental kinesiology from the University of Southern California and has published research exploring the relationship of physical strength to self-esteem. Holloway has served as chair of the women's committee and state director of Southern California for NSCA, and received the NSCA President's Award in 1988. She has also competed, coached, and officiated in the sport of Olympic-style weightlifting.

Gary R. Hunter, PhD, CSCS, has published over 100 papers focusing on body composition, high-intensity exercise, and metabolism. He is currently director of the Exercise Physiology Laboratory at the University of Alabama at Birmingham. Hunter earned his master's degree and doctorate from Michigan State University, and has been a coach, researcher, and educator for over 20 years.

William J. Kraemer, PhD, CSCS, is the director of research in the Center for Sports Medicine and an associate professor of applied physiology at the Pennsylvania State University. Kraemer is a past president of the NSCA, which also recognized him with the Outstanding Sport Scientist Award in 1992. He is a member of several other professional organizations and societies, including the American College of Sports Medicine (ACSM), of which he is a fellow and member of the board of trustees. He has published over 100 scientific manuscripts and two books.

Fred Roll, BS, CSCS, has been Strength and Conditioning Coordinator at the University of Kansas since 1989. He was coordinator at Tulane University from 1983 to 1989, and was Assistant Strength Coach at Clemson University prior to 1983. Roll earned his degree from East Carolina University, focusing his studies on health and physical education. He served on the CSCS Role Delineation Committee and has published several articles.

Douglas M. Semenick, MS, CSCS, currently runs his own health and wellness consulting firm, Semenick and Associates, Inc., in Louisville, Kentucky. He also has 12 years of college coaching experience, garnering the NSCA's Strength and Conditioning Coach of the Year Award in 1987. Semenick has published over 30 articles in the field of fitness and wellness and is currently working toward his doctorate of education.

Michael H. Stone, PhD, CSCS, is currently president-elect of the NSCA, chairman of the Sports Science and Medical Committee of the U.S. Weightlifting Federation, and a member of the International Weightlifting Federation's Sports Science and Research Committee. He is also a professor of exercise science at Appalachian State University in Boone, North Carolina. His research focuses primarily on strength/power performance with emphasis on the effects of strength/power performance on the endocrine system. Stone was a competitive weightlifter from 1965 to 1982, ranking in the top 10 in his weight class during the late 1970s and early 1980s. He was also the strength and conditioning coach at Louisiana State University from 1977 to 1980.

Dan Wathen, MS, ATC, CSCS, has published over 60 articles focusing on sports medicine and conditioning. He has been athletic trainer and conditioning coordinator at Youngstown State University in Youngstown, Ohio, since 1976. In 1989 Wathen was named Strength Coach of the Year by the NSCA membership.

Mark A. Williams, PhD, has authored 74 publications—including 2 books—focusing on cardiovascular disease, exercise training, the elderly, and exercise and cardiovascular medication interactions. He is an associate professor and director of cardiovascular disease prevention and rehabilitation at the Creighton University School of Medicine in Omaha, Nebraska. Williams is currently the president and a fellow of the American Association of Cardiovascular and Pulmonary Rehabilitation and is a fellow of the American College of Sports Medicine.

REVIEWERS

Damon Burton, PhD
University of Idaho

Donald A. Chu, PhD, PT, ATC, CSCS
Ather Sports Injury Clinic
Castro Valley, California

Roger Earle, MA, CSCS
Creighton University
Omaha, Nebraska

Steven J. Fleck, PhD, CSCS
U.S. Olympic Committee
Colorado Springs, Colorado

Andrew C. Fry, PhD, CSCS
Ohio University

Everett Harman, PhD, CSCS
U.S. Army Research Institute of Environmental
    Medicine
Natick, Massachusetts

Reed Humphrey, PhD
Medical College of Virginia
Virginia Commonwealth University
Richmond, Virginia

Robert E. Keith, PhD
Auburn University

William J. Kraemer, PhD, CSCS
The Pennsylvania State University

Jeffrey E. Lander, PhD
Life College
Marietta, Georgia

Carl M. Maresh, PhD
University of Connecticut

John P. McCarthy, PhD, CSCS
NASA Johnson Space Center
Houston, Texas

Bruno Pauletto, MS, CSCS
University of Tennessee

Ralph Rozenek, PhD
California State University, Long Beach

Per A. Tesch, PhD
Karolinska Institutet
Stockholm, Sweden

William T. Weinberg, PhD
University of Louisville

PREFACE

The ultimate goal for strength and conditioning professionals and other sports medicine specialists—athletic trainers, physical therapists, physician assistants, and physicians—is to help individuals achieve maximal physical performance without incurring injury. *Essentials of Strength Training and Conditioning* provides up-to-date information toward that goal. It serves not only undergraduate and graduate students preparing for careers in strength training and conditioning but also individuals who directly or indirectly work with athletes.

This text grew out of a realization that no one source on strength training and conditioning existed that captured the views of experts in physiology, exercise physiology, neurology, biochemistry, anatomy, biomechanics, and endocrinology, and related the principles of these disciplines to the challenge of designing safe and effective training programs. Early on, the scarcity of relevant, reliable studies hampered efforts to develop such a text. Even now there are more questions than answers—yet headway has been made. Although this text is not the ultimate answer, it is the best resource to date and will serve as a reference for further research and discussion. It will be an ideal resource for individuals preparing for both the Certified Strength and Conditioning Specialist (CSCS) and the NSCA–Certified Personal Trainer certification examinations.

It is important that such an organization as the NSCA takes the lead in developing a resource for strength and conditioning professionals. With more than 9,000 members in over 47 countries, including a sister association in Japan, the NSCA is an international clearinghouse for strength training and conditioning research, theories, and practices. It is the worldwide authority in this vital research. Furthermore, the CSCS Agency, which is the certifying body for the NSCA, has the only fitness-related certification programs to be accredited by the National Commission for Certifying Agencies, a nongovernmental, nonprofit agency (in Washington, DC) that sets national standards for certifying agencies.

Some of the world's most respected authors and reviewers contributed to this text, among them renowned researchers and practitioners. This is the first textbook on strength training and conditioning to pool such expertise. Whether used for learning the essentials of strength training and conditioning, preparing for a certification examination, or consulting a professional reference, *Essentials of Strength Training and Conditioning* will help practitioners to develop and administer sound, state-of-the-art training programs.

CREDITS

Figure 11.2 Reprinted from *Nutrition Research*, **10**, L. Bucci, J.F. Hickson, J.M. Pivarnik, I. Wolinsky, J.C. McMahon, and S.D. Turner, "Ornithine Ingestion and Growth Hormone Release in Bodybuilders," pp. 239-245, copyright 1990, with permission from Elsevier Science Ltd., Pergamon Imprint, The Boulevard, Langford Lane, Kidlington 0X5 1GB, United Kingdom.

Table 17.2 From "Testing and Evaluation" by D. Semenick, 1981, *NSCA Journal*, **2**(2), pp. 8-9. Adapted by permission of the National Strength and Conditioning Association.

Vertical Jump Test From "Tests and Measurements: Vertical Jump" by D. Semenick, 1990, *NSCA Journal*, **12**(3), pp. 68-69. Adapted by permission of the National Strength and Conditioning Association.

Figure 17.5 and Line Drill for Basketball Test From "Sport-Specific Test for Basketball: Line Drill Test" by D. Semenick, 1990, *NSCA Journal*, **12**(2), pp. 47-49. Adapted by permission of the National Strength and Conditioning Association.

Figure 17.6 and 300-Yard Shuttle Run Test From "300 Yard Shuttle Run" by G.M. Gilliam, 1983, *NSCA Journal*, **5**(5), p. 46. Adapted by permission of the National Strength and Conditioning Association.

Figure 17.7 and T-Test From "Tests and Measurements: The T-test" by D. Semenick, 1990, *NSCA Journal*, **12**(1), pp. 36-37. Adapted by permission of the National Strength and Conditioning Association.

Table 18.1 From Ted A. Baumgartner and Andrew S. Jackson, *Measurement for Evaluation in Physical Education and Exercise Science*, 3d ed. Copyright © 1987 Wm. C. Brown Communications, Inc., Dubuque, Iowa. All Rights Reserved. Reprinted by permission.

Table 20.3 From *Jumping Into Plyometrics* (p. 14) by D.A. Chu. Champaign, IL: Leisure Press. Copyright 1992 by Donald A. Chu. Reprinted by permission of Human Kinetics.

Table 22.2 From "Exercise and Training in Childhood and Adolescence" by H.C.G. Kemper. In *Current Therapy in Sports Medicine*, 2nd ed., by Torg, Welch, and Shepard (Eds.), 1990, St. Louis: Mosby. Reprinted by permission of Mosby.

Table 23.2 Adapted from *Sports Illustrated Strength Training* by John Garhammer. Copyright © 1987, Time, Inc. All rights reserved.

Table 24.2 From "Prevention of Anterior Cruciate Ligament Injuries" by J. Moore and G. Wade, 1989, *NSCA Journal*, **11**(3), pp. 35-40. Adapted by permission of the National Strength and Conditioning Association.

Figure 26.1 From *Designing Resistance Training Programs* (p. 61) by S.J. Fleck and W.J. Kraemer, Champaign, IL: Human Kinetics. Copyright 1987 by Stephen J. Fleck and William J. Kraemer. Reprinted by permission.

Table 26.3 From "Let's Talk Training #2: Intensity" by B. Pauletto, 1986, *NSCA Journal*, **8**(1), p. 37. Adapted by permission of the National Strength and Conditioning Association.

Table 26.4, Figure 27.1, Figure 27.2, and Table 28.1 From *Weight Training* by M. Stone and H. O'Bryant, 1987, Minneapolis: Burgess International. Adapted by permission.

Figures 30.3 and 30.4 From "Periodization Roundtable, Part 2" by A. Chargina, M. Stone, J. Piedmonte, H. O'Bryant, W.J. Kraemer, et al., 1987, *NSCA Journal*, **8**(6), pp. 17-24. Adapted by permission.

Weight Room Policies From *Huskies History Questionnaire* by University of Washington Athletic Department, 1991. Adapted by permission.

Shared Responsibility for Sport Safety From *Shared Responsibility Form for Sport Safety: Assumption of Risk* by University of Washington Athletic Department, 1993. Adapted by permission.

PAR-Q and You Reprinted in part from the 1994 revised version of the Physical Activity Readiness Questionnaire (PAR-Q and YOU) by special permission from the Canadian Society for Exercise Physiology. Copyright 1994, CSEP.

Risk Factor Questionnaire and **Health and Fitness History** From *The Stairmaster Fitness Handbook: A User's Guide* by J.A. Peterson and C.X. Bryant, 1992, Indianapolis, IN: Masters Press. Copyright 1992 by Masters Press. Adapted by permission.

Several figures throughout chapter 21 are reprinted from *Weight Training: Steps to Success* by T.R. Baechle and B.R. Groves, Champaign, IL: Leisure Press. Copyright 1992 by Leisure Press. Reprinted by permission of Human Kinetics. In order of appearance in this text, original figure numbers are 2.1, 2.2, 7.1a, 5.1b, A.3a, 4.1a-d, 4.3a-c, A.10b, 9.2a-c, 6.1a-c, 6.2a-c, and A.6a and c.

FROM THE EDITOR

The completion of this book could not have occurred without the significant commitment of many people. It was a project in which the authors willingly gave of their expertise and time to make a lasting contribution to the NSCA. All who read this book are indebted to them for their efforts.

Thanks also go to Janet Owens and Dan Brown, who helped sustain vital communication between Chris Drews at Human Kinetics, the authors, and myself. Chris Drews' expertise, patience, and intelligent decision-making provided the direction that was absolutely essential for this project.

As one might suspect by looking at the nature and scope of this text, it was an arduous task, and one that at times was not universally accepted as being important to complete. Nevertheless, strong leadership prevailed and the strength and conditioning profession now has another significant learning resource.

Through the process of developing and completing this project, I have gained an even greater appreciation of my friends, particularly Roger Earle, Dr. William Kraemer, Dr. Donald Chu, and Dan Wathen. These individuals not only provided needed expertise, but more importantly gave their unyielding support to the project. It was this support that ultimately made this text a reality. I dedicate this text to them and their families and to my very best friends—my wife, Susan, and sons, Todd and Clark.

PART I

CONCEPTS AND APPLICATIONS OF THE EXERCISE SCIENCES

CHAPTER 1

MUSCLE PHYSIOLOGY

Gary R. Hunter

This chapter provides an overview of how muscles work to create forces across joints and cause movement. Understanding the physiology of muscle is basic to developing and implementing training programs. At the simplest level, the strength and conditioning professional is concerned with the function of the muscle. Many systems, including the cardiovascular, nervous, and endocrine, affect the function of muscle, but muscle is the organ that creates movement.

MUSCLE MICROSTRUCTURE AND MACROSTRUCTURE

Each skeletal muscle is an organ that contains muscle tissue, connective tissue, nerves, and blood vessels. Fibrous connective tissue, or **epimysium**, covers the body's more than 430 skeletal muscles. The epimysium is continuous with the tendons at the ends of the muscle (Figure 1.1). The tendon is attached to bone **periosteum**, a specialized connective tissue covering all bones; any contraction of the muscle pulls on the tendon and, in turn, the bone. Limb muscles have two attachments to bone: **proximal** (closer to the trunk) and **distal** (farther from the trunk). The two attachments of trunk muscles are termed **superior** (closer to the head) and **inferior** (closer to the feet). By convention, the **origin** of a muscle is defined as the attachment of the muscle that is more proximal or superior, and the **insertion** is defined as the attachment that is more distal or inferior.

Muscle cells, often called **muscle fibers**, are long (sometimes running the entire length of a muscle), cylindrical cells 50 to 100 μm in diameter (about the diameter of a human hair). These fibers have many nuclei situated on the periphery of the cell and have a striated appearance under low magnification. Under the epimysium, the muscle fibers are grouped in bundles (called **fasciculi**) that may consist of up to 150 fibers, with the bundles surrounded by connective tissue called the **perimysium**. Each muscle fiber is surrounded by connective tissue called **endomysium**, which encircles and is continuous with the fiber's membrane, or **sarcolemma** (24). All the connective tissue—epimysium, perimysium, and endomysium—is continuous with the tendon, so tension developed in one muscle cell can develop tension in the tendon (see Figure 1.1).

The junction between a motor neuron (nerve cell) and the muscle fibers it innervates is called the motor end plate, or, more often, the **neuromuscular junction** (Figure 1.2). Each muscle cell has only one neuromuscular junction, although a single motor neuron innervates many muscle fibers, sometimes as many as several hundred. A motor neuron and the muscle fibers it innervates are called a **motor unit**. All the muscle fibers of a motor unit contract together when they are stimulated by the motor neuron.

The interior structure of a muscle fiber is depicted in Figure 1.3. The **sarcoplasm**—the term used for the cytoplasm of a muscle fiber—contains contractile components, which consist of protein filaments; other proteins; stored glycogen and fat particles; enzymes; and specialized structures such as mitochondria and the sarcoplasmic reticulum.

Hundreds to thousands of **myofibrils** (each about 1 μm in diameter, 1/100 the diameter of a hair) dominate the sarcoplasm. Myofibrils contain the apparatus that contracts the muscle cell, which consists primarily of two types of **myofilaments**: **myosin** and **actin**. The

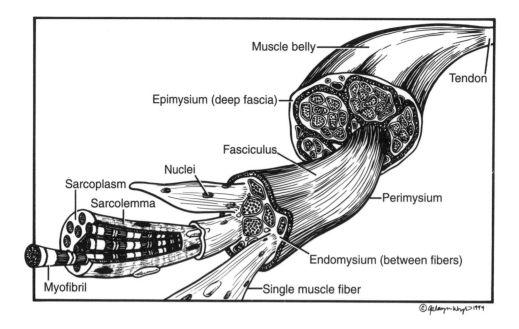

Figure 1.1 Schematic drawing of a muscle illustrating three types of connective tissue: epimysium (the outer layer), perimysium (surrounding each fasciculus, or group of fibers), and endomysium (surrounding individual fibers).

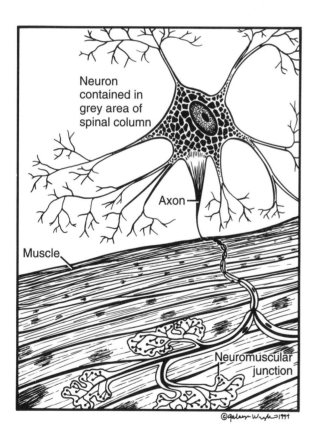

Figure 1.2 A motor unit, consisting of a motor neuron and the muscle fibers it innervates. There are typically many more than three muscle fibers in a single motor unit.

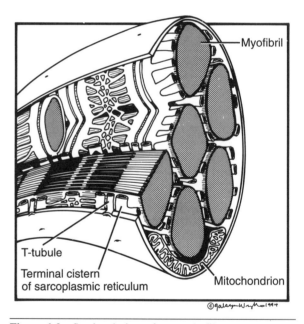

Figure 1.3 Sectional view of a muscle fiber.

myosin filaments (thick filaments about 16 nm in diameter, about 1/10,000 the diameter of a hair) contain up to 200 myosin molecules. Globular heads called **cross-bridges** protrude away from the myosin filament at regular intervals. The actin filaments (thin filaments about 6 nm in diameter) consist of two strands arranged in a double helix. Myosin and actin filaments are organized longitudinally in the smallest contractile unit of skeletal muscle, the **sarcomere**. Sarcomeres average

2.6 μm in length and are repeated the entire length of the muscle fiber.

Figure 1.4 shows the structure and orientation of the myosin and actin in the sarcomere. Adjacent myosin filaments anchor with each other at the M-bridge in the center of the sarcomere (center of the H-zone). Actin filaments are aligned at both ends of the sarcomere and are anchored at the Z-line. Z-lines are repeated through the entire myofibril. Six actin filaments surround each myosin filament and three myosin filaments surround each actin filament. A typical myofibril will contain about 450 myosin (thick) filaments in the center of a sarcomere and 900 actin (thin) filaments at either end of the sarcomere (19). There are additional filaments present in skeletal muscle that probably assist in maintaining the structural integrity of the muscle (23), but description of this filament system is beyond the scope of this chapter.

It is the arrangement of the mysoin and actin filaments and the Z-lines of the sarcomeres that gives skeletal muscle its alternating dark and light pattern—its striated appearance. The dark band (A-band) corresponds with the alignment of the myosin filaments, while the light band (I-band) corresponds with the areas in two adjacent sarcomeres that contain only actin filaments (2). The Z-line is in the middle of the I-band and causes the appearance of a thin dark line running longitudinally through the I-band (2). The H-zone is the area in the center of the sarcomere where only myosin filaments are present. During muscle contraction, the H-zone will decrease as the actin slides over the myosin toward the center of the sarcomere. The I-band will also decrease as the Z-lines are pulled toward the center of the sarcomere.

Parallel to and surrounding each myofibril is an intricate system of tubules called the **sarcoplasmic reticulum** that terminate as vesicles in the vicinity of the Z-lines (see Figure 1.3). Calcium ions are stored in the vesicles. It is through the regulation of calcium that muscular contraction is controlled. **T-tubules**, short for transverse tubules, run perpendicular to the sarcoplasmic reticulum and terminate in the vicinity of the Z-line and between two vesicles. This pattern of a T-tubule spaced between and perpendicular to two sarcoplasmic reticular vesicles is called a **triad**. Since the T-tubules run between outlying myofibrils and are open to the sarcolemma at the surface of the cell, discharge of an action potential (an electrical impulse) from the surface to all depths of the muscle fiber is nearly simultaneous. Thus, calcium is released throughout the muscle, producing a coordinated contraction.

SLIDING-FILAMENT THEORY OF MUSCULAR CONTRACTION

In its simplest form, the **sliding-filament theory** states that the actin filaments at each end of the sarcomere slide inward on myosin filaments, pulling the Z-lines toward the center of the sarcomere and thus shortening the muscle fiber (Figure 1.5); as actin filaments slide over myosin filaments, the H-zone and I-band shrink. The flexion of myosin cross-bridges as they pull on the actin filaments is responsible for the movement of the actin filament. Since only a very small displacement of the actin filament occurs with each flexion of the myosin cross-bridge, very rapid, repeated flexions must occur in many cross-bridges throughout the entire muscle for measurable movement to occur (19).

Before myosin cross-bridges can flex they must first attach to the actin filament. When the sarcoplasmic reticulum is stimulated to release calcium ions, they bind with **troponin**, a protein situated at regular intervals along the actin filament that has a high affinity for calcium ions (see Figure 1.4). This causes a shift to occur in another protein molecule, **tropomyosin**, which runs along the length of the actin filament in the groove of the double helix. The myosin cross-bridge head now attaches much more rapidly to the actin filament, allowing cross-bridge flexion to occur (3).

The energy for cross-bridge flexion comes from the hydrolysis (breakdown) of adenosine triphosphate (ATP) to adenosine diphosphate (ADP) and phosphate, a reaction catalyzed by the enzyme myosin ATPase. Another molecule of ATP must replace the ADP on the myosin cross-bridge head for the head to detach from the actin active site and recock. This allows the contraction process to be continued (if calcium is available to bind to the troponin molecule) or relaxation to occur (if calcium is not available). (It may be noted that calcium plays a role in regulating a large number of events in skeletal muscle besides contraction. These include glycolytic and oxidative energy metabolism, as well as protein synthesis and degradation [14].)

Measurable muscle shortening transpires only when this sequence of events—binding of calcium to troponin, coupling of the myosin cross-bridge with actin, cross-bridge flexion, dissociation of actin and myosin, and recocking of the myosin cross-bridge head—is repeated over and over again throughout the muscle fiber. This occurs as long as calcium is available in the myofibril, ATP is available to assist in uncoupling the myosin from the actin, and sufficient active myosin ATPase is available for catalysing the breakdown of ATP.

Resting Phase

Under normal resting conditions little calcium is present in the myofibril (most of it is stored in the sarcoplasmic reticulum), so very few of the myosin cross-bridges are bound to actin. No tension is developed in the muscle, so the muscle is said to be at rest.

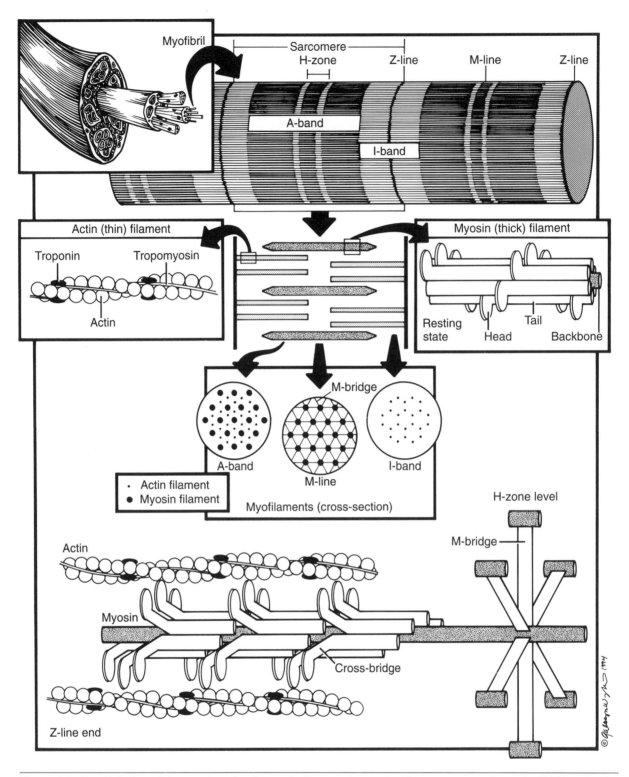

Figure 1.4 Detailed view of the myosin and actin protein filaments in muscle. The arrangement of myosin (thick) and actin (thin) filaments gives skeletal muscle its striated appearance.

TYPES OF MUSCLE ACTION

Concentric actions occur when the total tension developed in all the cross-bridges of a muscle is sufficient to overcome any resistance to shortening. During the upward phase of a biceps curl, for example, the cross-bridges in the biceps brachii and the other elbow flexors overcome the resistance of the barbell, arm, and hand.

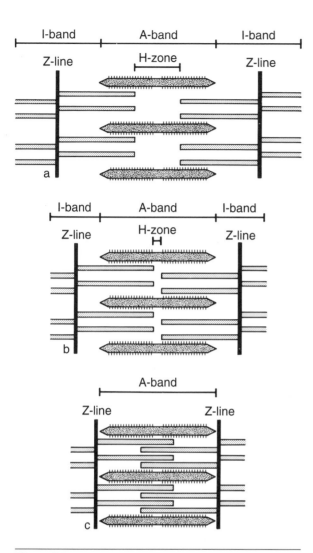

Figure 1.5 Contraction of a myofibril. (a) In stretched muscle, the I-bands and H-zone are elongated, and there is low force potential due to reduced cross-bridge–actin alignment. (b) When muscle contacts (here, partially), the I-bands and H-zone are shortened. There is high force potential due to optimal cross-bridge–actin alignment. (c) With completely contracted muscle, there is low force potential due to reduced cross-bridge–actin alignment.

Isometric actions* occur when the tension in the cross-bridges equals the resistance to shortening and the muscle length remains relatively constant. **Eccentric actions*** occur when the tension developed in the cross-bridges is less than the resistance, and the muscle lengthens despite contact between the myosin cross-bridge heads and the actin filaments (17). During the slow, controlled downward phase of the biceps curl, the cross-bridges within the elbow flexors exert enough force to slow the descent of the barbell, but exert insufficient force to stop the descent or raise the barbell.

Relaxation

Relaxation occurs when the stimulation of the motor nerve stops. Calcium is pumped back into the sarcoplasmic reticulum, which prevents the link between the actin and myosin molecules. Relaxation is brought about by the return of the actin and myosin filaments to their unbound state.

FORCE PRODUCTION

Several factors affect the generation of force within a muscle. The intent of this section is to provide strength and conditioning professionals with an introduction to some of the more salient factors.

Physiological Factors

In all likelihood, force production by a muscle is proportional to the number of cross-bridges that are attached to the actin filaments at any one time (22). A greater amount of calcium in a myofibril results in more myosin cross-bridge heads binding with actin filaments and thus more tension in that muscle. The amount of calcium released from the sarcoplasmic reticulum vesicles is related to how frequently the innervating motor neuron stimulates the muscle. Increased frequency of stimulation of a motor unit results in increased force production of that motor unit. The number of active motor units can also affect force production (the greater the number of active motor units, the greater the force production). In short, force production is controlled in two main ways: frequency of stimulation of motor units and number of motor units activated. It is possible that some training-induced increases in strength may occur because of increases in neural activation of motor units (16,21).

When we measure strength in a human we are measuring force output at the end of a lever (e.g., the hand during an arm curl). The measurement of force at the hand can be affected by activity of both the elbow flexors and antagonist elbow extensors. The flexors increase flexion force at the hand; the extensors decrease flexion force at the hand. Several recent studies have shown that antagonist muscle is active during human movement, presumably to maintain joint stability during muscular contraction (1,5,11). It is possible that training-mediated decreases in antagonist activity also affect strength (4).

---

*The NSCA chooses to avoid the use of the word *contraction* to describe eccentric and isometric muscle activity because *contraction* is defined as shortening, a phenomenon that occurs in neither of these types of muscle activity.

Although the release of the calcium ions and binding of myosin to actin occur very rapidly, the process does not occur instantaneously in all the motor units or at all the myosin cross-bridge heads. It takes some time for all the potential myosin cross-bridge heads to make contact with actin filaments. Variation in nerve conduction and in myosin cross-bridge cycling velocities between ''fast'' and ''slow'' muscle fibers (3) also affects the number of cross-bridge heads bound to actin filaments. This means that maximal force production in a muscle does not occur instantaneously. Consequently, maximal force production may not occur early in the range of motion, especially during fast movements.

Since high force development may be important in strength development, development of strength may be retarded under training conditions that do not allow high-tension development in the early part of the range of motion. High tension is developed in muscle even before movement occurs when lifting weights because the weights must be supported isometrically. This is called *preloading*. In addition, no movement can occur until sufficient force is developed in the muscle to overcome the inertia of the barbell. Preloading and inertia insure high tension development early in the range of motion. Accommodating-resistance apparatuses, such as hydraulic and isokinetic systems, do not load the muscle prior to the contraction. Research indicates that preloading during training may be important in the development of strength early in the range of motion (12).

Since neural activation controls calcium release from the sarcoplasmic reticulum, any factor that affects the neural activation of the muscle will influence the application of force within that muscle. For example, motivation, excitatory reflex activity, and inhibitory reflex activity all influence the activity of the motor neuron. These factors will be discussed in detail in chapter 2.

Cross-Sectional Area

The maximum force capability of a muscle is believed to be related to the cross-sectional area of the muscle. Muscles that have larger cross-sectional areas have larger numbers of sarcomeres in parallel, more potential cross-bridge heads in contact with actin molecules, and more potential for applying force. On the other hand, more sarcomeres in series (thus a longer muscle) increase the potential velocity of shortening (7), because all sarcomeres shorten at the same time (e.g., two sarcomeres in series could potentially shorten the ends of the muscle 2 times as far in the same amount of time as only one sarcomere).

Velocity of Shortening

Force production is inversely related to velocity of shortening during concentric actions (Figure 1.6); in other words, during faster movements, less force production is possible, and when lifting heavier loads, slower movements will occur (6). This is probably due to a smaller number of cross-bridge contacts on actin filaments at any instant as the velocity of shortening increases (3).

The relationship is different for eccentric actions. As the velocity of eccentric actions increases, maximal force production also increases. The force capabilities are typically 120% to 160% greater in eccentric actions than in concentric actions (10). This means that when overloading eccentrically, very heavy resistances may be needed, but when training for explosive concentric movements, relatively light resistance may be more suitable.

Angle of Pennation

Not all muscle has sarcomeres aligned along the long axis of the muscle (17,18). Some muscle is *pennate* (Figure 1.7), and the angle of pennation can affect the number of sarcomeres per cross-sectional area and thus the maximal force capabilities. Any factor that affects angle of pennation would thus affect strength and velocity of shortening as long as the cross-sectional area remains the same. Muscles with greater pennation have more sarcomeres in parallel and fewer sarcomeres in series; they are therefore better able to generate force but have a lower shortening velocity than nonpennate muscle (20). Angle of pennation may vary depending on hereditary factors and even training, which could help account for some of the differences in strength and speed seen in individuals who seem to have muscles of the same size.

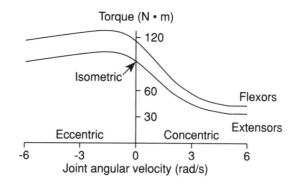

Figure 1.6 Force-velocity curve for eccentric and concentric actions. *Note.* From ''Force-Velocity Relationship in Human Elbow Flexors and Extensors'' by K. Jorgensen. In *Biomechanics V-A* (p. 147) by P.V. Komi (Ed.), 1976. Baltimore: University Park Press.

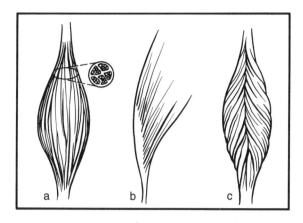

Figure 1.7 Three of the possible arrangements of muscle fibers. (a) Muscle fibers are parallel to the tendon. (b) Unipennate muscle. One set of muscle fibers is at an oblique angle to the tendon. (c) Bipennate muscle. Muscle fibers are aligned on either side of the muscle at an oblique angle to the tendon.

Sarcomere and Muscle Length

The number of myosin cross-bridge heads that can align with active sites on an actin filament at any given time is dependent on the relative length of the sarcomere or the relative length (percentage of contraction) of the muscle. When a sarcomere is very short, potential maximal force is reduced because actin filaments overlap, reducing the actin active sites that are available for myosin cross-bridge contact. When a sarcomere is relatively long, potential maximal force is also reduced because potential actin active sites are beyond the reach of the myosin cross-bridge heads. But when the sarcomere is at its approximate resting length, the optimal number of myosin cross-bridge heads can align with actin active sites and maximal force potential is greatest for that muscle (see Figure 1.5). This means the amount of force that a muscle can exert is related to its length. Peak force production is usually seen at resting or slightly greater than resting length. This is known as the **length-tension relationship** of muscle (8).

It has been speculated that the length-tension relationship is not constant and may adapt to specific demands. Indeed, recent comparison of the length-tension relationship of competitive cyclists and runners shows consistent differences. It is impossible to tell at this time whether the differences are due to adaptations of muscle to training or inherited differences (9).

Torque

The integration of the length-tension relationship and differences in mechanical advantage in the joint lever system contribute to variations in the maximal torque that can be produced through the range of motion of any joint. The *torque-position curve* (the graph of torque vs. position within a range of motion) is discussed in detail in chapter 3; however, it is pointed out here that an understanding of the relationship between torque and joint position is important for development of proper technique in all sport activities.

Prestretching

Prestretching a muscle just prior to a concentric action can enhance force production during the subsequent contraction (15). The increase in force production is called *stretch-shortening potentiation* or, more commonly, the **stretch-shortening cycle**. This enhancement is probably caused by the combined effects of the use of elastic energy in the muscle (primarily from stretching the myosin cross-bridges) and stretch-reflex potentiation (activation of the myotatic stretch reflex caused by a rapid stretch) of muscle (15). The stretch-shortening cycle is a very important phenomenon in sport, since it occurs so frequently and is an integral component of such activities as running, jumping, throwing, and striking (see chapter 20 for more information about the stretch-shortening cycle). Techniques and training programs for optimizing the use of the stretch-shortening cycle are important in developing superior performance in athletes.

Stretching a two-joint muscle at one joint may increase the muscle's ability to generate force at the other joint. For example, the hamstring not only is stronger but uses less energy during knee flexion with the hip flexed than with the hip extended (13). The improved function of the hamstring seems to be related not only to the length-tension relationship of the hamstring but to the use of elastic energy in the stretched muscle (13). It appears that muscle may use elastic energy gained even from a static stretch.

CONCLUSION

The strength and conditioning professional needs to be aware that many factors affect contraction of individual muscle fibers. Several questions should be answered before a sport-specific training program can be developed. What is the speed of the muscle action? Is the action concentric, isometric, or eccentric? Is the muscle stretched prior to the action? Through what range of motion does the action occur? Is the muscle preloaded prior to the action? Answering these questions should help the professional understand how the muscle functions in any sport and allow him or her to develop programs that will assist the athlete in obtaining specific training adaptations.

Key Terms

actin	3	motor unit	3	sarcoplasm	3
concentric action	6	muscle fiber	3	sarcoplasmic reticulum	5
cross-bridge	4	myofibril	3	sliding-filament theory	5
distal	3	myofilament	3	stretch-shortening cycle	9
eccentric action	7	myosin	3	superior	3
endomysium	3	neuromuscular junction	3	triad	5
epimysium	3	origin	3	tropomyosin	5
fasciculus	3	perimysium	3	troponin	5
inferior	3	periosteum	3	T-tubule	5
insertion	3	proximal	3		
isometric action	7	sarcolemma	3		
length-tension relationship	9	sarcomere	4		

Study Questions

1. Development of muscle force is controlled by

   a. the number of mitochondria surrounding a sarcomere
   b. movement of cross-bridges across the sarcomere
   c. frequency of motor neuron stimulation
   d. the chemical activity of the periosteum
   e. increases in calcium in the blood

2. Relaxation of a muscle fiber occurs when

   a. calcium is bound to troponin
   b. calcium is pumped into the sarcoplasmic reticulum
   c. cross-bridge heads are bound to actin filaments
   d. all the ATP in the myofilament has been used
   e. the transverse tubules are blocked by sodium ions

3. A motor unit consists of

   a. actin and myosin filaments
   b. all the motor neurons in a muscle
   c. the neuromuscular junction and T-tubules
   d. the neuromuscular junction and sarcoplasmic reticulum
   e. a motor neuron and all the muscle fibers it innervates

4. An eccentric action occurs when

   a. sufficient tension is developed in a muscle to cause shortening
   b. tension is developed in a muscle but outside forces cause it to lengthen
   c. calcium is pumped into the sarcoplasmic reticulum
   d. no movement occurs in the muscle
   e. troponin moves from the myofibril to the mitochondria

5. The maximum force capability of a muscle is inversely related to

   a. the velocity of a concentric contraction
   b. the angle of pennation
   c. the cross-sectional size of a muscle
   d. the size of the neuromuscular junction
   e. the number of cross-bridge heads bound to actin

6. Skeletal muscle fibers

   a. have multiple neuromuscular junctions
   b. normally are no longer than 1 cm in length
   c. have many nuclei situated on their surface
   d. are surrounded by periosteum
   e. are usually two sarcomeres in length

References

1. Baretta, R., B.H. Salononow, E.E. Zhou, D. Letson, R. Chunard, and R. D'Amdrosia. Muscular coactivation: The role of the antagonist musculative in maintaining knee stability. *Am. J. Sports Med.* 16:113-122. 1988.
2. Bergman, R.A., and A.K. Afifi. *Atlas of Microscopic Anatomy*. Philadelphia: Saunders. 1974.
3. Billeter, R., and H. Hoppeler. Muscular basis of strength. In: *Strength and Power in Sport*, P.V. Komi, ed. Boston: Blackwell Scientific. 1992. pp. 39-63.
4. Carolan, B.J., and E. Cararelli. Adaptation and coactivation after isometric resistance training. *J. Appl. Physiol.* 73(3):911-917. 1992.
5. Dragenich, L.F., R.T. Jarger, and A.R. Kradj. Coactivation of hamstring and quadriceps during extension of the knee. *J. Bone Joint Surg.* 71(7):1075-1081. 1989.
6. Edgerton, V.R., R.R. Roy, R.J. Gregor, C.L. Hager, and T.W. Wickiewicz. Muscle fiber activation and recruitment. In: *Biochemistry of Exercise*, vol. 13, H.G. Knuttgen, J.A. Vogel, and J. Poortmans, eds. Champaign, IL: Human Kinetics. 1983. pp. 31-49.
7. Edgerton, V.R., R.R. Roy, R.J. Gregor, and S. Rugg. Morphological basis of skeletal muscle power output. In: *Human Muscle Power*, N.L. Jones, N. McCartney, and A.J. McComas, eds. Champaign, IL: Human Kinetics. 1986. pp. 43-64.
8. Fox, E.L., R.W. Bowers, and M.L. Foss. *Physiological Basis of Physical Education and Athletics*. Philadelphia: Saunders. 1988.
9. Herzog, W., A.C. Guimaraes, M.G. Antona, and K.A. Carter-Erdman. Moment-length relationships of rectus femoris muscles of speed skaters/cyclists and runners. *Med. Sci. Sports Exerc.* 23(11):1289-1296. 1991.
10. Hortobagy, T., and F.I. Katch. Eccentric and concentric torque-velocity relationships during arm flexion and extension. *Eur. J. Appl. Physiol.* 60:395-401. 1990.
11. Hunter, G.R. Metabolic cost and antagonist EMG activity during low intensity arm curl exercise. *AAHPERD Journal.* 14(1):47-49. 1991.
12. Hunter, G.R., and M. Culpepper. Knee extension torque joint position relationships following isotonic fixed resistance and hydraulic resistance training. *Athl. Training* 23(1):16-20. 1988.
13. Hunter, G.R., T. Szabo, and A. Schnitzler. Metabolic cost/vertical work relationship during knee extension and knee flexion weight training exercise. *J. Appl. Sport Sci. Res.* 6(1):42-48. 1992.
14. Klug, G.A., and G.F. Tibbits. The effect of activity on calcium mediated events in striated muscle. In: *Exercise and Sport Science Reviews*, vol. 16, K.B. Pandolf, ed. New York: Macmillan. 1988. pp. 1-60.
15. Komi, P.V. The stretch-shortening cycle. In: *Strength and Power in Sport*, P.V. Komi, ed. Boston: Blackwell Scientific. 1992. pp. 169-179.
16. Komi, P.V. Training of muscle strength and power: Interaction of neuromotoric, hypertrophic, and mechanical factors. *Int. J. Sports Med.* 7[suppl.]:10-15. 1986.
17. Luttgens, K., and K.F. Wells. *Kinesiology: A Scientific Basis of Human Motion*, 7th ed. Philadelphia: Saunders. 1982.
18. Martini, F. *Fundamentals of Anatomy and Physiology*. Englewood Cliffs: Prentice Hall. 1989.
19. McArdle, W.D., F.I. Katch, and V.I. Katch. *Exercise Physiology*, 3rd ed. Philadelphia: Lea & Febiger. 1991.
20. Roy, R.R., and V.R. Edgerton. Skeletal muscle architecture and performance. In: *Strength and Power in Sport*, P.V. Komi, ed. Boston: Blackwell Scientific. 1992. pp. 115-129.
21. Sale, D.G. Neural adaptation in strength and power training. In: *Human Muscle Power*, N.L. Jones, N. McCartney, and A.J. McComas, eds. Champaign, IL: Human Kinetics. 1986. pp. 289-307.
22. Stone, M., and H. O'Bryant. *Weight Training: A Scientific Approach*. Minneapolis: Burgess International. 1987.
23. Waterman-Storer, C.M. The cytoskeleton of skeletal muscle: Is it affected by exercise? A brief review. *Med. Sci. Sports Exerc.* 23(11):1240-1249. 1991.
24. Witherspoon, J.D. *Human Physiology*. New York: Harper & Row. 1984.

CHAPTER 2

NEUROMUSCULAR ADAPTATIONS TO CONDITIONING

Gary A. Dudley
Robert T. Harris

One of the major goals of the strength and conditioning professional is to provide training programs for athletes that will increase muscular strength and power. Central to this goal is a sound understanding of the basic anatomy and physiology of the neuromuscular system. Equally important is knowing what adaptations occur in the neuromuscular system as a result of different training programs, for the nature of the athletic event determines the type of resistance training that should be undertaken to achieve the desired conditioning response. Accordingly, this chapter presents basic information on the functional unit of the human neuromuscular system, the motor unit; describes motor unit control; and explains the importance of proprioceptors. It then explains the basic adaptations of the neuromuscular system to different modes of training, with special reference to skeletal muscle.

NEUROMUSCULAR ANATOMY AND PHYSIOLOGY

As noted in chapter 1, skeletal muscles are composed of thousands of individual cells called muscle fibers held together with a network of connective tissue that fuses and becomes continuous with the tendons at each end of the muscle. Tendons serve to connect skeletal muscle to bones, and it is through this connection that muscle, by actively changing its length, produces force and results in limb movement.

Muscle fibers are innervated by motor neurons. A motor neuron can innervate as few as one muscle fiber or, as is generally the case, several hundred muscle fibers. When a motor neuron fires, all the fibers that it serves are simultaneously activated and develop force. A motor neuron and all of the muscle fibers that it innervates are referred to as a motor unit, the basic functional entity of muscular activity. The extent of control of a muscle is dependent on the number of muscle fibers within each motor unit. Muscles that must function with great precision, such as eye muscles, may have motor units with as few as one muscle fiber per motor neuron. In contrast, the quadriceps, which perform much less precise movements, may have several hundred fibers served by one motor neuron.

A motor neuron excites the muscle fiber or fibers that it innervates by chemical transmission. The action potential (electric current) that flows along the neuron is not capable of directly exciting the muscle fibers. Instead, the action potential causes release of a chemical, acetylcholine, which diffuses across the neuromuscular junction, causing excitation of the sarcolemma. Once an action potential causes release of sufficient acetylcholine to activate the sarcolemma, the fiber contracts. This behavior is known as the **all-or-none law**. The fact that a motor neuron innervates several fibers means that a motor unit also functions according to this all-or-none principle. The motor neuron makes all of the fibers within the unit contract and develop force at the same time.

Each action potential traveling down a motor neuron results in a short period of activation of the muscle fibers within the motor unit. This is referred to as a **twitch**. Activation of the sarcolemma results in the release of calcium ions within the fiber, and contraction proceeds as described in the previous chapter. Force develops if there is resistance to the pulling interaction of actin and myosin filaments. Although calcium release during a twitch is sufficient to allow optimal activation of actin and myosin, and thereby maximal force development by the fibers, calcium is removed before force reaches its maximum, and the muscle relaxes (Figure 2.1a). If a second twitch is elicited from the motor unit before the fibers completely relax, force from the two twitches summates, and the resulting force is greater than that produced by a single twitch (Figure 2.1b). Decreasing the time interval between the twitches results in greater summation of force. The stimuli may be delivered at so high a frequency that the twitches completely fuse, a condition called **tetanus** (Figure 2.1c and 2.1d). This is the maximal amount of force the motor unit can develop.

The fact that motor units are composed of skeletal muscle fibers with specific morphological and physiological characteristics has led to several different systems of classification, based on a variety of criteria. The most familiar approach is to classify fibers according to twitch time. A common classification scheme employs the terms **slow-twitch** (Type I) and **fast-twitch** (Type II) **fibers** (Table 2.1). A fast-twitch motor unit develops force rapidly and has a short twitch time. Slow-twitch fibers, in contrast, develop force rather slowly and have a long twitch time. This difference in mechanical characteristics is accompanied by a distinct difference in the ability to supply energy for contraction and to withstand fatigue. Slow-twitch motor units are generally fatigue-resistant and have a high aerobic capacity for energy supply, but they have limited potential for rapid force development and low anaerobic power. Fast-twitch motor units are essentially the opposite, characterized by fatigability, low aerobic power, rapid force development, and high anaerobic power. It is not surprising, then, that postural muscles, such as the soleus, have a high composition of slow-twitch fibers, and that large so-called locomotory muscles, such as the quadriceps, have a mixture of both fast-twitch and slow-twitch fibers to enable both low- and high-power output activities (such as jogging and sprinting, respectively).

Table 2.1   Major Characteristics of Fast-Twitch and Slow-Twitch Muscle Fibers

Variable	Fast-twitch fibers	Slow-twitch fibers
Contraction speed	Fast	Slow
Power output	High	Low
Endurance	Low	High
Aerobic enzymes	Low	High
Anaerobic enzymes	High	Low
Fatigue resistance	Low	High

MOTOR UNIT RECRUITMENT PATTERNS DURING EXERCISE

The force output of a muscle can vary over a wide range, a gradation that is essential for smooth, coordinated patterns of movement. Muscular force can be graded in two ways. One is by varying the **frequency of activation**. If a motor unit is activated once, a twitch arises and the force is not overly impressive. However, increasing the frequency of activation so that the twitch forces are allowed to summate results in greater force developed by the motor unit. This method of varying force output is generally used in small muscles, such as those of the hand. Most of the motor units are activated at low frequency even at low forces. Force output of the whole muscle is increased by increasing the frequency of firing of the individual motor units.

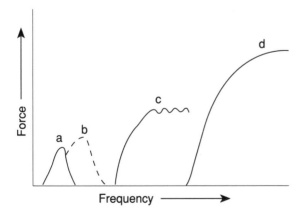

Figure 2.1   Twitch, twitch summation, and tetanus of a motor unit: (a) single twitch, (b) force resulting from summation of two twitches, (c) unfused tetanus, (d) fused tetanus.

The other means of achieving an increase in force is varying the number of motor units activated, a process known as **recruitment**. In large muscles such as those in the thigh, motor units are activated at near-fusion frequency when called on. Increases in force output by the muscle are achieved by recruiting additional motor units.

The type of motor unit recruited for a given activity is determined by its physiological characteristics (Table 2.2). For an activity such as distance running, slow-twitch motor units are engaged to take advantage of their remarkable endurance capacity and resistance to fatigue. If additional force development is needed, as in a sprint at the end of a race, the fast-twitch motor units are called into play to increase the pace; unfortunately, exercise at such an intensity cannot be maintained very long. If the activity requires near-maximal performance, such as in a power clean, most of the motor units are called into play, with fast-twitch units making the more significant contribution to the effort. Complete activation of the available motor neuron pool is probably not possible in untrained people. Although the large fast-twitch units may be recruited if the effort is substantial, they are probably not activated at a high enough frequency to realize tetanic tension.

Table 2.2   Relative Involvement of Fast-Twitch and Slow-Twitch Skeletal Muscle in Sport Events

Event	Fast-twitch	Slow-twitch
100-m sprint	High	Low
Marathon	Low	High
Olympic weightlifting	High	Low
Barbell squat	High	High
Soccer	High	High
Basketball	High	Low
Distance cycling	Low	High

ROLE OF PROPRIOCEPTORS IN LEARNING PHYSICAL SKILLS

Proprioceptors are specialized sensory receptors located inside muscles, joints, and tendons that monitor the length and tension of the musculotendonous complex. In doing so, they provide the central nervous system with information concerning **kinesthetic sense**, or conscious appreciation of the body in three-dimensional space. These receptors let us know without conscious thought the position of body parts. Such neural input is essential for executing coordinated movement and maintaining muscle tone and body posture.

Muscle spindles are proprioceptors that consist of several modified muscle fibers enclosed in a sheath of connective tissue. These *intrafusal fibers* run parallel to the normal, or *extrafusal*, muscle fibers. Muscles that perform precise movements have many spindles per unit of mass to help ensure exact control of their contractile activity. These receptors provide information on muscle length and the rate of change in length. When the muscle lengthens, spindles are stretched. This deformation activates the sensory neuron of the spindle, which sends an impulse to the spinal cord, where it synapses (connects) with alpha motor neurons. This results in the activation of motor neurons that innervate the same muscle. Spindles thus indicate the degree to which the muscle must be activated in order to overcome a given resistance. As a load increases, the muscle is stretched to a greater extent and activation of spindle fibers results in greater activation of the muscle. A simple example of this is the knee jerk reflex. Tapping on the tendon of the knee extensor muscle group below the patella stretches the muscle spindle fibers. This causes activation of extrafusal muscle fibers in the same muscle. There is a knee jerk as these fibers actively shorten. This, in turn, shortens the intrafusal fibers and causes their discharge to cease.

Golgi tendon organs (GTOs) are proprioceptors located in tendons near the myotendinous junction and are in series, that is, attached end to end, with extrafusal muscle fibers. These receptors are sensitive to stretch, but much less so than muscle spindles. In contrast to muscle spindles, activation of a GTO occurs most effectively when the muscle shortens. A GTO transmits information concerning tension rather than muscle length. Whereas spindles facilitate activation of the muscle, neural input from GTOs inhibit muscle activation, a process that is thought to provide a protective mechanism from development of excessive tension. Thus, when an extremely heavy load is placed on the muscle, the GTOs cause the muscle to relax. The ability to override this inhibition may be one of the fundamental adaptations to heavy resistance training.

NEUROMUSCULAR ADAPTATIONS TO EXERCISE CONDITIONING

Skeletal muscle adaptations to physical conditioning have generally been divided into those that occur as a result of the performance of either resistance or endurance exercise (Table 2.3). The text that follows emphasizes the major adaptations in skeletal muscle to these distinct types of training and how these responses relate to enhanced performance. Where appropriate, alterations in neural control of skeletal muscle will also be

Table 2.3 Major Adaptations to Resistance Versus Endurance Training

Variable	Resistance training	Endurance training
Size of muscle fibers	Increase	No change
Number of muscle fibers	No change	No change
Movement speed	Increase	No change
Endurance	No change	Increase
Strength	Increase	No change
Aerobic capacity	No change	Increase

explained. The goal is to provide strength and conditioning professionals with information that will enable them to develop an optimal conditioning program for enhancing athletic performance.

Adaptations to Resistance Training

One of the fundamental adaptations to resistance training is an increase in muscle mass. This occurs by enlargement of muscle fibers (**hypertrophy**), not by an increase in their number. The benefit of an increased cross-sectional area of the muscle fibers is an increased ability to develop force. Among a group of athletes, maximal isometric force of the knee extensors, for example, is highly correlated to cross-sectional area of the quadriceps.

Muscle fiber hypertrophy does not occur uniformly between the two major fiber types. It has been shown in several studies of conventional resistance training that fast-twitch fibers show greater increases in size than slow-twitch fibers (6). In fact, it has been argued that the ultimate potential for hypertrophy may reside in the relative proportion of fast-twitch fibers within a given person's muscles (3). Thus, people who possess a relatively low proportion of fast-twitch fibers may have limited potential to markedly increase muscle mass with resistance training. Differences in muscle fiber composition and number may partially explain the marked variability in the hypertrophic responses to training seen among a group of athletes.

Most studies of hypertrophic response to resistance training have been conducted on males. However, several recent studies have shown that females can also enjoy impressive increases in cross-sectional area of muscle fibers as a result of heavy resistance training (10,11). In fact, the relative increase in muscle fiber size in response to short-term training has been found to be comparable between males and females, even though this may not be visually obvious because of the

inherently greater proportion of body fat in females. Nevertheless, it seems that the enhanced athletic ability afforded males as a result of resistance training can in large part be enjoyed by females as well.

The extent of the hypertrophic response to resistance training is influenced by the time course of training. Increases in strength during the first 1 to 2 months of training performed by previously sedentary people are usually not accompanied by muscle fiber hypertrophy (9). Consequently, it has been hypothesized that neural factors must adapt in some way to allow for increased expression of strength. After this period, muscle fiber hypertrophy becomes obvious and contributes to increased strength. It is more difficult to demonstrate marked increases in muscle size and strength in weight-trained athletes. Athletes studied for 2 years of heavy resistance training showed increases in strength that paralleled optimization of training intensity, although muscle fiber hypertrophy contributed little to increased lifting performance (5). Thus, neural factors must again account for the improved performance. Accordingly, the contribution of training to optimal performance can only be realized if training intensity is maximal.

Unlike competitive weightlifters who train year-round, most athletes engage in separate protocols of in-season and out-of-season weight training in an effort to enhance performance. Although there is little data on the subject, it appears that 1 month of detraining results in minimal muscle fiber atrophy and strength loss (6,10). After this period, decreases in strength occur at a greater rate than decreases in fiber size. This suggests that it is the loss of the neural adaptations to resistance training that is mainly responsible for the decrease in strength over 2 to 3 months of detraining. Thus, it appears that if athletes are subjected to periods of 1 month of detraining, the benefits realized from the prior resistance training should not be seriously compromised.

The nature of the increases in muscle size and strength depends on the type of resistance training performed. Explosive training like that performed by Olympic weightlifters, where speed of movement is emphasized, results in substantial improvement in maximal power output (4). This occurs because of muscle fiber hypertrophy, but more significantly because of improvements in the maximal rate at which force can be developed. Such training may best serve, for example, wide receivers on an American-football team. In contrast, more conventional resistance training, in which lifting heavy loads is emphasized, induces greater hypertrophy and increases in strength but does not improve maximal power output as much (3). Such training may be especially attractive for linemen in rugby, in which great strength and muscle mass are crucial.

The benefits of resistance training can be realized by emphasizing training effort and not time. Significant increases in muscle strength and mass of the thighs can be induced by performing two to three intense training sessions per week, each no longer than 30 min. Three to five sets of two or three exercises with 6 to 12 repetitions per set are more than sufficient (6,10). When performed even once weekly, this regime is sufficient to maintain muscular strength and mass. Thus, it should be possible to conduct in-season training in such a way that muscle mass and strength do not decrease, thereby maintaining the gains that were made in the summer or winter during off-season or preseason periods. These points should be kept in mind by strength and conditioning professionals who must deal with constraints relative to student athletes' time and training facilities.

Resistance training does not enhance an athlete's maximal aerobic power or the aerobic power of his or her muscle tissue (12); neither does it appear to impair these variables. In fact, concurrent performance of resistance and endurance training does not abate the extent of the positive adaptations to endurance training (2,7). When competitive distance runners added lower body resistance training to their conditioning programs, several aspects of short-term endurance actually improved (8). Although the mechanisms responsible for the response have not been identified, it appears that resistance training may increase a distance runner's or cyclist's ability to sprint at the end of the race.

Adaptations to Endurance Training

One of the fundamental adaptive responses to endurance training is an increase in the aerobic capacity of the trained musculature. This allows the athlete to perform exercise at a given absolute intensity and, more impressively, at a given relative intensity with greater ease compared with pretraining intensities. For example, an endurance runner can perform a 6-min mile with less stress after training. In addition, he or she may also be able to run a 5:30 mile easier than a pretraining 6-min mile. This adaptation occurs as a result of glycogen sparing (less glycogen use during exercise) within the muscle, which prolongs performance and reduces lactic acid buildup. Moreover, increased fat utilization contributes to glycogen sparing.

The increase in the aerobic capacity of skeletal muscle that occurs after endurance training is expressed in both fast- and slow-twitch muscle fibers. Slow-twitch fibers have an inherently higher aerobic capacity than fast-twitch fibers and are preferentially recruited during endurance activities. However, if the intensity is sufficient, such as in running repeated 800-m intervals, fast-twitch fibers also make a significant contribution to the effort. Under such conditions their aerobic capacity also increases with training.

The concurrent performance of intense endurance and resistance training compromises the extent of the increase in strength that would have occurred if only resistance training had been performed (2,7). Thus, it does not seem wise to require strength-and-power athletes to perform intense endurance training. It has also been shown that elite endurance athletes, after cessation of training, actually show increases in muscular strength and power (1).

Performance of endurance training 3 days/week, 30 min/day is sufficient to increase aerobic power and the oxidative capacity of skeletal muscle. The recommended intensity is one that results in a heart rate of at least 70% of the athlete's maximum. Greater adaptive responses to training can be achieved if training frequency, daily duration, and intensity are increased, as would be necessary among athletes who are already endurance trained.

CONCLUSION

The fundamental unit of muscular performance in humans is the motor unit. The generation of force provided by a given motor unit depends on the frequency with which it is stimulated and the type and size of the muscle fibers themselves. A muscle is made up of numerous motor units; gradation in force in a muscle is achieved through variation in the frequency and number of motor units activated. The type and size of fibers in the activated units determines the speed and force developed by the muscle.

Adaptations to resistance training are specific to the type of exercise performed. Explosive training evokes marked increases in muscular power, whereas more conventional heavy resistance training mainly increases muscle size and strength. Neither type of training has meaningful impact on aerobic power. Resistance training, nevertheless, can be used to improve the "kick" that endurance athletes need at the end of the race. Aerobic training, in contrast, increases aerobic power; it does not enhance strength or muscle size. Intense endurance training, in fact, may actually compromise resistance training–induced increases in strength and muscle size when the two modes of training are performed simultaneously.

Key Terms

all-or-none law	13	hypertrophy	15	recruitment	14
fast-twitch fiber	13	kinesthetic sense	14	slow-twitch fiber	13
frequency of activation	13	muscle spindle	14	tetanus	13
Golgi tendon organ (GTO)	14	proprioceptor	14	twitch	13

Study Questions

1. Increases in strength as a result of resistance training

   a. are due to an increased number of muscle fibers
   b. reflect an increase in fiber size
   c. are relatively greater in males than females
   d. reflect hypertrophy during the first few weeks of training

2. During the first month after stopping resistance training,

   a. strength declines modestly, if at all
   b. the size of muscle fibers decreases to pretraining levels
   c. distribution of the two types of muscle fibers returns to pretraining values
   d. the aerobic enzyme content of skeletal muscle decreases

3. Concurrent endurance and resistance training might

   a. increase sprint ability in a distance cyclist
   b. augment increases in aerobic power
   c. augment increases in muscular strength
   d. compromise increases in aerobic power

4. Females, as compared to males,

   a. show modest increases in muscle size after resistance training
   b. reflect increases in strength mainly attributed to neural factors
   c. show greater muscle fiber hyperplasia after resistance training
   d. show the same or greater relative hypertrophy after resistance training

Applying Knowledge of Neuromuscular Adaptations

Problem 1

You have been asked to develop a resistance training program for the local high school football team, which has 75 players. The players have 45 min 3 days/week to train in a facility with five platforms, six squat racks, and three benches. What would you do?

Problem 2

The high school freshman football coach complains that he can see little progress in his players after 1 month of their first summer training program. They are no bigger than they were 1 month ago. He seriously questions their effort and the training program you designed. How would you respond?

References

1. Costill, D.L. The relationship between selected physiological variables and distance running performance. *J. Sports Med. Phys. Fitness* 7:61-66. 1967.

2. Dudley, G.A., and S.J. Fleck. Strength and endurance training: Are they mutually exclusive? *Sports Med.* 4:79-85. 1987.

3. Häkkinen, K., M. Alen, and P.V. Komi. Changes in isometric force- and relaxation-time, electromyographic and muscle fiber characteristics of human skeletal muscle during strength training and detraining. *Acta Physiol. Scand.* 125:573-585. 1985.

4. Häkkinen, K., P.V. Komi, and M. Alen. Effect of explosive type strength training on isometric force and relaxation time, electromyographic, and muscle fiber characteristics of leg extensors. *Acta Physiol. Scand.* 125:587-600. 1985.

5. Häkkinen, K., A. Pakarinen, M. Alen, H. Kauhanen, and P.V. Komi. Neuromuscular and hormonal adaptations in athletes to strength training in two years. *J. Appl. Physiol.* 65:2406-2412. 1988.

6. Hather, B.M., P.A. Tesch, P. Buchanan, and G.A. Dudley. Influence of eccentric actions on skeletal muscle adaptations to resistance training. *Acta Physiol. Scand.* 143:177-185. 1991.

7. Hickson, R.C. Interference of strength development by simultaneously training for strength and endurance. *Eur. J. Appl. Physiol.* 45:255-269. 1980.

8. Hickson, R.C., B.A. Dvorak, E.M. Gorostiga, T.T. Kurowski, and C. Foster. Potential for strength and endurance training to amplify endurance performance. *J. Appl. Physiol.* 65:2285-2290. 1988.

9. Komi, P.V. Training of muscle strength and power: Interactions of neuromotoric, hypertrophic, and mechanical factors. *Int. J. Sports Med.* 7:10-15. 1986.

10. Staron, R.S., M.J. Leonardi, D.L. Karapondo, E.S. Malicky, J.E. Falkel, F.C. Hagerman, and R.S. Kikada. Strength and skeletal muscle adaptations in heavy-resistance-trained women after detraining and retraining. *J. Appl. Physiol.* 70:631-640. 1991.

11. Staron, R.S., E.S. Mallicky, M.J. Leonardi, J.E. Falkel, F. Hagerman, and G.A. Dudley. Muscle hypertrophy and fast fiber type conversions in heavy resistance trained women. *Eur. J. Appl. Physiol.* 60:71-79. 1989.

12. Tesch, P.A. Acute and long-term metabolic changes consequent to heavy-resistance training. *Med. Sport Sci.* 26:67-89. 1987.

CHAPTER 3

THE BIOMECHANICS OF RESISTANCE EXERCISE

Everett Harman

Knowledge of musculoskeletal anatomy and biomechanics is important for understanding human movements, including those involved in sports and resistance exercise. **Anatomy** encompasses the study of components that make up the musculoskeletal "machine," and **biomechanics** focuses on the mechanisms through which these components interact to create movement. By providing insight into how body movements are carried out and what stresses movements place on the musculoskeletal system, both disciplines facilitate the design of safe and effective resistance training programs.

This chapter begins with an overview of the musculoskeletal system and body mechanics, followed by biomechanical principles related to the manifestation of human strength and power. Next are discussed the primary sources of resistance to muscle contraction used in exercise devices, including gravity, inertia, friction, fluid resistance, and elasticity. Then we turn to lifting safety (with special emphasis on the shoulders, back, and knees) and discuss the relationship of biomechanics to movement analysis and exercise prescription. Finally, examples are provided to show how biomechanical principles can be applied to training situations.

THE MUSCULOSKELETAL SYSTEM

The musculoskeletal system of the human body consists of bones, joints, and muscles configured so as to allow the great variety of movements characteristic of human activity. In this section, the various components of the musculoskeletal system are described both individually and in the context of how they function together in a system of levers.

The Skeleton

The muscles of the body do not act directly to exert force on the ground or other objects. Instead, they function by pulling against bones that rotate about joints and transmit force through the skin to the environment. Muscles can only pull, not push, but through the system of bony levers, muscle pulling forces can be manifested in either pulling or pushing forces against external objects (Figure 3.1).

There are approximately 206 bones in the body, though the number can vary. Figure 3.2 shows the human skeleton from the front and rear. The relatively light, strong structure provides leverage, support, and protection. The **axial skeleton** consists of the bones of the head, spinal column, and chest, and the **appendicular skeleton** consists of the bones of the arms, shoulders, legs, and pelvis (31).

Junctions of bones are called **joints**. **Fibrous joints** (e.g., sutures of the skull) allow virtually no movement, **cartilaginous joints** (e.g., intervertebral discs) allow limited movement, and **synovial joints** (e.g., elbow and knee) allow considerable movement. Sport and exercise movements occur mainly about the synovial joints, whose most important features are low friction and large

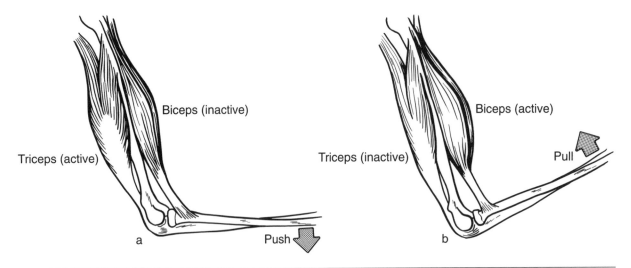

Figure 3.1 Triceps muscle activity (a) results in an external pushing force, whereas biceps muscle activity (b) results in an external pulling force. During actual body movements, particularly rapid ones, opposing muscle groups are usually both active, although one group predominates.

range of motion. Articulating bone ends are covered with smooth *hyaline cartilage*, and the entire joint is enclosed in a capsule filled with *synovial fluid*. There are usually additional supporting structures of ligament and cartilage.

Virtually all joint movement consists of rotation about points or axes. Joints can be categorized by the number of directions about which rotation can occur. **Uniaxial joints**, such as the elbow, operate as hinges, essentially rotating about only one axis. While the knee is often referred to as a hinge joint, its axis of rotation actually changes throughout the joint range of motion. **Biaxial joints**, such as the ankle and wrist, allow movement about two perpendicular axes. **Multiaxial joints**, including the shoulder and hip ball-and-socket joints as well as the knee, allow movement about all three perpendicular axes that define space.

The **spinal column** is made up of several vertebral bones separated by flexible spinal disks that allow movement to occur. The vertebrae are grouped into 7 **cervical vertebrae** in the neck region; 12 **thoracic vertebrae** in the middle to upper back; 5 **lumbar vertebrae**, which make up the lower back; 5 **sacral vertebrae**, which are fused together and make up the rear part of the pelvis; and 3 to 5 **coccygeal vertebrae**, which form a kind of vestigial internal tail extending downward from the pelvis.

Skeletal Musculature

The system of muscles that enables the skeleton to move is depicted in Figure 3.3. To cause movement or generate force against external objects, both ends of each skeletal muscle must be attached, by connective

tissue, to bone. Usually, the **proximal** attachment (toward the center of the body) is called the muscle **origin**, whereas the **distal** attachment (away from the center of the body) is called the **insertion**. In most cases muscle extends across one or more joints and causes rotation about the joint(s) when it contracts. For example, a straight-line movement of the hand is effected by rotations about the elbow and shoulder (Figure 3.4), and a straight-line movement of the foot is effected by rotations about the knee and hip.

Muscles are attached to bone in various ways. In **fleshy attachments**, which are most often found at the proximal end of a muscle, muscle fibers are directly affixed to the bone, usually over a wide area so that force is distributed rather than localized. **Fibrous attachments**, such as **tendons**, blend into and are continuous with both the muscle sheaths and the connective tissue surrounding the bone. They have additional fibers that extend into the bone itself, making for a very strong union. Tendons are capable of sustaining forces as high as 12,000 N (2,700 lb) per cm² of cross-sectional area (31).

Virtually all body movements involve the action of more than one muscle. The muscle most directly involved in bringing about a movement is called the prime mover, or **agonist**. A muscle that can slow down or stop the movement is called the **antagonist**. The antagonist assists in joint stabilization and in braking the limb towards the end of a fast movement, protecting ligamentous and cartilaginous joint structures from sustaining potentially destructive forces.

A muscle is called a **synergist** when it assists indirectly in a movement. For example, the muscles that stabilize the scapula act as synergists during upper arm

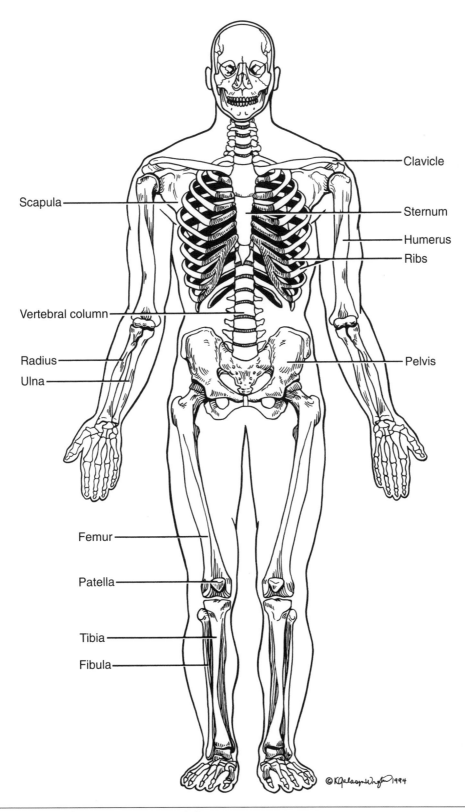

Figure 3.2a Front view of an adult male human skeleton.

Clavicle

Scapula

Sternum

Humerus

Ribs

Vertebral column

Radius

Ulna

Pelvis

Femur

Patella

Tibia

Fibula

©KGalagowright 1994

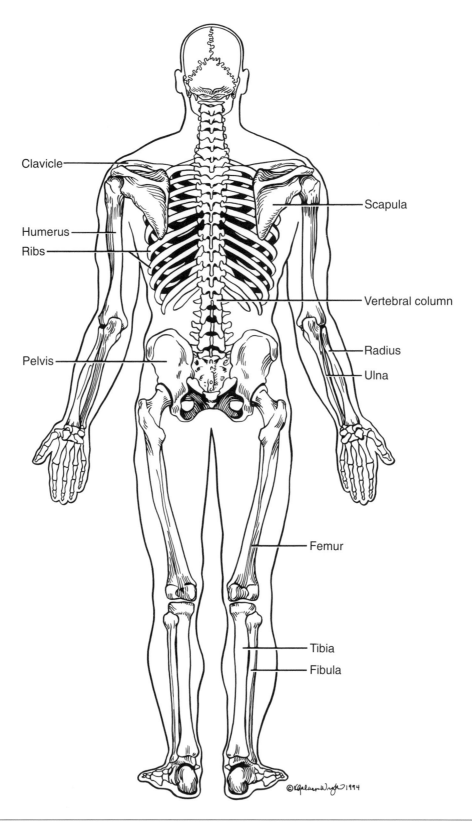

Clavicle

Humerus

Ribs

Pelvis

Scapula

Vertebral column

Radius

Ulna

Femur

Tibia

Fibula

©KGrahamWright 1994

Figure 3.2b   Rear view of an adult male human skeleton.

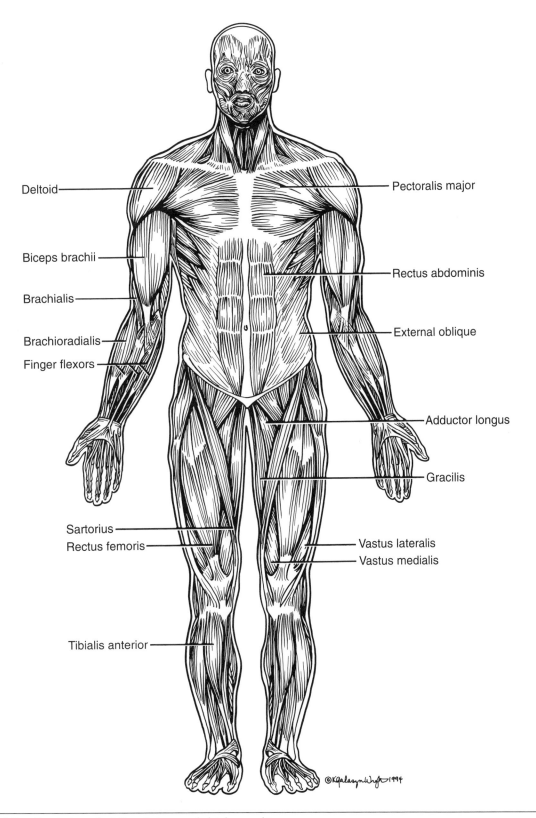

Deltoid

Biceps brachii

Brachialis

Brachioradialis

Finger flexors

Sartorius

Rectus femoris

Tibialis anterior

Pectoralis major

Rectus abdominis

External oblique

Adductor longus

Gracilis

Vastus lateralis

Vastus medialis

©KGalasynWryt 1994

Figure 3.3a Front view of adult male human skeletal musculature.

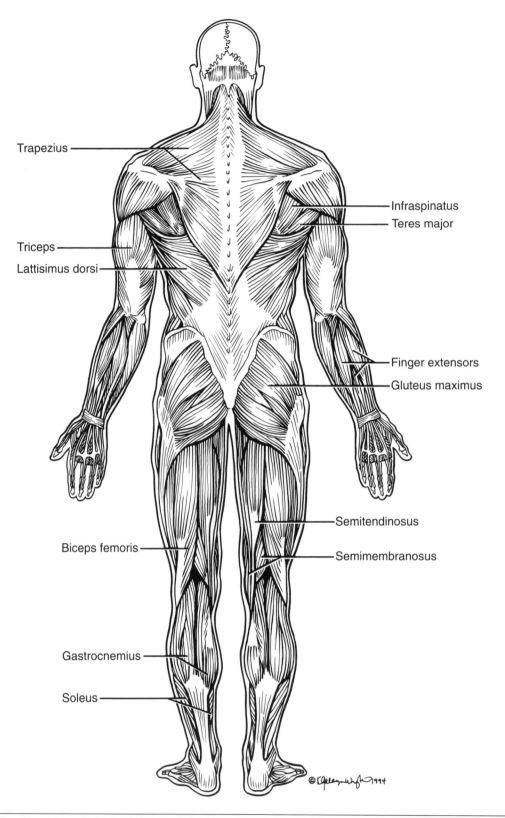

Figure 3.3b Rear view of adult male human skeletal musculature.

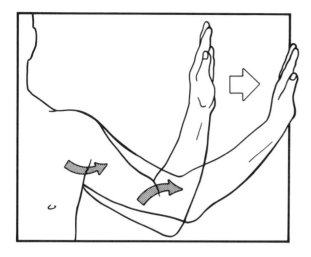

Figure 3.4 The depicted straight line movement of the hand is effected by clockwise rotation of the forearm about the elbow and counterclockwise rotation of the upper arm about the shoulder.

movement. Without these synergists, the muscles that move the upper arm (many of which originate on the scapula) would not be effective in bringing about this movement. Synergists are also required to control body motion when the agonist is a muscle that crosses two joints. For example, the rectus femoris muscle crosses the hip and knee, acting to flex the hip and extend the knee when contracting. Rising from a low squat involves both hip and knee extension. If the rectus femoris is to act to extend the knee as a person rises, then hip extensor muscles, such as the gluteus maximus, must act synergistically to counteract the hip flexion action of the rectus femoris.

Levers of the Musculoskeletal System

Understanding the musculoskeletal system requires a rudimentary knowledge of levers. Several basic definitions follow.

Lever—a rigid or semirigid body that, when subjected to a force whose line of action does not pass through its pivot point, exerts force on any object impeding its tendency to rotate (Figure 3.5)

Fulcrum—the pivot point of a lever

Moment arm (also called force arm, lever arm, or torque arm)—the perpendicular distance from the line of action of the force to the fulcrum. The line of action of a force is an infinitely long line passing through the point of application of the force, oriented in the direction in which the force is exerted.

Torque (also called moment)—the degree to which a force tends to rotate an object about a specified fulcrum; quantitatively defined as the magnitude of a force times the length of its moment arm

Muscle force—force generated by biochemical activity that tends to draw the opposite ends of a muscle towards each other

Resistive force—force generated by a source external to the body (e.g., gravity, inertia, friction) that acts contrary to muscle force

Mechanical advantage—the ratio of the moment arm through which an applied force acts to that through which a resistive force acts (Figure 3.6). For there to be a state of equilibrium between the applied and resistive torques, the product of the muscle force and the moment arm through which it acts must equal the product of the resistive force and the moment arm through which it acts. Therefore, a mechanical advantage greater than 1.0 allows the applied (muscle) force to be less than the resistive force to produce an equal amount of torque. A mechanical advantage of less than 1.0 is a *disadvantage* in the common sense of the term.

First-class lever—a lever for which the muscle force and resistive force act on opposite sides of the fulcrum (see Figure 3.6)

Second-class lever—a lever for which the muscle force and resistive force act on the same side of the fulcrum, with the muscle force acting through a moment arm longer than that through which the resistive force acts, as when the calf muscles work to raise the body onto the balls of the feet (Figure 3.7). Due to its mechanical advantage (i.e., the long moment arm), the required muscle force is smaller than the resistive force (body weight).

Third-class lever (Figure 3.8)—a lever for which the muscle force and resistive force act on the same side of the fulcrum, with the muscle force acting through a moment arm shorter than that through which the resistive force acts. The mechanical advantage is thus less than 1.0, so the muscle force has to be greater than the resistive force to produce torque equal to that produced by the resistive force.

Most human limbs are operated as third-class levers by the muscles that rotate the limbs about body joints. This is why internal muscle forces are much greater than the forces exerted by the body on external objects. For example, in Figure 3.6, because the resistance moment arm is 8 times longer than the muscle moment arm, muscle force must be 8 times the resistive force. The extremely high internal forces experienced by muscles and tendons account in large part for injury to these tissues.

During actual movement, the categorization of a lever as first, second, or third class often depends upon the somewhat arbitrary decision of where the fulcrum lies. Therefore, understanding the principle of mechanical

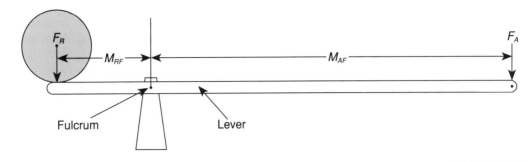

Figure 3.5 The lever can transmit force tangential to the arc of rotation from one contact point along the object's length to another. F_A = force applied to the lever; M_{AF} = moment arm of the applied force; F_R = force resisting the lever's rotation; M_{RF} = moment arm of the resistive force. The lever applies a force on the object equal in magnitude to but opposite in direction from F_R.

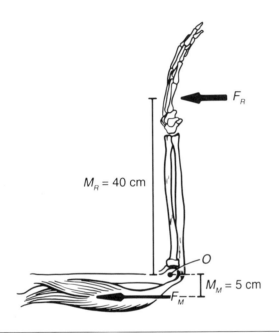

Figure 3.6 Elbow extension against resistance. O = fulcrum; F_M = muscle force; F_R = resistive force; M_M = moment arm of the muscle force; M_R = moment arm of the resistive force. Mechanical advantage = $M_M \div M_R$ = 0.125, which, being less than 1.0, is a *disadvantage* in the common sense. The depiction is of a first-class lever, because muscle force and resistive force act on opposite sides of the fulcrum. During isometric exertion or constant speed joint rotation, $F_M \times M_M = F_R \times M_R$. Because M_M is much smaller than M_R, F_M must be much greater than F_R; this illustrates the disadvantageous nature of this arrangement (i.e., a large muscle force is required to push against a relatively small resistance).

advantage is of much greater importance than being able to classify levers. Mechanical advantage often changes continuously during real-world activities. The following are examples of this:

- For movements such as knee extension and flexion, where the joint is not a true hinge, the location of

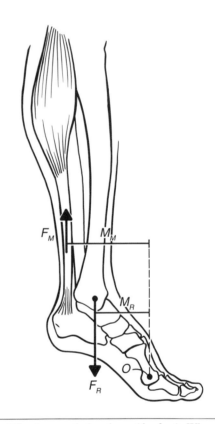

Figure 3.7 A second-class lever (the foot). When the body is raised, the ball of the foot, being the point about which the foot rotates, is the fulcrum (O). Because M_M is greater than M_R, F_M is less than F_R. (Abbreviations as in Figure 3.6.)

the axis of rotation changes continuously throughout the range of motion, affecting the length of the moment arm through which the quadriceps and hamstrings act (Figure 3.9). For knee extension, the patella, or kneecap, helps to prevent large changes in the mechanical advantage of the quadriceps muscle by keeping the quadriceps tendon from falling in close to the axis of rotation (Figure 3.10).

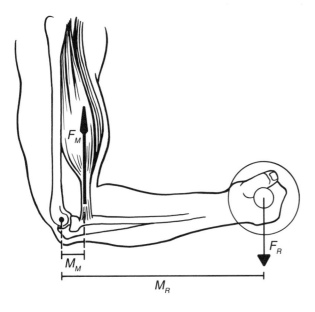

Figure 3.8 A third-class lever (the forearm). Because M_M is much smaller than M_R, F_M must be much greater then F_R. (Abbreviations as in Figure 3.6.)

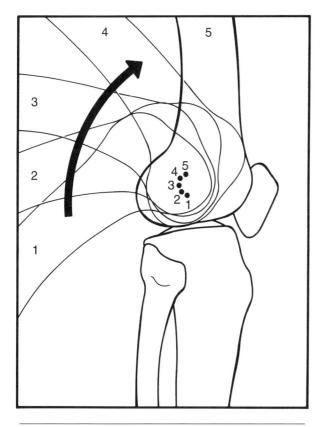

Figure 3.9 The location of the knee's axis of rotation changes continuously throughout the range of motion, affecting the length of the moment arm through which the quadriceps and hamstrings act.

- For movements such as knee and elbow flexion, there is no structure such as the patella to keep the perpendicular distance from the joint axis of rotation to the tendon's line of action relatively constant (Figure 3.11).
- During weight lifting, the moment arm through which the weight acts equals the horizontal distance from the weight to the body joint and varies throughout the movement (Figure 3.12).

Variations in Tendon Insertion

There is considerable variability in human anatomical structure, including the points at which tendons are attached to bone. A person whose tendons are inserted on the bone farther from the joint center should be able to lift heavier weights because muscle force acts through a longer moment arm and thus can produce greater torque around the joint. (In Figure 3.11, for example, consider how M would change if the tendon insertion were farther to the right.) However, it is important to recognize the tradeoff involved in tendon insertion. The mechanical advantage gained by having tendons insert farther from the joint center is accompanied by a loss of maximum speed, because with the tendon inserted farther from the joint center, the muscle has to contract more to make the joint move through a given range of motion. In other words, a given amount of muscle shortening results in a smaller angle of joint movement, which translates into a loss in movement speed. Figure 3.13a shows that, starting with the joint extended, when a hypothetical muscle shortens by a given amount the joint rotates by 37°. However, if the muscle were inserted further from the joint center, as in Figure 3.13b, the same amount of muscle shortening would bring about only 34° of joint rotation because of the geometry of the dynamic triangle formed by the muscle insertion and origin and the joint center of rotation.

To produce a given joint rotational velocity, a muscle inserted farther from the joint center must contract at a higher speed, at which it is less capable of generating force due to the inverse force-velocity relationship of muscle (43) described later in this chapter. Therefore such a tendon arrangement reduces the muscle's force capability during faster movements.

One can see how relatively subtle individual differences in structure can result in various advantages and disadvantages. For slow speed movements, such as in power lifting, tendon insertion farther from the joint than normal can be advantageous, while for athletic activities occurring at high speeds, such as tennis stroking, the arrangement can be disadvantageous.

HUMAN STRENGTH AND POWER

The terms *strength* and *power* are widely used to describe some important abilities that contribute to maximal

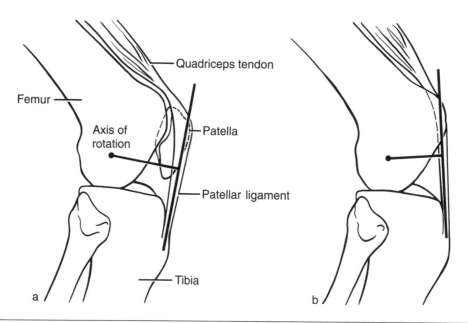

Figure 3.10   (a) The patella increases the mechanical advantage of the quadriceps muscle group by maintaining the quadriceps tendon's distance from the knee's axis of rotation. (b) Absence of the patella allows the tendon to fall closer to the knee's center of rotation, shortening the moment arm of the muscle force and thus the mechanical advantage.
Reprinted from reference 13, Gowitzke and Milner (1988).

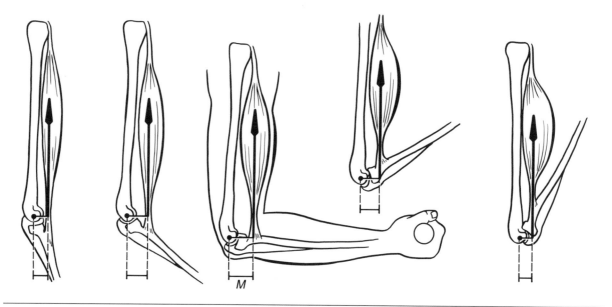

Figure 3.11   During elbow flexion with the biceps muscle, the perpendicular distance from the joint axis of rotation to the tendon's line of action varies throughout the range of joint motion. When the moment arm (*M*) is shorter, there is less mechanical advantage.

human efforts in sports and other physical activities. Unfortunately there is often little consistency in the way the terms are used. This section provides a scientific basis for understanding human strength and power and shows how various factors contribute to their manifestation.

Basic Definitions

While it is widely accepted that strength is the ability to exert force, there is considerable disagreement as to

how strength should be measured. The weight that a person can lift is probably the oldest quantitative measure of strength. Technological developments have popularized the use of isometric strength testing and, more recently, isokinetic strength testing.

All sports involve **acceleration** (change in velocity per unit time) of the body and, for some sports, an implement as well. Because of individual differences in the ability to exert force at different speeds (29),

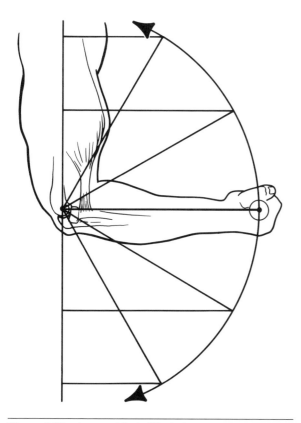

Figure 3.12 As a weight is lifted, the moment arm through which the weight acts, and thus the resistive torque, changes with the horizontal distance from the weight to the elbow.

strength scores obtained from isometric and low-speed lifting tests may have limited value in predicting performance in sports that involve acceleration at high speed. That is why Knuttgen and Kraemer (30) have suggested a more inclusive definition of **strength**: the maximal force that a muscle or muscle group can generate at a specified velocity. Although controlling and monitoring velocity during strength testing requires sophisticated equipment, the resulting strength scores are more meaningfully related to sports ability than static strength measures or maximum lifts.

The limited applicability of isometric and low-speed strength scores has led to a heightened interest in "power" as a measurement of the ability to exert force at higher speeds. Outside of the scientific realm, power is loosely defined as "force, energy, strength, and might" (39). However, in physics, **power** is precisely defined as "the time rate of doing work" (38), where **work** is the product of the force exerted on an object and the distance the object moves in the direction in which the force is exerted. Quantitatively, work and power are defined as

$$\text{Work} = \text{Force} \times \text{Distance} \tag{3.1}$$

and

$$\text{Power} = \frac{\text{Work}}{\text{Time}}. \tag{3.2}$$

Equation 3.2 can be rewritten as

$$\text{Power} = \frac{\text{Force} \times \text{Distance}}{\text{Time}} \tag{3.3}$$

$$= \text{Force} \times \frac{\text{Distance}}{\text{Time}},$$

so power can also be defined as

$$\text{Power} = \text{Force} \times \text{Velocity}. \tag{3.4}$$

More precisely, power is the product of the force exerted on an object and the velocity of the object in the direction in which the force is exerted.

For the above equations to work out correctly, consistent units must be used. In the Système International d'Unités (SI) (35), the worldwide standard, force is measured in newtons (N), distance in meters (m), work in joules (J, i.e., newton · meters, or N · m), time in seconds (s), and power in watts (W, i.e., J/s). The appropriate SI units for the equations can be obtained from other common units using the factors listed in Table 3.1.

Despite its definition as a unit of mass, the kilogram is widely used as a unit of force standardized as the gravitational force exerted on a kilogram of mass where the acceleration of gravity is 9.807 m/s² (e.g., central Europe). While a kilogram balance scale provides an accurate measure of an object's mass, a kilogram spring or electronic scale only determines the kilograms of force the mass exerts. An accurate mass in kilograms can be obtained by multiplying the object's kilogram weight by 9.807 divided by the local acceleration of gravity (Table 3.2).

The work and power equations just presented apply to an object moving from one place to another. Work and power are also required to start an object rotating

Table 3.1 Factors for Conversion of Common Measures to SI Units

To get	Multiply	By
newtons (N)	pounds (lb)	4.448
newtons (N)	kilograms mass (kg)	local acceleration of gravity (Table 3.2)
newtons (N)	kilograms force (kg)	9.807
meters (m)	feet (ft)	0.3048
meters (m)	inches (in)	0.02540
radians (rad)	degrees (°)	0.01745

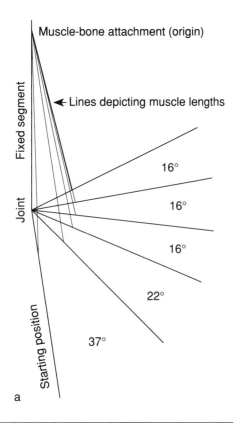

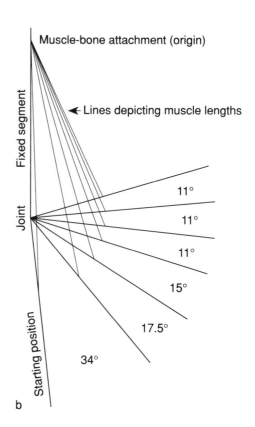

Figure 3.13   Changes in joint angle with equal increments of muscle shortening when the tendon is inserted (a) closer and (b) farther from the joint center. Configuration (b) has a larger moment arm and thus greater torque for a given muscle force, but less rotation per unit of muscle contraction and thus slower movement speed.
Reprinted from reference 13, Gowitzke and Milner (1988).

Table 3.2   Acceleration Due to Gravity at Sea Level, by Latitude

Latitude	Acceleration due to gravity (m/s^2)	Sample location
0°	9.780	Nairobi, Kenya
10°	9.782	Caracas, Venezuela
20°	9.786	Honolulu, Hawaii
30°	9.793	Houston, Texas
40°	9.802	Denver, Colorado
50°	9.811	Bonn, Germany
60°	9.819	Anchorage, Alaska

Note. A more complete table can be found in the *Handbook of Chemistry and Physics* (51).

about an axis or to change the velocity at which it rotates, even if the object as a whole doesn't move through space at all. The angle through which an object rotates is called **angular displacement**, the SI unit for which is the radian (rad); 1 rad = 180° ÷ π = 57.3°. **Angular velocity** is the object's rotational speed, measured in rad/s. Torque is expressed in N · m. Just as for

movement through space, the work done in rotating an object is in J, and power is in W (35). The equations for **rotational work** and **rotational power** are

$$\text{Work} = \text{Torque} \times \text{Angular Displacement} \quad (3.5)$$

and

$$\text{Power} = \frac{\text{Work}}{\text{Time}}. \quad (3.6)$$

Equation 3.6 can be rewritten as

$$\text{Power} = \frac{\text{Torque} \times \text{Angular Displacement}}{\text{Time}} \quad (3.7)$$

$$= \text{Torque} \times \frac{\text{Angular Displacement}}{\text{Time}},$$

so power can also be defined as

$$\text{Power} = \text{Torque} \times \text{Angular Velocity}. \quad (3.8)$$

The discrepancy between the common and scientific definitions of power has led to misunderstandings. For example, in so-called powerlifting, which involves high forces but relatively low movement speeds, less mechanical power is produced than in several other sports, including Olympic lifting (12). One cannot expect the sport of powerlifting to be renamed. However, the strength and conditioning professional should use the word *power* in all other contexts only in its scientific sense to avoid ambiguity.

Furthermore, although the word *strength* is often associated with slow speeds and the word *power* with high speeds of movement, both variables reflect the ability to exert force at a given speed. Power is a direct mathematical function of force and velocity. Therefore, if at any instant, any two of the variables force, velocity, and power are known, the third can be calculated. If at a particular velocity of movement an individual can generate high force or high power, precisely the same ability is being described; that is the ability to accelerate a mass at that particular speed. Therefore, it is not correct to associate strength with low speed and power with high speed. Strength is the capacity to exert force at any given speed, and power the mathematical product of force and velocity at whatever the speed. What is critical is the ability to exert force at speeds characteristic of the sport to overcome gravity and accelerate the body or an implement. For a sports movement made relatively slow by high resistance, low-speed strength is critical, whereas for a movement that is very fast due to low resistance, high-speed strength is important.

Biomechanical Factors in Human Strength

There are several biomechanical factors involved in the manifestation of human strength including neural control, muscle cross-sectional area, muscle fiber arrangement, muscle length, body joint angle, muscle contraction velocity, joint angular velocity, and body size. These factors are discussed below as are the three-dimensional strength relationship and the strength-to-mass ratio.

Neural Control.
Neural control affects the maximal force output of a muscle by determining which and how many motor units are involved in a muscle contraction (**recruitment**) and the rate at which the motor units are fired (**rate coding**) (10). Generally, muscle force is greater when (1) more motor units are involved in a contraction, (2) the motor units are greater in size, or (3) the rate of firing is faster. Much of the improvement in strength evidenced in the first few weeks of resistance training is attributable to neural adaptations (41).

Muscle Cross-Sectional Area.
All else being equal, the force a muscle can exert is related to its cross-sectional area rather than to its volume (26). For example, if two athletes of similar percent body fat but different height have the same biceps circumference, their upper arm muscle cross-sectional areas are about the same. While the taller (and therefore heavier) athlete's longer muscle makes for greater muscle volume, the strength of their biceps should be about the same. With the same strength but greater body weight, the taller athlete has less ability to lift and accelerate his own body, as when performing calisthenics or gymnastics.

Arrangement of Muscle Fibers.
Maximally contracting muscles have been found capable of generating forces of 16 to 100 N/cm^2 of muscle cross-sectional area (1, 20, 21, 37). This wide range can be partially accounted for by the arrangement of fibers within a muscle (Figure 3.14) (15, 21). A **pennate muscle** is one in which the fibers have a featherlike arrangement. The **angle of pennation** is defined as the angle between the muscle fibers and an imaginary line between the muscle's origin and insertion; 0° corresponds to no pennation. Many human muscles are pennate (15), but few have angles of pennation in excess of 15°. Actually, the angle of pennation does not remain constant for a given muscle, but increases as the muscle shortens. Pennation appears to provide some enhancement of force capability for muscle contracting at high speed, particularly at the extremes of the range of muscle motion, but pennation can be somewhat disadvantageous for generating eccentric, isometric, or low-speed concentric force (described later) (45). While there is a trade-off associated with pennation, and it is not the most advantageous arrangement for all muscles, many skeletal muscles are pennate (15).

Muscle Length.
When a muscle is at its resting length, a maximal number of cross-bridge sites are available between the actin and myosin filaments (see Figure 1.5). However, when the muscle is shorter or longer than its resting length there are fewer available sites. Thus, the muscle can generate the most force around its resting length and less force when it is in an elongated or shortened state.

Joint Angle.
Because all body movements, even those occurring in a straight line, take place by means of rotation about a joint, the forces that muscles produce must be manifested as torques (recall that a higher torque value indicates a greater tendency for the applied force to rotate the limb, etc., about a joint); consequently, we speak in terms of torque versus joint angle, rather than force versus joint angle. The amount of torque that can be exerted about a given body joint varies throughout the joint range of motion largely because of the force versus muscle length relationship as well as the geometric arrangement of muscles, tendons, and joint structures. Additional factors include the type of exercise (isotonic, isometric, etc.), the body joint in question, the muscles used at that joint (i.e., whether for extension or flexion), and the speed of contraction (Figure 3.15).

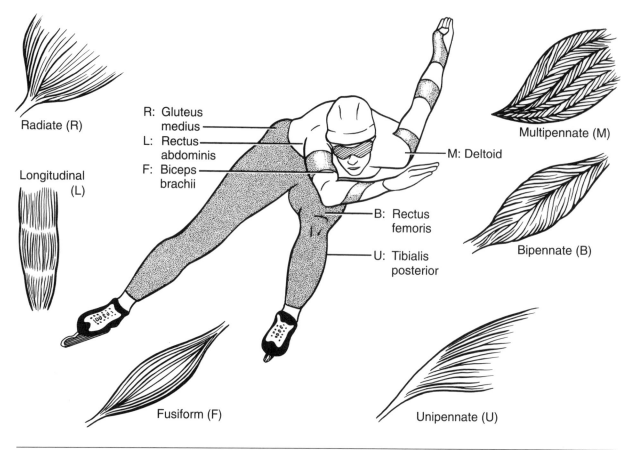

Figure 3.14 Muscle fiber arrangements and an example of each.
Reprinted from Hay and Reid (1988).

For a given body movement, curves for higher contraction speeds are lower in amplitude but similar in shape to those for lower contraction speeds (compare the several isokinetic curves in Figure 3.15a, for example).

Additionally, the shape of a curve of maximal muscle torque versus joint angle may or may not be the same as that of a curve of maximal muscle force versus muscle length, for several reasons:

- Because of changes in pivot point location and tendon position throughout the movement, the moment arm through which the muscle acts can vary.
- More than one muscle usually act together to cause movement about a given body joint. At any joint angle, the different muscles are at different points in their force-versus-length curves.
- The length of a muscle crossing two body joints (e.g., biceps, triceps, rectus femoris, hamstrings) is affected by both joint angles.

Muscle Contraction Velocity. Classic experiments by A.V. Hill on isolated animal muscle have shown that muscles can produce less force as the velocity of contraction increases (25). The relationship is not

linear; the decline in force capability is steepest over the range of lower movement speeds.

Joint Angular Velocity. There are three basic types of muscle action, during which contractile force acts to pull a muscle's ends toward each other (the term *muscle action* is preferable to *contraction*, which means "shortening" and does not accurately describe the second and third actions here):

- **Concentric muscle action**—when the muscle shortens because the contractile force is greater than the resistive force
- **Isometric muscle action**—when muscle length does not change because the contractile force is equal to the resistive force
- **Eccentric muscle action**—when the muscle lengthens because the contractile force is less than the resistive force

Muscle torque varies with joint angular velocity according to the type of muscular action (Figure 3.16). Tests have shown that, during isokinetic (constant speed) concentric exercise by human subjects, torque capability

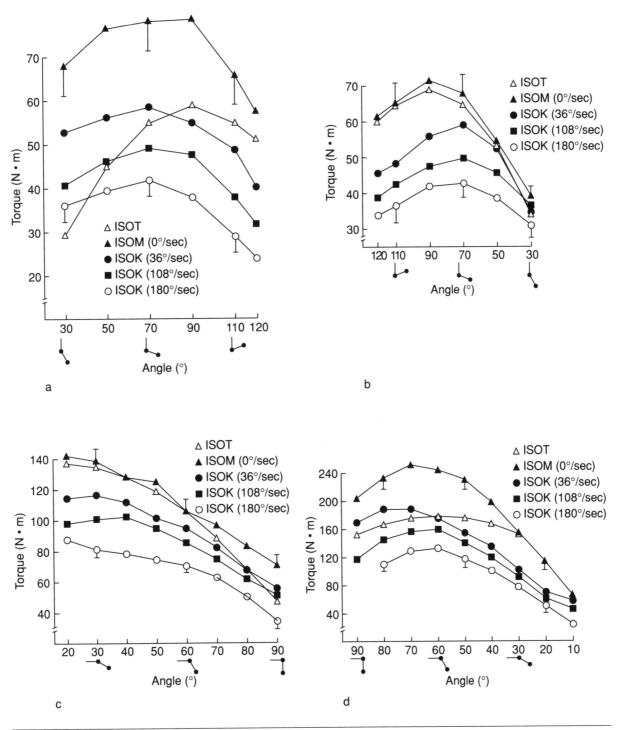

Figure 3.15 Torque versus joint angle curves for (a) elbow flexion, (b) elbow extension, (c) knee flexion, and (d) knee extension. ISOT = isotonic (weight lifting); ISOM = isometric; ISOK = isokinetic.
Reprinted from Knapik, Wright, Mawdsley, and Braun (1983).

declines as angular velocity increases. In contrast, during eccentric exercise, as joint angular velocity increases, maximal torque capability increases until about 90°/s (1.57 rad/s), after which it declines gradually (29).

Owing to joint geometry, there are differences in shape between curves of muscle force versus contraction

velocity and muscle torque versus joint angular velocity. Joint geometry also explains why, during isokinetic exercise, joint angle changes at a constant rate while the muscle length changes at a variable rate. For example, as the arm starts flexing from a straight position, the muscle contracts only a small amount for a given change in

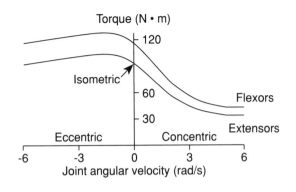

Figure 3.16   Maximal torque capability as a function of joint angular velocity. *Note.* From reference 29.

elbow angle; as the elbow flexes through the 90° position, much more muscle shortening is required to produce the same change in elbow angle.

The Three-Dimensional Strength Relationship Among Torque, Joint Angle, and Angular Velocity.

It is important to note that each torque versus joint angle curve depicted in Figure 3.15 resulted from testing at one angular velocity. Similarly, torque versus angular velocity curves (as in Figure 3.16) generally result from testing at one joint angle. A more comprehensive view of strength can be obtained when maximal torque capability is depicted as a function of both joint angle and angular velocity in a three-dimensional plot (Figure 3.17). Such a depiction allows one to visualize relative force capability at various combinations of joint angle and angular velocity for a particular body movement.

Strength-to-Mass Ratio.

In such sport activities as sprinting and jumping, the ratio of the strength of the muscles involved in the movement to the mass of the body parts being accelerated is critical. According to Newton's second law (38),

$$\text{Force} = \text{Mass} \times \text{Acceleration.} \qquad (3.9)$$

It follows that

$$\text{Acceleration} = \frac{\text{Force}}{\text{Mass}}. \qquad (3.10)$$

Thus, the strength-to-mass ratio directly reflects an athlete's ability to accelerate his or her body. If, after training, an athlete increases body mass by 15% but increases force capability by only 10%, then the strength-to-mass ratio, and thus the athlete's ability to accelerate, is reduced. A runner or jumper may benefit by experimenting with muscle mass to determine the highest strength-to-mass ratio, which should result in the best possible performance.

In sports involving weight classification, the strength-to-mass ratio is extremely important. If all competitors have the same body mass, the strongest one has a decided advantage. It is normal for the strength-to-mass ratio of larger athletes to be lower than that for smaller athletes (4). Trial and error can help an athlete determine the weight category in which his or her strength is highest relative to other athletes in the weight class. Once an athlete finds his or her most competitive weight class, the object is to get as strong as possible without exceeding the class weight limit.

Body Size.

It has long been observed that, all else being equal, smaller athletes are stronger ''pound-for-pound'' than larger athletes. The reason for this is that a muscle's maximal contractile force is fairly proportional to its cross-sectional area, which is related to the *square* of linear body dimensions, whereas a muscle's mass is proportional to its volume, which is related to the *cube* of linear body dimensions. Therefore, as body size increases, body mass increases more rapidly than does muscle strength. Given constant body proportions, the smaller athlete has a higher strength-to-mass ratio than does the larger athlete (4).

There has always been interest in comparing the performances of lifters in different weight categories. The most obvious method for doing so is to divide the weight lifted by the athlete's body weight. However, such an adjustment is biased against larger athletes because it does not take into account the expected drop in the strength-to-mass ratio with increasing body size. Various formulas have been derived to compare lifts more equitably. In the **classical formula**, the lift is divided by body weight to the two-thirds power, thus accounting for the cross-sectional area versus volume relationship. Other formulas have since been developed because the classical formula seemed to favor athletes of middle body weight over lighter and heavier athletes (23). However, the classical formula's determination that the performances of medium-weight lifters are usually the best may indeed be unbiased; one would expect the weight category with the largest number of competitors to produce the best performers.

SOURCES OF RESISTANCE TO MUSCLE CONTRACTION

The most common sources of resistance for strength training exercises are gravity, inertia, friction, fluid resistance, and elasticity. This section provides information on the force and power required to overcome these forms of resistance.

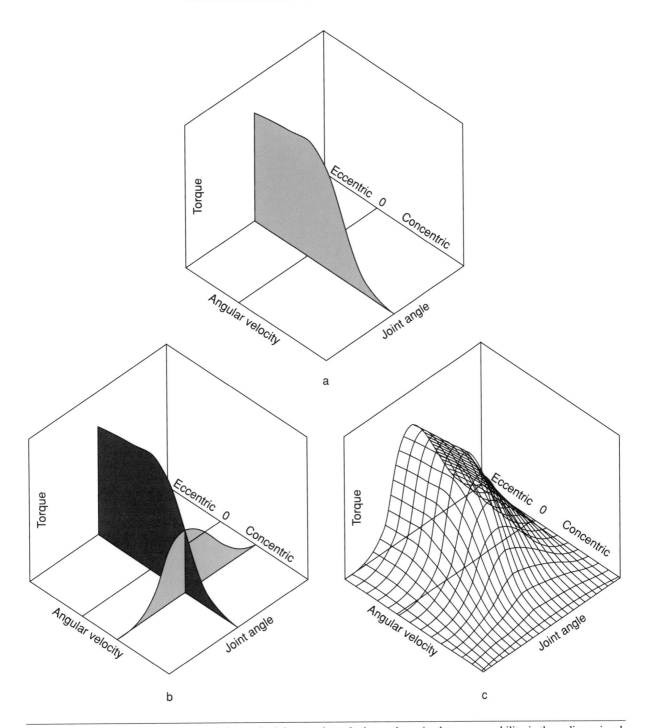

Figure 3.17   The relationship between joint angle, joint angular velocity, and maximal torque capability is three-dimensional. (a) The two-dimensional curve of maximal torque versus joint angular velocity is derived from testing at only one joint angle. (b) The two-dimensional curve of maximal torque versus joint angle (lighter shade) is derived from testing at one angular velocity. The height of the line of intersection of the two curves represents the maximal torque at one particular combination of joint angle and angular velocity. (c) Testing at several joint angles and angular velocities produces data describing the three-dimensional relationship.

Gravity

The downward force on an object due to gravity, otherwise called the object's **weight**, is equal to the object's mass times the local acceleration of gravity:

$$F_g = m \cdot a_g \qquad (3.11)$$

where F_g = force due to gravity (same as the object's weight), m = the object's mass, and a_g = the local acceleration of gravity (see Table 3.2).

Because the earth rotates and is not exactly spherical, the acceleration of gravity can vary as much as 1% according to geographic location, which is enough to affect world records in lifting and jumping. Weighing a barbell on a calibrated spring or electronic scale shows its actual weight. A balance scale determines only the object's mass, so its weight must be calculated using Equation 3.11 if a spring or electronic scale is not available.

The Earth's gravitational force on an object is inversely proportional to the square of the distance between the object and the center of the Earth. Because the bulging of the Earth at its equator contributes much more to that distance than does land height relative to sea level, geographical latitude is much more relevant to gravitational force than is terrestrial altitude.

The microgravity conditions in space reduce resistive force experienced by the muscles, resulting in both muscle atrophy (7) and loss of bone minerals, particularly in the weight-bearing bones (50). In an effort to reduce mineral loss, exercise programs aboard spacecraft using devices that provide resistance other than gravitational force have been implemented (7).

Popular terminology for weight and mass is often incorrect. For example, some barbell or stack machine plates are labeled in pounds. The pound is a unit of force, not mass. In actuality, only the mass of a barbell plate stays constant while its weight varies according to the local acceleration of gravity. The kilogram designation on a weight plate refers to its mass. It is not correct to say that an object weighs a certain number of kilograms, since weight refers to force, not mass. Instead, one can say something like ''The mass of the barbell is 85 kg.''

Applications to Resistance Training.

The gravitational force on an object always acts downward. Since, by definition, the moment arm by which a force produces torque is perpendicular to the line of action of the force, the moment arm of a weight is always horizontal. Thus, torque due to an object's weight is the product of the weight and the horizontal distance from the weight to the pivot point (joint). During a lift, although the weight does not change, its horizontal distance from a given joint axis changes constantly. When the weight is horizontally closer to the joint, it exerts less resistive torque, but when it is horizontally farther from a joint, it exerts more resistive torque. For example, in an arm curl (Figure 3.18), the horizontal distance from the elbow to the barbell is greatest when the forearm is horizontal. Thus, in that position the lifter must exert the greatest muscle torque to support the weight. The moment arm decreases as the forearm rotates either upward or downward away from the horizontal, decreasing the resistive torque due to the weight. When the weight is

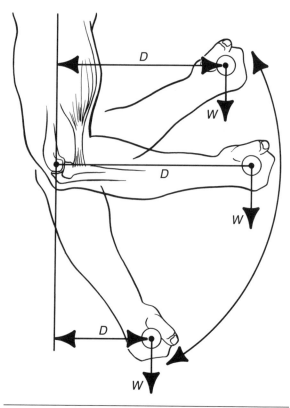

Figure 3.18 While the weight of the object (*W*) remains constant, the horizontal distance (*D*) from the weight to the elbow changes throughout a curl movement, directly affecting the resistive torque.

directly above or below the elbow pivot point there is no resistive torque due to the weight.

Lifting technique can affect the resistive torque pattern during a lift. In the squat, for example, a more forward inclination of the trunk brings the weight horizontally closer to the knee, thus reducing the resistive torque about the knee that the quadriceps must counteract. At the same time, the weight is horizontally farther from the hip, increasing the resistive torque about the hip that the gluteus and hamstring muscles must counteract. Lifting technique can thus be modified to shift stress among muscle groups; a competitive lifter may wish to adjust his or her lifting technique to shift resistance from muscles that are relatively weak to those that are relatively strong. While general lifting principles apply to everyone, the details of optimal lifting technique can vary among individuals.

Weight Stack Machines.

As with free weights, gravity is the source of resistance for weight stack machines. However, by means of pulleys, cams, cables, and gears, the machines provide increased control over the direction and pattern of resistance. Both free weights and stack machines have advantages and disadvantages.

Some of the advantages of the stack machine include the following:

- *Safety.* The likelihood of injury as a result of being hit by, tripping over, or being trapped under a weight is reduced. It requires less skill to maintain control of a weight stack than a free weight.
- *Design flexibility.* Machines can be designed to provide resistance to body movements that are difficult to resist with free weights (e.g., hip adduction and abduction). To some extent, the pattern of resistance can be engineered into a machine.
- *Ease of use.* It is quicker and easier to select a weight by insertion of a pin in a stack than by mounting plates on a bar.

Advantages of free weights include the following:

- *Whole body training.* Free weight exercises are often performed in the standing position with the weight supported by the entire body, taxing a larger portion of the body's musculature than a weight stack machine would. Such weight-bearing exercise promotes bone mineralization, helping to prevent osteoporosis in later life (46). Moreover, the movement of a free weight is constrained by the lifter rather than by a machine, requiring muscles to work in stabilization as well as support. "Structural" lifts, such as cleans and snatches, are particularly useful in providing training stimulus for a major portion of the body's musculature.
- *Simulation of real life activities.* The lifting and acceleration of objects are a major part of sports and other physically demanding activities. Machines tend to isolate single muscle groups; the lifting of free weights involves the more natural coordination of several muscle groups.

Nautilus Sports/Medical Industries popularized the concept of engineering resistive torque through the range of joint motion by creating an exercise machine that uses a cam of variable radius that changes the length of the moment arm through which the weight stack acts (Figure 3.19). The rationale was to provide more resistance in the range of motion in which the muscles could exert greater torque, and less resistance where the muscles could apply less torque. However, in order for the system to work as planned, the lifter has to move at a constant slow angular velocity, which is difficult to do consistently. Also, current cam-based machines don't always match normal human torque capability patterns (16, 27).

Inertia

In addition to gravitational force, a barbell or weight stack, when accelerated, exerts **inertial force** on the

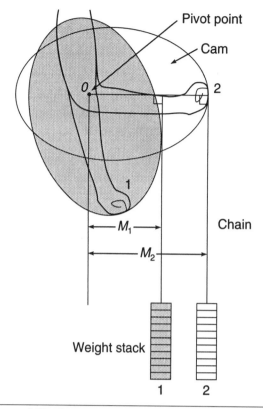

Figure 3.19 In cam-based weight stack machines the moment arm (M) of the weights (horizontal distance from the chain to the cam pivot point) varies during the exercise movement. When the cam is rotated in the direction shown from position 1 to position 2, the moment arm of the weights, and thus the resistive torque, increases.

lifter. While the force of gravity acts only downward, inertial force can act in any direction. The upward force a lifter exerts equals the weight lifted plus any inertial force, which is the mass times the upward acceleration of the bar (Equation 3.9). Horizontal bar acceleration reflects front-to-back or side-to-side forces.

Deceleration, or slowing down of a weight, also called negative acceleration, requires net force in the direction opposite to that in which the weight is moving. For a weight moving upward, the lifter can reduce upward force on the bar and let the force of gravity decelerate the weight. If the weight is moving horizontally, as at the top of a standing curl, the lifter must exert force in the direction opposite to that in which the weight is moving in order to decelerate it. If the weight is moving downward, as when lowering a weight, the lifter must exert upward force greater than the weight in order to decelerate it.

While acceleration changes the nature of an exercise and makes resistance patterns less predictable, acceleration in lifting is not necessarily undesirable. Because acceleration is characteristic of natural movements in sports and daily life, weight training exercises involving acceleration probably produce desirable neuromuscular training effects. Olympic lifting exercises such as the snatch and the clean-and-jerk are effective for improving the ability to produce high accelerations against heavy resistance (12).

All lifts involve some acceleration at the beginning to bring the bar from a zero to an upward velocity and some deceleration near the top of the lift to bring the bar's velocity back to zero. With this acceleration pattern the agonist muscles receive resistance in excess of bar weight early in the range of motion but resistance less than bar weight towards the end of the range of motion (32). The lifter decelerates the bar by either (1) reducing upward force on the bar to below bar weight in order to let some or all of the bar's weight decelerate it, or (2) pushing down against the bar using the antagonist muscles. In either case, the deceleration has the effect of providing less resistance to the agonist muscles late in the range of motion.

For a given weight, compared with a slow lift with minimal acceleration, a lift involving higher acceleration ("explosive lift") provides greater resistance to muscles involved early in the lift and less resistance to the muscles involved toward the end of the lift. However, heavier weights can be handled in accelerative lifts than in slow lifts, allowing near-maximal resistance to be attained for all muscles involved in the lift. During a power clean of a heavy weight, for example, the strong leg and back muscles accelerate the bar vertically to a high enough velocity so that even though the weaker upper body muscles cannot exert vertical force equal to the bar's weight, the bar continues to travel upwards until the force of gravity decelerates the bar to zero velocity at the top of the lift.

Friction

Friction is the resistive force encountered when one attempts to move two objects in contact with each other. Exercise devices that use friction as the main source of resistance include belt- or brake pad–resisted cycle ergometers and wrist-curl devices. For such devices,

$$F_R = kF_N, \qquad (3.12)$$

where F_R = the resistive force, k = the coefficient of friction for the two particular substances in contact, and F_N = the normal force, which presses the objects against each other.

The coefficients of friction for initiating and for maintaining movement are different. All else being equal, it takes more force to initiate movement between two substances in contact than to maintain previously initiated movement. Thus, a friction-resisted exercise device requires a relatively high force to initiate movement and a relatively constant force after movement has begun, no matter what the movement speed. Resistance provided by some such devices is adjusted using some mechanism to alter the normal force.

Fluid Resistance

The resistive force encountered by an object moving through a fluid (liquid or gas) or by a fluid moving past or around an object or through an orifice is called **fluid resistance**. Fluid resistance is a significant factor in such sports activities as swimming, golf, sprint running, discus throwing, and baseball pitching (except for swimming, in which the fluid is water, all these involve air resistance). The phenomenon has become important in resistance training with the advent of hydraulic (liquid) and pneumatic (gas) exercise machines and with the increasing popularity of swimming pool exercise routines, particularly among older people and pregnant women.

The two sources of fluid resistance are **surface drag**, which results from the friction of a fluid passing along the surface of an object, and **form drag**, which results from the way in which a fluid presses against the front or rear of an object passing through it. Cross-sectional (frontal) area has a major effect on form drag.

Fluid-resisted exercise machines most often use cylinders in which a piston forces fluid through an orifice as the exercise movement is performed. The resistive force is greater when the piston is pushed faster, the orifice is smaller, or the fluid is more viscous. All else being equal, resistance is roughly proportional to the velocity of piston movement (24):

$$F_R \approx kv, \qquad (3.13)$$

where F_R = the resistive force; k = a constant that reflects the physical characteristics of the cylinder and piston, the viscosity of the fluid, and the number, size, and shape of the orifices; and v = piston velocity relative to the cylinder.

Because they provide resistance that increases with speed, fluid cylinders allow rapid acceleration early in the exercise movement and little acceleration after higher speeds are reached. Movement speed is thus kept within an intermediate range. However, while such machines limit changes in velocity to a certain extent, they are not isokinetic (constant speed), as is often claimed. Some of the machines have adjustment knobs that allow the orifice size to be changed. A larger orifice allows a higher movement speed to be reached before the fluid resistive force curtails the ability to accelerate.

Fluid-resisted machines do not provide an eccentric exercise phase. With a free weight, a muscle group acts concentrically while raising the weight and eccentrically while lowering it. With fluid-resisted machines, a muscle group acts concentrically while performing the primary exercise movement, and the antagonist muscle group acts concentrically while returning to the starting position. In other words, whereas free weights or weight machines involve alternate concentric and eccentric actions of the same muscle with little or no rest in between, fluid-resisted machines involve alternate concentric actions of antagonistic muscle groups; each muscle group rests while its antagonist works. The lack of eccentric muscle action with fluid-resisted machines probably means that such exercise does not provide optimal training for the many sports movements that involve eccentric muscle actions (e.g., running, jumping, and throwing).

Elasticity

A number of exercise devices, particularly those designed for home use, have elastic components, such as springs or bands, as their source of resistance. The resistance provided by a standard elastic component is proportional to the distance it is stretched:

$$F_R = kx, \qquad (3.14)$$

where F_R = the resistive force, k = a constant that reflects the physical characteristics of the elastic component, and x = the distance the elastic component is stretched beyond its resting length.

The most obvious characteristic of elastic resistance is that the more the elastic component is stretched, the greater the resistance. The problem with devices using elastic resistance is that every exercise movement begins with low resistance and ends with high resistance. This is contrary to the force capability patterns of virtually all human muscle groups, which show a substantial drop-off of force capability toward the end of the range of motion. Another problem with elasticity-resisted machines is that the adjustability of resistance is usually limited by the number of bands that can be affixed to the device. An effective resistance exercise device must incorporate enough variation in resistive force so that the number of repetitions that the trainee can perform is kept within a desirable range.

There are products that provide resistance to vertical jumping with elastic bands as a means of developing jumping power. However, the elastic bands provide little resistance early in the jump, when the large muscles exert great force. The bands provide the greatest resistance while the jumper is in the air, where they serve mainly to pull the jumper back to the ground rather than to resist the muscles. Consequently, jumping with a weighted belt or vest is probably more effective for the development of jumping power.

Electronically Controlled Devices

Various resistance training devices are electronically controlled. The actual source of resistance may be one of those described above or a motor or pump. The distinguishing characteristic of these machines is that they can regulate the degree of resistance during an exercise movement through feedback and control technology. For example, isokinetic dynamometers match resistive force to muscle force in order to maintain constant joint angular velocity. Some devices allow eccentric exercise as well. Other machines control such parameters as power output and acceleration. It is difficult to generalize about electronically controlled exercise machines because of the great variety of such products; each device must be evaluated individually. However, they are generally much more expensive than other exercise apparatuses, and, as yet, there is no solid evidence that they provide superior training stimuli.

POWER OUTPUT DURING RESISTANCE EXERCISE

Because power is the product of both force and velocity, a knowledge of how various types of exercise devices provide resistive force is not sufficient for determining the power output elicited during training. Below are descriptions of how the constraints of both force and velocity affect human power output for various exercise modes.

Weight-Lifting Exercise

Since work equals force times distance, it takes the same amount of work to lift a particular weight a given distance, no matter how fast the weight is lifted. However, because power equals work per unit time, when the weight is lifted faster, the average power is higher. Peak power can be very high as the weight is accelerated. Whereas the force capability of muscle declines with increasing speed of contraction, muscle power increases (Figure 3.20) (43).

Friction-Resisted Exercise

Since the coefficient of friction does not change with the speed of sliding, the resistive force of a friction-resisted device stays constant regardless of the movement speed. Power output is then directly proportional to the speed of movement (see Equation 3.4).

Fluid-Resisted Exercise

For fluid-resisted exercise, as velocity of movement increases, the resistive force increases proportionately.

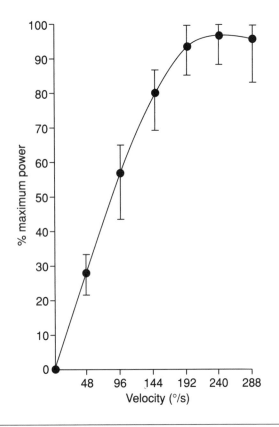

Figure 3.20 Muscle power as a function of muscle contraction speed.
Reprinted from Perrine and Edgerton (1978).

Since power is the product of force and velocity, power output is related to the square of velocity for such machines. Because power output increases so rapidly with movement speed, it is difficult to attain high velocity on these devices.

Elasticity-Resisted Exercise

Because resistance is proportional to the distance the elastic component is stretched, elasticity-resisted exercises are always easy to perform early in the movement and difficult at the end. If the exercise movement is performed at a constant velocity, the power output is highest furthest into the movement, where resistive force is greatest. As with the other forms of exercise, average power output increases when the exercise is performed faster.

Electronically Controlled Exercise

Because of the variety of electronically controlled exercise machines available, and the fact that they may be made to simulate the force and power patterns of other exercise modes, one cannot generalize about the power output required to exercise on all such devices.

Some electronically controlled exercise machines can be set for isokinetic operation wherein the body joint can flex or extend only at an operator-selected constant speed no matter how much torque is exerted on the machine; power output at a particular speed setting is directly proportional to the torque exerted by the athlete. To obtain a record of power output during the exercise, each torque data point is multiplied by the angular velocity at which the machine is set (see Equation 3.8). For the kind of isokinetic machine that moves at constant linear velocities, a record of power output during exercise can be obtained by multiplying each force data point by the linear velocity at which the machine is set (see Equation 3.4).

Some electronically controlled exercise machines can be set to operate at constant power output, no matter how the speed of movement varies. The machines accomplish this by constantly monitoring angular velocity and immediately adjusting the resistive torque to keep the product of force and velocity constant.

Negative Work and Power

Because power equals the product of force and velocity, when force is exerted on a weight in the direction opposite to the one in which the weight is moving, as when a weight is lowered in a controlled manner, calculated power has a negative sign, as does calculated work. All such "negative" power and work occurs during eccentric muscle activity, such as lowering a weight or decelerating at the end of a rapid movement.

Strictly speaking, there is no such thing as negative work or power. The term "negative work" really refers to work performed on, rather than by, a muscle. When a weight is lifted, muscles perform work on the weight, increasing the weight's potential energy. When the weight is lowered, its potential energy is used to perform an equal amount of work on the lifter. Thus, while lifting repetitions are performed, the lifter and weight alternately perform work on each other, rather than the lifter alternately performing positive and negative work. The rate at which the repetitions are performed determines the power output.

LIFTING SAFETY

As with any physical activity there is a degree of risk involved with resistance training. However, the risks involved are generally lower than for many sports. Nevertheless, it is desirable to minimize the likelihood of injury through prudent risk management. Below are discussed several factors to be considered in avoiding lifting injury with particular attention given to the back, shoulder, and knee.

The Back

Back Injury.   Back injury can be extremely debilitating, persistent, and difficult to remedy. Thus, every effort should be made to avoid back injury during lifting. The lower back is particularly vulnerable. It has been observed that 85% to 90% of all spinal-disk herniations occur at the disks between the lowest two lumbar vertebrae (L4 and L5) or between the lowest lumbar and the top sacral vertebra (L5 and S1) (Figure 3.21) (6). This is not surprising, given the extremely high compressive forces on the disks during lifting. When a weight is supported in the hands or on the shoulders and the trunk is inclined forward, there is great torque about the lower spinal disks due to the large horizontal distance between the lower back and the weight. The back muscles operate at an extremely low mechanical advantage because the perpendicular distance from the line of action of the spinal erector muscles to the spinal disks is much lower (about 5 cm) than the horizontal distance from the weight to the disks. As a result, the muscles must exert forces that frequently exceed 10 times the weight lifted. These forces act to squeeze the spinal disks between the adjacent vertebral bodies.

The spinal disks of larger people can generally support greater loads than those of smaller people. Also, as people age, the amount of force spinal disks can withstand decreases dramatically, as evidenced by compressive testing of the spines of cadavers (6). Disks of people under 40 years of age can typically withstand without damage more than twice the compressive force that would damage disks of people over 60.

The flat-back lifting posture has been found to be better overall than a rounded (opposite of arched) back in minimizing L5/S1 compressive forces and ligament strain (3). An arched back (**lordosis**) has been found to be superior to a rounded back for avoiding injury to vertebrae, disks, facet joints, ligaments, and muscles of the back. In addition, the low back muscles are capable of exerting considerably higher forces when the back is arched rather than rounded (22).

The spinal column is naturally S-shaped, being rounded in the upper back and arched in the lower back (see Figure 3.21). The wedged shape of the vertebrae give the spine its natural curve. However, the intervertebral disks are flat when the back is in its S-shape. When the lower back is rounded, the **ventral** (towards the belly) edges of the vertebral bodies squeeze the front portions of the spinal disks. In contrast, extreme arching of the back results in squeezing the **dorsal** (towards the back) portions of the disks. Such uneven squeezing of the spinal disks likely increases the risk of disk rupture. Thus, lifting should generally be performed with the lower back in a moderately arched position.

Intraabdominal Pressure and Lifting Belts.
When the diaphragm and the deep muscles of the torso contract, pressure is generated within the abdominal cavity. Because the abdomen is composed mainly of fluid and normally contains very little gas, it is virtually incompressible. The abdominal fluids and tissue kept under pressure by surrounding muscle (deep abdominal muscles and diaphragm) under tension have been described as a ''fluid ball'' (Figure 3.22) that aids in supporting the spinal column during lifting. Such support may significantly reduce both the forces required by the erector spinae muscles to perform a lift and the associated compressive forces on the disks (5, 42).

Weightlifting belts have been shown to increase intraabdominal pressure during lifting and are therefore probably effective in improving lifting safety (19, 33, 34). It has been cautioned, however, that if all lifting is done with a belt, the abdominal muscles that produce intraabdominal pressure might not get enough training stimulus to develop optimally (19). It is particularly risky for a person who has become accustomed to wearing a belt to suddenly perform a lift without one, because

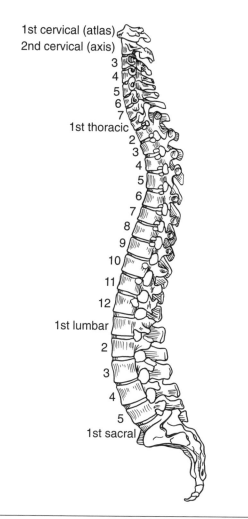

1st cervical (atlas)
2nd cervical (axis)
3
4
5
6
7
1st thoracic
2
3
4
5
6
7
8
9
10
11
12
1st lumbar
2
3
4
5
1st sacral

Figure 3.21 The spinal column.

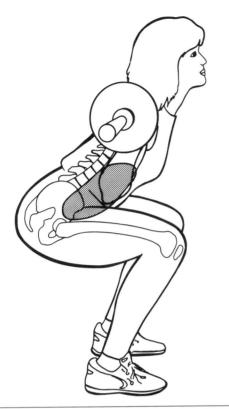

Figure 3.22 The "fluid ball" resulting from contraction of the deep abdominal muscles and the diaphragm.

the abdominal musculature might not be capable of generating enough intraabdominal pressure to significantly reduce erector spinae muscle forces. The resulting excessive compressive forces on the disks could increase the chance of back injury. Conservative recommendations are as follows:

- For exercises not stressing the back, do not wear a belt at all.
- For exercises directly stressing the back, refrain from wearing a belt during lighter sets but wear one for near-maximal and maximal sets. The belt-less sets allow the deep abdominal muscles, which generate intraabdominal pressure, to receive a training stimulus without placing excessive compressive forces on the spinal disks.

The Shoulders

The shoulder is particularly prone to injury during weight training, due both to its structure and to the forces to which it is subjected during lifting. Like the hip, the shoulder is capable of rotating in any direction. However, although the hip is a stable ball-and-socket joint, the glenoid cavity of the shoulder, which holds the head of the humerus, is not a true socket and is quite loose.

The looseness of the shoulder gives it a wide range of movement. It is so loose that the head of the humerus can actually move 2.5 cm out of the glenoid cavity during normal movement (14). Yet the joint's looseness contributes to its vulnerability, as does the close proximity of its bones, muscles, tendons, ligaments, and bursae.

The stability of the shoulder is largely dependent upon ligaments, joint capsules, and muscles. The rotator cuff muscles (supraspinatus, infraspinatus, subscapularis, and teres minor) and the pectorals are particularly instrumental in keeping the ball of the humerus in place (6). With the shoulder's great range of motion, its various structures easily impinge upon one another, causing tendinitis as well as inflammation and degeneration of contiguous tissue. High forces during lifting can result in tearing of ligaments, muscles, and tendons. Particular care must be taken when performing the various forms of the bench, incline, and military presses because of the great stresses they place on the shoulder.

The Knees

The knee is prone to injury because of its location between two long levers (the upper and lower leg). Flexion and extension about the knee occur almost exclusively in the **sagittal plane**. (Figure 3.23 indicates the three planes of the body in the **anatomical position**:

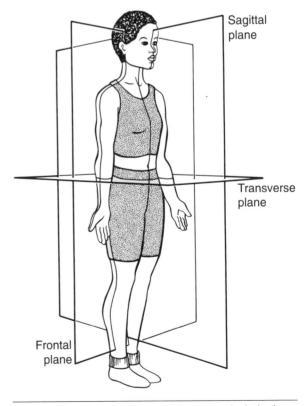

Figure 3.23 The three planes of the human body in the anatomical position.

body erect, arms down at sides, palms forward.) Rotation in the **frontal plane** and **transverse plane** is prevented mainly by ligamentous and cartilaginous stabilizing structures. Yet it does not take a great amount of torque about the knee in the frontal plane to cause serious damage. Frontal-plane torque on the knee occurs, for example, when a football player is hit at mid-leg from the side while his foot is planted firmly on the ground. Fortunately, in lifting, torques occur almost exclusively within the knee's normal plane of rotation.

Of the various components of the knee, the patella and surrounding tissue are most susceptible to the kinds of forces encountered in resistance training (9). The patella's main function is to hold the quadriceps tendon away from the knee axis, thereby increasing the moment arm of the quadriceps group and its mechanical advantage (see Figure 3.10). The high forces encountered by the patellar tendon during lifting can lead to tendinitis, which is characterized by tenderness and swelling.

Knee Wraps. It is not unusual for lifters to use knee wraps during training or competition. The wraps vary from the thin elastic pull-on variety that can be purchased in drug stores to the heavy, specialized wraps sold only through weightlifting supply houses. The use of knee wraps, particularly the heavy ones, is most prevalent among power lifters.

There has been very little research done on the efficacy of knee wraps. However, a number of professionals working with lifters have noted some detrimental side effects of heavy wraps, including skin damage and chondromalacia patellae, the wearing down and roughening of the posterior surface of the patella (17).

While there is no available evidence that wraps protect the knee against injury, a recent experiment showed that wraps can improve lifting performance (17). Through a spring effect alone, heavy wraps added an average of 25 lb (110 N) to the lifting force. The notion that wraps work only by either stabilizing the knee, lessening the lifter's fear of injury, or providing a kinesthetic cue is incorrect. The wraps actually provide direct help in extending the knee. Based on the lack of evidence that they prevent injury, and the opinion of a number of health practitioners working with lifters that they can actually cause injury, lifters should probably minimize the use of wraps.

Avoiding Injury During Weight Training

The following activities and procedures have been recommended to reduce the likelihood of injury during weight training:

- Perform one or more warm-up sets with relatively light weights, particularly for exercises that involve extensive use of the shoulder or knee. This stimulates blood flow to the muscles effecting the movement, increasing the temperature and pliability of ligaments, tendons, and other structures. Massage may provide additional benefit (49).

- Perform basic exercises through a full range of motion (49). Perform only specialized supplementary exercises through limited ranges of motion.

- Use relatively light weights when you introduce a new exercise to a program or resume lifting after a layoff of 2 or more weeks.

- Don't ignore pain in or around the joints. ''Working through'' pain can lead to chronic injury. Often, an athlete can continue lifting by using lighter weights with more repetitions, using different exercises, or both. If pain is severe and persistent, it may be necessary to temporarily suspend all lifting that affects the painful joint and to have the injury examined and treated medically. It is usually not necessary to discontinue resistance exercise completely.

- Never attempt maximal lifts without proper preparation, which includes technique instruction and a minimum of several weeks of training in the exercise movement. It is also prudent to phase into periods of maximal lifting a few times a year at most.

- Postworkout icing of superficial joints under heavy stress may aid in prevention of injury as well as in recuperation (9, 49).

- The inclusion of supplementary exercises in a workout may help to promote joint stability as well as balance within the muscles of a group and between those of opposing groups. For example, heavy squats can be accompanied by knee extension and flexion exercises on a weight stack machine (49). Lack of balance between muscles has been cited as a cause of athletic injury. It has been recommended that athletes perform exercise routines that maintain a ratio of knee flexion torque to extension torque of 0.67 to 0.77 at slow speed (60°/s), 0.80 to 0.91 at medium speed (180°/s), and 0.95 to 1.11 at fast speed (300°/s) (40).

- Avoid bouncing at the bottom of the squat exercise (49). The high eccentric force produced during such movements is a primary cause of muscle injury (47).

- Take care when incorporating plyometrics into a training program. It is generally agreed that athletes should be strong in the squat before beginning a lower-body plyometric program. Also, high-intensity plyometrics should not be performed year-round (44).

- During squatting, deviation of the knee from a vertical plane through the foot and hip can place potentially dangerous and unnecessary torques about the knee and should be avoided (49).

- Use knee and elbow wraps with great caution. If used at all, they should be limited to the heaviest lifts (49). Heavy and tight wraps can cause joint injury. If used, put them on immediately before and remove them immediately after each lift.
- Performing several variations of an exercise results in more complete muscle development and joint stability (e.g., a series or combination of the flat bench press, incline bench press, and decline bench press to train the chest and shoulders) (49).
- Do not attempt explosive exercises such as cleans, jerks, and snatches without qualified instruction, because minor flaws in technique can place extremely high and potentially destructive forces on muscles, ligaments, and tendons. Emphasize correct technique and mental concentration.

Flexibility and Stretching. Although it is frequently recommended that stretching can help prevent injury, evidence from research is lacking. The small amount of research relating flexibility to injury has focused on runners. A study of 583 habitual runners showed that those who regularly stretched before running had no fewer injuries than those who did not stretch (36).

People with relatively high flexibility, either naturally or through stretching, have not been shown to be at lower risk for injury. In fact, high flexibility as well as low flexibility can increase risk. Among 335 male recruits in army basic training, the most flexible 20% of the recruits and the least flexible 20% had more than twice as many injuries as those of average flexibility (8, 28). There is some evidence that low flexibility may increase the risk of muscle and tendon injury and that high flexibility may increase the risk for ligament and cartilage injury (2). Tight muscles, which protect cartilage and ligaments by limiting a joint's range of motion, are susceptible to tearing. People who are naturally loose-muscled should not engage in more than mild stretching. Naturally tight-muscled people probably benefit most from stretching. The most effective stretching occurs when a muscle is warm. Warming can be accomplished through either exercise or external heating; appropriate clothing allows muscles and tendons to warm up faster in cool weather. The key point is that, for improvement in flexibility that is not merely transient, most stretching should be done after exercise when the muscles are warm and can be most readily stretched without injury. Little pre-exercise stretching is needed before exercise that does not involve extreme ranges of motion. However, before engaging in sports that do require extreme ranges of motion, the most appropriate sequence is: light stretching, full warm-up using exercises not involving extreme ranges of motion, then comprehensive stretching to extreme ranges of motion.

Stretching is probably most important for athletes engaged in sports that involve extreme ranges of joint motion (e.g., gymnastics). The athlete should be flexible enough to move easily through the range of joint motion required by the sport.

MOVEMENT ANALYSIS AND EXERCISE PRESCRIPTION

The concept of **specificity**, widely recognized in the field of resistance training (11), holds that training is most effective when resistance exercises are similar to the sports activity in which improvement is sought (the target activity). Although all athletes should use well-rounded, whole-body exercise routines, supplementary exercises specific to the sport can provide a training advantage and lessen the likelihood of injury. The simplest and most straightforward way to implement the principle of specificity is to select exercises similar to the target activity with regard to the joints about which movements occur and the directions of movement. In addition, joint ranges of motion in the training exercises should be at least as great as those in the target activity.

Biomechanical analysis of human movement can be used to quantitatively analyze the target activity. However, in the absence of the requisite equipment and expertise, simple visual observation is adequate for identifying the basic features of a sports movement. Exercises can then be selected that involve similar movement around the same joints. Slow-motion film or videotape can facilitate the necessary observation.

A simplified list of possible body movements that provides a manageable framework for a movement-oriented exercise prescription is illustrated in Figure 3.24. Only movements in the frontal, sagittal, and transverse planes (see Figure 3.23) are considered because, whereas few body movements occur only in these three major planes, there is enough overlap of training effects so that exercising muscles within the planes also strengthens them for movements between the planes.

Movement-Oriented Exercise Prescription

Although a program providing resistance exercise for all the movements in Figure 3.24 would be both comprehensive and balanced, some of the movements are commonly omitted from standard exercise programs, while others receive particular emphasis. Important sports movements not usually exercised in standard weight training programs include shoulder internal and external rotation (throwing, pulling), knee flexion (sprinting),

Wrist—sagittal

Flexion
Exercise: wrist curl
Sport: tennis serve

Extension
Exercise: reverse wrist curl
Sport: racquet backhand

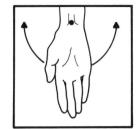

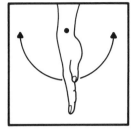

Wrist—frontal

Ulnar deviation
Exercise: specific wrist curl
Sport: baseball batting

Radial deviation
Exercise: specific wrist curl
Sport: golf backswing

Elbow—sagittal

Flexion
Exercise: arm curl
Sport: rowing

Extension
Exercise: triceps pushdown
Sport: boxing jab

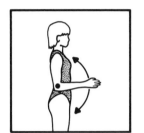

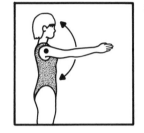

Shoulder—sagittal

Flexion
Exercise: medium-grip military press
Sport: softball pitch

Extension
Exercise: narrow-grip row
Sport: freestyle swimming

Shoulder—frontal

Adduction
Exercise: wide-grip pulldown
Sport: gymnastic rings

Abduction
Exercise: wide-grip military press
Sport: springboard diving

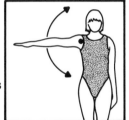

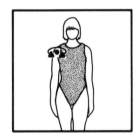

Shoulder—transverse

Internal rotation
Exercise: arm wrestle movement (with dumbbell or cable)
Sport: baseball pitch

External rotation
Exercise: reverse arm wrestle movement
Sport: karate block

Shoulder—transverse

(upper arm 90° to trunk)

Adduction
Exercise: wide-grip bench press
Sport: boxing hook

Abduction
Exercise: row (elbows high)
Sport: tennis backhand

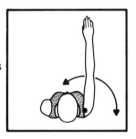

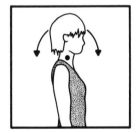

Neck—sagittal

Flexion
Exercise: neck machine
Sport: somersault

Extension
Exercise: neck machine
Sport: wrestling bridge

Neck—transverse

Left rotation
Exercise: neck machine
Sport: wrestling

Right rotation
Exercise: neck machine
Sport: wrestling

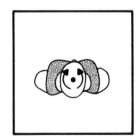

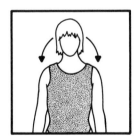

Neck—frontal

Left tilt
Exercise: neck machine
Sport: wrestling

Right tilt
Exercise: neck machine
Sport: wrestling

(continued)

Figure 3.24 Major body movements. Planes of movement are relative to the body in the anatomical position unless stated otherwise. Common exercises that provide resistance to the movements and related sports activities are listed.
Reprinted from reference 18, Harman, Johnson, and Frykman (1992).

hip flexion (kicking, sprinting), ankle dorsiflexion (running), hip internal and external rotation (pivoting), hip adduction and abduction (lateral movement), torso rotation (throwing), and all the neck movements (impact absorption). Yet a resistance training program designed around sport-specific exercise movements is important for both improving performance and lessening the likelihood of injury.

Figure 3.24 can assist in designing comprehensive and balanced training programs, determining deficiencies

Lower back—sagittal

Flexion
Exercise: weighted sit-up
Sport: somersault

Extension
Exercise: reverse sit-up
Sport: rowing

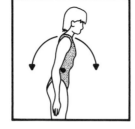

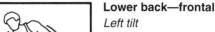

Lower back—frontal

Left tilt
Exercise: side bend
Sport: gymnastics side aerial

Right tilt
Exercise: side bend
Sport: gymnastics side aerial

Lower back—transverse

Left rotation
Exercise: torso machine
Sport: baseball batting

Right rotation
Exercise: torso machine
Sport: baseball batting

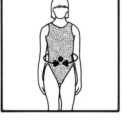

Hip—sagittal

Flexion
Exercise: leg raise
Sport: football punt

Extension
Exercise: squat
Sport: jumping

Hip—frontal

Adduction
Exercise: adduction machine
Sport: lateral movement

Abduction
Exercise: abduction machine
Sport: skating

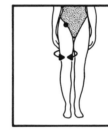

Hip—transverse

Internal rotation
Exercise: friction rotation
Sport: pivot movement

Extension
Exercise: friction rotation
Sport: pivot movement

Hip—transverse

(upper leg 90° to trunk)
Adduction
Exercise: adduction machine
Sport: karate in-sweep

Abduction
Exercise: abduction machine
Sport: karate out-sweep

Knee—sagittal

Flexion
Exercise: leg curl
Sport: sprint running

Extension
Exercise: leg extension
Sport: bicycling

Ankle—sagittal

Dorsiflexion
Exercise: dorsiflexion
(weight-resisted)
Sport: running

Plantarflexion
Exercise: calf raise
Sport: jumping

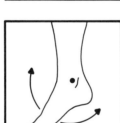
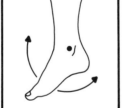

Ankle—frontal

Inversion
Exercise: inversion
Sport: ice skating

Eversion
Exercise: eversion (friction
resisted)
Sport: ice skating

Figure 3.24 *(continued)*

in existing programs, and identifying exercises that could improve performance in particular sports. Visual observation of a sport, with or without the assistance of high-speed film or video, allows the determination of which movements are particularly important to that sport. Sport-specific training exercises can be selected that provide resistance to relevant movements through the appropriate ranges of motion. Not only should the desired movement occur in an exercise, but the movement must be resisted (e.g., an arm curl involves both flexion and extension about the elbow, but only the flexion is resisted). Specificity of speed is important to consider as well. If a sport involves rapid application of force, then ''explosive'' exercises should be incorporated into the training program (48).

CONCLUSION

It is hoped that readers will apply the biomechanical principles provided in this chapter to the selection of resistance exercise equipment and the design of exercise programs. Knowledge of how different forms of resistance tax the body can aid in the tailoring of programs to suit the specific needs of various types of athletes and others who engage in resistance training for enhancement of physical performance, health, sense of well-being, and self-confidence.

Key Terms

acceleration	28	fleshy attachment	20	recruitment	31
agonist	20	fluid resistance	38	resistive force	25
anatomical position	42	form drag	38	rotational power	30
anatomy	19	friction	38	rotational work	30
angle of pennation	31	frontal plane	43	sacral vertebra	20
angular displacement	30	fulcrum	25	sagittal plane	42
angular velocity	30	inertial force	37	second-class lever	25
antagonist	20	insertion	20	specificity	44
appendicular skeleton	19	isometric muscle action	32	spinal column	20
axial skeleton	19	joint	19	strength	29
biaxial joint	20	lever	25	surface drag	38
biomechanics	19	lordosis	41	synergist	20
cartilaginous joint	19	lumbar vertebra	20	synovial joint	19
cervical vertebra	20	mechanical advantage	25	tendon	20
classical formula	34	moment arm	25	third-class lever	25
coccygeal vertebra	20	multiaxial joint	20	thoracic vertebra	20
concentric muscle action	32	muscle force	25	torque	25
distal	20	origin	20	transverse plane	43
dorsal	41	pennate muscle	31	uniaxial joint	20
eccentric muscle action	32	power	29	ventral	41
fibrous attachment	20	proximal	20	weight	35
fibrous joint	19	rate coding	31	work	29
first-class lever	25				

Study Questions

1. Which kind of joint is the knee?

   a. fibrous
   b. cartilaginous
   c. synovial
   d. appendicular
   e. multiaxial

2. Most human limbs are operated as which class of lever?

    a. first class
    b. second class
    c. third class

3. Power is the product of

    a. mass and acceleration
    b. force and angular velocity
    c. force and distance
    d. force and velocity
    e. torque and time

4. To compare performances of lifters of different body weights, the classical formula divides the lift by

    a. body weight
    b. body weight squared
    c. body weight to the two-thirds power
    d. body weight to the three-fourths power
    e. lean body weight

5. During free-weight exercise, resistive torque varies with

    a. the horizontal distance from the weight to the body joint
    b. the vertical distance from the weight to the body joint
    c. the movement velocity
    d. the square of movement velocity
    e. the inverse of movement velocity

6. A vertical jump involves knee, hip, and shoulder movement mainly in which plane?

    a. perpendicular
    b. orthogonal
    c. sagittal
    d. frontal
    e. transverse

7. Compared to other athletes of various sizes and body builds, an athlete with a high strength-to-mass ratio should be able to

    a. lift more
    b. change direction more quickly
    c. throw farther
    d. hit harder
    e. absorb impact better

Applying Knowledge
of the Biomechanics of Resistance Exercise

Problem 1
A student who has been engaging in bodybuilding for 3 years asks for help in modifying his training program to enable him to compete in high jumping. What would you recommend?

Problem 2
A tennis coach has funds available to purchase one or two pieces of equipment for the university weight room and asks advice on which equipment would be particularly beneficial for tennis players. What would you recommend?

Problem 3

A member of the football team asks if heavy elastic bands tightly wrapped about his knees before squat training should be used to improve his strength and football performance. How would you answer him?

References

1. Alexander, R., and A. Vernon. The dimensions of the knee and ankle muscles and the forces they exert. *J. Human Mvmt. Studies* 1:115-123. 1975.
2. Alter, M.J. *Science of Stretching*. Champaign, IL: Human Kinetics. 1988. pp. 8-9.
3. Anderson, C.K., and D.B. Chaffin. A biomechanical evaluation of five lifting techniques. *Appl. Ergon.* 2-7. March 1986.
4. Astrand, P., and K. Rodahl. *Textbook of Work Physiology*, 3rd ed. New York: McGraw-Hill. 1986.
5. Bartelink, D.L. The role of abdominal pressure in relieving the pressure on the lumbar intervertebral discs. *J. Bone Joint Surg.* 39B(4):718-725. 1957.
6. Chaffin, D.B., and G. Andersson. *Occupational Biomechanics*. New York: Wiley. 1984.
7. Convertino, V.A. Physiological adaptations to weightlessness: Effects on exercise and work performance. In: *Exercise and Sports Sciences Reviews*, vol. 18, K.B. Pandolf and J.O. Halloszy, eds. Baltimore: Williams & Wilkins. 1990. pp. 119-166.
8. Cowan, D., B. Jones, P. Tomlinson, J. Robinson, D. Polly, P. Frykman, and K. Reynolds. *The Epidemiology of Physical Training Injuries in U.S. Army Infantry Trainees, Technical Report T4-89.* Natick, MA: U.S. Army Research Institute of Environmental Medicine. 1988.
9. Ellison, A.E., A.L. Boland, P. Grace, and H. Calehuff, eds. *Athletic Training and Sports Medicine*. Chicago: American Academy of Orthopaedic Surgeons. 1986.
10. Enoka, R.M. *Neuromechanical Basis of Kinesiology*. Champaign, IL: Human Kinetics. 1988.
11. Fleck, S.J., and W.J. Kraemer. *Designing Resistance Training Programs*. Champaign, IL: Human Kinetics. 1987.
12. Garhammer, J. Weight lifting and training. In: *Biomechanics of Sport*, C. Vaughn, ed. Boca Raton, FL: CRC Press. 1989. pp. 169-211.
13. Gowitzke, B.A., and M. Milner. *Scientific Bases of Human Movement*, 3rd ed. Baltimore: Williams & Wilkins. 1988.
14. Gray, H. *Anatomy of the Human Body*, 28th ed. Philadelphia: Lea & Febiger. 1966.
15. Gregor, R.J. The structure and function of skeletal muscle. In: *Kinesiology and Applied Anatomy*, 7th ed., P.J. Rasch, ed. Philadelphia: Lea & Febiger. 1989. pp. 34-35.
16. Harman, E. Resistive torque analysis of 5 Nautilus exercise machines. *Med. Sci. Sports Exerc.* 15(2):113. 1983.
17. Harman, E., and P. Frykman. The effects of knee wraps on weightlifting performance and injury. *NSCA Journal* 12(5):30-35. 1990.
18. Harman, E.A., M. Johnson, and P.N. Frykman. A movement-oriented approach to exercise prescription. *NSCA Journal* 14(1):47-54. 1992.
19. Harman, E.A., R.M. Rosenstein, P.N. Frykman, and G.A. Nigro. Effects of a belt on intra-abdominal pressure during weight lifting. *Med. Sci. Sports Exerc.* 21(2):186-190. 1989.
20. Haxton, H.A. Absolute muscle force in the ankle flexors of man. *J. Physiol.* 103:267-273. 1944.
21. Hay, J.G., and J.G. Reid. *The Anatomical and Mechanical Bases of Human Motion*. Englewood Cliffs, NJ: Prentice Hall. 1982.
22. Herbert, L., and G. Miller. Newer heavy load lifting methods help firms reduce back injuries. *Occup. Health Saf.* 57-60. February 1987.
23. Hester, D., G. Hunter, K. Shuleva, and T. Kekes-Sabo. Review and evaluation of relative strength-handicapping models. *NSCA Journal* 12(1):54-57. 1990.
24. Higdon, A., W.B. Stiles, A.W. Davis, and C.R. Evces. *Engineering Mechanics*. Englewood Cliffs, NJ: Prentice Hall. 1976.
25. Hill, A.V. *First and Last Experiments in Muscle Mechanics*. London: Cambridge University Press. 1970.
26. Ikai, M., and T. Fukunaga. Calculation of muscle strength per unit cross-sectional area of human muscle by means of ultrasonic measurement. *Int. Z. Angew. Physiol. Arbeitphysiol.* 26:26-32. 1968.
27. Johnson, J.H., S. Colodny, and D. Jackson. Human torque capability versus machine resistive torque for four Eagle resistance machines. *J. Appl. Sport Sci. Res.* 4(3):83-87. 1990.
28. Jones, B., D. Cowan, P. Tomlinson, D. Polly, and J. Robinson. Risks for training injuries in army recruits. *Med. Sci. Sports Exerc.* 20(2):S42. 1988.
29. Jorgensen, K. Force-velocity relationship in human elbow flexors and extensors. In: *Biomechanics V-A*, P.V. Komi, ed. Baltimore: University Park Press. 1976.
30. Knuttgen, H., and W. Kraemer. Terminology and measurement in exercise performance. *J. Appl. Sport Sci. Res.* 1(1):1-10. 1987.
31. Landau, B.R. *Essential Human Anatomy and Physiology*. Glenview, IL: Scott, Foresman. 1976.
32. Lander, J.E., B.T. Bates, J.A. Sawhill, and J. Hamill. A comparison between free-weight and isokinetic bench pressing. *Med. Sci. Sports Exerc.* 17(3):344-353. 1985.

33. Lander, J.E., J.R. Hundley, and R.L. Simonton. The effectiveness of weight-belts during multiple repetitions of the squat exercise. *Med. Sci. Sports Exerc.* 24(5):603-609. 1990.

34. Lander, J.E., R.L. Simonton, and J.K.F. Giacobbe. The effectiveness of weight-belts during the squat exercise. *Med. Sci. Sports Exerc.* 22(1):117-126. 1990.

35. *Le Système International d'Unités (SI)*, 3rd ed. Sevres, France: Bureau International des Poids et Mesures. 1977.

36. Macera, C.A., R.R. Pate, K.E. Powell, K.L. Jackson, J.S. Kendrick, and T. Craven. Predicting lower extremity injuries among habitual runners. *Archives Intern. Med.* 149:2565-2568. November 1989.

37. McDonagh, M.J.N., and C.T.M. Davies. Adaptive response of mammalian skeletal muscle to exercise with high loads. *European J. Appl. Physiol.* 52:139-155. 1984.

38. Meriam, J. *Engineering Mechanics*, vol. 2: Dynamics. New York: Wiley. 1978.

39. Mish, F., ed. *Webster's Ninth New Collegiate Dictionary*. Springfield, MA: Merriam-Webster. 1984.

40. Moore, J.R., and G. Wade. Prevention of anterior cruciate ligament injuries. *NSCA Journal* 11(3):35-40. 1989.

41. Moritani, T., and H.A. deVries. Neural factors versus hypertrophy in the time course of muscle strength gain. *Am. J. Phys. Med.* 58(3):115-130. 1979.

42. Morris, J.M., D.B. Lucas, and B. Bresler. Role of the trunk in stability of the spine. *J. Bone Joint Surg.* 43A:327-351. 1961.

43. Perrine, J.J., and V.R. Edgerton. Muscle force-velocity and power-velocity relationships under isokinetic loading. *Med. Sci. Sports* 10(3):159-166. 1978.

44. Practical considerations for utilizing plyometrics, part 2. *NSCA Journal* 8(4):14-24. 1986.

45. Scott, S.H., and D.A. Winter. A comparison of three muscle pennation assumptions and their effect on isometric and isotonic force. *J. Biomech.* 24(2):163-167. 1991.

46. Smith, E.L. Exercise for the prevention of osteoporosis: A review. *Phys. Sportsmed.* 10:72-83. 1982.

47. Stauber, W.T. Eccentric action of muscles: Physiology, injury, and adaptation. In: *Exercise and Sports Sciences Reviews*, vol. 17, K.B. Pandolf, ed. Baltimore: Williams & Wilkins. 1989. pp. 157-185.

48. Stone, M. Explosive exercises/explosive training: NSCA position paper. *NSCA Journal* 15(3):7-15. 1993.

49. Totten, L. Knee wraps. *NSCA Journal* 12(5):36-38. 1990.

50. Vorobyov, E.I., O.G. Gazenko, A.M. Genin, and A.D. Egorov. Medical results of Salyut-6 manned space flights. *Aviat. Space Environ. Med.* 54(suppl. 1):S31-S40. 1983.

51. Weast, R., ed. *Handbook of Chemistry and Physics*, 54th ed. Cleveland, OH: CRC Press. 1973.

CHAPTER 4

BONE, MUSCLE, AND CONNECTIVE TISSUE ADAPTATIONS TO PHYSICAL ACTIVITY

Brian P. Conroy
Roger W. Earle

The three major components of the musculoskeletal system are bone, skeletal muscle, and intervening connective tissue. Each component contributes to the overall function of the entire system. Bone provides the structural support for the system, muscle contains the contractile units and converts stored chemical energy into the mechanical energy needed to produce movement, and connective tissue acts as a framework upon which the forces generated by the contracting musculature can be transmitted to the associated bony levers to elicit the desired movement. The three components are functionally inseparable relative to their role in athletic performance. Muscles cannot undergo even an isometric contraction without using bone and connective tissue for stabilization.

The ability to create, transmit, and sustain the forces required to successfully create movement depends on a predetermined balance of functional abilities among bone, muscle, and connective tissue. This intimate relationship suggests that when the system is stressed, as during physical activity, bone, muscle, and connective tissue must adapt in a coordinated manner to preserve the strength and integrity of the whole force-generating system. When an athlete repeatedly stresses the musculoskeletal system beyond its normal level of functioning, it is not uncommon that bone or connective tissue adaptations lag behind the development of the exercising muscle. This phenomenon needs to be recognized by the strength and conditioning professional so that injury is avoided and athletic performance maximized. Understanding how the individual components of the musculoskeletal system adapt to physical activity should provide a knowledge base upon which the strength and conditioning professional can predict the outcome of a specific training program.

This chapter will describe the adaptations that occur in bone, muscle, and connective tissue in response to various exercise programs. Background information regarding the essential structural features of bone and other connective tissues is included in this chapter to assist the reader in understanding the specific adaptations that occur within these tissues. (The structure of skeletal muscle was described in detail in chapter 1 and thus will not be presented here.)

ADAPTATION OF BONE TO EXERCISE

Bone is classified as a connective tissue. It is a unique connective tissue in that it becomes mineralized and thereby provides a rigid support structure. Interestingly, this rigid structure is actually a very active tissue that is sensitive to changes in the forces it experiences and has the capacity for growth and regeneration if damaged. Exercise creates mechanical forces that cause deformation of specific regions of the skeleton. These forces can be bending forces, compressive forces, torsional forces, or the forces created by muscular contractions on the tendinous insertion of a muscle into bone. The sections that follow will discuss how bone responds to mechanical forces, identify the types of forces that best stimulate new bone formation, and explore the response of bone to physical activity in untrained and aged populations.

The Biology of Bone Formation

In response to mechanical loading, bone cells called **osteoblasts** migrate to the bone surface that is experiencing the strain and begin the process of **bone modeling** (Figure 4.1). The osteoblasts manufacture and secrete proteins, primarily collagen molecules, that are deposited in the spaces between bone cells to increase the strength of the bone in that area. These proteins form a meshwork, called the **bone matrix**, between the bone cells. The proteins added to the matrix eventually become mineralized as calcium phosphate crystals (hydroxyapatite), precipitate from the extracellular fluid, and bind to the protein matrix. It is the mineralization of the matrix that gives bone its characteristic rigidity. (For further detail on bone formation, refer to reference 50.)

New bone formation occurs predominantly on the outer surface of the bone called the **periosteum** (86). Laying down new bone on the periphery to increase bone diameter is the most effective way of increasing bone strength without compromising the space requirements for the highly vascular bone marrow cavity at the center of the bone (18). Growth of bone in this manner is somewhat analogous to the growth of skeletal muscle in response to exercise. During the process of muscle hypertrophy, the addition of new myofilaments is to the periphery of the existing myofibril. The myofilaments are layered onto the outside of the existing myofibril rather than within the myofibril to avoid altering the geometric arrangement of myofilaments within the preexisting sarcomeres of the myofibril (43).

The adaptation of bone to mechanical loading occurs at different rates in the **axial skeleton** (spine and proximal femur) and the **appendicular skeleton** (long

bones), owing to differing amounts of **trabecular bone** (spongy) and **cortical bone** (compact). Cortical bone is dense and forms a compact outer shell that is bridged by interconnecting narrow and delicate plates of trabecular bone. The spaces between the trabecular plates are occupied by bone marrow, which consists of adipose tissue and blood products. Blood vessels from the marrow cavity extend into the dense cortical bone through a network of vertical and horizontal canals (Figure 4.2). Trabecular bone is able to respond more rapidly to stimuli than cortical bone. The bones of the vertebral column contain approximately 70% trabecular bone by volume, whereas trabecular bone is found only in the marrow cavities of long bones (50). Deposition of new collagen fibers in vertebral bone can be expected after 8 to 12 weeks of mechanical loading. Subsequent mineralization of the new bone matrix to give full strength to the new bone requires additional time and may take several weeks to complete (14,50).

The Stimulus for New Bone Formation

The term **minimal essential strain (MES)** is used to refer to the threshold stimulus that initiates new bone formation. A force that reaches or exceeds this threshold and is repeated often enough will signal osteoblasts to migrate to that region of the bone and lay down matrix proteins to increase the strength of the bone in that area. Forces that fall below the MES do not present a stimulus for new bone formation. Physical activities that generate forces exceeding the MES are those activities that represent an increase in intensity relative to normal daily activities. For example, in aged and sedentary individuals brisk walking may exceed the MES, while for younger, more active people the activities may need to be of higher intensity—such as sprinting, jumping, and heavy resistance exercise—to exceed the MES. Regardless of the population and their loading history, it is clear that the activities chosen need to be weight bearing—that is, having the additional stress of one's body weight involved—to provide the most effective stimulus for bone formation.

Bone cells regulate the quantity of the bone in each area to ensure that forces that are experienced on a regular basis do not exceed the MES. This regulation of bone mass establishes a margin of safety in the bone against fracture. The strain registered by the bone is a function of the force per unit area of bone. The MES is thought to be a level of strain approximately one tenth of the force required to fracture the bone (18). If a large force is regularly applied to a bone, the area of the bone supporting the load will need to be large enough to dissipate the forces and prevent damage consequent to loading. Increasing the diameter of the bone by laying down new bone at the periosteum allows the force to

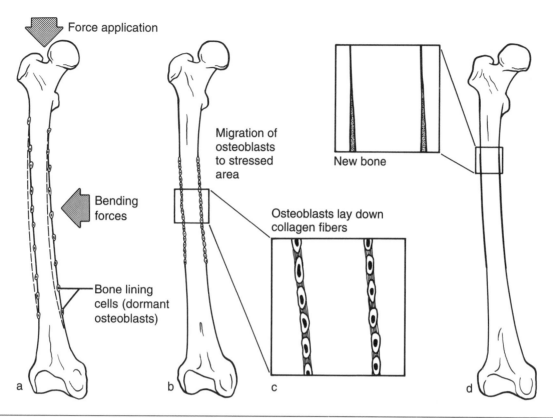

Figure 4.1 Bone modeling in response to mechanical loading. (a) Application of a longitudinal weight bearing force causes the bone to bend (as depicted by the dotted line), creating a stimulus for new bone formation at the regions experiencing the greatest deformation. (b) Previously dormant osteoblasts migrate to the area experiencing the strain. (c) Osteoblasts lay down additional collagen fibers at the site. (d) The collagen fibers become mineralized and the bone diameter has effectively increased.

be distributed over a larger surface area. Thus, there is a decrease in the amount of force per unit area across the bone surface. After bone growth occurs, the same force that previously exceeded the MES will now be below the MES threshold and not present a threat to the bone (18).

Effects of Physical Activity on Bone

The total mass of a muscle reflects the forces that the muscle is capable of exerting on the bones to which it is attached. The force capabilities of larger and better trained muscles are greater; consequently, the related regions of connective tissue and bone must increase their mass and strength to provide a sufficient support structure for the hypertrophied muscles. To generalize, an increase or decrease in muscle strength or mass through training or periods of reduced activity will result in a corresponding increase or decrease in connective tissue and bone (11).

Immobility

The loss of bone matrix and **bone mineral density** (the quantity of mineral deposited in a given area of bone)

following a period of reduced loading or immobility appears to occur at a much more rapid rate than the formation and mineralization of new bone. Rapid removal of calcium from bone, which results in a net loss of bone mineral content, occurs after only a few weeks of bed rest (33,38). Interestingly, the absence of weight-bearing forces on the spine during bed rest has a greater influence on the vertebral bone loss than the absence of muscular contractions (33,38). This information underlines the importance of loading the spine with compressive forces associated with weight bearing during an exercise program designed to increase bone mass.

Important Training Concepts for Stimulating New Bone Formation

Numerous studies have demonstrated a significant positive correlation between bone mineral density values and the strength of the attached musculature (27,63,64). Activities that stimulate muscle hypertrophy and strength gains also appear to stimulate the growth of bone and associated connective tissue. It is currently thought that training programs designed to stimulate bone growth need to incorporate specificity of loading, progressive overload, and variation (5).

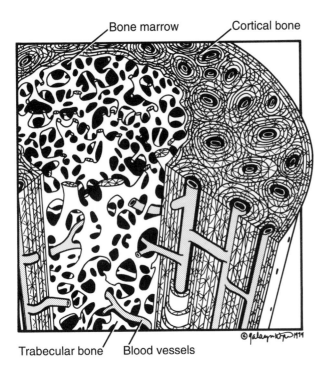

Figure 4.2 Bone architecture—cortical and trabecular bone.

Specificity refers to employing exercises that directly load a particular region of the skeleton. The forces created by exercise are directed through the supporting skeletal structures. If the body interprets these forces as new or unusual they will stimulate bone growth in the area receiving the strain. To provide a practical example: Running may be a good stimulus for increasing bone mineral density in the femur, but the wrong choice for loading the wrist. More appropriate exercises for stimulating bone growth of the wrist might include bench presses or overhead presses.

The concept of specificity of loading becomes particularly important when a professional prescribes exercises to increase the bone mass in the regions of the skeleton most commonly affected in osteoporosis. **Osteoporosis** is a disease in which bone mineral density and bone mass become reduced to critically low levels. When the bone becomes this compromised, forces that would normally be absorbed by the skeleton now result in bone fractures. The sites of fracture that are the most devastating are in the axial skeleton (the spine and hip). In order to minimize the risk of developing critically low levels of bone mineral density in late adulthood, current thinking suggests that people maximize their peak bone mineral density in the axial skeleton in early adulthood when they are most capable of performing the intense physical activities that increase bone mineral density (5,42).

Because bone and connective tissue respond to mechanical forces that threaten the supporting structures of the contracting musculature, the principle of **progressive overload**—progressively placing greater-than-normal demands on the exercising musculature—applies to training to increase bone mass as well as training to improve muscle strength (27,57,87). Although the maximal strength of bone and connective tissue is maintained well above the voluntary force capabilities of the associated musculature (18), these tissues respond to dramatic or unusual forces that are repetitively presented to the skeleton. The adaptive response is to ensure that the forces do not exceed a specific critical level that would place the bone or the connective tissue at risk for damage.

Stress fractures—microfractures in bone due to structural fatigue—and soft tissue injuries can occur when a force is routinely applied to the bone and related connective tissues before they have had a chance to adapt to the new exercise stimulus. This occurs, for example, when previously sedentary recruits undergo rigorous physical training following arrival at a military training center (51). This training often includes running with a weighted backpack. The dramatic change in the intensity and quantity of daily physical activity necessitates rapid adaption of bone and connective tissue. Recruits either make the adaption very quickly or sustain daily musculoskeletal damage that becomes cumulative when it cannot be repaired quickly enough. The end result of such damage can include stress fractures, tendinitis, and muscle injuries, all of which can be quite painful and take weeks or months to heal.

Appropriate application of the principles of overloading the musculoskeletal system and progressively increasing the load as the tissues become accustomed to the stimulus are the keys to increasing bone and connective tissue strength. Support for this concept comes from studies that have compared the bone mineral density of various groups of athletes with the mass and strength of the associated musculature and with the bone mineral content in nonathletes (12,16,27,56). In fact, elite adolescent weightlifters have been found to possess levels of bone mineralization that far exceed the typical values found in untrained adults with fully mature bone status (6,87). This observation is interesting because it indicates that young bone may be more responsive to **osteogenic stimuli**—factors that stimulate new bone formation—than mature bone. The enhanced sensitivity of young bone to mechanical forces has been repeated in other human studies (42) and various investigations involving experimental animals (40). The result of these studies has led to a hypothesis that in order to avoid dangerously low bone mass in old age, people should train to maximally elevate their **peak bone mass**—the maximum bone mass achieved—during early adulthood when the mechanisms for bone growth still function at optimal levels.

World-class powerlifters have made some unique contributions to the knowledge of the bone response to extreme external loading. Competitors at the 1983 World Powerlifting Championships were assessed for the bone mineral content of their lumbar vertebrae (27). As expected, the bone mineral content was very high and correlated positively with the overall loads each competitor lifted during the previous year (Figure 4.3). However, the magnitude of the forces sustained by the vertebrae of the powerlifters during deadlifts exceeded the predicted fracture threshold of the vertebral bone as calculated from the bone mineral content. (Normally, the relationship between bone mineral content and bone strength is linear.) This finding demonstrates that, at very high strength levels, bone strength is disproportionately greater than bone mineral content. It also suggests that vertebral bone in such highly trained athletes must undergo significant structural adaptations of the internal bone architecture to create such a resistance to fracture.

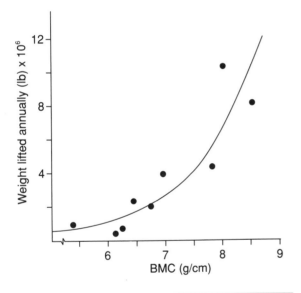

Figure 4.3 The relationship between the bone mineral content (BMC) in the third lumbar vertebrae in eight world-class powerlifters and the amount of weight lifted annually ($r^2 = 0.815$).
Reprinted from Granhed, Jonson, and Hansson (1987).

The Essential Components of Mechanical Loading

The components of the mechanical load that stimulate bone growth in laboratory animals are (a) the magnitude of the load (intensity) (67), (b) the rate (speed) of loading (59), (c) the direction of the forces (66), and (d) the volume of loading (number of repetitions) (66). The first three components have been shown to exert a powerful

influence on new bone formation in the following manner: The greater the magnitude of the load, the greater the stimulus for bone growth; higher rates of contraction (high–power output activities) enhance the stimulus for new bone growth; and alteration of the normal pattern of bone loading (direction of force) with other variables held constant stimulates bone growth. If the magnitude of the load and/or the rate of force application is sufficient, then there is no need to perform more than a total of 30 to 35 repetitions as a greater volume of loading will not provide any additional stimulus for bone growth (66).

A few longitudinal training studies have been performed using resistance exercise as the stimulus for new bone formation. These studies have reported variable results, with some studies showing gains in bone mineral density (9,72) and others showing little or no changes consequent to training (19,57). No resistance training studies designed to increase new bone formation have been performed to date that incorporate the relative magnitude of loading, rate of loading, and type of exercises typically used by competitive strength athletes.

In training for improvements in muscle strength and size, strength athletes incorporate into their training programs all the components of mechanical loading necessary to stimulate new bone formation. A summary of the exercise variables common to the training program of athletic populations found to have high bone mineral density values is seen in Table 4.1. This table is intended to be a guideline for designing resistance exercise programs to promote increases in bone mass. Until further studies are performed, the guidelines described in Table 4.1 must be viewed as preliminary because they arise from the observation of the strong correlation between muscular strength and bone mineral density, rather than from a documented cause and effect relationship.

Exercise Selection

The selection of the appropriate exercises to elicit a maximal osteogenic response at a specific skeletal site

Table 4.1 Exercise Prescription Guidelines for Stimulating Bone Growth

Variables	Specific recommendations
Volume	3-6 sets of up to 10 repetitions
Load	1-10RM
Rest	1-4 min
Variation	Typical periodization schemes designed to increase muscle strength and size
Exercise selection	Structural exercises: squats, deadlifts, cleans, bench press, shoulder press

has been a common source of error in the exercise literature. The choice of exercises should be based on exercises that involve many muscle groups in one exercise (**structural exercises**), direct the force vectors through the axial skeleton (spine and hip), and allow greater absolute loads to be utilized in training. Use of body part or isolation exercises should be limited because they isolate a single muscle group by bracing and stabilizing the rest of the body with the use of equipment supports rather than by using the body's synergistic muscle groups for support during the movement. For example, performing a leg extension rather than a squat eliminates the compressive forces of the bar on the person's back and the muscular contractions of the synergistic muscle groups acting on the vertebral column for stabilization during the exercise. The only forces experienced by the lower limb during the leg extension are those at the point of muscle attachment of the knee extensors; the longitudinally directed compressive (bending) forces experienced through the lower limb as one supports the load during a squat exercise are missing. Thus, structural exercises such as squats, cleans, deadlifts, snatches, and jerks (for the axial skeleton) and bench presses and overhead presses (for the upper limbs) are recommended for increasing the muscle and bone strength.

Body part exercises may be useful for gently introducing untrained people to resistance exercise. Increased kinesthetic awareness and initial muscle conditioning should be priority goals at the beginning of a new conditioning program for previously untrained people. Progression to structural exercises will require proper instruction and practice to establish the necessary coordination and to develop the baseline levels of strength needed to safely and effectively execute the more complex structural movements.

Another important consideration in selecting exercises to increase bone mass is the adaptability of the internal architecture of the human skeleton. To optimally dissipate the imposed forces, the direction of the collagen fibers within the bone matrix may change to conform to the lines of stress experienced by the bone. Thus, changing the distribution of the force vectors by using a variety of exercises continually presents a unique stimulus for new bone formation within a common region of bone.

Aerobic Exercise

The selection of different forms of aerobic exercise have met with some success in bringing about improvements in bone mass. The aerobic training programs that are the most successful in stimulating bone growth involve more intense physical activities such as rowing, stair climbing, running, and running with weight packs or vests (9). The key to the success of an aerobic exercise program in stimulating new bone formation is that the aerobic activity be significantly more intense than the normal daily activities typically experienced by the person. Thus, brisk walking may stimulate bone growth in previously sedentary individuals who are not accustomed to that level of activity. The intensity of the activity must systematically increase in order to continually overload the bone. Eventually, it may become difficult to overload bone through aerobic exercise when the progression to a new exercise intensity is restricted by the person's oxygen transport system rather than limitations of the musculoskeletal system. Bone responds to the magnitude and rate of external loading; therefore, to enhance the stimulus to the musculoskeletal system it is also necessary to increase the rate of limb movement. Utilizing interval training techniques is one method of providing a greater osteogenic stimulus while still providing the benefits associated with regular aerobic exercise.

Untrained and Aged People

In designing exercise programs to increase bone strength in untrained or aged people, one must use the same precautionary guidelines that would apply to prescribing resistance exercise to that population: a proper patient history and physical exam and an analysis of joint stability, flexibility, and muscular strength. An additional precaution needs to be implemented for people who are suspected of having low bone mass. If bone mass drops to an extremely low level and remains there for an extended period of time, the internal structure of the bone can deteriorate, or essentially collapse (61), and may not be able to be rebuilt. Mineral may be deposited in the area, but if the internal structure of the bone has been significantly compromised previous bone strength will not be regained. When dealing with people suspected of having low bone mass (i.e., amenorrheic athletes, postmenopausal women, and older men and women) it would be wise to have some form of bone imaging, such as dual energy x-ray absorptiometry, performed prior to applying specific forces through the bone, to gain as much information as possible about the skeletal regions that will be receiving the dynamic loading. Noninvasive techniques such as bone imaging provide valuable information about the bone mineral density, but a bone biopsy would be necessary to delineate the competency of the internal bone structure.

ADAPTATION OF MUSCLE TO EXERCISE

An athlete trains the various physiological systems to encourage adaptation and improve performance. This training must be specific to the desired outcome, since the body can be subjected to large variations in exercise intensity and duration. At one extreme, resistance training can involve very heavy loads with minimal repetitions; at the other, long-distance cycling or running requires a very submaximal muscular effort but it is extended over a period of time. Due to this large diversity of possible exercise stimuli, adaptations in muscle tissue are similarly variable. A given activity dictates which types of muscle fibers—the subcomponents of muscle, each with differing structural and functional characteristics—will be recruited. This section will discuss the muscular adaptations to strength (such as Olympic weightlifting), hypertrophy (bodybuilding), and endurance (aerobic) training.

Muscle Growth

The muscular enlargement that results from a resistance training program is called **hypertrophy** and is primarily a result of an increase in the cross-sectional area of the existing fibers (20,45,70). The process of hypertrophy involves an increase in the synthesis of the contractile proteins actin and myosin (the primary components of two respective types of myofilaments) within the myofibril (43,48,62) as well as an increase in the number of myofibrils within a muscle fiber (21,26,46). The new myofilaments are added to the external layers of the myofibril (43), resulting in an increase in its diameter. These adaptations create the cumulative effect of enlarging the fiber and the associated muscle group. It is also theorized that there is an increase in the number of muscle fibers, which increases the overall size of the muscle. Here the initial muscle undergoes **hyperplasia**—longitudinal fiber splitting—as a response to high-intensity weight training. Hyperplasia has been found to occur in animals (13,24,25,30), but studies both reject (45,46) and support (44,47,81) hyperplasia in humans.

Training Programs

In general, the mode of exercise dictates the changes in the muscle or other structure. As noted in the discussion of bones, this relationship is known as specificity (4). The three common modes of exercise pertaining to muscular adaptation are strength, hypertrophy, and aerobic endurance training.

Training for Strength.
A strength training program is characterized by high-resistance, near-maximal muscle contractions extended over a small number of repetitions with a full recovery period between each set (76). Therefore, the relative intensity of an exercise is high and the overall volume (total number of repetitions) of exercise is low. This type of training elicits increases in the cross-sectional area of the exercised muscles (32), with Type II fiber areas increasing more readily (22,58,71) and at a faster rate (52) than Type I fibers. The degree and rate of hypertrophy of Type II fibers demonstrate their greater recruitment during strength training than other modes of exercise; this is a desired response, since Type II motor units produce a greater force output and contract with greater velocity than Type I motor units (75). Additionally, an initial dominance of Type II fibers is an advantage to increasing muscular strength (10,28) because their growth results in an increase in lean body mass, one of the most influential factors in determining maximum strength (69).

The biochemical adaptations to strength training lie in the significant increases in muscle glycogen, creatine phosphate, and adenosine triphosphate (ATP) substrate stores (35,49). There is also an increase in the quantity and activity of the glycolytic enzymes myokinase and creatine kinase (15,22); the higher level of substrates requires additional enzymatic activity to speed reactions so that energy stores can be used efficiently. (See chapter 5 for definitions of terms related to biochemical adaptations.)

Training for Muscle Size.
A hypertrophy, or bodybuilding, training program involves using lighter loads, which allows the athlete to perform more repetitions than is typical of a strength training program, but heavy enough to elicit concentric or eccentric contraction failure (inability of the muscle to shorten or lengthen under control) within 6 to 12 repetitions (76,81). The rest period is of short to moderate duration, since it is important to begin the next set of the exercise before full recovery has been achieved. Also, it is not unusual for the athlete to perform 12 to 20 (or more) successive sets that focus on one muscle group during a single training session. This higher overall training volume coupled with a moderate relative intensity (expressed as a percent of 1RM), although lower than for strength training, appears to be optimal to increase muscle girth (81). A significant observation made in research studies is that there is a relative lack of individual-fiber hypertrophy in bodybuilders who possess substantial limb girths. Thus, researchers conclude that larger muscles may be caused by an increase in the number of muscle fibers. Additional research indicates that bodybuilders exhibit a larger absolute amount of collagen and other noncontractile connective tissue, which also contribute to increases in overall muscle size (45). Other cross-sectional studies have revealed a percentage of Type II fibers in bodybuilders lower than that found in other anaerobic athletes (Table 4.2) and a larger number and size of Type I fibers (81). Note that these characteristics are similar to those found in endurance athletes (23, 80,82).

Table 4.2 Proportion of Type II Fibers in Athletes Who Perform Anaerobic Activities

Type of athlete	Type II fibers
Bodybuilders	44%
Javelin throwers	50%
800-m runners	52%
Weightlifters	60%
Shot-putters	62%
Discus throwers	62%
Sprinters and jumpers	63%

Data from references 65 and 85.

The biochemical adaptations to hypertrophy training programs are similar to those resulting from strength training programs, in that both regimes result in Type II fiber hypertrophy. There is discussion, however, that the increases in creatine phosphate levels do not benefit maximal strength training activities, because the duration of actual exercise (i.e., a set) is too short (43). Increased creatine phosphate levels would possibly influence the total power output that can be extended over the 20- to 30-s durations that are typically seen in higher repetition and lower resistance bodybuilding training programs (43).

Training for Muscular Endurance Using Aerobic Exercise. The muscular component of an aerobic endurance training program involves submaximal muscle contractions extended over a large number of repetitions with little recovery allowed between each "set." Therefore, the relative intensity is very low and the overall volume is very high. This type of training encourages a similar relative increase in aerobic potential in Type I and Type II fibers; however, the increase in aerobic potential in Type I fibers adds to the preexisting high initial aerobic capacity of Type I fibers relative to Type II fibers (23). Thus, Type I fibers are said to possess an **oxidative capacity** greater than that of Type II fibers both before and after training.

Whereas strength and hypertrophy training produce somewhat similar muscular adaptations, aerobic training adaptations are different (12,29). Endurance training reduces the concentration of glycolytic enzymes and can reduce the overall muscle mass of the hypertrophied (and nonhypertrophied) Type II fibers (41). Conversely, there is selective hypertrophy of Type I muscle fibers (8) due to their increased recruitment during endurance activities, although the resulting cross-sectional diameter is not as great as seen in Type II fibers. There is little evidence to show that Type II fibers change into Type I fibers as a result of chronic aerobic training, but

there may be a gradual conversion of Type IIb fibers to Type IIa fibers, the two major Type II fiber subgroups (3). This type of adaptation is significant, in that Type IIa fibers, or **fast oxidative glycolytic fibers**, possess a greater oxidative capacity than Type IIb fibers, also called **fast glycolytic fibers**, as well as functional characteristics more similar to Type I fibers. The result of this conversion is a greater number of muscle fibers that can contribute to endurance performance.

At the cellular level, aerobic exercise adaptations include an increase in the size and number of mitochondria and a greater myoglobin content (17). **Mitochondria** are the organelles in cells that are responsible for aerobically producing ATP via oxidation of glycogen. When the larger and more prevalent mitochondria are combined with an increase in the quantity of oxygen that can be delivered to mitochondria by higher levels of **myoglobin** (a protein that transports oxygen within the cell), the aerobic capacity of the muscle tissue is enhanced. This adaptation is further augmented by the increase in the level and activity of the enzymes involved in the aerobic metabolism of glucose (31) and a parallel increase in glycogen (22,23) and triglyceride (55) stores.

ADAPTATION OF CONNECTIVE TISSUE TO EXERCISE

The primary structural component of all connective tissues encountered in the musculoskeletal system is the **collagen** fiber. The strength of tendons and ligaments is derived from the internal architecture of collagen fibers (Figure 4.4; see references 2 and 74 for further detail). A protein, **procollagen**, is synthesized and secreted by a spindle-shaped connective tissue support cell called a **fibroblast**. Procollagen molecules consist of three protein strands (strings of amino acids) twisted around each other in a triple helix. The procollagen molecule leaves the cell with protective extensions on the ends of the molecule to prevent collagen fibers from forming prematurely within the cell. Cleavage of the procollagen extensions results in the formation of the active or mature collagen molecule that will align end-to-end with other collagen molecules to form a long filament. As the molecules line up they do not actually connect end-to-end; rather, a slight gap is left between the ends of the molecules within a single filament. The complete filament then aligns itself side-by-side with neighboring filaments in such a manner that the collagen molecules in one filament overlap the gaps between molecules in the adjacent filaments. The parallel arrangement of filaments is called a *microfibril*. The microfibrils become arranged into fibers and the fibers into longer bundles.

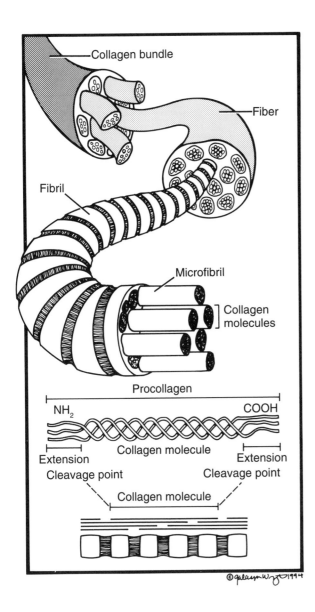

Figure 4.4 Formation of a collagen fiber.

Collagen has a striated (striped) appearance under a light microscope, somewhat like skeletal muscle, owing to the orderly alignment of the gaps between the collagen molecules within a microfibril. The true strength of collagen comes from the strong chemical bonding called **covalent cross-linking** that forms between adjacent collagen molecules throughout the collagen bundles. Finally, the collagen bundles can be bunched together longitudinally to form tendons or ligaments or arranged into sheets with the layers oriented in different directions as found in bones and the fascia located in skeletal muscle.

The primary type of collagen found in bones, tendons, ligaments, and fascia is called Type I collagen. The only collagen found in the cartilage at the articulating surfaces of bone is Type II collagen. The two forms are similar in appearance; they differ in amino acid sequence, which results in differences in their functional properties.

The organization of collagen fibers and their incorporation into connective tissue is similar to the organization of muscle fibers in skeletal muscle. It is important to remember, however, a key difference between the two types of fibers. The muscle fiber is a cell with a membrane (sarcolemma) that seals the cell off as an individually existing fluid-filled unit with its own microenvironment. Found within the boundaries of the sarcolemma are nuclei, myofibrils, organelles, and various molecules, such as glycogen, all suspended in the sarcoplasm of the muscle cell. In contrast, a collagen fiber is not a cell. It is in the extracellular space, not within the cells, that the collagen molecules align to form collagen fibers. Thus, a complete collagen fiber is not enclosed by a cell membrane but rather is just a parallel arrangement of protein strands that have bunched together in the extracellular space because of mutual attraction and subsequently chemically cross-link to form a stable structure. The cells that originally produced the collagen molecules become compressed between the bundles of collagen.

Biology of Tendons, Ligaments, and Fascia

Tendons and ligaments are composed primarily of tightly packed parallel arrangements of collagen bundles. Mature tendons and ligaments contain relatively few cells. The small number of metabolically active cells in tendons and ligaments make the requirement for oxygen and nutrients in these tissues relatively low. However, tendons and ligaments do have a direct blood supply.

Ligaments contain elastic fibers in addition to collagen. These fibers contain **elastin**, an extensible protein: A certain amount of stretch must be permitted within a ligament to allow normal joint motion, the degree of elasticity being specific to the functional requirement of the joint. Thus, ligaments contain fibers that provide strong structural support (collagen) and fibers that confer a degree of flexibility to the ligament (elastin).

Tendons and ligaments attach directly to either cartilage or bone. This union is well designed to resist separation. For example, connective tissue support cells at a bone-tendon junction produce both collagen fibers and other essential structural components needed for the formation of tendons and bone tissue, thus creating a blend of the structure at the site of insertion. As the bone grows in diameter, the tendon or ligament insertion becomes buried in the bone surface increasing the strength of this junction.

The fibrous connective tissues that surround and separate the different organizational levels within skeletal muscle are referred to as **fascia**. Fascia have sheets of fibrocollagenous support tissue containing bundles of collagen fibers arranged in different planes to provide resistance to forces from several different directions. Individual muscle fibers are surrounded by a layer of connective tissue called **endomysium**, which consists of several layers of proteins that serve to anchor the muscle cell to the extracellular matrix proteins found between the muscle cells. The extracellular matrix proteins are part of a fascia layer called **perimysium**, which connects muscle fibers together into distinct bundles, or **fasciculi**. Finally, all the fasciculi of muscle are bound together by the fascia layer termed the **epimysium**, which surrounds the entire muscle. The different fascial layers found within muscles converge together near the end of the muscle to form a tendon. It is the tendon rather than the muscle fibers that attach directly to the bone surface. Thus, the force of muscle contraction is transmitted to the bone through the arrangement of fascia located throughout the muscle.

Biology of Cartilage

Cartilage is a dense connective tissue consisting of cells embedded in a firm matrix. The unique composition of the cartilage matrix renders cartilage capable of withstanding considerable force without damage to its structure. The main functions of cartilage are

- to provide a smooth articulating surface at the interface of bones in a joint,
- to act as a shock absorber for forces directed through the joint, and
- to aid in the attachment of muscle to the skeleton.

A feature unique to cartilage tissue is that it lacks its own blood supply. This means that the cells that produce cartilage, the **chondrocytes**, must depend on diffusion of oxygen and nutrients from synovial fluid for survival. This unique feature is the main reason that cartilage does not easily repair itself after sustaining a substantial injury.

Two primary types of cartilage are significant as they relate to physical activity: hyaline cartilage and fibrous cartilage. **Hyaline cartilage** is found on the articulating surfaces of bones and thus is often referred to as *articular cartilage*. The collagen fibers in hyaline cartilage arise from the bone surface perpendicular to the articulating surface of the bone and curve to become parallel to it. The number of collagen fibers present in cartilage is only about one-half the number found in a comparable quantity of tendons or ligaments. The internal environment of the cartilage tissue (cartilage matrix), within which the collagen fibers traverse, exists as a gellike

material called **ground substance**. Ground substance is composed of large carbohydrate molecules (glycoaminoglycans) and carbohydrate-protein molecules (proteoglycans), which attract a great deal of fluid into the cartilage matrix. Each proteoglycan molecule acts as a compressed spring within the matrix. The loose packing of the collagen fibers, the spring action of the carbohydrate molecules, and the aqueous environment of the cartilage matrix allow cartilage to accept a large force—by temporarily changing shape to dissipate the force—and then return to the original form. This characteristic allows the cartilage to be compressed during weight bearing or joint movement and then spring back to its original shape when the stress is removed.

Fibrous cartilage is a very tough form of cartilage found in the intervertebral disks of the spine and at the junctions where tendons attach to bone. It consists of prominent bundles of Type I and Type II collagen fibers arranged in parallel to provide resistance to extreme forces. Each intervertebral disk is a thick rubbery pad of concentrically arranged fibrous cartilage layers. The outer, articulating surface of the disk is lined with a thin layer of hyaline cartilage, and the deep part of the disk is a soft gelatinous matrix. Intervertebral disks function as shock absorbers and permit limited movement between vertebrae.

Effects of Physical Activity on Connective Tissue

The primary stimulus for connective tissue growth in the mature adult is the mechanical forces created during physical activity. The degree of tissue adaptation appears to be on a continuum with the intensity of the exercise stimulus. As with bone and muscle, intensities of exercise that exceed the strain placed on the connective tissues during normal daily activities stimulate connective tissue changes if the stimulus is repeated on a regular basis.

Local and systemic hormonal and metabolic responses to exercise may also influence the growth of connective tissue. Intense exercise elicits peak secretion of two anabolic hormones, growth hormone and testosterone, which enter the general circulation and become available to act on muscle, bone, and other connective tissues (37). Connective tissues respond to anabolic hormones by secreting growth factors (e.g., insulinlike growth factor I [IGF-I]), which can act locally, act on adjacent tissues such as muscle, or enter the systemic circulation (37). The specific responses of connective tissues to the hormonal surges that occur in response to exercise are not known, although these responses probably provide a strong stimulus for adaptations in connective tissues consequent to exercise training.

Empirical evidence suggests that connective tissues must increase their functional capabilities in response to the enhanced contractile forces created by a hypertrophied muscle. The sites where connective tissues can increase strength and thus load-bearing capacity are

- at the junctions between the tendon (or ligament) and bone surface,
- within the body of the tendon or ligament, and
- in the network of fascia within skeletal muscle.

Stronger muscles pull harder on their bony attachments and cause an increase in bone mass at the tendon-bone junction and along the line over which the forces are distributed. Such adaptation occurs in the collateral knee ligaments of experimental animals following several weeks of treadmill running (83,84). Additionally, animals exercised on treadmills with uneven surfaces have shown even greater tendon-bone junction strength compared with animals trained on smooth surfaces (1). The adaptation that occurs at the tendon-bone junction is quite effective. The point of ligament rupture in animals moves from the tendon-bone junction in untrained animals to within the body of the tendon or ligament after chronic exercise training (7).

A general connective tissue response to endurance exercise is increased collagen metabolism, meaning that damaged collagen fibrils are being replaced without a net gain in the amount of collagen in the remodeled tissue (36,77,78). This response indicates that training of low to moderate intensity does not markedly change the collagen content in connective tissue (36). Conversely, high-intensity loading of the musculoskeletal system will result in net growth of the involved connective tissues. Work-induced muscle hypertrophy in animals having followed extreme loading regimes relates to an increase in the number and size of fibroblast cells within the connective tissue of the hypertrophied muscle and raises fibroblast activity, resulting in a greater supply of the total collagen available for incorporation into the fascia of the growing muscle. Interestingly, activation of fibroblasts and the subsequent growth of the connective tissue network are prerequisites for hypertrophy of the active muscle (34,85). An enhanced connective tissue network is probably necessary to withstand the greater force capabilities of the growing muscle. This relationship may explain why biopsy studies on trained athletes have shown that hypertrophied muscle contains greater total collagen, but that the collagen content remains proportionate to the existing muscle mass (53).

Specific changes that occur within a tendon that contribute to the increase in its cross-sectional area and strength in response to a functional overload include

- an increase in collagen fibril diameter,
- a greater number of covalent cross-links present within a fiber of increased diameter,
- an increase in the number of collagen fibrils, and
- an increase in collagen fibril packing density.

Together these adaptations enhance the tendon's ability to withstand greater tensional forces (39,54,79).

The response of articular cartilage to physical activity may seem less obvious. However, the fact that articular cartilage gets its nutrient supply by diffusion from synovial fluid links joint mobility to joint health. Movement about a joint creates changes in pressure in the joint capsule that drive nutrients from the synovial fluid toward the articular cartilage of the joint (73). Immobilization of a joint prevents proper diffusion of oxygen and essential nutrients throughout the joint, resulting in the death of the chondrocytes and resorption of the cartilage matrix. These changes may become irreversible if a joint is immobilized for too long without periodic passive mobilization of the joint through its range of motion. However, mobilization of a joint prior to healing of the articular surfaces can be damaging to the joint (53,73). A more encouraging finding is that long-term adherence to treadmill exercise in experimental animals thickens the cartilage and increases the number of cells and later the total ground substance present in articular cartilage (61,68). Further support for the positive effects of weight-bearing activity on articular cartilage is evidenced in a typical knee joint where the surfaces of the joint that experience the greatest degree of weight bearing are thicker than the non-weight-bearing surfaces (60). Complete movement throughout the range of motion of a joint and weight-bearing forces seem to be essential to maintaining tissue viability (73).

CONCLUSION

The musculoskeletal system is sensitive to changes in a person's level of physical activity. Exercise training has positive effects on bone, muscle, and associated connective tissue; the entire musculoskeletal system undergoes a coordinated adaptation to exercise. Because the overall function of the system is based on the intimate linkage of contractile tissue (muscle) and non-contractile support tissues that establish the framework through which the forces created by muscle contractions are transmitted, healthy people experience changes in the force-generating capabilities of muscle resulting in a coordinated and proportional increase in the load-bearing capacity of bone and other connective tissue.

Exercise training can increase skeletal muscle mass, force-generating capability, and metabolic capacity. Changes in the collective properties of muscle fibers are specific to the metabolic and force requirements of the activity. Some of the most important ways in which muscle fibers increase in aerobic and anaerobic capacity are an enhanced enzyme profile, an increase in the number of key organelles (such as mitochondria), an increase in the storage of various substrates, and an increase in the amount of contractile proteins within the cell.

Bone and other connective tissues show a more general response to increased physical activity. The extent of tissue adaptation is related to the degree of deformation experienced by the tissue involved in the activity, that is, the intensity of training. Connective tissue changes consequent to high-intensity exercise training include an increase in the number of collagen fibers and the strengthening of individual collagen fibers though an increase in the number of covalent cross-links within the fiber. In bone, there is an increase in the amount of mineral deposited in the collagen matrix.

Key Terms

appendicular skeleton	52	fast glycolytic fiber	58	osteogenic stimulus	54
axial skeleton	52	fast oxidative glycolytic fiber	58	osteoporosis	54
bone matrix	52			oxidative capacity	58
bone mineral density	53	fibroblast	58	peak bone mass	54
bone modeling	52	fibrous cartilage	60	perimysium	60
chondrocyte	60	ground substance	60	periosteum	52
collagen	58	hyaline cartilage	60	procollagen	58
cortical bone	52	hyperplasia	57	progressive overload	54
covalent cross-linking	59	hypertrophy	57	specificity	54
elastin	59	minimal essential strain (MES)	52	stress fracture	54
endomysium	60	mitochondrion	58	structural exercise	56
epimysium	60	myoglobin	58	trabecular bone	52
fascia	60	osteoblast	52		
fasciculus	60				

Study Questions

1. Resistance exercise programs designed to stimulate new bone formation should emphasize all of the following except

   a. metabolic specificity
   b. specificity of loading
   c. progressive overload
   d. variation in exercise selection

2. Which of the following exercises should most effectively stimulate new bone formation in the axial skeleton?

   a. squat
   b. leg extension
   c. bench press
   d. lat pull-down

3. Which of the following factors is least effective in creating an effective osteogenic stimulus?

   a. volume of exercise
   b. magnitude of the load
   c. rate of force application
   d. variation of exercise selection

4. Increases in Type II muscle fiber diameter from training for strength are associated with increases in all of the following except

   a. phosphagen levels
   b. glycogen levels
   c. triglyceride levels
   d. myokinase

5. Muscle size increases are caused by all of the following except

   a. a higher proportion of Type II fibers
   b. a greater amount of intermuscular collagen fibers
   c. an increase in diameter of Type I fibers
   d. greater substrate stores

6. Increases in the endurance capability of muscle tissue are caused by all of the following except

   a. conversion of Type IIb to Type IIa fibers
   b. hypertrophy of Type I fibers
   c. greater myoglobin content
   d. conversion of Type II to Type I fibers

7. Which of the following is the connective tissue support cell found in cartilage?

   a. chondrocyte
   b. osteoblast
   c. fibroblast
   d. myocyte

8. Which of the following is not a specific change that occurs within tendons or ligaments in response to chronic resistance exercise training?

   a. a switch from Type II to Type I collagen
   b. an increase in collagen fibril diameter
   c. an increase in collagen fibril packing density
   d. an increase in covalent cross-links present in collagen fibrils

9. Which tissue has the poorest blood supply?

   a. cartilage
   b. bone
   c. muscle
   d. tendon

Applying Knowledge
of Bone, Muscle, and Connective Tissue

Problem 1

A 27-year-old woman has requested your advice regarding development of a resistance training program that will improve her physique. An interview with this person reveals the following information.

1. Past activity profile: participated in intramural sports during college 4 years ago.
2. Present activity profile: rides an exercise bike three times/week for 20 min/session.
3. Contraindications for exercise: none; family history positive for high blood pressure and osteoporosis.
4. Physical data: height, 170 cm (5 ft 7 in); weight, 55 kg (121 lb); body fat, 26%; heart rate, 72; blood pressure, 102/60 mm Hg.

Using this information, design a resistance training program that will satisfy her immediate goal; the program should consist of at least one basic exercise for each muscle group. Also, augment her program by addressing any factors that will encourage increases in the peak bone mineral density of her axial skeleton, to minimize her risk for developing osteoporosis.

Problem 2

If an individual decides to begin a 3-year resistance training program with 1 year devoted to each training outcome (muscular strength, hypertrophy, and muscular endurance), how would his or her muscular system respond? What are the typical changes experienced by each outcome?

References

1. Adams, A. Effect of exercise upon ligament strength. *Res. Q.* 37:163-176. 1976.
2. Alberts, B., D. Bray, J. Lewis, M. Raff, K. Roberts, and J.D. Watson. *Molecular Biology of the Cell*, 2nd ed. New York: Garland. 1989.
3. Andersen, P., and J. Henriksson. Training induced changes in the subgroups of human Type II skeletal muscle fibers. *Acta Physiol. Scand.* 99:123-125. 1975.
4. Baechle, T.R., and R.W. Earle. *Weight Training: A Text Written for the College Student*. Omaha: Creighton University. 1989.
5. Conroy, B.P., W.J. Kraemer, C.M. Maresh, and G.P. Dalsky. Adaptive responses of bone to physical activity. *Med. Exerc. Nutr. Health* 1:64-74. 1992.
6. Conroy, B.P., W.J. Kraemer, C.M. Maresh, S.J. Fleck, M.H. Stone, A.C. Fry, P.D. Miller, and G.P. Dalsky. Bone mineral density in elite junior Olympic weightlifters. *Med. Sci. Sports Exerc.* 25:1103-1109. 1993.
7. Conwall, M.W., and B.F. Leveau. The effect of physical activity on ligamentous strength: An overview. *J. Orthop. Sports Phys. Ther.* 5(5):275-277. 1984.
8. Costill, D.L., J. Daniels, W. Evans, W. Fink, G. Krahenbuhl, and B. Saltin. Skeletal muscle enzymes and fiber composition in male and female track athletes. *J. Appl. Physiol.* 40(2):149-154. 1976.
9. Dalsky, G.P., K.S. Stocke, A.A. Ehsani, E. Slatoplsky, W.C. Lee, and S.J. Birge. Weight-bearing exercise training and lumbar bone mineral content in post menopausal women. *Ann. Intern. Med.* 108:824-828. 1988.
10. Dons, B., K. Bollerup, F. Bonde-Peterson, and S. Hancke. The effect of weightlifting exercise related to muscle fiber composition and muscle cross-sectional area in humans. *Eur. J. Appl. Physiol.* 40:95-106. 1979.
11. Doyle, F., J. Brown, and C. Lachance. Relation between bone mass and muscle weight. *Lancet* 1:391-393. 1970.
12. Dudley, G.A., and R. Djamil. Incompatibility of endurance and strength training modes of exercise (abstract). *Med. Sci. Sports Exerc.* 17:184. 1985.
13. Edgerton, V. Morphology and histochemistry of the soleus muscle from normal and exercised rats. *Am. J. Anat.* 127:81-88. 1970.
14. Eriksen, E.F., H.J.G. Gundersen, F. Melsen, and L. Mosekilde. Reconstruction of the formative site in iliac trabecular bone in 20 normal individuals employing a kinetic model for matrix and mineral apposition. *Metab. Bone Dis. Relat. Res.* 5:243-252. 1984.
15. Eriksson, B., P. Gollnick, and B. Saltin. Muscle metabolism and enzyme activities after training in boys 1-13 years old. *Acta Physiol. Scand.* 87:485-497. 1973.
16. Fiore, C.E., E. Cottini, C. Fargetta, D.S. Giuseppe, R. Foti, and M. Raspagliesi. The effects of muscle-building exercise on forearm bone mineral content and osteoblast activity in drug-free and anabolic steroids self-administering young men. *Bone Miner.* 13:77-83. 1991.
17. Fox, E.L., R.W. Bowers, and M.L. Foss. *The Physiological Basis of Physical Education and Athletics*. Dubuque, IA: Brown. 1989.
18. Frost, H.M. Skeletal structural adaptations to mechanical usage (SATMU): 1. Redefining Wolff's Law: The bone modeling problem. *Anat. Rec.* 226:403-413. 1990.
19. Gleeson, P.B., E.J. Protas, A.D. LeBlanc, V.S. Schneider, and H.J. Evans. Effects of weight lifting on bone mineral density in premenopausal women. *J. Bone Miner. Res.* 5(2):153-158. 1990.
20. Goldberg, A.L., J.D. Etlinger, L.F. Goldspink, and C. Jablecki. Mechanism of work-induced hypertrophy of skeletal muscle. *Med. Sci. Sports Exerc.* 7:248-261. 1975.
21. Goldspink, G. The combined effects of exercise and reduced food intake on skeletal muscle fibers. *J. Cell Comp. Physiol.* 63:209-216. 1964.
22. Gollnick, P., R. Armstrong, B. Saltin, C. Saubert, W. Sembrowich, and R. Shepard. Effects of training on enzyme activity and fiber composition of human skeletal muscle. *J. Appl. Physiol.* 34(1):107-111. 1973.
23. Gollnick, P.R., C. Armstrong, K.P. Saubert, and B. Saltin. Enzyme activity and fiber composition in skeletal muscle of untrained and trained men. *J. Appl. Physiol.* 33(3):312-319. 1972.
24. Gonyea, W.J. The role of exercise in inducing skeletal muscle fiber number. *J. Appl. Physiol.* 48(3):421-426. 1980.
25. Gonyea, W.J., G.C. Erikson, and F. Bonde-Petersen. Skeletal muscle fiber splitting induced by weightlifting exercise in cats. *Acta Physiol. Scand.* 99:105-109. 1977.

26. Gordon, E. Anatomical and biochemical adaptations of muscle to different exercises. *JAMA* 201:755-758. 1967.

27. Granhed, H., R. Jonson, and T. Hansson. The loads on the lumbar spine during extreme weight lifting. *Spine* 12(2):146-149. 1987.

28. Häkkinen, K., and P.V. Komi. Specificity of training-induced changes in strength performance considering the integrative functions of the neuromuscular system. *World Weightlifting* 3:44-46. 1982.

29. Hickson, R. Interference of strength development by simultaneous training for strength and endurance. *Eur. J. Appl. Physiol.* 45:255-263. 1980.

30. Ho, K., R. Roy, J. Taylor, W. Heusner, W. Van Huss, and R. Carrow. Muscle fiber splitting with weightlifting exercise. *Med. Sci. Sports Exerc.* 9(1):65. 1977.

31. Holloszy, J. Effects of exercise on mitochondrial oxygen uptake and respiratory enzyme activity in skeletal muscle. *J. Biol. Chem.* 242:2278-2282. 1967.

32. Ikai, M., and T. Fukunaga. Calculations of muscle strength per unit cross-sectional area of human muscle by means of ultrasonic measurements. *Int. Z. Angew. Physiol.* 26:26-32. 1968.

33. Issekutz, B., J.J. Blizzard, N.C. Birkhead, and K. Rodahl. Effect of prolonged bed rest on urinary calcium output. *J. Appl. Physiol.* 21(3):1013-1020. 1966.

34. Jablecki, C.K., J.E. Heuser, and S. Kaufman. Autoradiographic localization of new RNA synthesis in hypertrophying skeletal muscles. *J. Cell Bio.* 57:743-759. 1973.

35. Karlsson, J., L. Nordesjo, L. Jorfeldt, and B. Saltin. Muscle lactate, ATP, and CP levels during exercise after physical training in man. *J. Appl. Physiol.* 33(2):199-203. 1972.

36. Kovanen, V., H. Suominen, and E. Heikkinen. Connective tissue of "fast" and "slow" skeletal muscle in rats—effects of endurance training. *Acta Physiol. Scand.* 108:173-180. 1980.

37. Kraemer, W.J., L. Marchitelli, S.E. Gordon, E. Harman, J.E. Dziados, R. Mello, P. Frykman, D. McCurry, and S.J. Fleck. Hormonal and growth factor responses to heavy resistance exercise protocols. *J. Appl. Physiol.* 69(4):1442-1450. 1990.

38. Krolner, B., and B. Toft. Vertebral bone loss: An unheeded side effect of therapeutic bed rest. *Clin. Sci.* 64:537-540. 1983.

39. Kruggel, W.B., and R.A. Field. Crosslinking of collagen in active and quiescent bovine muscle. *Growth* 38:495-499. 1974.

40. Lanyon, L.E. Functional strain on bone tissue as an objective and controlling stimulus for adaptive remodeling. *J. Biomech.* 20(11): 1083-1093. 1987.

41. Lemon, W.R., and F.J. Nagle. Effects of exercise on protein and amino acid metabolism. *Med. Sci. Sports Exerc.* 13:141-149. 1981.

42. Loucks, A.B. Osteoporosis prevention begins in childhood. In: *Competitive Sports for Children and Youth*, E.W. Brown and C.F. Branta, eds. Champaign, IL: Human Kinetics. 1988: pp. 213-224.

43. MacDougall, J.D. Morphological changes in human skeletal muscle following strength training and immobilization. In: *Human Muscle Power*, N.L. Jones, N. McCarthy, and A.J. McComas, eds. Champaign, IL: Human Kinetics. 1986. pp. 269-288.

44. MacDougall, J.D., G.C.B. Elder, D.G. Sale, and J.R. Sutton. Effects of strength training and immobilization on human muscle fibers. *Eur. J. Appl. Physiol.* 43:25-34. 1980.

45. MacDougall, J.D., D.G. Sale, S.E. Alway, and J.R. Sutton. Muscle fiber number in biceps brachii in bodybuilders and control subjects. *J. Appl. Physiol.* 57:1399-1403. 1984.

46. MacDougall, J.D., D.G. Sale, G. Elder, and J.R. Sutton. Ultrastructural properties of human skeletal muscle following heavy resistance exercise and immobilization. *Med. Sci. Sports Exerc.* 8(1):72. 1976.

47. MacDougall, J.D., D.G. Sale, G.C.B. Elder, and J.R. Sutton. Muscle ultrastructural characteristics of elite powerlifters and bodybuilders. *Med. Sci. Sports Exerc.* 2:131. 1980.

48. MacDougall, J.D., D.G. Sale, J.R. Moroz, G.C.B. Elder, J.R. Sutton, and H. Howald. Mitochondrial volume density in human skeletal muscle following heavy resistance training. *Med. Sci. Sports Exerc.* 11(2):164-166. 1979.

49. MacDougall, J.D., G.R. Ward, D.G. Sale, and J.R. Sutton. Biochemical adaptation of human skeletal muscle to heavy resistance exercise and immobilization. *J. Appl. Physiol.* 43:700-703. 1977.

50. Marcus, R. Skeletal aging: Understanding the functional and structural basis of osteoporosis. *Trends Endocrinol. Metab.* 2:53-58. 1991.

51. Margulies, J.K., A. Simkin, I. Leichter, A. Bivas, R. Steinberg, K. Kashtan, and C. Milgrom. Effects of intense physical activity on bone mineral content in the lower limbs of young adults. *J. Bone Joint Surg.* 68A:1090-1093. 1986.

52. McDonach, M.J.N., and C.T.M. Davies. Adaptive response of mammalian skeletal muscle to exercise with high loads. *Eur. J. Appl. Physiol.* 52:139-155. 1984.

53. McDonough, A.L. Effects of immobilization and exercise on articular cartilage—a review of literature. *J. Orthop. Sports Phys. Ther.* 3(1):2-5. 1981.

54. Minchna, H., and G. Hantmann. Adaptation of tendon collagen to exercise. *Int. Orthop.* 13:161-165. 1989.

55. Morgan, T., L. Cobb, F. Short, R. Ross, and D. Gunn. Effects of long-term exercise on human muscle mitochondria. In: *Muscle Metabolism During Exercise*, B. Pernow and B. Saltin, eds. New York: Plenum Press. 1971. pp. 87-95.

56. Nilsson, B.E., and N.E. Westlin. Bone density in athletics. *Clin. Orth.* 77:179-182. 1971.

57. Notelovitz, M., D. Martin, R. Tesar, F.Y. Khan, C. Probart, C. Fields, and L. McKenzie. Estrogen therapy and variable-resistance weight training increase bone mineral in surgically menopausal women. *J. Bone Miner. Res.* 6:583-590. 1991.

58. O'Bryant, H., and M.H. Stone. Ultrastructure of human muscle among Olympic-style weightlifters. Poster presentation to Southeastern American College of Sports Medicine Convention at Virginia Tech., Blacksburg, VA, Feb. 5-6. 1982.

59. O'Connor, J.A., and L.E. Lanyon. The influence of strain rate on adaptive bone remodeling. *J. Biomech.* 15(10):767-781. 1982.

60. Oettmeier, R., J. Arokoski, A.J. Roth, A.J. Helminen, M. Tammi, and K. Abendroth. Quantitative study of articular cartilage and subchondral bone remodeling in the knee joint of dogs after strenuous running training. *J. Bone Miner. Res.* 7:5419-5423. 1992.

61. Parfitt, A.M., C.H.E. Mathews, A.R. Villanueva, M. Kleenekopen, B. Frame, and D.S. Rao. Relationships between surface, volume and thickness of iliac trabecular bone in aging and in osteoporosis: Implications for the microanatomic and cellcular mechanisms of bone loss. *J. Clin. Invest.* 72:1346-1409. 1983.

62. Penman, K. Ultrastructural changes in human striated muscle using three methods of training. *Res. Q.* 40:764-772. 1969.

63. Pirnay, F., M. Bodeux, J.M. Crielaard, and P. Franchimont. Bone mineral content and physical activity. *Int. J. Sports Med.* 8:331-335. 1987.

64. Pocock, N.A., J. Eisman, T. Gwinn, P. Sambrook, P. Kelley, J. Freund, and M. Yeates. Muscle strength, physical fitness, and weight but not age to predict femoral neck bone mass. *J. Bone Miner. Res.* 4(3):441-448. 1989.

65. Powers, S.K., and E.T. Howley. *Exercise Physiology.* Dubuque, IA: Brown. 1990.

66. Rubin, C.T., and L.E. Lanyon. Regulation of bone formation by applied dynamic loads. *J. Bone Joint Surg.* 66(3):397-402. 1984.

67. Rubin, C.T., and L.E. Lanyon. Regulation of bone mass by mechanical strain magnitude. *Calcif. Tissue Int.* 37:411-417. 1985.

68. Saaf, R.B. Effect of exercise on adult cartilage. *Acta Orthop. Scand. [Suppl.]* 7(1):1-83. 1950.

69. Sale, D.G., J.D. MacDougall, S.E. Alway, and J.E. Sutton. Muscle cross-sectional area, fiber type distribution, and voluntary strength in humans (abstract). *Can. J. Appl. Sport Sci.* 2:21. 1983.

70. Sale, D.G., J.D. MacDougall, S.E. Alway, and J.R. Sutton. Voluntary strength and muscle characteristics in untrained men and women and bodybuilders. *J. Appl. Physiol.* 62:1786-1793. 1987.

71. Schmidtbleicher, D., and G. Haralambie. Changes in contractile proteins of muscle after strength training in man. *Eur. J. Appl. Physiol.* 46:221-228. 1981.

72. Simkin, A., J. Ayalon, and I. Leichter. Increased trabecular bone density due to bone loading exercises in post menopausal women. *Calcif. Tissue Int.* 40:59-63. 1987.

73. Staff, P.H. The effects of physical activity on joints, cartilage, tendons, and ligaments. *Scand. J. Med. [Suppl.]* 29:59-63. 1982.

74. Stevens, A., and J. Lowe. *Histology.* New York: Grower Medical. 1992.

75. Stone, M., and H. O'Bryant. *Weight Training: A Scientific Approach.* Minneapolis: Bellwether Press. 1987.

76. Stone, M.H., H. O'Bryant, and J.G. Garhammer. A hypothetical model for strength training. *J. Sports Med. Phys. Fitness.* 21:342-351. 1981.

77. Suominen, H., and E. Heikkinen. Effect of physical training on collagen. *Ital. J. Biochem.* 24:64-65. 1975.

78. Suominen, H., E. Heikkinen, and T. Parkattio. Effect of eight weeks' physical training on muscle and connective tissue of the M. vastus lateralis in 69-year-old men and women. *J. Gerontol.* 32(1):33-37. 1977.

79. Suominen, H., A. Kiiskinen, and E. Heikkinen. Effects of physical training on metabolism of connective tissues in young mice. *Acta Physiol. Scand.* 108:17-22. 1980.

80. Tesch, P.A., J. Karlsson, and B. Sjodin. Muscle fiber type distribution in trained and untrained muscles of athletes. In: *Exercise and Sport Biology*, V. Komi, ed. Champaign, IL: Human Kinetics. 1982. pp. 79-83.

81. Tesch, P.A., and L. Larsson. Muscle hypertrophy in bodybuilders. *Eur. J. Appl. Physiol.* 49:310. 1982.

82. Thorstensson, A., L. Larsson, P.A. Tesch, and J. Karlsson. Muscle strength and fiber composition in athletes and sedentary men. *Med. Sci. Sports Exerc.* 9:26-30. 1977.

83. Tipton, C.M., R.D. Matthes, J.A. Maynard, and R.A. Carey. The influence of physical activity on ligaments and tendons. *Med. Sci. Sports Exerc.* 7(3):165-175. 1975.

84. Tipton, C.M., R.D. Matthes, and D.S. Sandage. In-situ measurements of junction strength and ligament elongation in rats. *J. Appl. Physiol.* 37(5):758-761. 1974.

85. Turto, H., S. Lindy, and J. Halme. Procollagen proline hydroxylase activity in work-induced hypertrophy of rat muscle. *Am. J. Physiol.* 226(1):63-65. 1974.

86. Uhthoff, H.K., and Z.F.G. Jaworski. Periosteal stress-induced reactions resembling stress fractures: A radiologic and histologic study in dogs. *Clin. Orthop.* 199:284-291. 1985.

87. Virvidakis, K., E. Georgion, A. Konkotsidis, K. Ntalles, and C. Proukasis. Bone mineral content of junior competitive weightlifters. *Int. J. Sports Med.* 11:214-246. 1990.

CHAPTER 5

BIOENERGETICS

Michael H. Stone
Michael S. Conley

The metabolic basis for specificity of exercise and training is based on an understanding of the production and use of energy in biological systems. More efficient and productive training programs can be designed through an understanding of how energy is produced for specific types of exercise and how energy production can be modified by specific training regimens.

Energy may be defined as the ability or capacity to perform work. Various forms of energy exist: mechanical, chemical, electromagnetic, heat, and nuclear energy, for example. The transformation of energy from one form to another is essential to almost every activity. In a biological system, the conversion of chemical energy to mechanical energy is necessary for many functions, including movement. **Bioenergetics**, or the flow of energy in a biological system, is concerned primarily with the conversion of food—large carbohydrate, protein, and fat molecules, which contain chemical energy—into biologically usable forms of energy. The breakdown of chemical bonds in these molecules releases the energy necessary to perform work, such as muscular contraction.

The breakdown of large molecules into smaller molecules associated with the release of energy is termed **catabolism**. The synthesis of larger molecules from smaller molecules can be accomplished using the energy released from catabolic reactions; this building-up process is termed **anabolism**. The breakdown of proteins into amino acids is an example of catabolism, while the formation of proteins from amino acids is an anabolic process. **Exergonic** reactions are energy-releasing reactions and are generally catabolic. **Endergonic**

reactions require energy and include anabolic processes and the contraction of muscle. **Metabolism** is the total of all the catabolic/exergonic and anabolic/endergonic reactions in a biological system. Figure 5.1 illustrates the basic concept of metabolism: Energy derived from catabolic/exergonic reactions is used to drive anabolic/endergonic reactions, through an intermediate molecule, **adenosine triphosphate (ATP)**. ATP allows for the transfer of energy from exergonic to endergonic reactions.

ADENOSINE TRIPHOSPHATE

ATP is composed of adenine, a nitrogen-containing base; ribose, a five-carbon sugar; and three phosphate groups (Figure 5.2). The removal by hydrolysis of one phosphate group yields adenosine diphosphate (ADP); the hydrolysis of a second phosphate group yields adenosine monophosphate (AMP).

In essence, ATP provides the energy for muscular contraction and thus human movement. ATP is classified as a high-energy molecule because it stores large amounts of energy in the chemical bonds of the two terminal phosphate groups. The breaking of these chemical bonds releases energy to drive various reactions in the body (86,118). Because muscle cells store ATP only in limited amounts and because muscular activity requires a constant supply of ATP to provide the energy needed for contraction, ATP-producing processes must exist in the cell.

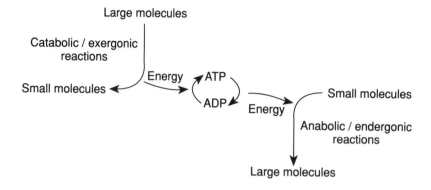

Figure 5.1   General scheme of metabolism.

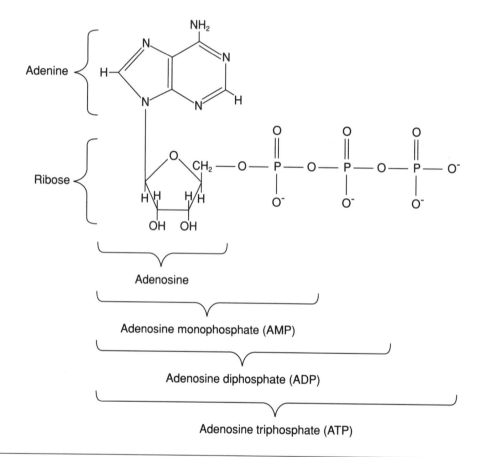

Figure 5.2   Chemical structures of ATP, ADP, and AMP.

BIOLOGICAL ENERGY SYSTEMS

Three energy systems exist in mammalian muscle cells to replenish ATP (102,115):

- The phosphagen system (an **anaerobic** process, i.e., one that occurs in the absence of molecular oxygen)
- Glycolysis, of which there are two types, fast glycolysis and slow glycolysis

- The oxidative system (an **aerobic** process, i.e., one that requires molecular oxygen)

Of the three main food components—carbohydrates, fats, and proteins—only carbohydrates can be metabolized for energy without the direct involvement of oxygen (12). Therefore, the importance of carbohydrates in anaerobic metabolism cannot be underestimated. All three energy systems are active at a given time; however, the extent to which each is used depends primarily on the intensity of the activity and secondarily on its duration (29,115).

The Phosphagen System

The **phosphagen system** provides ATP primarily for short-term, high-intensity activities (e.g., weight training and sprinting) and is active at the start of all exercise regardless of intensity (12). This energy system relies on the chemical reactions of ATP and creatine phosphate—two phosphagens—as well as the enzymes myosin ATPase and creatine kinase. Myosin ATPase catalyzes the hydrolysis of ATP to form ADP and inorganic phosphate (P_i) and release energy. Creatine kinase catalyzes the synthesis of ATP from creatine phosphate and ADP; creatine phosphate supplies a phosphate group that combines with ADP to form ATP.

$$ATP \xrightarrow{\text{Myosin ATPase}} ADP + P_i + Energy$$

$$ADP + Creatine\ phosphate \xrightarrow{\text{Creatine kinase}}$$
$$ATP + Creatine$$

These reactions provide energy at a high rate; however, because ATP and creatine phosphate are stored in muscle in small amounts, the phosphagen system cannot supply energy for continuous, long-duration activities (18). Approximately 5 millimoles (mmols) of ATP and 16 mmols of creatine phosphate are stored in each kilogram of muscle (16,59). Generally, Type II (fast-twitch) muscle fibers contain greater concentrations of phosphagens than Type I (slow-twitch) fibers (22,65).

Another important reaction of the phosphagen system is the *myokinase reaction*:

$$2ADP \xrightarrow{\text{Myokinase}} ATP + AMP$$

This reaction provides an immediate source of ATP. It is also important because AMP is a powerful stimulant of glycolysis (12,79).

Control of the Phosphagen System.
Creatine kinase activity primarily regulates the breakdown of creatine phosphate. An increase in the sarcoplasmic concentration of ADP promotes creatine kinase activity; an increase in ATP concentration inhibits it (102). At the beginning of exercise, ATP is hydrolyzed to ADP, releasing energy for muscular contraction. This increase in ADP concentration activates creatine kinase to catalyze the formation of ATP from the breakdown of creatine phosphate. Creatine kinase activity remains elevated if exercise is continued at a high intensity. If exercise is discontinued, or continues at an intensity low enough to allow glycolysis or the oxidative system to supply an adequate amount of ATP for the muscle

cells' energy demands, the sacroplasmic concentration of ATP will likely increase. This increase in ATP will then result in a decrease in creatine kinase activity.

Glycolysis

Glycolysis is the breakdown of carbohydrates—either glycogen stored in the muscle or glucose in the blood—to produce ATP (12,79). The process of glycolysis involves nine enzymatically catalyzed reactions (Figure 5.3). The enzymes for glycolysis are located in the cytoplasm of the cells (in muscle cells this is referred to as the sarcoplasm). The glycolytic system supplements the energy supply from the phosphagen system for high-intensity muscular activity (115).

As seen in Figure 5.3, the process of glycolysis may go in one of two ways, termed fast glycolysis and slow glycolysis. During **fast glycolysis** pyruvate is converted to lactic acid, providing energy (ATP) at a fast rate compared with **slow glycolysis**, in which pyruvate is transported to the mitochondria for use in the oxidative system. (Fast glycolysis has commonly been called "anaerobic glycolysis," and slow glycolysis "aerobic glycolysis," as a result of the ultimate fate of the pyruvate. However, because glycolysis itself does not depend on oxygen, these terms are not practical for describing the process [12].) The fate of the end products is controlled by the energy demands within the cell. If a high rate of energy supply is needed, such as during resistance training, fast glycolysis is primarily used. If the energy demand is not as high and oxygen is present in sufficient quantities in the cell, slow glycolysis is activated.

Fast Glycolysis.
Fast glycolysis occurs during periods of reduced oxygen availability in the muscle cells and results in the formation of **lactic acid**. Muscular fatigue experienced during exercise is often associated with high tissue concentrations of lactic acid (47). Lactic acid accumulation in tissue is the result of an imbalance between production and utilization (74). As lactic acid accumulates, there is a corresponding increase in hydrogen ion concentration, which is believed to inhibit glycolytic reactions and directly interfere with muscle excitation-contraction coupling, possibly by inhibiting calcium binding to troponin (40,96) or by interfering with cross-bridge formation (35,40,50,96,122). Also, the decrease in pH inhibits the enzymatic activity of the cell's energy systems (5,50). The cumulative effect is a decrease in available energy and muscle contractile force during exercise (47,50).

Lactic acid is converted to its salt, **lactate**, by buffering systems in the muscle and blood (10,12). Unlike lactic acid in the muscle, lactate is not believed to be a fatigue-producing substance (12). Instead, lactate is often utilized as an energy substrate, especially in Type I and cardiac muscle fibers (6,87,135). It is also used

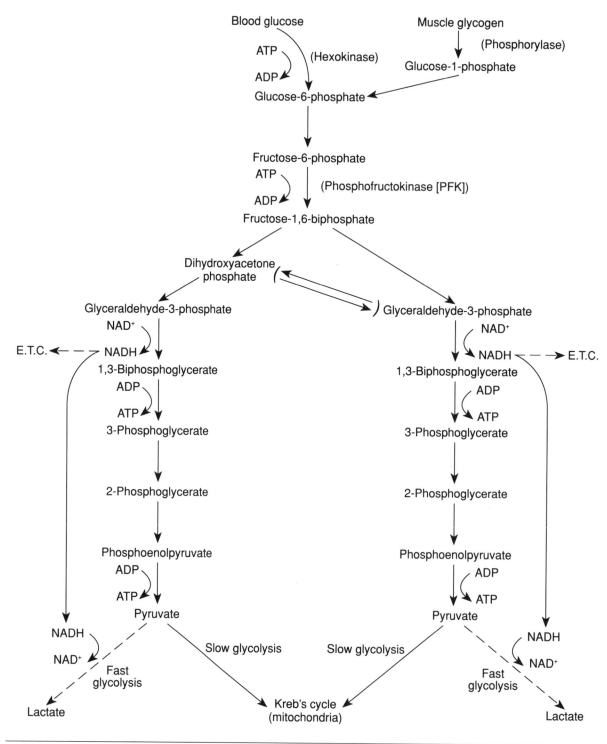

Figure 5.3 Glycolysis.

in **gluconeogenesis**, the formation of glucose from lactate and noncarbohydrate sources, during extended exercise and recovery (10,87,97).

Normally there is a low concentration of lactate in blood and muscle. At rest the reported normal range of lactate concentration in blood is 0.5 to 2.2 mmol/L (44,90), and also 0.5 to 2.2 mmol in muscle for each kg of wet muscle (muscle that has not been desiccated) (44). Lactic acid production increases with exercise intensity (44,106) and appears to be dependent upon muscle fiber type. Researchers have reported that the maximal rate of lactic acid production for Type II muscle fibers is 0.5 mmol · g^{-1} · s^{-1} (30,84) and for Type I muscle is 0.25 mmol · g^{-1} · s^{-1} (95). The higher rate of lactic acid production by Type II muscle fibers may reflect a higher concentration and/or activity of glycolytic enzymes compared to Type I muscle fibers (6,15,75,98). Although the highest possible concentration of lactate accumulation is not known, complete fatigue may occur at blood concentrations between 20 and 25 mmol/L (84); one study, however, reported blood lactate concentrations of greater than 30 mmol/L following multiple bouts of dynamic exercise (51). Along with exercise intensity and muscle fiber types, lactate accumulation can also be influenced by exercise duration (44), state of training (43), and initial glycogen levels (44).

Blood lactate concentrations reflect lactic acid production and clearance and exercise intensity (102). The clearance of lactate from the blood reflects a return to homeostasis and thus a person's ability to recover. Gollnick et al. (44) have reported that blood lactate concentrations normally return to preexercise values within an hour after the activity. Light activity during the postexercise period has been shown to increase lactate clearance rates (39,44,51,101), and aerobically trained (44,101) and anaerobically trained (93,99) athletes have faster lactate clearance rates compared with untrained people. Peak blood lactate concentrations occur approximately 5 min after the cessation of exercise (44), a delay frequently attributed to the time required to buffer and transport lactic acid from the tissue to the blood (67).

Blood lactate accumulation is greater following high-intensity intermittent exercise (e.g., weight training and sprints) than following lower intensity continuous exercise (51,77,127). Jacobs (62) reported highest blood lactate concentrations after maximal bouts of anaerobic exercise. Stone et al. (116) observed that multiple sets of resistance exercise (squats), with increases in resistance to failure, resulted in higher blood lactate concentrations in trained individuals and that the time to failure and total work accomplished was greater in trained people compared to untrained. However, trained people experienced lower blood lactate concentrations compared to untrained when exercising at an absolute work load (same resistance). This indicates that resistance training results in alterations in lactate response to exercise similar to those found in aerobic training (44,62,120). These alterations include a lower blood lactate concentration at a given workload in trained individuals and higher blood lactate concentrations in trained individuals during maximal exercise (44, 62,120).

The net reaction for fast glycolysis may be summarized as follows:

$$\text{Glucose} + 2P_i + 2ADP \longrightarrow 2 \text{ Lactate} + 2ATP + H_2O$$

Slow Glycolysis. If oxygen is present in sufficient quantities in the **mitochondria** (specialized cellular organelles where the reactions of aerobic metabolism occur), the end product of glycolysis, pyruvate, is not converted to lactic acid but is transported to the mitochondria. Also transported there are two molecules of **reduced nicotinamide adenine dinucleotide (NADH)** produced during glycolytic reactions (*reduced* refers to the hydrogen added to nicotinamide adenine dinucleotide, or NAD$^+$). When pyruvate enters the mitochondria it is converted to acetyl-CoA (CoA stands for coenzyme A) by the pyruvate dehydrogenase complex (86). Acetyl-CoA can then enter the Krebs cycle (discussed on p. 72) for further ATP production. The NADH molecules enter the electron transport system (discussed on p. 72), where they can also be used to produce ATP (78,86,118).

The net reaction for slow glycolysis may be summarized as follows:

$$\text{Glucose} + 2P_i + 2ADP + 2NAD^+ \longrightarrow 2 \text{ Pyruvate} + 2ATP + 2NADH + 2H_2O$$

Energy Yield of Glycolysis. Glycolysis produces a net two molecules of ATP from one molecule of glucose. However, if **glycogen** (the storage form of glucose) is used, there is a net production of three ATPs because the reaction of phosphorylating (adding a phosphate group to) glucose, which requires one ATP, is bypassed (see Figure 5.3) (115).

Control of Glycolysis. Glycolysis is stimulated by ammonia, inorganic phosphate, and ADP and a slight decrease in pH and is strongly stimulated by AMP (12,78,119). It is inhibited by markedly lowered pH and increased levels of ATP, creatine phosphate, citrate, and free fatty acids (12,50,79). The phosphorylation of glucose by hexokinase primarily controls glycolysis (12,73,75,78,79,91); the rate of glycogen breakdown to glucose, which is catalyzed by phosphorylase, must also be considered in the regulation of glycolysis (12, 100,103).

Another important consideration in the regulation of any series of reactions is the rate-limiting step, that is, the slowest reaction in the series. The rate-limiting step in glycolysis is the conversion of fructose-6-phosphate to fructose-1,6-biphosphate, a reaction catalyzed by the enzyme **phosphofructokinase (PFK)**. Thus, the activity of PFK is of particular importance in the regulation of the rate of glycolysis. Activation of the phosphagen energy system and the production of AMP through the myokinase reaction stimulates glycolysis (by stimulating PFK) to contribute to the energy production of high-intensity exercise (12,92,123). Ammonia produced during high-intensity exercise as a result of AMP or amino acid deamination can stimulate PFK. This effect may partially offset the results of the lowered pH that is experienced during high-intensity exercise, which inhibits both phosphorylase and PFK activities.

Lactate Threshold and Onset of Blood Lactate. Recent evidence suggests that there are specific break points in the lactate accumulation curve (Figure 5.4) as exercise intensity increases (22,25,70,72). The exercise intensity or relative intensity at which blood lactate begins an abrupt increase above the baseline concentration has been termed the **lactate threshold (LT)** (134). The LT represents an increasing reliance on anaerobic mechanisms. The LT typically begins at 50% to 60% of maximal oxygen uptake in untrained subjects and at 70% to 80% in trained subjects (17,36). A second increase in the rate of lactate accumulation has been noted at higher relative intensities of exercise. This second point of inflection has been termed the **onset of blood lactate accumulation (OBLA)** and generally occurs when the concentration of blood lactate is near 4 mmol/L (55,111,121). The breaks in the lactate accumulation curve may correspond to the points at which intermediate and large motor units are recruited during increasing exercise intensities (66). The muscle cells associated with large motor units are typically Type II fibers, which are particularly suited for anaerobic metabolism and lactic acid production.

Some studies suggest that training at intensities near or above the LT or OBLA pushes the LT and OBLA to the right (i.e., lactate accumulation occurs later at a higher exercise intensity). This shift probably occurs as a result of changes in hormone release, particularly reduced catecholamine release at high exercise intensities. The shift allows the athlete to perform at higher

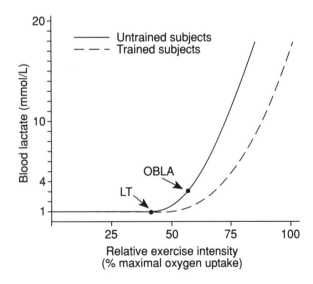

Figure 5.4 Lactate threshold (LT) and onset of blood lactate accumulation (OBLA).

percentages of maximal oxygen uptake without as much lactate accumulation in the blood (12,25).

Endurance performance can vary greatly among individuals with similar maximal oxygen uptakes. Endurance, especially at high percentages of maximal oxygen uptake, may be more related to lactate production and removal and glycogen utilization than to maximal oxygen uptake. High-volume weight training has been shown to increase high-intensity work time without increasing maximal oxygen uptake (53,54,117). This suggests that some types of weight training may modify the LT and OBLA, allowing greater endurance (115). Marcinik et al. (85) have recently provided evidence that resistance training can beneficially alter the LT and increase endurance on a cycle ergometer.

The Oxidative (Aerobic) System

The **oxidative system** uses primarily carbohydrates and fats as substrates. Protein is normally not metabolized significantly, except during long-term starvation and very long bouts (>90 min) of exercise (27,80). At rest approximately 70% of the ATP produced is derived from fats and 30% from carbohydrates. Following the onset of activity, there is a shift in substrate preference from fats to carbohydrates as the intensity of the exercise is increased because carbohydrates are a more efficient fuel and as a result of hormonal stimulations. During high-intensity aerobic exercise, almost 100% of the energy is derived from carbohydrates, if an adequate supply is available. However, during prolonged, submaximal, steady-state work there is a gradual shift from carbohydrates back to fats and protein as energy substrates (12,102,132).

The oxidative metabolism of blood glucose and muscle glycogen begins with glycolysis. If oxygen is present in sufficient quantities, the end product of glycolysis, pyruvate, is not converted to lactic acid, but is transported to the mitochondria where it is taken up and enters the **Krebs cycle**, or citric acid cycle (102). The Krebs cycle is a series of reactions that continues the oxidation of the substrate begun in glycolysis and produces two ATPs indirectly from guanine triphosphate (GTP) for each molecule of glucose (Figure 5.5). Also produced from one molecule of glucose are six molecules of reduced nicotinamide adenine dinucleotide (NADH) and two molecules of **reduced flavin adenine dinucleotide (FADH₂)**. These molecules transport hydrogen atoms to the electron transport chain to be used to produce ATP from ADP (12,88). The **electron transport chain** uses the NADH and $FADH_2$ molecules to rephosphorylate ADP to ATP (Figure 5.6). The hydrogen atoms are passed down the chain, a series of electron carriers known as cytochromes, to form a proton concentration gradient to provide energy for ATP production,

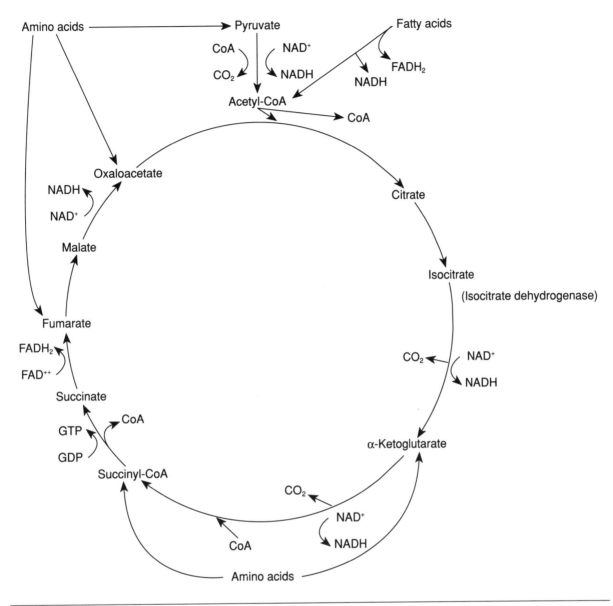

Figure 5.5 The Krebs cycle. CoA = coenzyme A; FAD⁺⁺/FADH₂ = flavin adenine dinucleotide; GDP = guanine diphosphate; GTP = guanine triphosphate; NAD⁺/NADH = nicotinamide adenine dinucleotide.

Figure 5.6 The electron transport chain. CoQ = coenzyme Q; cyt = cytochrome.

with oxygen serving as the final electron acceptor (resulting in the formation of water) (79,86,118). Because NADH and FADH₂ enter the electron transport chain at different sites, they differ in their ability to produce ATP. One molecule of NADH can produce three molecules of ATP, whereas one molecule of FADH₂ can produce only two molecules (79,86,118). The production of ATP during this process is referred to as **oxidative phosphorylation**. The oxidative system, beginning with glycolysis, results in the production of approximately 38 ATPs from the degradation of 1 glucose molecule (12,115).

Fats can also be used by the oxidative energy system. Triglycerides stored in fat cells can be broken down by an enzyme, hormone-sensitive lipase. This releases free fatty acids from the fat cells into the blood, where they can be circulated and enter muscle fibers (12,60,79,100). Additionally, limited quantities of triglycerides are stored within the muscle along with a form of hormone-sensitive lipase to produce an intramuscular source of free fatty acids (12,31). Free fatty acids enter the mitochondria, where they undergo **beta oxidation**, a series of reactions in which the free fatty acids are broken down, resulting in the formation of acetyl-CoA and hydrogen atoms. The acetyl-CoA enters the Krebs cycle directly, and the hydrogen atoms are carried by NAD^+ and FAD^{++} to the electron transport chain (12,86).

Although not a significant source of energy for most activities, protein can be broken down into its constituent amino acids by various metabolic processes. These amino acids can then be converted into glucose (in a process known as *gluconeogenesis*), pyruvate, or various Krebs cycle intermediates to produce ATP. The nitrogenous waste products of amino acid degradation are eliminated through the formation of urea and small amounts of ammonia (12,75). The elimination of ammonia is crucial because it is toxic and is associated with fatigue (79,115).

Control of the Oxidative System. The rate-limiting step in the Krebs cycle (see Figure 5.5) is the conversion of isocitrate to α-ketoglutarate, a reaction catalyzed by the enzyme isocitrate dehydrogenase. Isocitrate dehydrogenase is stimulated by ADP and normally inhibited by ATP. The reactions that produce NADH or $FADH_2$ also influence the regulation of the Krebs cycle. If NAD^+ and FAD^{++} are not available in sufficient quantities to accept hydrogen, the rate of the Krebs cycle is reduced. Also, when GTP accumulates, the concentration of succinyl-CoA increases, which inhibits the initial reaction (Oxaloacetate + Acetyl-CoA → Citrate + CoA) of the Krebs cycle. The electron transport chain is inhibited by ATP and stimulated by ADP (12,78,79).

Energy Production Power and Capacity

The phosphagen, glycolytic, and oxidative energy systems differ in their ability to supply energy for activities of various intensities and durations (Tables 5.1 and 5.2). Exercise intensity is defined as a level of muscular activity that can be quantified in terms of power (work performed per unit of time) output (71). A recent study has shown that power at maximal oxygen uptake is

Table 5.1 Rankings of Rate and Capacity of ATP Production

System	Rate of ATP production	Capacity of ATP production
Phosphagen	1	5
Fast glycolysis	2	4
Slow glycolysis	3	3
Oxidation of carbohydrates	4	2
Oxidation of fats and proteins	5	1

Note. 1 = fastest/greatest; 5 = slowest/least.

Table 5.2 Effect of Event Duration on Primary Energy System Used

Duration of event	Intensity of event	Primary energy system(s)
0-6 s	Very intense	Phosphagen
6-30 s	Intense	Phosphagen and fast glycolysis
30 s–2 min	Heavy	Fast glycolysis
2-3 min	Moderate	Fast glycolysis and oxidative system
> 3 min	Light	Oxidative system

approximately 20% to 30% of peak power on a cycle ergometer (20). Therefore, exercise primarily supported by aerobic mechanisms, even at 100% of maximal oxygen uptake, should not be classified as high-intensity exercise. Activities such as weight training, that are high-intensity, thus having a high power output, require a rapid rate of energy supplied; they rely almost entirely on the energy supplied by the phosphagen system. Activities that are of low intensity (but long duration), such as marathon running, require a high capacity for energy supplied; they rely on the supply of energy from the oxidative energy system. The primary source of energy for activities between these two extremes shifts depending on the intensity and duration of the event (Table 5.2). In general, short, high-intensity activities (e.g., weight training and sprinting) rely on the phosphagen energy system and fast glycolysis. As the intensity decreases and the duration increases, the emphasis gradually shifts to slow glycolysis and the oxidative energy system (12,29,115).

The duration of the activity also influences which energy system is being used. Athletic events range in duration from 1 to 3 s (e.g., snatch and shot-put) to greater than 4 hr (e.g., triathlons and ultramarathons). If a best effort (effort that will result in the best possible performance for a given event) is being made, the time considerations shown in Table 5.2 are reasonable (12,32,50,75,104,122,124).

At no time, during either exercise or rest, does any one energy system provide the complete supply of energy. During exercise, the degree to which anaerobic and oxidative systems contribute to the energy being produced is primarily determined by the exercise intensity and secondarily by exercise duration (12,29,32,75,91).

SUBSTRATE DEPLETION AND REPLETION

Energy substrates—molecules that provide starting materials for bioenergetic reactions, including phosphagens (ATP and creatine phosphate), glucose, glycogen, lactate, free fatty acids, and amino acids—may be selectively depleted during the performance of activities of various intensities and durations. Subsequently, the energy that can be produced by the bioenergetic systems is reduced. Fatigue experienced during many activities is frequently associated with the depletion of phosphagens (43,58) and glycogen (11,12,50,63,108); the depletion of substrates such as free fatty acids, lactate, and amino acids, however, typically does not occur to the extent that performance is limited. Consequently, the depletion and repletion pattern of phosphagens and glycogen following physical activity is important in exercise and sport bioenergetics.

Phosphagens

Fatigue during exercise appears to be at least partially related to the decrease in phosphagens. Phosphagen muscle concentrations are more rapidly depleted as a result of high-intensity anaerobic exercise than of aerobic exercise (43,58). Creatine phosphate can decrease markedly (50%-70%) during the first stage (5-30 s) of high-intensity exercise and can be almost eliminated as a result of very intense exercise to exhaustion (56,64, 68,89). However, muscle ATP concentrations do not decrease more than about 60% from initial values, even during very intense exercise (56,68). It should also be noted that dynamic muscle actions, which produce external work, use more metabolic energy and typically deplete phosphagens to a greater extent than do isometric muscle actions (9).

The intramuscular ATP concentration is largely spared during exercise as a consequence of creatine phosphate depletion and because of the contribution of additional ATP from the myokinase reaction and other

energy sources, such as glycogen and free fatty acids. Postexercise phosphagen repletion can occur in a relatively short period; complete resynthesis of ATP appears to occur within 3 to 5 min and complete creatine phosphate resynthesis can occur within 8 min (48,58). Repletion of phosphagens is largely accomplished as a result of aerobic metabolism (48), although fast glycolysis can contribute to recovery after high-intensity exercise (17,26).

The effects of training on concentrations of phosphagens are not well studied or understood. Aerobic training may increase resting concentrations of phosphagens (33,69) and decrease their rate of depletion at a given (same absolute power output) submaximal power output (21,69) but not at a relative (percent of maximum) submaximal power output (21). Although researchers have noted indications of increased resting concentrations of phosphagens (105), short-term (8-week) studies of sprint training have not shown alterations in resting concentrations of phosphagens (8,125). However, total phosphagen content can be larger following sprint training due to increases in muscle mass (125). Weight training has been shown to increase the resting concentrations of phosphagens in the triceps brachii after 5 weeks of training (83). The increases in phosphagen concentration may have occurred due to selective hypertrophy of Type II fibers, which can contain a higher phosphagen concentration than Type I fibers (81).

Glycogen

Limited stores of glycogen are available for exercise. Approximately 300 to 400 g of glycogen are stored in the body's total muscle and about 70 to 100 g in the liver (97,110). Resting concentrations of liver and muscle glycogen can be influenced by training and dietary manipulations (see chapter 12) (38,110). Research suggests that both anaerobic training, including sprinting and weight training (8,83), and typical aerobic training (41,42) can increase resting muscle glycogen concentration.

The rate of glycogen depletion is related to exercise intensity (110). Muscle glycogen is a more important energy source than is liver glycogen during moderate- and high-intensity exercise; liver glycogen appears to be more important during low-intensity exercise, and its contribution to metabolic processes increases with duration of exercise. Increases in relative exercise intensity of 50%, 75%, and 100% of maximal oxygen uptake result in increases in the rate of muscle **glycogenolysis** (the breakdown of glycogen) of 0.7, 1.4, and 3.4 mmol $\cdot$ kg^{-1} $\cdot$ min^{-1}, respectively (108). At relative intensities of exercise above 60% of maximal oxygen uptake, muscle glycogen becomes an increasingly important energy substrate; the entire glycogen content of some muscle cells can become depleted during exercise (107).

Relatively constant blood glucose concentrations are maintained at very low exercise intensities (<50% of maximal oxygen uptake) as a result of low muscle glucose uptake (2); as duration increases, blood glucose concentrations fall after 90 min but rarely fall below 2.8 mmol/L. Long-term exercise (>90 min) at higher intensities (>50% of maximal oxygen uptake) may result in substantially decreased blood glucose concentrations as a result of liver glycogen depletion. Hypoglycemic reactions may occur in some people with exercise-induced blood glucose values of less than 2.5 mmol/L (3,23). A decline in blood glucose to around 2.5 to 3.0 mmol/L results from reduced liver carbohydrate stores and causes decreased carbohydrate oxidation and eventual exhaustion (19,23,110).

Very high intensity intermittent exercise, such as weight training, can cause substantial depletion of muscle glycogen (20%-50%) with relatively few sets of exercise (low total work loads) (76,82,104,122). Although phosphagens may be the primary limiting factor during resistance exercise with few repetitions or few sets (82), muscle glycogen may become the limiting factor for resistance training with many total sets and larger total amounts of work (104,115). This type of exercise could cause selective muscle fiber glycogen depletion (more depletion in Type II fibers), which can also limit performance (34,104). As with other types of dynamic exercise, the rate of muscle glycogenolysis during resistance exercise is dependent on intensity. The rate of muscle glycogenolysis during six sets of six repetitions of leg extensions at 70% of 1RM (repetition maximum) was double that of six sets at 35% of 1RM (0.46 ±0.05 mmol · kg^{-1} · s^{-1} vs. 0.21 ±0.03 mmol · kg^{-1} · s^{-1}). However, it appears that equal amounts of total work produced equal amounts of glycogen depletion regardless of relative exercise intensity (104). These findings for the rate of muscle glycogenolysis during resistance training exercise are similar to those observed during electrical stimulation of the vastus lateralis and maximal intermittent isokinetic cycling (89,112).

Repletion of muscle glycogen during recovery is related to postexercise carbohydrate ingestion. Repletion appears to be optimal if 0.7 to 3.0 g of carbohydrate per kg body weight are ingested every 2 hr following exercise (38,110). This level of carbohydrate consumption can maximize muscle glycogen repletion at 5 to 6 µmol per g of wet muscle mass per hr during the first 4 to 6 hr following exercise. Muscle glycogen may be completely repleted within 24 hr provided sufficient carbohydrate is ingested (see chapter 12) (38,110). However, if the exercise has a high eccentric component (associated with exercise-induced muscle damage), more time may be required to completely replenish muscle glycogen.

BIOENERGETIC LIMITING FACTORS IN EXERCISE PERFORMANCE

Factors limiting maximal performance (12,14,33,50, 59,61,75,80,91,115) must be considered in the mechanisms of fatigue experienced during exercise and training. Understanding the possible limiting factors associated with a particular athletic event is required when one is designing training programs and attempting to delay fatigue and possibly enhance performance. Table 5.3 depicts examples of various limiting factors based on depletion of energy source and increases in muscle hydrogen ions.

Glycogen depletion can be a limiting factor both for long-duration, low-intensity exercise supported primarily by aerobic metabolism and for repeated very high intensity exercise supported primarily by anaerobic mechanisms. Of importance to weight training, sprinting, and other primarily anaerobic activities is the possible effect of lactic acid and increased tissue hydrogen

Table 5.3   Ranking of Bioenergetic Limiting Factors

Degree of exercise (example)	ATP and creatine phosphate	Muscle glycogen	Liver glycogen	Fat stores	Lower pH
Light (marathon)	1	5	4-5	2-3	1
Moderate (1500-m run)	1-2	3	2	1-2	2-3
Heavy (400-m run)	3	3	1	1	4-5
Very intense (discus)	2-3	1	1	1	1
Very intense, repeated	4-5	4-5	1-2	1-2	4-5
(Example: sets of 10 repetitions in the power snatch with 60% of 1RM.)					

Note. 1 = least probable limiting factor; 5 = most probable limiting factor.

ion concentration in both indirectly and directly limiting contractile force (50).

OXYGEN UPTAKE AND ANAEROBIC CONTRIBUTION TO WORK

Oxygen uptake (or consumption) is a measure of a person's ability to function aerobically. During low-intensity exercise of a constant power output, oxygen uptake increases for the first few minutes until a steady state (oxygen demand equals oxygen consumption) of uptake is reached (Figure 5.7) (4,55). However, at the start of the exercise bout, some of the energy must be supplied through anaerobic mechanisms (129). This anaerobic contribution to the total energy cost of exercise is termed the **oxygen deficit** (55,88). After exercise, oxygen uptake remains above preexercise levels for a period of time that varies according to the intensity and length of the exercise. Postexercise oxygen uptake has been termed the **oxygen debt** (55,88) or the **excess postexercise oxygen consumption (EPOC)** (12). The EPOC is the oxygen uptake above resting values used to restore the body to the preexercise condition (113). Only small to moderate relationships have been observed between the oxygen deficit and the EPOC (7,49); the oxygen deficit may influence the size of the EPOC, but they are not equal. The possible factors affecting the EPOC are listed in Table 5.4 (11-13,88,115).

Anaerobic mechanisms provide much of the energy for work if the exercise intensity is above the maximal oxygen uptake that a person can attain (Figure 5.8). Generally, as the contribution of anaerobic mechanisms

supporting the exercise increases, the exercise duration decreases (4,45,130,131). The approximate contribution of anaerobic and aerobic mechanisms to maximal sustained efforts on a cycle ergometer is shown in Table 5.5 (126,133). Contributions from anaerobic mechanisms are primary for about 30 to 60 s, after which aerobic metabolism becomes the primary energy-supplying mechanism. Thus, maximal sustained efforts to exhaustion may greatly depend upon aerobic metabolism. The contribution of anaerobic mechanisms to this type of exercise represents the maximal anaerobic capacity (94,126).

Table 5.4 Possible Factors Increasing Excess Postexercise Oxygen Consumption

Resynthesis of ATP and creatine phosphate stores
Resynthesis of glycogen from lactate (20% of lactate accumulation)
Oxygen resaturation of tissue water
Oxygen resaturation of venous blood
Oxygen resaturation of skeletal muscle blood
Oxygen resaturation of myoglobin
Redistribution of ions within various body compartments
Repair of damaged tissue
Additional cardiorespiratory work
Residual effects of hormone release and accumulation
Increased body temperature

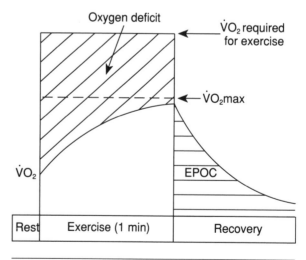

Figure 5.8 High-intensity non–steady-state exercise metabolism (80% of maximum power output). The "required $\dot{V}O_2$" (oxygen uptake) here is the oxygen uptake that would be required to sustain the exercise *if* such an uptake were possible to attain. Since it is not, the oxygen deficit lasts for the duration of the exercise. EPOC = excess postexercise oxygen uptake; $\dot{V}O_2$max = maximal oxygen uptake.

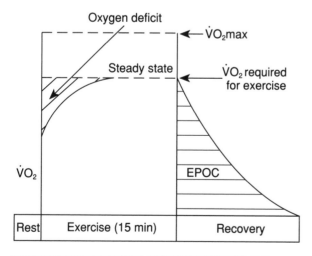

Figure 5.7 Low-intensity steady-state exercise metabolism (75% of maximal oxygen uptake [$\dot{V}O_2$max]). EPOC = excess postexercise oxygen uptake; $\dot{V}O_2$ = oxygen uptake.

Table 5.5   Contribution of Anaerobic and Aerobic Mechanisms to Maximal Sustained Efforts

	Duration of effort (s)			
	0-5	30	60	90
Exercise intensity (% of maximum power output)	100	55	35	31
Contribution of anaerobic mechanisms (%)	96	75	50	35
Contribution of aerobic mechanisms (%)	4	25	50	65

Power output decreases as the contribution of energy from aerobic mechanisms increases. On a cycle ergometer, the power output that can be briefly sustained at maximal oxygen uptake is typically less than 35% of the peak power output. Thus, exercise primarily supported by aerobic metabolism must proceed at low exercise intensities relative to maximum power output capabilities. It should be noted that different types of training may enhance either anaerobic or aerobic capacity. Enhancement of either aerobic or anaerobic capacity can increase endurance and the total amount of work accomplished during sustained maximal effort to exhaustion (90,94,126).

METABOLIC SPECIFICITY OF TRAINING

Appropriate exercise intensities and rest intervals can permit the "selection" of specific energy systems during training for specific athletic events (12,37,75). Few sports or physical activities require maximum sustained-effort exercise to exhaustion or near exhaustion. Most sports and training activities (such as football, interval jumping, sprinting, and weight training) produce metabolic profiles that are very similar to a series of high-intensity constant or near-constant effort exercise bouts interspersed with rest periods. In this type of exercise the required exercise intensity (power output) that must be met during each exercise bout is much greater than the maximal power output that can be sustained using aerobic energy sources. Increasing aerobic power through primarily aerobic training while simultaneously compromising or neglecting anaerobic power and anaerobic-capacity training is of little benefit to athletes in these sports (52,94). (Refer again to the section entitled "Energy Production Power and Capacity," p. 74.)

Interval Training

One method of training that allows appropriate metabolic systems to be stressed is **interval training**. Interval training is based on the concept that more work can be performed at higher exercise intensities with the same or less fatigue compared to continuous training. The theoretical metabolic profile for exercise and rest intervals stressing aerobic metabolism, fast glycolysis, and the phosphagen system is based on the knowledge of which energy system predominates during exercise and time of substrate recovery. Table 5.6 represents the authors' proposed exercise and rest intervals based on exercise relative to maximum attainable power and substrate (phosphagen) recovery times.

By choosing appropriate exercise intensities, exercise durations, and rest intervals, the appropriate energy system(s) can be trained (see also reference 99 and chapter 22 for additional details on training modes and methods). It should be noted that exercise-rest intervals may change as physiological adaptations are made during a training program or as a result of changes in extended programming of training (i.e., periodization).

Weight training, sprint training, and other forms of anaerobic training can increase stores of phosphagens and glycogen, enhance the myokinase reaction (13,83), and generally enhance anaerobic metabolism (1,12), especially considering the faster hypertrophy rates of fast-twitch fibers (45,57).

Combination Training

Some authors have suggested that aerobic training should be added to the training of "anaerobic athletes" (a process that can be termed **combination training**) to enhance recovery (101) because recovery primarily relies on aerobic mechanisms. However, aerobic training may reduce anaerobic performance capabilities, particularly high-strength, high-power performance (52). Aerobic training has been shown to reduce anaerobic

Table 5.6   Proposed Exercise : Rest Intervals

% of maximum power	Primary system stressed	Typical exercise time	Range of exercise to rest period ratios
90-100	Phosphagen	5-10 s	1:12–1:20
75-90	Fast glycolysis	15-30 s	1:3–1:5
30-75	Fast glycolysis and oxidative	1-3 min	1:3–1:4
20-35	Oxidative	> 3 min	1:1–1:3

energy production capabilities in rats (128). Additionally, combined anaerobic and aerobic training can reduce the gain in muscle girth (24), maximum strength (24,46,52), and especially speed- and power-related performance (28), although the exact mechanism is not known (114). It does not appear that the opposite holds true; some studies and reviews suggest that anaerobic training (strength training) can improve low-intensity exercise endurance (53,54,114). Although oxidative metabolism is important in recovery from heavy anaerobic exercise (e.g., weight training, sprint training) (12,109), care must be used in prescribing aerobic training for anaerobic sports. In this context it should be noted that specific anaerobic training can stimulate increases in aerobic power and enhance markers of recovery (114,116,129). Thus, extensive aerobic training to enhance recovery from anaerobic events is not necessary and may be counterproductive in most strength and power sports.

CONCLUSION

Training programs with increased productivity can be designed through an understanding of how energy is produced during various types of exercise and how energy production can be modified by specific training regimens. Which energy system is used to supply energy for muscular contraction is primarily determined by the intensity of exercise and secondarily by the duration of exercise. Metabolic responses and training adaptations are largely regulated by exercise characteristics (e.g., intensity, duration, and recovery intervals). How these responses and adaptations occur following physical activity forms the basis of specificity of exercise and training. This principle allows for enhanced athletic performance through the implementation of improved training programs.

Key Terms

adenosine triphosphate (ATP)	67	fast glycolysis	69	oxidative phosphorylation	72
aerobic	68	gluconeogenesis	70	oxidative system	72
anabolism	67	glycogen	71	oxygen debt	77
anaerobic	68	glycogenolysis	75	oxygen deficit	77
beta oxidation	74	glycolysis	69	oxygen uptake	77
bioenergetics	67	interval training	78	phosphofructokinase (PFK)	71
catabolism	67	Krebs cycle	72	phosphagen system	69
combination training	78	lactate	69	reduced flavin adenine dinucleotide (FADH$_2$)	72
electron transport chain	72	lactate threshold (LT)	72	reduced nicotinamide adenine dinucleotide (NADH)	71
endergonic	67	lactic acid	69		
energy	67	metabolism	67		
excess postexercise oxygen consumption (EPOC)	77	mitochondrion	71	slow glycolysis	69
exergonic	67	onset of blood lactate accumulation (OBLA)	72		

Study Questions

1. The ultimate source of energy for muscular contraction is

    a. GTP
    b. oxygen
    c. NADH
    d. ATP

2. Which of the following can be metabolized anaerobically?

   a. protein
   b. carbohydrate
   c. fat
   d. all of the above

3. Which energy system is used depends primarily on

   a. exercise intensity
   b. exercise duration
   c. state of training
   d. body composition

4. The activation of ____ results in the production of lactic acid.

   a. the phosphagen system
   b. slow glycolysis
   c. fast glycolysis
   d. the oxidation of carbohydrates

5. Which of the following has the highest rate of energy production?

   a. the phosphagen system
   b. fast glycolysis
   c. oxidation of fats
   d. oxidation of carbohydrates

6. The oxidative system results in the production of approximately ___ ATPs from the degradation of 1 glucose molecule.

   a. 36
   b. 27
   c. 41
   d. 38

7. Which of the following supports the initiation of all exercise?

   a. the oxidative system
   b. the phosphagen system
   c. slow glycolysis
   d. fast glycolysis

8. Which enzyme catalyzes the rate-limiting step of glycolysis?

   a. PFK
   b. isocitrate dehydrogenase
   c. phosphorylase
   d. lactate dehydrogenase

Applying Knowledge of Bioenergetics

Problem 1

Two 5,000-m runners (A and B) have similar maximal oxygen uptakes. However, Runner A consistently performs better than Runner B. What bioenergetic factors may explain the differences in performance between the two runners? How could Runner B alter her training to possibly improve her performance?

Problem 2

A competitive weightlifter (age, 24 years; height, 178 cm; weight, 90 kg; body fat, 8%) is considering adding low-intensity aerobic exercise to his current weight training program. Will this likely improve his weightlifting performance? Why or why not?

Problem 3

A collegiate wrestler is unable to maintain intensity throughout the duration (6 min) of his matches. His current training program consists of jogging 3 miles in the morning, 1.5 hr of practice in the afternoon, and another 3-mile jog in the evening. Is his current training program appropriate for the metabolic demands of wrestling? What would you suggest he do to improve his endurance during wrestling matches?

References

1. Abernathey, P.J., R. Thayer, and A.W. Taylor. Acute and chronic responses of skeletal muscle to endurance and sprint exercise. *Sports Med.* 10(6):365-389. 1990.
2. Ahlborg, G., and P. Felig. Influence of glucose ingestion on the fuel-hormone response during prolonged exercise. *J. Appl. Physiol.* 41:683-688. 1967.
3. Ahlborg, G., and P. Felig. Lactate and glucose exchange across the forearm, legs and splanchnic bed during and after prolonged leg exercise. *J. Clin. Invest.* 69:45-54. 1982.
4. Astrand, P.O., and K. Rodahl. *Textbook of Work Physiology*, 2nd ed. New York: McGraw-Hill. 1970.
5. Barany, M., and C. Arus. Lactic acid production in intact muscle, as followed by ^{13}C and ^{1}H nuclear magnetic resonance. In: *Human Muscle Power*, N.L. Jones, N. McCartney, and A.J. McComas, eds. Champaign, IL: Human Kinetics. 1990. pp. 153-164.
6. Barnard, R.J., V.R. Edgerton, T. Furakawa, and J.B. Peter. Histochemical, biochemical and contractile properties of red, white and intermediate fibers. *Am. J. Physiol.* 220:410-441. 1971.
7. Berg, W.E. Individual differences in respiratory gas exchange during recovery from moderate exercise. *Am. J. Physiol.* 149:507-530. 1947.
8. Boobis, I., C. Williams, and S.N. Wooten. Influence of sprint training on muscle metabolism during brief maximal exercise in man. *J. Physiol.* 342:36-37P. 1983.
9. Bridges, C.R., B.J. Clark III, R.L. Hammond, and L.W. Stephenson. Skeletal muscle bioenergetics during frequency-dependent fatigue. *Am. J. Physiol.* 29:C643-C651. 1991.
10. Brooks, G.A. The lactate shuttle during exercise and recovery. *Med. Sci. Sports Exerc.* 18:360-368. 1986.
11. Brooks, G.A., K.E. Brauner, and R.G. Cassens. Glycogen synthesis and metabolism of lactic acid after exercise. *Am. J. Physiol.* 224:1162-1186. 1973.
12. Brooks, G.A., and T.D. Fahey. *Exercise Physiology: Human Bioenergetics and Its Applications.* New York: Wiley. 1984.
13. Brooks, G.A., K.J. Hittelman, J.A. Faulkner, and R.E. Beyer. Temperature, skeletal muscle mitochondrial functions and oxygen debt. *Am. J. Physiol.* 220:1053-1068. 1971.
14. Brouha, L. Training. In: *Science and Medicine of Exercise and Sports*, W. Johnson and E.R. Buskirk, eds. New York: McGraw-Hill. 1974. pp. 276-283.
15. Burke, R.E., and V.R. Edgerton. Motor unit properties and selective involvement in movement. In: *Exercise and Sports Science Reviews*, J. Wilmore and J. Drough, eds. New York: Academic Press. 1975. pp. 31-81.
16. Cain, D.F., and R.E. Davis. Breakdown of adenosine triphosphate during a single contraction of working muscle. *Biochem. Biophys. Res. Commun.* 8:361-466. 1962.
17. Cerretelli, P., G. Ambrosoli, and M. Fumagalli. Anaerobic recovery in man. *Eur. J. Appl. Physiol.* 34:141-148. 1975.
18. Cerretelli, P., D. Rennie, and D. Pendergast. Kinetics of metabolic transients during exercise. *Int. J. Sports Med.* 55:178-180. 1980.
19. Coggan, A.R., and E.F. Coyle. Reversal of fatigue during prolonged exercise by carbohydrate infusion or ingestion. *J. Appl. Physiol.* 63:2388-2395. 1987.
20. Conley, M.S., M.H. Stone, H.S. O'Bryant, R.L. Johnson, D.R. Honeycutt, and T.P. Hoke. Peak power versus power at maximal oxygen uptake (abstract). *J. Strength and Cond. Res.* 7(4):253. 1993.
21. Constable, S.H., R.J. Favier, J.A. McLane, R.D. Feil, and M. Chen. Energy metabolism in contracting rat skeletal muscle: Adaptation to exercise training. *Am. J. Physiol.* 253:316-322. 1987.
22. Coyle, E.F., A.R. Coggan, M.K. Hemmart, and T.J. Walters. Glycogen usage performance relative to lactate threshold (abstract). *Med. Sci. Sports Exerc.* 16:120. 1984.
23. Coyle, E.F., J.M. Hagberg, B.F. Hurley, W.H. Martin III, A.A. Ehsani, and J.O. Holloszy. Carbohydrate feeding during prolonged strenuous exercise can delay fatigue. *J. Appl. Physiol.* 55:230-235. 1983.
24. Craig, B.W., J. Lucas, R. Pohlman, and H. Stelling. The effects of running, weightlifting and a combination of both on growth hormone release. *J. Appl. Sport Sci. Res.* 5(4):198-203. 1991.
25. Davis, J.A., M.H. Frank, B.J. Whipp, and K. Wasserman. Anaerobic threshold alterations caused by endurance training in middle-aged men. *J. Appl. Physiol.* 46:1039-1046. 1979.
26. diPrampero, P.E., L. Peeters, and R. Margaria. Alactic O_2 debt and lactic acid production after exhausting exercise in man. *J. Appl. Physiol.* 34:628-632. 1973.
27. Dohm, G.L., R.T. Williams, G.J. Kasperek, and R.J. VanRij. Increased excretion of urea and *N*-methylhistidine by rats and humans after a bout of exercise. *J. Appl. Physiol.* 52:27-33. 1982.

28. Dudley, G.A., and R. Djamil. Incompatibility of endurance- and strength-training modes of exercise. *J. Appl. Physiol.* 59(5):1446-1451. 1985.

29. Dudley, G.A., and T.F. Murray. Energy for sport. *NSCA Journal.* 3(3):14-15. 1982.

30. Dudley, G.A., and R. Terjung. Influence of aerobic metabolism on IMP accumulation in fast-twitch muscle. *Am. J. Physiol.* 248:C37-C42. 1985.

31. DuFax, B., G. Assmann, and W. Hollman. Plasma lipoproteins and physical activity: A review. *Int. J. Sports Med.* 3:123-136. 1982.

32. Edington, D.E., and V.R. Edgerton. *The Biology of Physical Activity.* Boston: Houghton Mifflin. 1976.

33. Ericksson, B.O., P.D. Gollnick, and B. Saltin. Muscle metabolism and enzyme activities after training in boys 11-13 years old. *Acta Physiol. Scand.* 87:485-497. 1973.

34. Essen, B. Glycogen depletion of different fibre types in man during intermittent and continuous exercise. *Acta Physiol. Scand.* 103:446-455. 1978.

35. Fabiato, A., and F. Fabiato. Effects of pH on the myofilaments and sarcoplasmic reticulum of skinned cells from cardiac and skeletal muscle. *J. Physiol.* 276:233-255. 1978.

36. Farrel, P.A., J.H. Wilmore, E.F. Coyle, J.E. Billing, and D.L. Costill. Plasma lactate accumulation and distance running performance. *Med. Sci. Sports.* 11(4):338-344. 1979.

37. Fox, E.L., and D.K. Mathews. *The Physiological Basis of Physical Education and Athletics*, 3rd ed. Philadelphia: Saunders. 1981.

38. Friedman, J.E., P.D. Neufer, and L.G. Dohm. Regulation of glycogen synthesis following exercise. *Sports Med.* 11(4):232-243. 1991.

39. Freund, H., and P. Gendry. Lactate kinetics after short strenuous exercise in man. *Eur. J. Appl. Physiol.* 39:123-135. 1978.

40. Fuchs, F., Y. Reddy, and F.N. Briggs. The interaction of cations with calcium binding site of troponin. *Biochim. Biophys. Acta* 221:407-409. 1970.

41. Gollnick, P.D., R.B. Armstrong, B. Saltin, W. Saubert, and W.L. Sembrowich. Effect of training on enzyme activity and fibre composition of human muscle. *J. Appl. Physiol.* 34:107-111. 1973.

42. Gollnick, P.D., R.B. Armstrong, W. Saubert, K. Piel, and B. Saltin. Enzyme activity and fibre composition in skeletal muscle of untrained and trained men. *J. Appl. Physiol.* 33:312-319. 1972.

43. Gollnick, P.D., and W.M. Bayly. Biochemical training adaptations and maximal power. In: *Human Muscle Power*, N.L. Jones, N. McCartney, and A.J. McComas, eds. Champaign, IL: Human Kinetics. 1986. pp. 255-267.

44. Gollnick, P.D., W.M. Bayly, and D.R. Hodgson. Exercise intensity, training diet and lactate concentration in muscle and blood. *Med. Sci. Sports Exerc.* 18:334-340. 1986.

45. Gollnick, P.D., and L. Hermansen. Significance of skeletal muscle oxidative enzyme enhancement with endurance training. *Clin. Physiol.* 2:1-12. 1982.

46. Hadmann, R. The available glycogen in man and the connection between rate of oxygen intake and carbohydrate usage. *Acta Physiol. Scand.* 40:305-330. 1957.

47. Häkkinen, K. Effects of fatiguing heavy resistance loading on voluntary neural activation and force production in males and females. In: *Proc. Second North American Congress on Biomechanics.* Chicago. 1992. pp. 567-568.

48. Harris, R.C., R.H.T. Edwards, E. Hultman, L.O. Nordesjo, B. Nylind, and K. Sahlin. The time course of phospho-creatinine resynthesis during recovery of the quadriceps muscle in man. *Pfluegers Arch.* 97:392-397. 1976.

49. Henry, F.M. Aerobic oxygen consumption and alactic debt in muscular work. *J. Appl. Physiol.* 3:427-450. 1957.

50. Hermansen, L. Effect of metabolic changes on force generation in skeletal muscle during maximal exercise. *Human Muscle Fatigue.* London: Pittman Medical. 1981.

51. Hermansen, L., and I. Stenvold. Production and removal of lactate in man. *Acta Physiol. Scand.* 86:191-201, 1972.

52. Hickson, R.C. Interference of strength development by simultaneously training for strength and endurance. *Eur. J. Appl. Physiol.* 215:255-263. 1980.

53. Hickson, R.C., B.A. Dvorak, E.M. Gorostiaga, T.T. Kurowski, and C. Foster. Potential for strength and endurance training to amplify endurance performance. *J. Appl. Physiol.* 65(5):2285-2290. 1988.

54. Hickson, R.C., M.A. Rosenkoetter, and M.M. Brown. Strength training effects on aerobic power and short-term endurance. *Med. Sci. Sports Exerc.* 12:336-339. 1980.

55. Hill, A.V. Muscular exercise, lactic acid and the supply and utilization of oxygen. *Proc. R. Soc. Lond. [Biol.]* 96:438. 1924.

56. Hirvonen, J., S. Ruhunen, H. Rusko, and M. Harkonen. Breakdown of high-energy phosphate compounds and lactate accumulation during short submaximal exercise. *Eur. J. Appl. Physiol.* 56:253-259. 1987.

57. Houston, M.E., and J.A. Thomson. The response of endurance-adapted adults to intense anaerobic training. *Eur. J. Appl. Physiol.* 36:207-213. 1977.

58. Hultman, E., and H. Sjoholm. Biochemical causes of fatigue. In: *Human Muscle Power*, N.L. Jones, N. McCartney, and A.J. McComas, eds. 1986. pp. 215-235.

59. Hultsmann, W.C. On the regulation of the supply of substrates for muscular activity. *Bibl. Nutr. Dieta.* 27:11-15. 1979.

60. Hurley, B.F., D.R. Seals, J.M. Hagberg, A.C. Goldberg, S.M. Ostrove, J.O. Holloszy, W.G. Wiest, and A.P. Goldberg. Strength training and lipoprotein lipid profiles: Increased HDL cholesterol in body builders versus powerlifters and effects of androgen use. *JAMA* 252:507-513. 1984.

61. Jacobs, I. Lactate, muscle glycogen and exercise performance in man. *Acta Physiol. Scand.* 495:1-35. 1981.

62. Jacobs, I. Blood lactate: Implications for training and sports performance. *Sports Med.* 3:10-25. 1986.

63. Jacobs, I., P. Kaiser, and P. Tesch. Muscle strength and fatigue after selective glycogen depletion in human skeletal muscle fibers. *Eur. J. Appl. Physiol.* 46:47-53. 1981.

64. Jacobs, I., P.A. Tesch, O. Bar-Or, J. Karlsson, and R. Dotow. Lactate in human skeletal muscle after 10 and 30 s of supramaximal exercise. *J. Appl. Physiol.* 55:365-367. 1983.

65. Jansson, E., C. Sylven, and E. Nordevang. Myoglobin in the quadriceps femoris muscle of competitive cyclists and in untrained men. *Acta Physiol. Scand.* 114:627-629. 1982.

66. Jones, N., and R. Ehrsam. The anaerobic threshold. In: *Exercise and Sport Sciences Review*, vol. 10. R.L. Terjung, ed. Philadelphia: Franklin Press. 1982. pp. 49-83.

67. Juel, C. Intracellular pH recovery and lactate efflux in mouse soleus muscles stimulated in vitro: The involvement of sodium/proton exchange and a lactate carrier. *Acta Physiol. Scand.* 132:363-371. 1988.

68. Karlsson, J. Lactate and phosphagen concentrations in working muscle of man. *Acta Physiol. Scand.* 485:358-365. 1971.

69. Karlsson, J., L.O. Nordesco, L. Jorfeldt, and B. Saltin. Muscle lactate, ATP and CP levels during exercise and after physical training in man. *J. Appl. Physiol.* 33(2):194-203. 1972.

70. Kindermann, W., G. Simon, and J. Jeul. The significance of the aerobic-anaerobic transition for the determination of work load intensities during endurance training. *Eur. J. Appl. Physiol.* 42:25-34. 1979.

71. Knuttgen, H.G., and P.V. Komi. Basic definitions for exercise. In: *Strength and Power in Sport*, P.V. Komi, ed. Oxford: Blackwell Scientific. 1992. pp. 3-8.

72. Komi, P.V., A. Ito, B. Sjodin, and J. Karlsson. Lactate breaking point and biomechanics of running (abstract). *Med. Sci. Sports Exerc.* 13:114. 1981.

73. Krebs, H.A. The Pasteur effect and the relation between respiration and fermentation. *Essays in Biochem.* 8:2-34. 1972.

74. Kreisberg, R.A. Lactate homeostasis and lactic acidosis. *Ann. Intern. Med.* 92(2):227-237. 1980.

75. Lamb, D.R. *Physiology of Exercise: Responses and Adaptations*. New York: Macmillan. 1984.

76. Lambert, C.P., M.G. Flynn, J.B. Boone, T.J. Michaud, and J. Rodriguez-Zayas. Effects of carbohydrate feeding on multiple-bout resistance exercise. *J. Appl. Sport Sci. Res.* 5(4):192-197. 1991.

77. Lehmann, M., and J. Keul. Free plasma catecholamines, heart rates, lactate levels, and oxygen uptake in competition weightlifters, cyclists, and untrained control subjects. *Int. J. Sports Med.* 7:18-21. 1986.

78. Lehninger, A.L. *Bioenergetics*. New York: W.A. Banjamin, 1973.

79. Lehninger, A.L. *Biochemistry*, 2nd ed. New York: Worth. 1975.

80. Lemon, P.W., and J.P. Mullin. Effect of initial muscle glycogen levels on protein catabolism during exercise. *J. Appl. Physiol. Res. Env. Exerc. Physiol.* 48:624-629. 1980.

81. MacDougall, J.D. Morphological changes in human skeletal muscle following strength training and immobilization. In: *Human Muscle Power*, N.L. Jones, N. McCartney, and A.J. McComas, eds. Human Kinetics: Champaign, IL. 1986. pp. 269-288.

82. MacDougall, J.D., S. Ray, N. McCartney, D. Sale, P. Lee, and S. Gardner. Substrate utilization during weight lifting (abstract). *Med. Sci. Sports Exerc.* 20:S66. 1988.

83. MacDougall, J.D., G.R. Ward, D.G. Sale, and J.R. Sutton. Biochemical adaptations of human skeletal muscle to heavy resistance training and immobilization. *J. Appl. Physiol.* 43:700-703. 1977.

84. Mainwood, G., and J. Renaud. The effect of acid-base on fatigue of skeletal muscle. *Can. J. Physiol. Pharmacol.* 63:403-416. 1985.

85. Marcinik, E.J., G. Potts, G. Schlabach, S. Will, P. Dawson, and B.F. Hurley. Effects of strength training on lactate threshold and endurance performance. *Med. Sci. Sports Exerc.* 23(6):739-743. 1991.

86. Mathews, C.K., and K.E. van Holde. *Biochemistry*. Redwood City, CA: Benjamin/Cummings. 1990.

87. Mazzeo, R.S., G.A. Brooks, D.A. Schoeller, and T.F. Budinger. Disposal of blood [$1-^{13}C$] lactate in humans during rest and exercise. *J. Appl. Physiol.* 60(10):232-241. 1986.

88. McArdle, W.D., F.I. Katch, and V.L. Katch. *Exercise Physiology: Energy, Nutrition, and Human Performance*, 2nd ed. Philadelphia: Lea & Febiger. 1986.

89. McCartney, N., L.L. Spriet, G.J.F. Heigenhauser, J.M. Kowalchuk, J.R. Sutton, and N.L. Jones. Muscle power and metabolism in maximal intermittent exercise. *J. Appl. Physiol.* 60:1164-1169. 1986.

90. McGee, D.S., T.C. Jesse, M.H. Stone, and D. Blessing. Leg and hip endurance adaptations to three different weight-training programs. *J. Appl. Sport Sci. Res.* 6(2):92-95. 1992.

91. McGilvery, R.W. *Biochemical Concepts*. Philadelphia: Saunders. 1975.

92. McGilvery, R.W. *Biochemistry: A Functional Approach*. Philadelphia: Saunders. 1979.

93. McMillan, J.L., M.H. Stone, J. Sartin, R. Keith, D. Marple, C. Brown, and R.D. Lewis. 20-hour physiological responses to a single weight-training session. *J. Strength and Cond. Res.* 7(1):9-21. 1993.

94. Medboe, J.I., and S. Burgers. Effect of training on the anaerobic capacity. *Med. Sci. Sports Exerc.* 22(4):501-507. 1991.

95. Meyer, R.A., and R.L. Terjung. Differences in ammonia and adenylate metabolism in contracting fast and slow muscle. *Am. J. Physiol.* 237:C111-C118. 1979.

96. Nakamura, Y., and A. Schwartz. The influence of hydrogen ion concentration on calcium binding and release by skeletal muscle sarcoplasmic reticulum. *J. Gen. Physiol.* 59:22-32. 1972.

97. Newsholme, E.A. Application of principles of metabolic control to the problem of metabolic limitations in sprinting, middle distance and marathon running. In: *Human Muscle Power*, N.L. Jones, N. McCartney, and A.J. McComas, eds. Champaign, IL: Human Kinetics. 1986. pp. 169-174.

98. Opie, L.J., and E.A. Newsholme. The activities of fructose-1,6-diphosphate, phosphofructokinase, and phospho-enolpyruvate carboxykinase in white and red muscle. *Biochem. J.* 103:391-399. 1967.

99. Pierce, K., R. Rozenek, M. Stone, and D. Blessing. The effects of weight training on plasma cortisol, lactate, heart rate, anxiety and perceived exertion (abstract). *J. Appl. Sports Sci. Res.* 1(3):58. 1987.

100. Pike, R.L., and M. Brown. *Nutrition: An Integrated Approach*, 2nd ed. New York: Wiley. 1975.

101. Plisk, S.S. Anaerobic metabolic conditioning: A brief review of theory, strategy and practical application. *J. Appl. Sport Sci. Res.* 5(1):22-34. 1991.

102. Powers, S.K., and E.T. Howley. *Exercise Physiology: Theory and Application to Fitness and Performance*. Dubuque, IA: Brown. 1990.

103. Richter, E.A., H. Galbo, and N.J. Christensen. Control of exercise-induced muscular glycogenolysis by adrenal medullary hormones in rats. *J. Appl. Physiol.* 50:21-26. 1981.

104. Robergs, R.A., D.R. Pearson, D.L. Costill, W.J. Fink, D.D. Pascoe, M.A. Benedict, C.P. Lambert, and J.J. Zachweija. Muscle glycogenolysis during differing intensities of weight-resistance exercise. *J. Appl. Physiol.* 70(4):1700-1706. 1991.

105. Roberts, A.D., R. Billeter, and H. Howald. Anaerobic muscle enzyme changes after interval training. *Int. J. Sports Med.* 3:18-21. 1982.

106. Rozenek, R., L. Rosenau, P. Rosenau, and M.H. Stone. The effect of intensity on heart rate and blood lactate response to resistance exercise. *J. Strength and Cond. Res.* 7(1):51-54. 1993.

107. Saltin, B., and P.D. Gollnick. Skeletal muscle adaptability: Significance for metabolism and performance. In: *Handbook of Physiology*, L.D. Peachey, R.H. Adrian, and S.R. Geiger, eds. Baltimore: Williams & Wilkins. 1983. pp. 540-555.

108. Saltin, B., and J. Karlsson. Muscle glycogen utilization during work of different intensities. In: *Muscle Metabolism During Exercise*, B. Pernow and B. Saltin, eds. New York: Plenum Press. 1971. pp. 289-300.

109. Scala, D., J. McMillan, D. Blessing, R. Rozenek, and M.H. Stone. Metabolic cost of a preparatory phase of training in weightlifting: A practical observation. *J. Appl. Sport Sci. Res.* 1(3):48-52. 1987.

110. Sherman, W.M., and G.S. Wimer. Insufficient carbohydrate during training: Does it impair performance? *Sports Nutr.* 1(1):28-44. 1991.

111. Sjodin, B., and I. Jacobs. Onset of blood lactate accumulation and marathon running performance. *Int. J. Sports Med.* 2:23-26. 1981.

112. Spriet, L.L., M.L. Lindinger, R.S. McKelvie, G.J.F. Heigenhausser, and N.L. Jones. Muscle glycogenolysis and H^+ concentration during maximal intermittent cycling. *J. Appl. Physiol.* 66:8-13. 1989.

113. Stainsby, W.M., and J.K. Barclay. Exercise metabolism: O_2 deficit, steady level O_2 uptake and O_2 uptake in recovery. *Med. Sci. Sports.* 2:177-195. 1970.

114. Stone, M.H., S.J. Fleck, W.J. Kraemer, and N.T. Triplett. Health and performance related adaptations to resistive training. *Sports Med.* 11(4):210-231. 1991.

115. Stone, M.H., and H.S. O'Bryant. *Weight Training: A Scientific Approach*. Minneapolis: Burgess International. 1987.

116. Stone, M.H., K. Pierce, R. Godsen, D. Wilson, D. Blessing, R. Rozenek, and J. Chromiak. Heart rate and lactate levels during weight-training in trained and untrained men. *Phys. Sportsmed.* 15(5):97-105. 1987.

117. Stone, M.H., G.D. Wilson, D. Blessing, and R. Rozenek. Cardiovascular responses to short-term Olympic style weight training in young men. *Can. J. Appl. Sport Sci.* 8:134-139. 1983.

118. Stryer, L. *Biochemistry*. New York: Freeman. 1988.

119. Sugden, P.H., and E.A. Newsholme. The effects of ammonium, inorganic phosphate and potassium ions on the activity of phosphofructokinase from muscle and nervous tissues of vertebrates and invertebrates. *Biochem. J.* 150:113-122. 1975.

120. Sutton, J. Hormonal and metabolic responses to exercise in subjects of high and low work capacities. *Med. Sci. Sports.* 10:1-6. 1978.

121. Tanaka, K., Y. Matsuura, S. Kumagai, A. Matsuzaka, K. Hirakoba, and K. Asano. Relationships of anaerobic threshold and onset of blood lactate accumulation with endurance performance. *Eur. J. Appl. Physiol.* 52:51-56. 1983.

122. Tesch, P. Muscle fatigue in man, with special reference to lactate accumulation during short intense exercise. *Acta Physiol. Scand.* 480:1-40. 1980.

123. Tesch, P.A., B. Colliander, and P. Kaiser. Muscle metabolism during intense, heavy resistance exercise. *Eur. J. Appl. Physiol.* 55:362-366. 1986.

124. Thorstensson, P. Muscle strength, fibre types and enzymes in man. *Acta Physiol. Scand.* 102:443. 1976.

125. Thorstensson, P., B. Sjodin, and J. Karlsson. Actinomyosin ATPase, myokinase, CPK and LDH in human fast and slow twitch muscle fibres. *Acta Physiol. Scand.* 99:225-229. 1975.

126. Vandewalle, H., G. Peres, and H. Monod. Standard anaerobic exercise tests. *Sports Med.* 4:268-289. 1987.

127. VanHelder, W., M. Radomski, R. Goode, and K. Casey. Hormonal and metabolic response to three types of exercise of equal duration and external work output. *Eur. J. Appl. Physiol.* 54:337-342. 1985.

128. Vihko, V., A. Salmons, and J. Rontumaki. Oxidative and lysomal capacity in skeletal muscle. *Acta Physiol. Scand.* 104:74-81. 1978.

129. Warren, B.J., M.H. Stone, J.T. Kearney, S.J. Fleck, G.D. Wilson, and W.J. Kraemer. The effects of short-term overwork on performance measures and blood metabolites in elite junior weightlifters. *Int. J. Sports Med.* 13(5):372-376. 1992.

130. Wells, J., B. Balke, and D. Van Fossan. Lactic acid accumulation during work. A suggested standardization of work classification. *J. Appl. Physiol.* 10:51-55. 1957.

131. Whipp, B.J., C. Scard, and K. Wasserman. O_2deficit–O_2debt relationship and efficiency of aerobic work. *J. Appl. Physiol.* 28:452-458. 1970.

132. Wilmore, J.H., and D.L. Costill. *Training for Sport and Activity: Physiological Basis of the Conditioning Process*, 3rd ed. Dubuque, IA: Brown. 1988.

133. Withers, R.T., W.M. Sherman, D.G. Clark, P.C. Esselbach, S.R. Nolan, M.H. Mackay, and M. Brinkman. Muscle metabolism during 30, 60 and 90 s of maximal cycling on an airbraked ergometer. *Eur. J. Appl. Physiol.* 63:354-362. 1991.

134. Yoshida, I. Effect of dietary modifications on lactate threshold and onset of blood lactate accumulation during incremental exercise. *Eur. J. Appl. Physiol.* 53:200-205. 1984.

135. York, J., L.B. Oscai, and D.G. Penny. Alterations in skeletal muscle lactate dehydrogenase isozymes following exercise training. *Biochem. Biophys. Res. Commun.* 61:1387-1393. 1974.

CHAPTER 6

NEUROENDOCRINE RESPONSES TO RESISTANCE EXERCISE

William J. Kraemer

Strength and conditioning specialists need a basic appreciation of the neuroendocrine system in order to better understand physical stress and adaptation to exercise. Hans Selye, a Canadian endocrinologist, laid the basis for "periodization of training" with his work on adrenal gland stress hormones long before the concept was ever applied to exercise training. Using Selye's work on stress, distress, illness, and death and their relationship to adrenal function, sport scientists and coaches from the former Eastern bloc countries forged a training theory that is still used today in strength training programs.

It is important for strength and conditioning professionals to have a basic understanding of the hormonal responses to resistance exercise (81, 82). Such knowledge provides them with greater insight into how an exercise prescription can enable hormones to mediate optimal adaptations to resistance training. Although resistance training is the only natural stimulus that causes increases in lean tissue mass, dramatic differences exist among resistance training programs in their ability to produce increases in muscle and connective tissue size. The type of resistance training workout used dictates the hormonal responses (81, 82). Tissue adaptations are influenced by the changes in circulating hormonal concentrations following exercise (8, 10, 12, 39). Thus, understanding this natural anabolic activity that takes place in the athlete's body is fundamental to successful recovery, adaptation, program design, training progression, and ultimately athletic performance (71, 74, 76, 112).

BASIC CONCEPTS

Resistance exercise can represent a potent stimulus to various neuroendocrine glands to secrete or release their hormones. Not all exercise protocols elicit increases in the circulating concentrations of hormones in the body (80, 81). Thus, hormonal responses to resistance exercise are not general in nature. This fact again supports the basic principle of "specificity" in resistance training. Furthermore, it makes resistance exercise stress a very specific tool for remodeling various tissues in the body. This can only be accomplished by creating an effective exercise stimulus. This stimulus must be based upon specific program design variables that define the configuration of an exercise stimulus (70). This stimulus

The preparation of this manuscript was supported in part by a grant from the Robert F. and Sandra M. Leitzinger Research Fund in Sports Medicine to the Center for Sports Medicine at The Pennsylvania State University. I would also like to thank Joann Ruble and Carol Glunt for their help in the preparation of the manuscript.

will require monitoring and change as training progresses. A workout's effectiveness is dependent upon its ability to stimulate adaptations and all adaptations will have an upper limit for change.

Synthesis, Storage, and Secretion of Hormones

Hormones are chemical messengers that are synthesized, stored in, and released by **endocrine glands**—body structures specialized for secretion—and certain other cells (Figure 6.1; Table 6.1). Similarly, neurons synthesize, store, and secrete neurotransmitters, which may have hormonal functions. Thus, the relatively new term **neuroendocrinology** has been used to describe the close integration of chemical substances that have both neural and hormonal functions. Typically, endocrine glands are stimulated to release hormones by a chemical signal received by receptors on the gland or by neural stimulation. For example, the hormone epinephrine is released from the adrenal medulla (the internal part of the adrenal gland) upon neural stimulation from the brain (62, 83, 84). The adrenal cortex (the outer part of the adrenal gland) synthesizes and secretes the hormone cortisol after stimulation by another hormone, adrenocorticotropic hormone, released from the pituitary gland (85). Following stimulation, glands release hormones into the circulation, which carries the

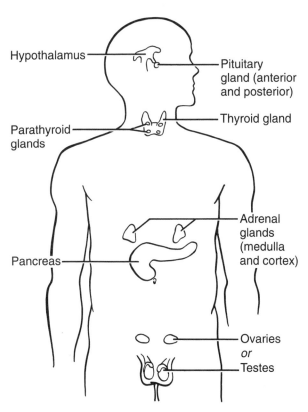

Figure 6.1 The principal endocrine glands of the body.

Hypothalamus

Pituitary gland (anterior and posterior)

Thyroid gland

Parathyroid glands

Adrenal glands (medulla and cortex)

Pancreas

Ovaries *or* Testes

response information to hormone-specific receptors on **target tissues** and ultimately to the nucleus of the cell (5-7, 9, 28, 38).

A variety of binding proteins that carry hormones are found in the blood (5, 7). These binding proteins also can act as storage sites within the circulation and are not active unless separated from the binding protein. In addition, binding proteins can have their own biological activity with cells, acting as a type of hormone. Thus, binding proteins, whether circulating or bound to a cell, are major players in endocrine function. They can extend the life of a hormone, act as a storage reservoir, reduce any degradative effects on the circulating hormone, and even create a hormone/binding-protein combined signal.

Many hormones affect multiple tissues in the body (2, 55, 57-59). Testosterone, for example, interacts with almost every tissue. In this chapter we will focus upon muscle tissue as the primary target of hormonal interactions, but many other tissues, such as bone, kidney, and liver, are just as important as muscle to the adaptive changes observed with resistance training.

Hormones are responsible for regulating many different physiological systems, and most hormones play multiple physiological roles, acting to regulate metabolic function through control of energy substrates and nutrient uptake into cells.

Hormones interact in complex ways with each other. A particular hormone may function in either an independent or dependent manner, depending upon its role in a given physiological mechanism. This complexity and flexibility allows the neuroendocrine system to respond in proper magnitude to a physiological challenge and to interact differently with each physiological system or target tissue simultaneously.

Muscle Fiber Remodeling

Hormonal mechanisms that interact with skeletal muscle are a part of an integrated system that mediates the changes made in the metabolic and cellular processes of muscle as a result of resistance training. Remodeling of muscle involves the synthesis of new proteins and their orderly incorporation into or creation of new sarcomere (3). The most prominent resistance training adaptation in muscle is an increase in the amount of a muscle's contractile proteins, actin and myosin. Other changes in these proteins are also significant; for example, heavy-chain myosin proteins can go through a change in their molecular structure from IIB to IIA heavy-chain proteins. Furthermore, the synthesis of noncontractile proteins is needed for structural integrity and orientation of the contractile proteins within the sarcomere. Stimulation of protein synthesis by heavy

Table 6.1 Endocrine Glands and Hormones

Endocrine gland	Hormone	Physiological actions
Anterior pituitary gland	Growth hormone	Stimulates insulinlike growth factor I, protein synthesis, growth, and metabolism
	Andrenocorticotropic hormone	Stimulates glucocorticoids in the adrenal cortex
	Thyroid-stimulating hormone	Stimulates thyroid hormone synthesis and secretion
	Follicle-stimulating hormone	Stimulates growth of follicles in ovary and seminiferous tubules in testes; stimulates ovum and sperm production
	Luteinizing hormone	Stimulates ovulation and secretion of sex hormones in ovaries and testes
	Prolactin	Stimulates milk production in mammary glands; maintains corpora lutea and secretion of progesterone
	Melanocyte-stimulating hormone	Stimulates melanocytes, which contain the dark pigment melanin
Posterior pituitary gland	Antidiuretic hormone	Increases contraction of smooth muscle and reabsorption of water by kidneys
	Oxytocin	Stimulates uterine contractions and release of milk by mammary glands
Thyroid gland	Thyroxine	Stimulates oxidative metabolism in mitochondria and cell growth
	Calcitonin	Reduces calcium phosphate levels in blood
Parathyroid glands	Parathyroid hormone	Increases blood calcium; decreases blood phosphate; stimulates bone formation
Pancreas	Insulin	Stores glycogen and promotes glucose entry into cells; involved in protein synthesis
	Glucagon	Increases blood glucose levels
Adrenal cortex	Glucocoritcoids (cortisol, cortisone, etc.)	Inhibits or retards amino acid incorporation into proteins; stimulates conversion of proteins into carbohydrates; maintains normal blood sugar level; conserves glucose; promotes use of fat
	Mineralocorticoids (aldosterone, deoxycorticosterone, etc.)	Sodium-potassium metabolism increases body fluids
Liver	Insulinlike growth factors	Increases protein synthesis in cells
Adrenal medulla	Epinephrine	Increases cardiac output; increases blood sugar and glycogen breakdown and fat mobilization
	Norepinephrine	Has properties of epinephrine; also constricts blood vessels
Ovaries	Estrogens	Stimulates development of female sex characteristics
	Progesterone	Stimulates development of female sex characteristics and mammary glands; maintains pregnancy
Testes	Testosterone	Stimulates growth, increased protein anabolism, and development and maintenance of male sex characteristics

resistance training allows for both the quality and the quantity of muscle to be altered over a period of time.

The increase in protein synthesis and decrease in protein degradation are the first steps in muscle growth.

Hormones are intimately involved with these mechanisms. The production of the contractile proteins actin and myosin, and ultimately the incorporation of these proteins into the sarcomere, completes the process at the molecular level. A multitude of hormones—including **anabolic hormones** (hormones that promote tissue building) such as insulin, insulinlike growth factors, testosterone, and growth hormone—all contribute to various aspects of this process. Blocking the cell effects of **catabolic hormones**, such as cortisol and progesterone, that attempt to degrade cell proteins is also important for this process. The remodeling of muscle fiber involves the changes in protein metabolism and the structural alterations and additions that take place after an exercise stress. The more muscle fibers involved with the performance of the exercise, the greater the extent of remodeling observed in the whole muscle. The relationship between hormones and muscle fibers and the subsequent changes in functional capabilities of muscle cells provide the basis for the adaptive influence of hormones.

The Role of Receptors in Mediating Hormonal Changes

Receptors are found in every cell, from muscle fibers to brain cells. One of the basic principles in neuroendocrinology is that a given hormone interacts with a specific receptor, a phenomenon known as the **lock-and-key theory** (where the receptor is the lock and the hormone is the key) (Figure 6.2). However, whereas only one hormone has exactly the right characteristics needed to interact with the receptor, there are cases of **cross-reactivity**, in which a certain receptor accepts hormones that are not specifically designed for it. When this occurs, the resulting biological actions are different from those induced by the primary hormone.

Receptors can have **allosteric binding sites** on them, at which substances other than hormones can enhance or reduce the cellular response to the primary hormone. Receptors may also have a number of domains. This means that part of the receptor may be outside the cell membrane, internalized within it (part inside the membrane, part outside), and/or within the cell membrane. Receptors are also observed in the nuclear portion of the cell for some hormones (e.g., steroid hormones).

It is usually the receptor or the hormone-receptor complex that transmits the message to the nucleus of the cell. The genetic material within the nucleus ultimately translates the hormonal message into either inhibition or facilitation of protein synthesis. When an adaptation is no longer possible (e.g., maximal amount of pain accretion), receptors become nonresponsive to the specific hormone that is trying to stimulate that response from the cell. This inability of a hormone to interact with a receptor is called **down regulation** of receptor function. Therefore, receptors have the ability to increase or decrease their binding sensitivity, and the

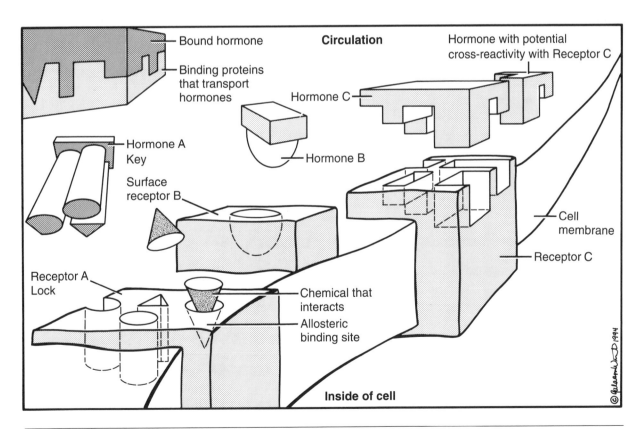

Figure 6.2 A geometrical representation of the classical lock-and-key theory for hormonal action at the cell receptor level.

actual number of receptors there are to bind with can be altered. Alterations in the receptor binding characteristics or number of receptors can be as dramatic an adaptation as the release of increased amounts of hormone from an endocrine gland. Obviously, if a receptor is not responsive to the hormone, little or no alteration in cell metabolism will result.

Hormone-Receptor Interactions

In terms of molecular structure there are two main categories of hormones, steroid and polypeptide hormones. Each interacts with muscle cells in different ways.

Steroid Hormone Interactions. Steroid hormones, which include the adrenal cortex hormones and those secreted by the gonads, are fat soluble and thus diffuse across the sarcolemma of a muscle fiber. Some scientists have hypothesized the presence of transport proteins in the sarcolemma that facilitate this movement. The location of steroid receptors in the cell is still controversial; they may be in the cytosol and/or bound to the nuclear membrane. Regardless of the location of the receptor, the basic series of events is the same. After diffusing across the sarcolemma, the hormone binds with its receptor to form a **hormone-receptor complex (H-RC)**, causing a conformational shift in the receptor and activating it. The H-RC arrives at the genetic material in the cell's nucleus and "opens" it in order to expose transcriptional units that code for the synthesis of specific proteins. The H-RC then recognizes specific enhancers, or upstream regulatory elements of the genes. RNA polymerase II then binds to the promoter that is associated with the specific upstream regulatory elements for the H-RC. The RNA polymerase II then transcribes the gene by coding for the protein dictated by the steroid hormone. Messenger RNA is processed and then moves into the sarcoplasm of the cell where it is translated into protein. Thus, the action of the steroid hormone is complete with its interaction at the genetic level of the cell (100).

Polypeptide Hormone Interactions. Polypeptide hormones are made up of amino acids; examples are growth hormone and insulin. Polypeptide hormones bind to the receptors on the surface of the cell or to receptors that have domains integrated into the sarcolemma. Since polypeptide hormones are not fat soluble and thus cannot penetrate the sarcolemma, they rely on **second messengers** to get their message to the cell nucleus. Second messengers are activated by the conformational change in the receptor induced by the hormone. The second messenger directs its actions to specific areas in the cell, where the hormone's message is amplified. The subsequent cascade of intracellular events

eventually leads up to the physiological response ascribed to the hormone.

In a muscle fiber, for example, a hormone arrives at the sarcolemma, forming a hormone-receptor complex. Adenyl cyclase, an enzyme bound to the cytoplasmic leaflet of the sarcolemma, is then activated, catalyzing the formation of cyclic adenosine monophosphate (cAMP), which then activates a protein kinase (an enzyme involved in energy transfer). In turn, the protein kinase may phosphorylate and activate an enzyme that stimulates protein synthesis. This shows only one of the many second messengers systems that peptide hormones stimulate by binding to a receptor.

Heavy Resistance Exercise and Hormonal Increases

Heavy resistance exercise brings about significant adaptive responses that result in enhanced size, strength, and power of trained musculature (32). The increase in anabolic hormone levels observed consequent to the performance of heavy resistance exercise protocols can result in increased interactions with various cellular mechanisms and enhance the development of muscle protein contractile units. Upon neural stimulation from an alpha motor nerve to initiate a muscle action, various signals are sent from the brain and from activated muscles to a number of endocrine glands.

Hormones are secreted under the physiological stress of resistance exercise. Acute hormonal secretions provide an abundant amount of information to the body regarding such things as the amount and type of physiological stress (e.g., epinephrine), the metabolic demands of the exercise (e.g., insulin response), and the need for subsequent changes in resting metabolism. Thus, with specific patterns of nervous system stimulation from resistance exercise, certain hormonal changes are simultaneously activated for specific purposes related to the acute exercise stress. The pattern of stress and hormonal responses integrate into an adaptive response of the tissues to a training program.

Hormonal increases in response to resistance exercise take place in a physiological environment that is unique to this type of exercise stress. Significant amounts of force are produced that require the activation of high-threshold motor units not typically stimulated by other types of exercise, such as endurance exercise. The muscle fibers of the activated motor units are stimulated, and forces are placed upon the sarcolemmas of the muscle fibers due to the heavy external loads being lifted. Among many different responses to the force production stress, alterations in sarcolemma permeability to nutrients and sensitivity and synthesis of receptors in the muscle cell membrane are affected. In addition, local inflammatory processes related to tissue damage and repair mechanisms are activated with stress and run their time course with recovery (17). Ultimately, it is the specific force produced in the activated fibers that stimulates receptor and membrane sensitivities to anabolic factors, including hormones, which lead to muscle growth and strength changes in the intact muscle.

Following the exercise session, remodeling of the muscle tissue is undertaken in the environment of hormonal secretions that provide for anabolic actions. Increases in protein synthesis of actin and myosin and a reduction in protein degradation take place. Conversely, if the stress is too great, catabolic actions in the muscle may occur as a result of the inability of anabolic hormones to bind to receptors or by the down regulation of receptors in the muscle tissue (87). Thus, hormonal actions are important both during and after exercise in response to the exercise stress. The magnitude of the hormonal response depends on the amount of tissue stimulated, the amount of tissue remodeling, and repair required consequent to the exercise (9). Thus, the characteristics of the exercise stimulus are again paramount to the response of the body to the exercise protocol.

In highly hypertrophied muscle fibers, protein synthesis is not the primary mechanism for muscle growth because little growth is possible. Reductions in protein degradation is of greater importance. Nevertheless, only muscle fibers that are activated by the resistance training are affected. Thus, some fibers may be close to genetic ceilings for cell-size increases while others may have a great potential for growth. It is clear that the extent of hormonal interactions with growth of muscle fibers is directly related to the adapted size of the fibers (i.e., potential for size increases) that is dictated by the loads and exercise angles used in a resistance training program. Thus, if a specific program uses the same exercise, only a specific set of muscle fibers associated with that movement will be activated and then stimulated to grow. This could leave many fibers in the muscle unaffected and without any significant interactions with hormonal factors. The same can be said of various load patterns and progression schemes. It is only the activated fiber that realizes the benefits of the resistance exercise program and utilizes physiological mechanisms, including hormonal mechanisms, to adapt.

Mechanisms of Hormonal Interactions

The mechanisms of hormonal interaction with muscle tissue are dependent on several factors. First, when exercise acutely increases the blood concentrations of hormones, a greater probability of interaction with receptors is possible. However, if the physiological function to be affected is already close to a genetic maximum (i.e., with little adaptive potential left), the receptor will not be sensitive to the increased hormonal exposure.

For example, a muscle cell that has already reached its maximum size with long-term training may not be sensitive to hormonal signals from the body to stimulate further protein accretion. How and when this reduction in receptor sensitivity to hormonal increases occurs in human muscle is unknown; however, increases in size are ultimately limited by genetic predisposition. Second, since adaptations to heavy resistance exercise typically are anabolic in nature, the recovery mechanisms involved are related to increases in the size of cells. Third, mistakes in exercise prescriptions can result in a greater catabolic effect or an ineffective exercise program. Accordingly, hormonal mechanisms will either adversely affect cellular development or minimally activate mechanisms that augment the hypertrophy initiated by the neural recruitment and the force production demands of heavy-intensity resistance exercise.

The combination of many different mechanisms is thought to stimulate the phenomenon of exercise-induced hypertrophy. However, not all force production can be explained just by muscle tissue mass increases alone. Neural factors interact with this process too. The integration of the nervous system and the various hormonal mechanisms is different in trained and untrained people (44, 104). In addition, certain hormonal mechanisms, such as those mediated by testosterone, may not be operational in males and females or fully operational at all ages (78, 80). It now appears that a wide array of hormonal mechanisms with differential effects based on program design, training level, gender, age, genetic predisposition, and adaptational potential appear to provide a myriad of possible adaptation strategies needed for the maintenance or improvement of muscle size and strength (44, 65).

Hormonal Changes in Peripheral Blood

Blood can be drawn from athletes at various stages of training and hormone concentrations in the blood samples determined. Integration can be difficult, however, because many hormones can change their secretory patterns almost continuously, and assaying the responses to exercise stress has to be done properly for each hormone. Consequently, while one has to carefully interpret peripheral hormonal responses, they do provide an indication of the status or responsibilities of the glands or functional status of the mechanisms controlled by the hormone. It should be noted that peripheral concentrations of hormones in the blood do not indicate the status of the various receptor populations or the effects of a hormone within the cell. It is typically assumed, however, that if large increases in hormone concentration are observed, higher probabilities for interactions with receptors exist.

Many different physiological mechanisms may contribute in varying degrees to the observed changes in peripheral blood concentrations of hormones. These include the following:

• *Fluid volume shifts.* Body fluid tends to shift from the blood to the cells as a result of exercise. This shift can increase hormone concentrations in the blood without any changes of secretion from endocrine glands. It has been hypothesized that regardless of the mechanism of increase, such concentration changes increase receptor interaction probabilities.

• *Tissue, especially liver, clearance rates of a hormone,* that is, the time it takes a hormone to go through the circulation of the tissue. Hormones circulate through various tissues and organs, the liver being one of the major processing organs in the body. Time delays are seen as the hormone goes through the circulation in the liver and other tissues (e.g., lungs). The clearance time of a tissue keeps the hormone out of the circulation and away from contact with target receptors in other parts of the body or can degrade it and make it nonfunctional.

• *Hormonal degradation,* that is, breakdown of the hormone itself.

• *Venous pooling of blood.* Blood flow back to the heart is slowed by pooling of blood in veins; the blood is delayed in the peripheral circulation due to intense muscle activity (muscle contractions greater than 45% of maximal). Thus, blood flow must recover during intervals when muscle activity is reduced. The pooling of the blood can increase the concentrations of hormones in the venous blood and also increase time of exposure to target tissues.

• *Interactions with binding proteins in the blood.* Hormones bind with specialized proteins in the blood that help with transport (5, 7). Free hormones and bound hormones all interact differently with tissue; ultimately, it is the free hormone that interacts with the membrane or other cellular receptors.

• *Receptor interactions.* All these mechanisms interact to produce a certain concentration of a hormone in the blood, which influences the potential for interaction with the receptors in target tissue and their subsequent secondary effects, leading to the final effect of the hormone on a cell.

Adaptation of the Neuroendocrine System

While organs such as muscle and connective tissue are the ultimate target of most resistance training programs, many adaptations occur within the neuroendocrine system as well. These changes are temporally related to changes in the target organs and the toleration of exercise stress. The potential for adaptation in the neuroendocrine system is great with so many different sites and mechanisms that can be affected. The following kinds of adaptation are possible:

• Amount of synthesis and storage of hormones
• Transport of hormones via binding proteins
• Time needed for the clearance of hormones through hepatic and extrahepatic tissues
• Amount of hormonal degradation that takes place over a given period of time
• How much of a blood-to-tissue fluid shift occurs with exercise stress
• How tightly the hormone binds to its receptor (receptor affinity), which is an uncommon response to exercise training
• How many receptors are in the tissue
• The magnitude of the signal sent to the cell nucleus by the hormone-receptor complex or second messenger
• The degree of interaction with the cell nucleus (which would dictate how much muscle protein is to be produced)

Hormones are secreted in response to a need for homeostatic alterations in the body; indeed, the endocrine system is a part of an overall strategy to bring physiological functions back into normal ranges (37). These homeostatic mechanisms controlled by the neuroendocrine system can be activated in response to an acute resistance exercise stress or be altered after a chronic period of resistance training (65, 66). The mechanisms that mediate acute homeostatic changes typically respond to acute resistance exercise stress with a sharp increase or decrease in hormonal concentrations, in order to regulate a physiological variable such as glucose level. A more subtle increase or decrease usually occurs in chronic resting hormonal concentrations in response to resistance training. For example, the subtle increases in testosterone over the course of a resistance training program may help to mediate changes in protein synthesis, thus leading to increased muscle fiber size.

THE PRIMARY ANABOLIC HORMONES

The primary anabolic hormones involved in muscle tissue growth and remodeling are testosterone, growth hormone, and insulinlike growth factors (IGF), discussed in detail in this section, as well as insulin and the thyroid hormones, previously examined in great detail (33, 34).

Testosterone

Testosterone has been used as a physiological marker to evaluate the anabolic status of the body (50, 87). The hormonal control of testosterone release has been previously reviewed in detail (38, 65, 67). The direct effects of testosterone on skeletal muscle growth in culture are not as dramatic as IGF. In addition to the direct effects of testosterone on muscle tissue, testosterone may indirectly affect the protein content of the muscle fiber by promoting growth hormone release, which leads to IGF synthesis and release from the liver (42). In addition, the effects of testosterone on development of strength and muscle size are related to the influence of testosterone on the nervous system (10, 61). For example, testosterone can interact with receptors on neurons and increase the amount of neurotransmitters and influence structural protein changes leading to size changes of the neuromuscular junction. Each of these can enhance the force production capabilities of the muscle it innervates. These potential interactions with other hormones demonstrate the highly interdependent nature of the neuroendocrine system in influencing the expression of strength in the intact muscles.

How testosterone exactly interacts with the nucleus of the muscle cell remains a point of inquiry.

Following secretion, testosterone is thought to be transported to target tissues by a transport protein, e.g., sex hormone–binding globulin, after which it associates with a membrane-bound protein or cytosolic receptor, is activated, and subsequently migrates to the cell nucleus, where interactions with nuclear receptors take place, resulting in protein synthesis (33, 41, 96, 103, 106, 121).

Increases in peripheral blood concentrations of testosterone have been observed during and following many types of high-intensity endurance exercise (37); thus, variations in testosterone's cellular actions may be due to differences in the cell membrane consequent to resistance exercise. This could be due to the forces placed on membranes with resistance exercise or different feedback mechanisms sending signals to the higher brain centers (e.g., higher levels of testosterone feeding back in the brain to decrease leutinizing hormone secretion). Furthermore, receptor interactions may be quite different under different exercise conditions due to the differential force on membranes. One must keep in mind that high-intensity endurance exercise can have a very dramatic catabolic tissue response, and increases in testosterone may be related to the need for maintaining protein synthesis to keep up with protein loss (116, 117). Hypertrophy does not typically take place with endurance training. In fact, oxidative stress may actually promote a decrease in muscle fiber size in order to optimize oxygen transport kinetics into the cell. It therefore appears that the muscle fiber is merely trying to maintain its optimal size for oxidative metabolism. Without the proper exercise stimulus, the cellular mechanisms that mediate increased cell growth are not activated.

In young males, several factors appear to influence the acute serum testosterone concentrations and may play a role in determining if significant increases are observed during or following exercise. Independently or in various combinations several exercise variables can increase serum testosterone concentrations (65, 81):

- Large–muscle group exercises (e.g., deadlift, power clean, squats)
- Heavy resistance (85%-95% of 1RM [repetition maximum])
- Moderate to high volume of exercise, achieved with multiple sets and/or multiple exercises
- Short rest intervals (30 s to 1 min)

Increases in serum total testosterone are evident when blood is sampled before and immediately after exercise protocols that utilize large–muscle group exercise (e.g., deadlifts, but not bench presses) (29, 43, 47, 49, 122). When blood is sampled, say, 4 hr or more after exercise and not immediately following it, other factors, such as diurnal variations (normal fluctuations in hormone levels throughout the day) or recovery phenomena, can affect the magnitude or direction of the acute stress response (Figure 6.3). Additionally, possible rebounds or decreases in testosterone blood values over time may reflect augmentation or depression of diurnal variations (81), making interpretation of "late" blood samples that much more difficult.

A wide variety of exercise protocols have been shown to elicit increases in testosterone in response to the acute exercise stress of the protocol. Any lack of change can typically be attributed to one of the previously discussed factors (size of muscle group, intensity, etc.). Fahey et al. (29) were unable to demonstrate significant increases among high school–aged males in serum concentrations of total testosterone. This was thought to be due to the nonresponsiveness of cells in testes of young males. A recent report by Kraemer et al. (79) suggests that increases may occur if the resistance training experience of high school–aged males (14-18 years) is 2 years or more. This initial report supports the possibility that resistance exercise training may alter physiological release and/or concentrating mechanisms (e.g., clearance times and plasma volume shifts) of the hypothalamic-pituitary-testicular axis (hormones from the brain stimulate the testes to produce and secrete testosterone) in younger males. Only recently have more advanced resistance exercise training programs in younger children become acceptable in both the scientific and medical

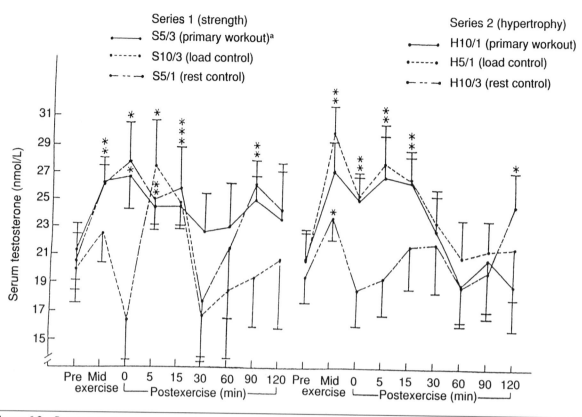

Figure 6.3 Serum testosterone responses to various resistance exercise protocols. All sessions consisted of eight identically ordered resistance exercises that exercised each of the main muscle groups of the body. Series 1 (lower total work) was a 5RM (repetition maximum)–based workout of three to five sets/exercise and made up the primary workout (S5/3). Total work for the load control (5RM to 10RM) (S10/3) and the rest control (3 min reduced to 1 min) (S5/1) was identical to that of the primary workout. For Series 2 (higher total work, same exercises and order), the primary workout (H10/3) was three sets of 10RM for the eight identical exercises. Again, total work for the load control (10RM to 5RM) (H5/1) and the rest control (1 min increased to 3 min) (H10/3) was identical to that of the primary workout. *Significantly above preexercise levels. Reprinted from Kraemer et al. (1990).

communities (78). Such programs may be more effective in causing changes in testosterone secretion patterns. The consistent use of a wide range of advanced protocols may influence the responses of testosterone in younger males. Exactly how this is related to pubertal growth and development remains to be studied.

Free Testosterone and Sex Hormone–Binding Globulin. Scant data are available concerning the acute exercise responses of free testosterone (testosterone not bound to a protein, such as sex hormone–binding globulin, for transport). Häkkinen and co-workers (45, 46, 47) have observed that free testosterone remains unaltered or decreases after resistance exercise training sessions. The so-called free-hormone hypothesis says that it is only the free hormone that interacts with target tissues. Still, the bound hormone could significantly influence the rate of hormone delivery to a target tissue, such as muscle (26).

The role, regulation, and interaction of binding proteins and their interactions with cells also present interesting possibilities, especially with women, whose total

amount of testosterone is very low in comparison with males. In fact, the binding protein itself may act as a hormone with biological activity (103). The biological role of various binding proteins appears to be an important factor in tissue interactions (45, 46, 47, 103). Their observations have demonstrated that changes in sex hormone–binding globulin and the ratio of this protein to testosterone are correlated to isometric leg strength and reflect the patterns of force production improvements in leg musculature.

Testosterone Responses in Women. For the most part, the majority of data on hormonal responses to resistance exercise and training have utilized college-aged male subjects. The testosterone hormonal response patterns during growth and development have traditionally been credited as the responsible factors in differences in muscular development and strength between men and women. To date, the majority of studies have shown that women typically do not demonstrate an exercise-induced increase in testosterone consequent to various forms of heavy resistance exercise (29, 54, 77, 80, 122). This may vary with individual women when high adrenal androgen release is possible. In one report, changes were observed in baseline levels of testosterone compared to inactive controls (20). Still, other studies have been unable to demonstrate changes in serum concentrations of testosterone with training (123). Recently, Häkkinen et al. (51) have shown that changes in total and free-testosterone levels during strength training were correlated with muscle force production characteristics but that no significant increases were observed. The response of testosterone in females in response to two different workouts is seen in Figure 6.4.

Training Adaptations of Testosterone

still learning about the responses of testostero tance training (48, 110, 123). It appears t' time and experience may be very important factoı₃ ꞏ altering the resting and exercise-induced concentrations of this hormone. In adult males, acute increases in testosterone are observed if the exercise stimulus is adequate (i.e., multiple sets, 5-10RM, adequate amount of muscle mass used). Häkkinen et al. (47) have demonstrated that over the course of 2 years of training in elite weightlifters, increases in resting serum testosterone concentrations do occur, even in elite power athletes. This was concomitant to increases in follicle-stimulating

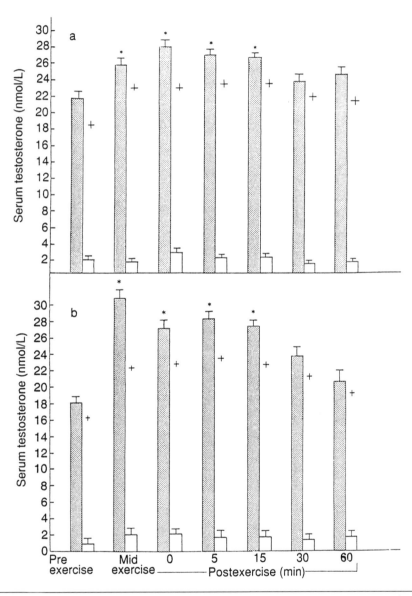

Figure 6.4 Male (shaded bars) and female (unshaded bars) serum testosterone responses to two exercise programs. The protocol in (a) entailed eight exercises using 5RM and 3-min rest periods between sets and exercises. The program in (b) called for eight exercises using 10RM and 1-min rest periods between sets and exercises. The total work for the second protocol was higher. *Significantly above preexercise levels. ⁺Significantly above the other group.
Reprinted from Kraemer et al. (1991).

hormone and leutinizing hormone, which are the higher brain regulators of testosterone production and release. Such changes augment the neural adaptations that occur for strength gain in highly trained power athletes.

In the Häkkinen study, whereas the testosterone changes showed remarkable similarities to the patterns of strength changes, the ratio of sex hormone–binding globulin to testosterone mirrored strength changes even more closely. It is interesting to hypothesize that in those athletes among whom little adaptive potential exists for changes in muscle hypertrophy (i.e., highly trained strength athletes), changes in testosterone cybernetics may be a part of a more advanced adaptive strategy for increasing the force capabilities of muscle via neural factors. This may occur by the potentiation of other hormonal mechanisms in tissue development or by the enhancement of neural factors (34). Such differences in adaptational strategies appear essential to providing for further gains in performance over the course of a long-term training program. This may reflect the interplay of different neural and hypertrophic factors involved in mediating strength and power changes as training time is extended into years (104).

Growth Hormone

It has long been recognized that growth hormone, a polypeptide hormone secreted in pulsatile (burstlike) manner from the anterior pituitary gland, is intimately involved with the growth process of skeletal muscle and many other tissues in the body. Not only is it important for normal development of a child but it also appears to play a vital role in adapting to the stress of resistance training. The main physiological roles of growth hormone are listed here:

- Decreases glucose utilization
- Decreases glycogen synthesis
- Increases amino acid transport across cell membranes
- Increases protein synthesis
- Increases utilization of fatty acids
- Increases lipolysis (fat breakdown)
- Increases availability of glucose and amino acids
- Increases collagen synthesis
- Stimulates cartilage growth
- Increases retention of nitrogen, sodium, potassium, and phosphorus
- Increases renal plasma flow and glomerular filtration
- Promotes compensatory renal hypertrophy

The secretion of growth hormone is regulated by a complex system of neuroendocrine feedback mechanisms (18, 30, 94, 102, 109, 124). Many of the hormone's actions may be mediated by a secondary set of hormones, the IGFs (discussed in the next section) (34). Growth hormone stimulates both the release of IGFs and the availability of amino acids for protein synthesis. This results in conditions that promote tissue repair in general and, perhaps, recovery following resistance exercise. There are reports of IGF being released from non-hepatic tissues (e.g., fat) including muscle itself which may not produce as much endogenous IGF as other body tissues (22, 34, 52). Still, growth hormone plays a crucial role in augmenting IGF release which in its own right is one of the most potent anabolic factors. Because IGF stores cannot be released from the liver without the stimulation of growth hormone, its importance in the augmentation of the body's own natural "anabolic" response cannot be minimized (34). Thus, growth hormone promotes IGF release from liver sources which interacts with the various cells and in addition, growth hormone may stimulate synthesis and release of IGF from within the various cells to influence growth promoting actions and metabolic regulation.

The secretion of growth hormone and thus the amount in the blood varies according to time of day, with the highest levels observed at night during sleep (31, 109). Secreting pulses also have different amplitudes throughout the day, and exercise appears to increase their amplitude. It has been hypothesized that nocturnal increases are involved in various tissue repair mechanisms in the body. Thus, it is possible that growth hormone secretion and release may directly influence adaptations of the contractile unit of muscle and subsequent expression of strength. Various external factors, such as age, gender, sleep, nutrition, alcohol consumption, and exercise, all alter growth hormone release patterns (13, 14, 16, 97, 109, 119, 120).

Release and Binding of Growth Hormone.
Growth hormone is released into the peripheral circulation, where it attaches to specific binding proteins which represent the extracellular domain of the growth hormone receptor (88). Growth hormone acts by binding to plasma membrane-bound receptors on the target cells. A glycosylated single polypeptide appears to be important for growth hormone binding. It is not known how extracellular domain binding of the receptor leads to a signal transduction in the cytosolic domain via such a short transmembrane sequence (18). Growth hormone binding may produce aggregates of receptors that traverse laterally in the fluid plasma membrane. Subsequently, the cell membrane-bound receptor also interacts and binds specifically with growth hormone.

Because of the fact that growth hormone has so many roles in metabolism, including growth-promoting actions in tissues (18, 34, 109), the pharmacological use of growth hormone has unknown and unpredictable results, especially in people with normal pituitary glands.

It appears that the role of growth hormone in muscle tissue is not related to events involving immature muscle fibers, since it has few direct effects on embryonic muscle tissue cultures (34). The enhancement of the contractile unit by such interactions would appear to contribute to the development of the intact muscle and subsequent force production characteristics. Still, further research is needed to clarify exactly how growth hormone is involved with exercise-induced hypertrophy. In a review by Rogol (102) it was shown that the growth hormone treatment alone is not effective in causing strength increases and that the total motor unit involvement is probably necessary. Although size increases are possible, the quality of the muscle may be compromised owing to limitations in the activation and control. Any apparent ergogenic effects may be outweighed by a wide variety of secondary effects not related to strength changes in muscle tissue (102). It seems plausible that the endogenous mechanisms related to the exercise stimulus have greater specificity and are more effective than growth hormone injections in mediating the specific mechanisms related to strength and hypertrophy development. In fact, exercise-induced hypertrophy is apparently quite different from hypertrophy resulting from injections of growth hormone, with force production in muscle fibers superior consequent to exercise-induced size increases (39, 101, 102). Furthermore, biological timing of cellular events in muscle and release of growth hormone may be crucial for optimal interactions between the exercise-stressed muscle and growth hormone.

Growth Hormone Responses to Stress.
Growth hormone has been found to be responsive to a variety of exercise stressors, including resistance exercise (37, 63, 65). Growth hormone levels increase in response to breath holding and hyperventilation alone (25), as well as to hypoxia (115). It appears that the stimulus for growth hormone release is increased hydrogen ion concentrations; Gordon et al. (40) have demonstrated that it is not increased lactate per se. Thus, the higher the lactate concentrations (which are associated with higher hydrogen ion concentrations) in the blood, the greater the growth hormone concentrations.

Not all resistance exercise protocols demonstrate increased serum growth hormone concentration. VanHelder et al. (120) observed that when a light load (28% of 7RM) was utilized with a high number of repetitions in each set, no changes in the serum concentration of growth hormone occurred. This suggests that in resistance exercise a threshold probably exists for intensity when longer rest periods (>3 min) are used to elicit a significant stimulatory response of growth hormone to resistance exercise.

Resistance loads utilized can span a wide continuum and operationally define the resistance exercise protocols. Thus, it may be characterized as a very light (e.g., 15RM or greater) to a very heavy (e.g., <10RM) resistance exercise protocol. Typically, heavy resistance exercise protocols utilize loads ranging from 1 to 10RM (32). Lighter resistances, while increases in strength are observed, are typically directed toward improving local muscular endurance rather than maximal strength and power (4, 32). In more advanced resistance training programs periodization techniques are used which vary the loads and the volume (sets × repetitions × loads) of exercise over the course of training (32, 89, 107, 111). Therefore, depending upon load, rest, and volume of exercise, differential growth hormone responses will occur.

Kraemer et al. (81) found serum increases in growth hormone are differentially sensitive to different resistance exercise protocols (see Figure 6.5). When the intensity utilized was 10RM (heavy resistance) with three sets performed for each exercise (high total work, approximately 60,000 J)—combined with short (1-min) rest periods—large increases were observed in serum concentrations of growth hormone. Thus, the most dramatic increases occurred in response to a decrease in rest period length (1 min) when the duration of exercise was longer (10RM vs. 5RM). With such differences being related to the exercise configuration (e.g., rest period length) of the exercise session, it appears that greater attention needs to be given to program design variables when evaluating physiological adaptations to resistance training. Future studies will need to explore the use of various exercise protocols and their associated growth hormone changes to determine where muscle tissue hypertrophy and strength-and-power adaptations are optimized for individuals of different training levels.

Growth Hormone Responses in Women.
Throughout the menstrual cycle women have higher blood levels of growth hormone compared with men due to greater frequency and amplitude of secretion. Hormone concentrations and hormone responses to exercise vary with menstrual phase (24), although the mechanisms of this variation are unclear. Kraemer et al. (77) found that during the early follicular phase of the menstrual cycle, females had significantly higher growth hormone concentrations at rest compared to males. Furthermore, when using a heavy resistance exercise protocol characterized by longer rest periods (3 min) and heavy loads (5RM), growth hormone levels did not increase above resting concentrations. However, when a short-rest (1-min) and moderate-resistance (10RM) resistance exercise protocol was used, significant increases in serum growth hormone levels were observed. This suggests that hormonal response patterns

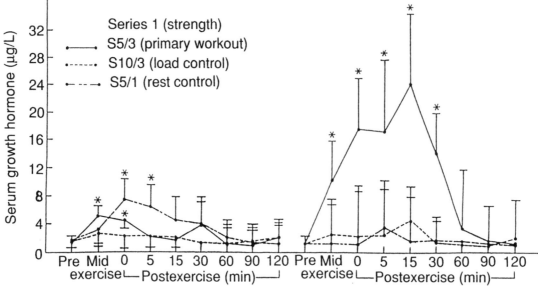

Figure 6.5   Serum growth hormone responses to various resistance exercise protocols. (See Figure 6.3 for an explanation of the graphs.)

Reprinted from Kraemer et al. (1990).

to different resistance exercise routines may not be similar over the course of the menstrual cycle, owing to alterations in resting levels (80).

The possibility of periodizing resistance training over the course of the menstrual cycle remains to be examined, but more research is needed to elucidate any gender-related neuroendocrine adaptational mechanisms. At present, the reduced levels of testosterone and differential resting hormonal levels over the course of the menstrual cycle appear to be the most striking neuroendocrine differences between males and females. How such differences are related to the training adaptations and the development of muscle tissue and expression of strength and power remains to be demonstrated (Figure 6.6).

Training Adaptations of Growth Hormone.   It appears that longer time periods (2-24 hr) will need to be measured in order to see if changes in growth hormone levels exist with resistance exercise. It is the area under the time curve, which includes an array of pulsatile effects, that tells if changes in release have occurred. The responses of growth hormone to resistance training have not been extensively studied but observations of normal single measures of resting concentrations of growth hormone in elite lifters suggest little change (47).

It is likely that differences in feedback mechanisms, changes in receptor sensitivities, insulinlike growth factor potentiation, diurnal variations, and maximal exercise concentrations may mediate and be representative of growth hormone alterations with resistance training.

Insulinlike Growth Factors

Many of the effects of growth hormone are mediated through small polypeptides called insulinlike growth factors (IGFs), or somatomedins (21, 28, 34). IGF-I is a 70–amino acid polypeptide and IGF-II a 67–amino acid polypeptide; the function of the latter is less clear. IGFs are secreted by the liver, after growth hormone stimulates liver cell DNA to synthesize them, a process that takes about 8 to 29 hr. Typical of many polypeptide hormones, both growth factors are synthesized as larger precursor molecules, which then undergo processing to the hormones themselves. IGFs travel in the blood attached to binding proteins (of which there are at least five types) and are released as free hormones to interact with receptors (1, 113, 114), and are regulated by various factors (125-127). Measures of blood levels of IGFs are usually either total levels (bound and free) or free-IGF levels.

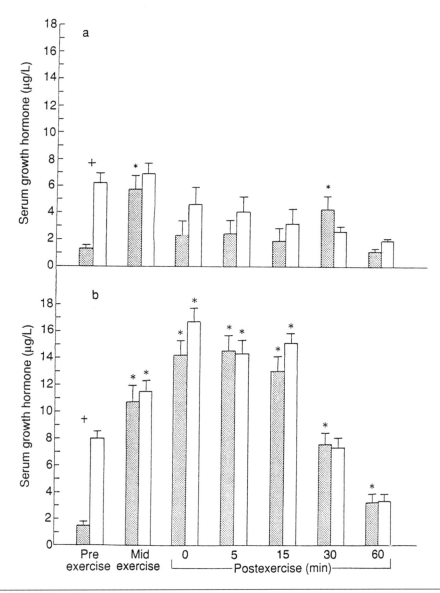

Figure 6.6 Male (shaded bars) and female (unshaded bars) serum growth hormone responses to two exercise programs. (See Figure 6.4 for an explanation of the graphs.)
Reprinted from Kraemer et al. (1991).

The reasons for acute increases in blood levels of IGF are unknown but are probably related to the disruption of various cells, including fat and muscle cells, since these cells manufacture and store IGF (118). Fat cells contain relatively high levels of IGF; skeletal muscle has very little of its own. It is possible that IGF may be released from nonliver cells without the mediation of growth hormone (1, 3, 34, 52, 55, 56). In addition, cells may produce and keep IGF, where they work without entering the peripheral circulation.

Circulating IGFs are associated with binding proteins. At least five circulating binding proteins have been identified and regulate the amount of IGF which is available in the plasma. Binding proteins are important

factors in the transport and physiological mechanisms related to IGF (18, 19, 36). IGF has been shown to stimulate the secretion of its own binding proteins from within the muscle cell itself, thus modulating the cell's responsiveness to IGF (95). The circulating IGF binding proteins play an important role in restricting access of the IGF peptides to receptors and are influenced by growth hormone concentrations. Other factors, such as nutritional status and insulin levels, also have been shown to be an important signal mechanism for IGF release. The nutritional influence on IGF transport, production, and regulatory control is a dramatic variable affecting cellular interactions. Acute changes in nitrogen balance and protein intake, and nutritional status all affect a variety of mechanisms and have been previously reviewed (18, 92, 102). It also appears that binding proteins act as a reservoir of IGF, and release from the binding protein is signaled by the availability of a receptor on the cell. Thus, free IGF is released from the binding protein to interact with the cell receptor (11). This could theoretically reduce the amount of degradation of IGF. It allows IGF to be viable for a longer period of time.

In strength training, many of these mechanisms would be influenced by the exercise stress, acute hormonal responses, and the need for muscle, nerve, and bone tissue remodeling at the cellular level (53, 56, 108). The dramatic interactions of multiple hormones and receptors provide powerful adaptive mechanisms in response to resistance training and can contribute to the subsequent changes in muscular strength and size.

Exercise Responses of IGFs. Few data are available concerning the acute responses of IGF to exercise. Variable responses in total serum concentrations of IGF-I have been observed consequent to endurance exercise (60). How acute changes occur with exercise is a bit of a mystery. As mentioned previously, it takes 8 to 29 hr for IGF to be produced following stimulation by growth hormone. This seems to indicate that IGF is

being released from storage sources other than the liver, that release is due to cellular disruption of cells that already contain IGF, or that growth hormone-mediated release of IGF with certain types of exercise has a different time course from injection-response studies. Kraemer et al. (81) showed that, for almost all of a variety of resistance exercise protocols, concentrations of total IGF-I rose at some point over the 2 hr following exercise. In a recent study examining changes in levels of total IGF with the same types of exercise protocols, this time with female subjects, no changes were observed (77). Systematic alterations in circulatory concentrations of IGF to various types of exercise protocols appear to be closely related to regulatory factors of IGF release and transport (11). Evaluation of serum changes over longer periods may be necessary to evaluate specific effects and relationships to growth hormone in the serum (33). Figure 6.7 shows total IGF-I responses to various heavy resistance exercise protocols in men and women.

Training Adaptations of IGFs. Responses of IGF-I to heavy resistance training remain unclear (35). As with growth hormone, training-induced adaptations in IGF are probably reflected in a variety of release,

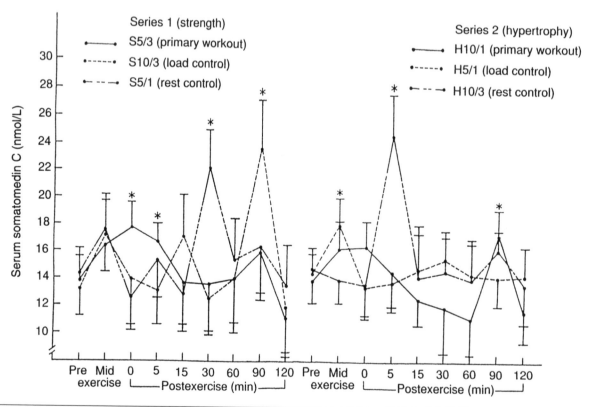

Figure 6.7 Serum insulinlike growth factor (somatomedin C) responses to various resistance exercise protocols. (See Figure 6.3 for an explanation of the graphs.)
Reprinted from Kraemer et al. (1990).

transport, and receptor interaction changes. Such adaptations need further examination in response to heavy resistance exercise.

ADRENAL HORMONES

The adrenal gland has two major divisions, the cortex and the medulla. Both divisions respond to exercise stress. The adrenal medulla is stimulated by the nervous system and thus provides the faster response; the cortex is stimulated by adrenocorticotropic hormone from the anterior pituitary. The adrenal gland plays a crucial role in the fight-or-flight phenomenon. The adrenal hormones most important to training and conditioning are cortisol, a glucocorticoid from the adrenal cortex, and the catecholamines, from the adrenal medulla, and enkephalin-containing polypeptides (e.g., peptide F) (23, 68, 73, 75, 86).

Cortisol

In a classic sense, glucocorticoids and more specifically cortisol in humans have been viewed as a catabolic hormone in skeletal muscle (34,87). The major catabolic effects of cortisol in muscle are as follows:

- Converts amino acids to carbohydrates
- Increases levels of proteolytic enzymes (enzymes that break down proteins)
- Inhibits protein synthesis

Cortisol has a greater catabolic effect in fast-twitch muscle fibers than in slow-twitch fibers.

In situations of disease, joint immobilization, or injury, an elevation in cortisol mediates a nitrogen-wasting effect with a net loss of contractile protein. This results in muscle atrophy, with associated reductions in force production capability (34, 90). In the muscle, cortisol's catabolic effects are countered by the anabolic effects of testosterone and insulin. If a greater number of receptors are bound with insulin, or if testosterone blocks the genetic element in the DNA for cortisol, protein is conserved or enhanced. Conversely, if a greater number of receptors are bound to cortisol, protein is degraded and lost. The balance of anabolic and catabolic activities in the muscle affects the protein contractile unit, directly influencing strength.

Although the cellular mechanisms and the molecular biology of catabolism remain to be completely elucidated, a number of possibilities exist (105). The catabolic activities appear to be mediated at the glucocorticoid-receptor complex level (64). Also, glucocorticoids may influence mRNA mechanisms for production of proteolytic enzymes (34). Additionally,

the acute increases in circulating cortisol following exercise also implicate acute inflammatory response mechanisms in the tissue remodeling processes.

Resistance Exercise Responses of Cortisol. Cortisol responds to resistance exercise protocols that create a dramatic stimulus to anaerobic metabolism. As with growth hormone, resistance exercise protocols that utilize high volume, large muscle groups, and shorter rest periods result in elevations in serum cortisol values. It is interesting that the acute exercise protocols that produce the highest catabolic responses in the body also produce the greatest growth hormone response. Thus, while chronic high levels of cortisol may have adverse effects, acute increases may be a part of a larger remodeling process in muscle tissue. Muscle must be disrupted to a certain extent (below injury levels) to remodel itself and enlarge; acute elevations in cortisol would help in this process.

Because of the catabolic role attributed to cortisol, athletes and training professionals have exhibited much interest in its potential as a whole-body marker of tissue breakdown. Furthermore, the testosterone-cortisol ratio has been used in the attempt to mark the anabolic-catabolic status of the body (50). However, although such markers are attractive conceptually, the use of serum cortisol and the testosterone-cortisol ratio has met with only limited success in predicting or monitoring changes in strength and power capabilities. Problems with these tests probably have to do with the multiple roles of cortisol and other hormones. Further study is required.

It is very probable that vast differences are observed in the physiological role of cortisol in acute (immediate response) versus chronic (response which happens with longer periods of training time) exercise responses to resistance exercise. Acutely, cortisol may reflect the metabolic stress of the exercise and in chronic aspects be primarily involved with tissue homeostasis involving protein metabolism (34). Thus, its role in overtraining, detraining, or injury may be critical as muscle tissue atrophy as well as decreases in force production capabilities are observed (90). Such roles remain to be demonstrated.

Catecholamines

The catecholamines—epinephrine, norepinephrine, and dopamine—are probably more important for the acute expression of strength than any of the other hormones (84). Their role in growth-promoting actions of muscle tissue is less clear but may be important during prenatal development in accelerating the growth process (15, 33, 34). It may be that catecholamines again augment the production of growth-promoting hormones in the system. The physiological functions of epinephrine and norepinephrine in muscle are listed here:

- Increases force production
- Increases muscle contraction rate
- Increases blood pressure
- Increases energy availability
- Augments secretion rates of other hormones, such as testosterone

Catecholamines appear to reflect the acute demands and physical stress of resistance exercise protocols (82, 93). A high-intensity (10RM), short-rest (10-60 s between sets and exercises) heavy resistance exercise routine (10 exercises, three sets) typically utilized by bodybuilders for development of strength and hypertrophy was shown to maintain increased plasma norepinephrine, epinephrine, and dopamine levels for 5 min into recovery (82). These data demonstrate how different configurations of an exercise stimulus can produce dramatic physiological stress that only highly trained individuals can tolerate.

Training Adaptations of Catecholamines.

Heavy resistance training has been shown to increase the ability of an athlete to secrete greater amounts of epinephrine during maximal exercise (62). It has also been suggested that training reduces epinephrine responses to a single bench press exercise workout (43). Since epinephrine is involved in metabolic control, force production, and the potentiation of the response mechanisms of other hormones, such as testosterone and IGFs, stimulation of catecholamines is probably one of the first neuroendocrine mechanisms to occur in response to resistance exercise.

OTHER HORMONAL CONSIDERATIONS

A host of different hormones are involved in the maintenance of normal body function, as well as in adaptive responses of the body to resistance training (27, 69, 91, 99). Although we might focus on one or two hormones for their roles in a particular physiological function, there are actually other hormones that create an optimal environment for the primary hormonal actions to take place. Hormones such as insulin, thyroid hormones, and beta-endorphin have been implicated in growth, repair, and exercise stress mechanisms; unfortunately, few data are available concerning their responses and adaptations to resistance exercise or training (72). Owing to the relatively tight homeostatic control surrounding both insulin and thyroid hormone secretion, alterations in circulating resting concentrations of these hormones resulting from chronic training adaptations would not be expected. It is more likely that changes in 24-hr secretion rates, sensitivity of the receptors, and binding interactions would be affected. Pakarinen et al. (98) have demonstrated only slight, nonsignificant decreases in serum concentrations of total and free thyroxine (a thyroid hormone) after 20 weeks of strength training. The permissive effects of such hormones in metabolic control, amino acid synthesis, and augmentation of other hormonal release mechanisms are the essence of such interactions with resistance training.

CONCLUSION

Hormonal mechanisms are responsive to resistance exercise and training (65, 66). Hormones interact with a variety of tissues to mediate changes with resistance training. It is evident that muscle fibers benefit from these hormonal interactions. Neuroendocrine mechanisms appear to be intimately involved with both the acute exercise response and chronic training adaptations. A greater physiological understanding of muscle hypertrophy and subsequent strength and power performances may well be elucidated by studies that examine the molecular biology of various neuroendocrine mechanisms. Performance can only be enhanced with optimal stimulation of the neuroendocrine system using proper configurations of resistance exercise stress. Optimal training of endogenous anabolic factors may well enhance training adaptations in resistance training.

Key Terms

allosteric binding site	89	endocrine gland	87	neuroendocrinology	87
anabolic hormone	89	hormone	87	second messenger	90
catabolic hormone	89	hormone-receptor complex (H-RC)	90	target tissue	87
cross-reactivity	89	lock-and-key theory	89		
down regulation	89				

Study Questions

1. Which of the following hormones enhance muscle tissue growth?

   I. growth hormone
   II. cortisol
   III. IGF-I
   IV. progesterone

   a. I and III only
   b. I and IV only
   c. I, II, and III only
   d. I, II, and IV only

2. Which hormone has the greatest influence on changes in nerves?

   a. growth hormone
   b. testosterone
   c. cortisol
   d. IGF

3. Which hormone is higher in women than men at rest?

   a. cortisol
   b. insulin
   c. testosterone
   d. growth hormone

4. What type of workout promotes the highest growth hormone increases following the exercise session?

   a. short rest (1 min), high volume, multiple sets
   b. single set, low volume
   c. sets of 5RM
   d. long rest (3 min), low volume, multiple sets

Applying Knowledge of Neuroendocrine Responses

Problem 1

List the primary anabolic and catabolic hormones for muscle. Design a program that will acutely elevate these hormones. Design a program that may elevate testosterone but not growth hormone and explain why. Determine when in a training cycle each program would be performed.

References

1. Adem, A., S.S. Jossan, R. D'Argy, P.G. Gillberg, A. Nordberg, B. Windbald, and V. Sara. Insulin-like growth factor I (IGF-1) receptors in the human brain: Quantitative autoradiographic localization. *Brain Res.* 503(2):299-303. 1989.
2. Allen, R.E., and L.K. Boxhorn. Regulation of skeletal muscle satellite cell proliferation and differentiation by transforming growth factor-beta, insulin-like growth factor I, and fibroblast growth factor. *J. Cell Physiol.* 138(2):311-315. 1988.
3. Allen, R.E., R.A. Merkel, and R.B. Young. Cellular aspects of muscle growth: Myogenic cell proliferation. *J. Anim. Sci.* 49(1):115-127. 1979.
4. Atha, J. Strengthening muscle. In: *Exercise Sport Sciences Reviews*, D.I. Miller, ed. Philadelphia: The Franklin Institute Press. 1981. pp. 1-73.
5. Bartalena, L. Recent achievements in studies on thyroid hormone binding proteins. *Endocr. Rev.* 11:47-64. 1990.

6. Baxter, R.C., and J.L. Martin. Stricture of the M_r 140000 growth hormone–dependent insulin-like growth factor binding protein complex: Determination by reconstitution affinity-labeling. *Proc. Nat. Acad. Sci. U.S.A.* 86(18): 6898-6902. 1989.

7. Baxter, R.C., J.L. Martin, and V.A. Beniac. High molecular weight insulin-like growth factor binding protein complex: Purification and properties of the acid-labile subunit from human serum. *J. Biol. Chem.* 264(20):11843-11848. 1989.

8. Ben-Ezra, V., R.G. McMurray, and A. Smith. Effects of exercise or diet on plasma somatomedin-C (abstract). *Med. Sci. Sports Exerc.* 17(2):209. 1985.

9. Biró, J., and E. Endröczi. Nuclear RNA content and synthesis in anterior pituitary in intact, castrated and androgen sterilized rats. *Endocrinol. Exp.* 11:164-168. 1977.

10. Bleisch, W., V.N. Lunie, and F. Nottebohm. Modification of synapses in androgen-sensitive muscle. Hormonal regulation of acteylcholine receptor number in the songbird. Syrinx. *J. Neurosci.* 4:786-792. 1984.

11. Blum, W.F., E.W. Jenne, F. Reppin, K. Kietzmann, M.B. Ranke, and J.R. Bierich. Insulin-like growth factor I (IGF-I)–binding protein complex is a better mitogen than free IGF-I. *Endocrinology* 125:766-772. 1989.

12. Borer, K.T., D.R. Nicoski, and V. Owens. Alteration of pulsatile growth hormone secretion by growth-inducing exercise: Involvement of endogenous opiates and somatostatin. *Endocrinology* 118:844-850. 1986.

13. Buckler, J.M. The effect of age, sex, and exercise on the secretion of growth hormone. *Clin. Sci.* 37:765-774. 1969.

14. Buckler, J.M.H. The relationship between exercise, body temperature and plasma growth hormone levels in a human subject. *J. Physiol.* 214:25-26. 1971.

15. Carmichael, S.W. *The Adrenal Medulla*, vol. 4. Cambridge, England: Cambridge University Press. 1987.

16. Chang, F., W. Dodds, M. Sullivan, M. Kim, and W. Malarkey. The acute effects of exercise on prolactin and growth hormone secretion: Comparison between sedentary women and women runners with normal and abnormal menstrual cycles. *J. Clin. Endocrinol. Metab.* 62:551-556. 1985.

17. Clarkson, P., and I. Tremblay. Exercise-induced muscle damage, repair, and adaptation in humans. *J. Appl. Physiol.* 65(1):1-6. 1988.

18. Clemmons, D.R., H.W. Busby, and L.E. Underwood. Mediation of the growth promoting actions of growth hormone by somatomedin-C/insulin-like growth factor I and its binding protein. In: *The Physiology of Human Growth*, J.M. Tanner and M.A. Preece, eds. Cambridge, England: Cambridge University Press. 1989. pp. 111-128.

19. Clemmons, D.R., J.P. Thissen, M. Maes, J.M. Ketelslegers, and L.E. Underwood. Insulin-like growth factor-I (IGF-I) infusion into hypophysectomized or protein-deprived rats induces specific IGF-binding proteins in serum. *Endocrinology* 125(6):2967-2972. 1989.

20. Cumming, D.C., S.R. Wall, M.A. Galbraith, and A.N. Belcastro. Reproductive hormone responses to resistance exercise. *Med. Sci. Sports Exerc.* 19:234-238. 1987.

21. Czech, M.P. Signal transmission by the insulin-like growth factors. *Cell* 59:235-238. 1989.

22. Daughaday, W.H., and P. Rotwein. Insulin-like growth factors I and II. Peptide, messenger ribonucleic acid and gene structures, serum and tissue concentrations. *Endocr. Rev.* 10:68-91. 1989.

23. DeSouza, M.J., M.S. Maguire, C.M. Maresh, W.J. Kraemer, K. Ruben, and A.B. Loucks. Adrenal activation and the prolactin response to exercise in eumenorrheic and amenorrheic runners. *J. Appl. Physiol.* 70(6):2378-2387. 1991.

24. DeSouza, M.J., C.M. Maresh, M.S. Maguire, W.J. Kraemer, G.F. Ginter, and K.L. Goetz. Menstrual status and plasma vasopressin, renin activity and aldosterone exercise responses. *J. Appl. Physiol.* 67:736-743. 1989.

25. Djarova, T., A. Ilkov, A. Varbanova, A. Nikiforova, and G. Mateev. Human growth hormone, cortisol, and acid-base balance changes after hyperventilation and breath-holding. *Int. J. Sports Med.* 7:311-315. 1986.

26. Ekins, R. Measurement of free hormones in blood. *Endocr. Rev.* 11:5-45. 1990.

27. Elloit, D., L. Goldberg, and W. Watts. Resistance exercise and plasma beta-endorphin/beta-lipotrophin immuno-reactivity. *Life Sci.* 35:515-518. 1984.

28. Fagin, J.A., C. Fernandez-Mejia, and S. Melmed. Pituitary insulin-like growth factor-I gene expression: Regulation by triodothyronine and growth hormone. *Endocrinology* 125(5):2385-2391. 1989.

29. Fahey, T.D., R. Rolph, P. Moungmee, J. Nagel, and S. Mortar. Serum testosterone, body composition, and strength of young adults. *Med. Sci. Sports* 8:31-34. 1976.

30. Faria, A.C.S., J.D. Veldhuis, M.O. Thorner, and M.L. Vance. Half-time of endogenous growth hormone (GH) disappearance in normal man after stimulation of GH secretion by GH-releasing hormone and suppression with somatostatin. *J. Clin. Endocrinol. Metab.* 68(3):535-541. 1989.

31. Finkelstein, J.W., H.P. Roffwarg, R.M. Boyar, J. Kream, and L. Hellman. Age related change in the twenty-four hour spontaneous secretion of growth hormone. *J. Clin. Endocrinol. Metab.* 35:665-670. 1972.

32. Fleck, S.J., and W.J. Kraemer. *Designing Resistance Training Programs*. Champaign, IL: Human Kinetics. 1987.

33. Florini, J.R. Hormonal control of muscle cell growth. *J. Anim. Sci.* 61:21-37. 1985.

34. Florini, J.R. Hormonal control of muscle growth. *Muscle Nerve* 10:577-598. 1987.

35. Florini, J.R., P.N. Prinz, M.V. Vitiello, and R.L. Hintz. Somatomedin-C levels in healthy young and old men: Relationship of peak and 24 hour integrated levels of growth hormone. *J. Gerontol.* 40:2-7. 1985.

36. Forbes, B., L. Szabo, R.C. Baxter, F.J. Ballard, and J.C. Wallace. Classification of the insulin-like growth factor binding proteins into three distinct categories according to their binding specificities. *Biochem. Biophys. Res. Commun.* 157:196-202. 1988.

37. Galbo, H. *Hormonal and Metabolic Adaptation to Exercise*. Stuttgart: Georg Thieme Verlay. 1983.

38. Gharib, S.D., M.E. Wioerman, M.A. Shupnik, and W.W. Chin. Molecular biology of the pituitary gonadotropins. *Endocr. Rev.* 71:177-199. 1990.

39. Goldberg, A.L., and H. Goodman. Relationship between growth hormone and muscular work in determining muscle size. *J. Appl. Physiol.* 200:655-666. 1969.

40. Gordon, S.E., W.J. Kraemer, N. Vos, and J.M. Lynch. Acid base manipulation: Effect on serum human growth hormone concentration after acute high intensity cycle exercise. *J. Appl. Physiol.* In press.

41. Griggs, R.C., D. Halliday, W. Kingston, and R.T. Moxley, III. Effect of testosterone on muscle protein synthesis in myotonic dystrophy. *Ann. Neurol.* 20:590-596. 1986.

42. Griggs, R.C., W. Kingston, R.F. Jozefowicz, B.E. Herr, G. Forbes, and D. Halliday. Effect of testosterone on muscle mass and muscle protein synthesis. *J. Appl. Physiol.* 66(1):498-503. 1989.

43. Guezennec, Y., L. Leger, F. Lhoste, M. Aymonod, and P.C. Pesquies. Hormone and metabolite response to weight-lifting training sessions. *Int. J. Sports Med.* 7:100-105. 1986.

44. Häkkinen, K. Neuromuscular and hormonal adaptations during strength and power training. *J. Sports Med. Phys. Fitness* 29:9-24. 1989.

45. Häkkinen, K., P.V. Komi, M. Alén, and H. Kauhanen. EMG, muscle fibre and force production characteristics during a one year training period in elite weightlifters. *Eur. J. Appl. Physiol.* 56:419-427. 1987.

46. Häkkinen, K., A. Pakarinen, M. Alén, H. Kauhanen, and P.V. Komi. Relationships between training volume, physical performance capacity, and serum hormone concentrations during prolonged training in elite weight lifters. *Int. J. Sports Med.* (8):61-65. 1987.

47. Häkkinen, K., A. Pakarinen, M. Alén, H. Kauhanen, and P.V. Komi. Daily hormonal and neuromuscular responses to intensive strength training in 1 week. *Int. J. Sports Med.* 9:422-428. 1988.

48. Häkkinen, K., A. Pakarinen, M. Alén, H. Kauhanen, and P.V. Komi. Neuromuscular and hormonal adaptations in athletes to strength training in two years. *J. Appl. Physiol.* 65(6):2406-2412. 1988.

49. Häkkinen, K., A. Pakarinen, M. Alén, H. Kauhanen, and P.V. Komi. Neuromuscular and hormonal responses in elite athletes to two successive strength training sessions. *Eur. J. Appl. Physiol.* 57:133-139. 1988.

50. Häkkinen, K., A. Pakarinen, M. Alén, and P.V. Komi. Serum hormones during prolonged training of neuromuscular performance. *Eur. J. Appl. Physiol.* 53:287-293. 1985.

51. Häkkinen, K., A. Pakarinen, H. Kyrolainen, S. Cheng, D.H. Kim, and P.V. Komi. Neuromuscular adaptations and serum hormones in females during prolonged power training. *Int. J. Sports Med.* 11:91-98. 1990.

52. Han, V.K.M., A.J. D'Ercole, and P.K. Lund. Cellular localization of somatomedin (insulin-like growth factor) messenger RNA in the human fetus. *Science* 236:193-196. 1987.

53. Hansson, H.A., C. Brandsten, C. Lossing, and K. Petruson. Transient expression of insulin-like growth factor I immunocreactivity by vascular cells during angionenesis. *Exp. Mol. Pathol.* 50(1):125-138. 1989.

54. Hetrick, G.A., and J.H. Wilmore. Androgen levels and muscle hypertrophy during an eight-week training program for men/women (abstract). *Med. Sci. Sports* 11:102. 1979.

55. Hill, D.J., C. Camacho-Hubner, P. Rashid, A.J. Strain, and D.R. Clemmons. Insulin-like growth factor (IGF)–binding protein release by human fetal fibroblasts: Dependency on cell density and IGF peptides. *J. Endocrinol.* 122(1):87-98. 1989.

56. Horikawa, R., K. Asakawa, N. Hizuka, K. Takano, and K. Shizume. Growth hormone and insulin-like growth factor I stimulate Leydig cell steroikogensis. *Eur. J. Pharmacol.* 166(1):87-93. 1989.

57. Housley, P.R., E.R. Sanchez, and J.F. Grippo. Phosphorylation and reduction of glucocorticoid components. In: *Receptor Phosphorylation*, V.M. Moudgil, ed. Boca Raton, FL: CRC Press. 1989. pp. 289-314.

58. Ikeda, T., K. Fujiyama, T. Takeuchi, M. Honda, O. Mokuda, M. Tominaga, and H. Mashiba. Effect of thyroid hormone on somatomedin-C release from perfused rat liver. *Experientia* 45(2):170-171. 1989.

59. Ishii, D.N. Relationship of insulin-like growth factor II gene expression in muscle to synaptogenesis. *Proc. Nat. Acad. Sci. U.S.A.* 86(8):2898-2902. 1989.

60. Jahreis, G., V. Hesse, H.E. Schmidt, and J. Scheibe. Effect of endurance exercise on somatomedin-C/insulin-like growth factor I concentration in male and female runners. *Exp. Clin. Endocrinol.* 94:89-96. 1989.

61. Kelly, A., G. Lyongs, B. Gambki, and N. Robinstein. Influences of testosterone on contractile proteins of the guinea pig temporalis muscle. *Adv. Exp. Med. Biol.* 182:155-168. 1985.

62. Kjaer, M., and G. Henrik. Effect of physical training on the capacity to secrete epinephrine. *J. Appl. Physiol.* 64:11-16. 1988.

63. Klimes, I., M. Vigas, J. Jurcovicová, and S. Németh. Lack of effect of acid-base alterations on growth hormone secretion in man. *Endocrinol. Exp.* 11:155-162. 1977.

64. Konagaya, M., P.A. Bernar, and S.R. Max. Biocade of glucocorticoid receptor binding and inhibition of dexamethasone-induced muscle atrophy in the rat by RU38486, a potent glucocorticoid antagonist. *Endocrinology* 119:375-380. 1986.

65. Kraemer, W.J. Endocrine responses to resistance exercise. *Med. Sci. Sports Exerc.* 20 (suppl.):S152-S157. 1988.

66. Kraemer, W.J. Endocrine responses and adaptations to strength training. In: *The Encyclopaedia of Sports Medicine: Strength and Power*, P.V. Komi, ed. Oxford, UK: Blackwell Scientific. 1992. pp. 291-304.

67. Kraemer, W.J. Hormonal mechanisms related to the expression of muscular strength and power. In: *The Encyclopaedia of Sports Medicine: Strength and Power*, P.V. Komi, ed. Oxford, UK: Blackwell Scientific. 1992. pp. 64-76.

68. Kraemer, W.J., L.E. Armstrong, K.J. Marchitelli, R.W. Hubbard, and B.N. Leva. Plasma opioid peptide responses during heat acclimation in humans. *Peptides.* 8:715-719. 1987.

69. Kraemer, W.J., L.E. Armstrong, P. Rock, R.W. Hubbard, L.J. Marchitelli, N. Leva, and J.E. Dziados. Responses of humanatrial natriuretic factor to high intensity submaximal exercise in the heat. *Eur. J. Appl. Physiol.* 57:399-403. 1988.

70. Kraemer, W.J., and T.R. Baechle. Development of a strength training program. In: *Sports Medicine*, 2nd ed., A.J. Ryan and F.L. Allman, eds. San Diego: Academic Press. 1989. pp. 113-127.

71. Kraemer, W.J., M.R. Deschenes, and S.J. Fleck. Physiological adaptations to resistance exercise implications for athletic conditioning. *Sports Med.* 6:246-256. 1988.

72. Kraemer, W.J., J.E. Dziados, L.J. Marchitelli, S.E. Gordon, E.A. Harman, R. Mello, S.J. Fleck, P.N. Frykman, and N.T. Triplett. Effects of different heavy-resistance exercise protocols on plasma B-endorphin concentrations. *J. Appl. Physiol.* 74(1):450-459. 1993.

73. Kraemer, W.J., J.E. Dziados, S.E. Gordon, L.J. Marchitelli, A.C. Fry, J. Hoffman, and K. Reynolds. The effects of graded exercise on plasma catecholamines and proenkephalin Peptide F responses at sea level. *Eur. J. Appl. Physiol.* 61:214-217. 1990.

74. Kraemer, W.J., and S.J. Fleck. Resistance training: Exercise prescription. *Phys. Sportsmed.* 16(6):69-81. 1988.

75. Kraemer, W.J., S.J. Fleck, R. Callister, M. Shealy, G. Dudley, C.M. Maresh, L. Marchitelli, C. Cruthirds, T. Murray, and J.E. Falkel. Training responses of plasma beta-endorphin, adrenocorticotropin and cortisol. *Med. Sci. Sports Exerc.* 21(2):146-153. 1989.

76. Kraemer, W.J., S.J. Fleck, and M. Deschenses. A review: Factors in exercise prescription of resistance training. *NSCA Journal.* 10(5):36-41. 1988.

77. Kraemer, W.J., S.J. Fleck, J.E. Dziados, E.A. Harman, L.J. Marchitelli, S.E. Gordon, R. Mello, P.N. Frykman, L.P. Koziris, and N.T. Triplett. Changes in hormonal concentrations after different heavy-resistance exercise protocols in women. *J. Appl. Physiol.* 75(2):594-604. 1993.

78. Kraemer, W.J., A.C. Fry, P.N. Frykman, B. Conroy, and J. Hoffman. Resistance training and youth. *Pediatr. Exerc. Sci.* 1:336-350. 1989.

79. Kraemer, W.J., A.C. Fry, B.J. Warren, M.H. Stone, S.J. Fleck, J.T. Kearney, B.P. Conroy, C.M. Maresh, C.A. Weseman, N.T. Triplett, and S.E. Gordon. Acute hormonal responses in elite junior weightlifters. *Int. J. Sports Med.* 13(2):103-109. 1992.

80. Kraemer, W.J., S.E. Gordon, S.J. Fleck, L.J. Marchitelli, R. Mello, J.E. Dziados, K. Friedl, E. Harman, C. Maresh, and A.C. Fry. Endogenous anabolic hormonal and growth factor responses to heavy resistance exercise in males and females. *Int. J. Sports Med.* 12(2):228-235. 1991.

81. Kraemer, W.J., L. Marchitelli, D. McCurry, R. Mello, J.E. Dziados, E. Harman, P. Frykman, S.E. Gordon, and S.J. Fleck. Hormonal and growth factor responses to heavy resistance exercise. *J. Appl. Physiol.* 69(4):1442-1450. 1990.

82. Kraemer, W.J., B.J. Noble, M.J. Clark, and B.W. Culver. Physiologic responses to heavy-resistance exercise with very short rest periods. *Int. J. Sports Med.* 8:247-252. 1987.

83. Kraemer, W.J., B.J. Noble, B. Culver, and R.V. Lewis. Changes in plasma proenkephalin Peptide F and catecholamine levels during graded exercise in men. *Proc. Nat. Acad. Sci. U.S.A.* 82:6349-6351. 1985.

84. Kraemer, W.J., J.F. Patton, H.G. Knuttgen, C.J. Hannan, T. Kittler, S. Gordon, J.E. Dziados, A.C. Fry, P.N. Frykman, and E.A. Harman. The effects of high intensity cycle exercise on sympatho-adrenal medullary response patterns. *J. Appl. Physiol.* 70:8-14. 1991.

85. Kraemer, W.J., J.F. Patton, H.G. Knuttgen, L.J. Marchitelli, C. Cruthirds, A. Damokosh, E. Harman, P. Frykman, and J.E. Dziados. Hypothalamic-pituitary-adrenal responses to short duration high-intensity cycle exercise. *J. Appl. Physiol.* 66:161-166. 1989.

86. Kraemer, W.J., P.B. Rock, C.S. Fulco, S.E. Gordon, J.P. Bonner, C.D. Cruthirds, L.J. Marchitelli, L. Trad, and A. Cymerman. Influence of altitude and caffeine during rest and exercise on plasma levels of proenkephalin Peptide F. *Peptides.* 9:1115-1119. 1988.

87. Kuoppasalmi, K., and H. Adlercreutz. Interaction between catabolic and anabolic steroid hormones in muscular exercise. In: *Exercise Endocrinology*, K. Fotherby and S.B. Pal, eds. Berlin: Walter de Gruyter. 1985. pp. 65-98.

88. Leung, D.W., S.A. Spencer, G. Cachianes, R.G. Hammonds, C. Collins, W.J. Henzel, R. Barnard, M.J. Waters, and W.I. Wood. *Nature* 330:537-543. 1987.

89. Lukaszewska, J., B. Biczowa, D. Bobilewixz, M. Wilk, and B. Bouchowixz-Fidelus. Effect of physical exercise on plasma cortisol and growth hormone levels in young weight lifters. *Endokrynol. Pol.* 2:149-158. 1976.

90. MacDougall, J. Morphological changes in human skeletal muscle following strength training and immobilization. In: *Human Muscle Power*, N.L. Jones, N. McCartney, and A.J. McComas, eds. Champaign, IL: Human Kinetics. 1986. pp. 269-284.

91. Mahler, D.A., L.N. Cunningham, G.S. Skrinar, W.J. Kraemer, and G.L. Colice. Beta-endorphin activity and hypercapnic ventilatory responsiveness after marathon running. *J. Appl. Physiol.* 66(5):2431-2436. 1989.

92. Maiter, D., T. Fliesen, L.E. Underwood, M. Maes, G. Gerard, M.L. Davenport, and J.M. Ketelslegers. Dietary protein restriction decreases insulin-like growth factor I independent of insulin and liver growth hormone binding. *Endocrinology* 124(5):2604-2611. 1989.

93. Maresh, C.M., T.G. Allison, B.J. Noble, A. Drash, and W.J. Kraemer. Substrate and endocrine responses to race-intensity exercise following a marathon run. *Int. J. Sports Med.* 10(2):101-106. 1989.

94. Martin, J.B. Growth hormone releasing factor. In: *Brain Peptides*, D.T. Krieger, J.J. Brownstein, and J.B. Martin, eds. New York: Wiley. 1983. pp. 976-980.

95. McCusker, R.H., C. Camacho-Hubner, and D.R. Clemmons. Identification of the types of insulin-like growth factor-binding proteins that are secreted by muscle cells in vitro. *J. Biol. Chem.* 264(14):7795-7800. 1989.

96. Michel, G., and E. Baulieu. Androgen receptor in rat skeletal muscle: Characterization and physiological variations. *Endocrinology* 107:2088-2097. 1980.

97. Okayama, T. Factors which regulate growth hormone secretion. *Med. J.* 17(1):13-19. 1972.

98. Pakarinen, A., K. Häkkinen, and P. Komi. Serum thyroid hormones thyrotropin and thyroxine binding globulin during prolonged strength training. *Eur. J. Appl. Physiol.* 57:394-398. 1988.

99. Pruett, E.D. Insulin and exercise in non-diabetic and diabetic man. In: *Exercise Endocrinology*, K. Fotherby and S.B. Pal, eds. Berlin: Walter de Gruyter. 1985. pp. 1-24.

100. Rance, N.E., and S.R. Max. Modulation of the cytosolic androgen receptor in striated muscle by sex steroids. *Endocrinology* 115(3):862-866. 1984.

101. Riss, T., J. Novakofski, and P. Bechtel. Skeletal muscle hypertrophy in rats having growth hormone-secreting tumor. *J. Appl. Physiol.* 61(5):1732-1735. 1986.

102. Rogol, A.D. Growth hormone: Physiology, therapeutic use, and potential for abuse. In: *Exercise and Sport Sciences Reviews*, K.B. Pandolf, ed. Baltimore: Williams & Wilkins. 1989. pp. 353-377.

103. Rosner, W. The functions of corticosteroid-binding globulin and sex-hormone-binding globulin: Recent advances. *Endocr. Rev.* 11:80-91. 1990.

104. Sale, D.G. Neural adaptation to resistance training. *Med. Sci. Sport Exerc.* 20:135-145. 1988.

105. Schmidt, T.J., A.S. Miller-Diener, T.M. Kirsch, and G. Litwack. Association of phosphorylation reactions with glucocorticoid receptor. In: *Receptor Phosphorylation*, V.M. Moudgil, ed. Boca Raton, FL: CRC Press. 1989. pp. 315-332.

106. Sherman, M.R., and J. Stevens. Structure of mammalian steroid receptors: Evolving concepts and methodological developments. *Annual Reviews of Physiology*, vol. 46, 83-105. 1984.

107. Skierska, E., J. Ustupska, B. Biczowa, and J. Lukaszewska. Effect of physical exercise on plasma cortisol, testosterone and growth hormone levels in weight lifters. *Endokrynol. Pol.* 2:159-165. 1976.

108. Skottner, A., M. Kanie, E. Jennische, J. Sjögren, and L. Fryklund. Tissue repair and IGF-1. *Acta Paediatr. Scand.* 347:110-112. 1988.

109. Sonntag, W.E., L.J. Forman, N. Miki, and J. Meiters. Growth hormone secretion and neuroendocrine regulation. In: *Handbook of Endocrinology*, G.H. Gass and H.M. Kaplan, eds. Boca Raton, FL: CRC Press. 1982. pp. 35-39.

110. Stone, M.H., R. Byrd, and C. Johnson. Observations on serum androgen response to short term resistive training in middle age sedentary males. *NSCA Journal* 5:40-65. 1984.

111. Stone, M., and H. O'Bryant. *Weight Training, Scientific Approach*. Minneapolis: Burgess. 1987.

112. Stowers, T., J. McMillian, D. Scala, V. Davis, D. Wilson, and M. Stone. The short-term effects of three different strength-power training methods. *NSCA Journal* 5(3):24-27. 1983.

113. Suikkari, A.-M., V.A. Koivisto, R. Koistinen, M. Seppala, and H. Yki-Jarvinen. Dose-response characteristics for suppression of low molecular weight plasma insulin-like growth factor-binding protein by insulin. *J. Clin. Endocrinol. Metab.* 68(1):135-140. 1989.

114. Suikkari, A.-M., V.A. Koivisto, R. Koistinen, M. Seppala, and H. Yki-Jarvinen. Prolonged exercise increases serum insulin-like growth factor-binding protein concentrations. *J. Clin. Endocrinol. Metab.* 68(1):141-144. 1989.

115. Sutton, J.R. Effect of acute hypoxia on the hormonal response to exercise. *J. Appl. Physiol.: Respir. Env. Exerc. Physiol.* 39:587-592. 1977.

116. Tapperman, J. *Metabolic and Endocrine Physiology*. Chicago: Year Book Medical. 1980.

117. Terjung, R. Endocrine response to exercise. In: *Exercise and Sport Sciences*, R.S. Hutton and D.I. Miller, eds. 1979. pp. 153-180.

118. Turner, J.D., P. Rotwein, J. Novakofski, and P.J. Bechtel. Induction of messenger RNA for IGF-I and -II during growth hormone–stimulated muscle hypertrophy. *Am. J. Physiol.* 255(4):E513-E517. 1988.

119. VanHelder, W.P., R.C. Goode, and M.W. Radomski. Effect of anaerobic and aerobic exercise of equal duration and work expenditure on plasma growth hormone levels. *Eur. J. Appl. Physiol.* 52:255-257. 1984.

120. VanHelder, W.P., M.W. Radomski, and R.C. Goode. Growth hormone responses during intermittent weight lifting exercise in men. *Eur. J. Appl. Physiol.* 53:31-34. 1984.

121. Vermeulen, A. Physiology of the testosterone-binding globulin in man. *The New York Academy of Sciences*. R. Frairia, H.L. Bradlow, and G. Gaidano, eds. 103-111. 1988.

122. Weiss, L.W., K.J. Cureton, and F.N. Thompson. Comparison of serum testosterone and androstenedione responses to weight lifting in men and women. *Eur. J. Appl. Physiol.* 50(3):413-419. 1983.

123. Westerlind, K.C., W.C. Byrnes, P.S. Freedson, and F.I. Katch. Exercise and serum androgens in women. *Phys. Sportsmed.* 15:87-94. 1987.

124. Wolf, M., S.H. Ingbar, and A.C. Moses. Thyroid hormone and growth hormone interact to regulate insulin-like growth factor-I messenger RNA and circulating levels in the rat. *Endocrinology* 125(6):2905-2914. 1989.

125. Yeoh, S.I., and R.C. Baxter. Metabolic regulation of the growth hormone–independent insulin-like growth factor binding protein in human plasma. *ACTA Endocrinology* 119:465-473. 1988.

126. Young, I.R., S. Mesiano, R. Hintz, D.J. Caddy, M.M. Ralph, C.A. Browne, and G.D. Thorburn. Growth hormone and testosterone can independently stimulate the growth of hypophysectomized prepubertal lambs without any alteration in circulating concentrations of insulin-like growth factors. *J. Endocrinol.* 121(3):563-570. 1989.

127. Zorzano, A., D.E. James, N.B. Ruderman, and P.F. Pilch. Insulin-like growth factor I binding and receptor kinase red and white muscle. *Fed. Eur. Biochem. Soc.* 234(2):257-262. 1988.

CARDIOVASCULAR AND RESPIRATORY ANATOMY AND PHYSIOLOGY: RESPONSES TO EXERCISE

Mark A. Williams

This chapter summarizes cardiovascular and respiratory anatomy and physiology, both in conditions of rest and in response to exercise, so that appropriate and effective exercise programs can be designed.

CARDIOVASCULAR ANATOMY AND PHYSIOLOGY

A clear understanding of basic cardiovascular anatomy and physiology is critical for providing an appropriate strength and conditioning program. The function of the cardiovascular system is to provide and maintain an optimal environment for cellular function (2).

The Heart

The heart, a muscular organ (Figure 7.1), is actually two interconnected but separate pumps; the right side of the heart pumps blood through the lungs and the left side pumps blood through the rest of the body. Each pump has two chambers: an **atrium** and a **ventricle**. The right and left atria function principally as blood reservoirs, but also pump blood into the right and left ventricles. The right and left ventricles, respectively, supply the main force that propels the blood through the pulmonary and peripheral circulations (2, 3).

Valves. The **tricuspid valve** and **mitral valve** (collectively called **atrioventricular [AV] valves**) prevent the flow of blood from the ventricles back into the atria during ventricular contraction (**systole**). The **aortic valve** and **pulmonary valve (semilunar valves)**, prevent backflow from the aorta and pulmonary arteries into the ventricles during ventricular relaxation (**diastole**). Each valve opens and closes passively; that is, each closes when a backward pressure gradient pushes blood back into them, and they open when a forward pressure gradient forces blood in the forward direction. The thin AV valves require almost no backflow for closure, whereas the much thicker semilunar valves require stronger backflow (2, 3).

Conduction System. A specialized electrical conduction system (Figure 7.2) controls the mechanical contraction of the heart. The conduction system comprises

- the **sinoatrial (SA) node**, in which rhythmic electrical impulses are initiated;

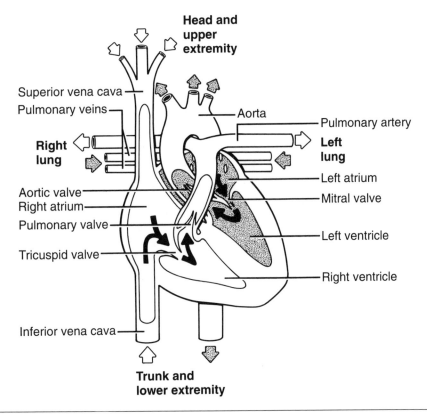

Figure 7.1   Structure of the human heart and course of blood flow through its chambers.

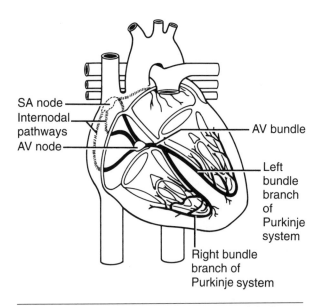

Figure 7.2   The electrical conduction system of the heart.

- the internodal pathways, which conduct the impulse from the SA node to the **atrioventricular (AV) node**;
- the AV node, in which the impulse is delayed before passing into the ventricles;

- the **atrioventricular (AV) bundle**, which conducts the impulse to the ventricles; and
- the left and right bundle branches of the **Purkinje fibers**, which conduct the impulse to all parts of the ventricle.

The SA node is a small strip of specialized muscle tissue located in the upper lateral wall of the right atrium. The fibers of the node are continuous with the muscle fibers of the atrium, with the result that each action potential (electrical impulse) that begins in the SA node normally spreads immediately into the atria. The conductive system is organized so that the cardiac impulse will not travel into the ventricles too rapidly; this allows time for the atria to empty their blood into the ventricles before ventricular contraction begins (Figure 7.3). It is primarily the AV node and its associated conductive fibers that delay each action potential from entering into the ventricles. The AV node is located in the posterior septal wall of the right atrium (2, 3).

The Purkinje fibers lead from the AV node through the AV bundle into the ventricles. Except for their initial portion, where they penetrate the AV barrier, the Purkinje fibers have functional characteristics quite the opposite of those of the AV nodal fibers; they are very large, even larger than the normal ventricular muscle fibers, and they transmit impulses at a much higher

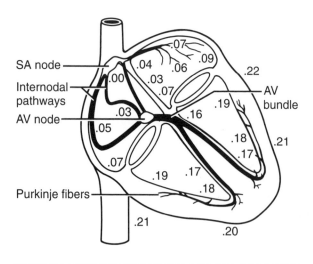

Figure 7.3 Transmission of the cardiac impulse through the heart, showing the time of appearance (in fractions of a second) of the impulse in different parts of the heart.

velocity than the AV nodal fibers. This allows almost immediate transmission of the cardiac impulse throughout the entire ventricular system.

Although the cardiac impulse normally arises in the SA node, this may not always be the case. Other parts of the heart, particularly the AV node and the Purkinje fibers, may generate electrical impulses in the same way the SA nodal fibers do. The SA node normally controls heart rhythmicity, however, because its discharge rate is considerably greater (70-80 times/min) than that of either the AV (40-60 times/min) or the Purkinje fibers (15-40 times/min). Each time the SA node discharges, its impulse is conducted into the AV node and the Purkinje fibers, discharging their excitable membranes. Thus, these potentially self-excitatory tissues are discharged before self-excitation can actually occur. Exceptions occur when some other part of the heart develops a rhythmic discharge rate that is more rapid than that of the SA node. Under these conditions, atrial or ventricular muscle can develop excessive excitability and become the pacemaker for a single discharge or more frequent discharges. A pacemaker elsewhere than the SA node is called an ectopic pacemaker and causes an abnormal sequence of contraction of the different parts of the heart (2, 6)

Although, as just mentioned, the normal discharge rate of the SA node ranges from 70 to 80 times/min, exercise training may result in a significantly slower discharge rate. It appears that physical training creates an imbalance between the activity of the sympathetic accelerator and parasympathetic depressor neurons in favor of parasympathetic dominance. Increased stroke volume (the amount of blood ejected per contraction) at rest resulting from chronic exercise may also impact

resting heart rate. These adaptations may account for the significant bradycardia (slower heart rate) observed in highly conditioned endurance athletes, with heart rates ranging from 40 to 60 beats/min not infrequent (1, 2, 7).

Electrocardiogram. The electrical activity of the heart just discussed can be recorded at the surface of the body; a graphic representation of this activity is called an **electrocardiogram (ECG)**. A normal electrocardiogram, seen in Figure 7.4, is composed of a *P wave*, a *QRS complex*, and a *T wave*. The QRS complex is often three separate waves; a Q wave, an R wave, and an S wave. The P wave is caused by the electrical potentials that depolarize the atria and result in atrial contraction. **Depolarization** is the reversal of the membrane potential, whereby the normally negative potential inside the membrane becomes slightly positive and the outside becomes slightly negative. The QRS complex is caused by the electrical potentials that depolarize the ventricles and result in ventricular contraction. The T wave is caused by electrical potentials generated as the ventricles recover from the state of depolarization; this process, called **repolarization**, occurs in ventricular muscle shortly after depolarization. Although atrial repolarization occurs as well, its wave formation usually occurs during the time of ventricular depolarization and is thus masked by the QRS complex (2, 3).

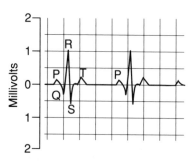

Figure 7.4 Normal electrocardiogram.

Blood Vessels

The central and peripheral circulation is a single closed-circuit system with two components: an arterial system, which carries blood away from the heart, and a venous system, which carries blood toward the heart (Figure 7.5). The blood vessels of each system are identified here (2).

Arteries. The function of **arteries** is to transport blood pumped from the heart under high pressure to tissues. For this reason, arteries have strong muscular walls. Blood flows relatively rapidly in the arteries. **Arterioles** are small branches of arteries that act as

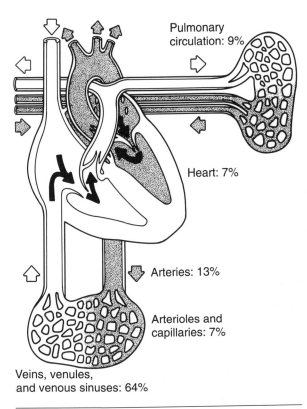

Pulmonary circulation: 9%

Heart: 7%

Arteries: 13%

Arterioles and capillaries: 7%

Veins, venules, and venous sinuses: 64%

Figure 7.5 The arterial (*right*) and venous components of the circulatory system. The percent values indicate the distribution of blood volume throughout the circulatory system at rest.

control valves through which blood enters the capillaries. Arterioles have strong muscular walls that are capable of closing the arteriole completely or allowing it to be dilated severalfold, thus vastly altering blood flow to the capillaries in response to the needs of the tissues. **Metarterioles** are vessels that serve either as conduits giving rise to capillaries and supplying the capillary bed or as thoroughfare channels bypassing the capillary bed, emptying into the venules (2).

Capillaries. The function of **capillaries** is to exchange oxygen, fluid, nutrients, electrolytes, hormones, and other substances between the blood and the interstitial fluid in the various tissues of the body. The capillary walls are very thin and are permeable to small molecular substances (2).

Veins. **Venules** collect blood from the capillaries, gradually coalescing into progressively larger **veins**, which function as conduits for transporting blood from tissues back to the heart. Because the pressure in the venous system is very low, venous walls are thin, although muscular. This allows them to contract or expand and thereby act as a reservoir for extra blood, either a

small or large amount, depending on the needs of the body (2).

Blood

The major function of blood is the transport of oxygen from the lungs to the tissues and carbon dioxide from the tissues to the lungs. The transport of oxygen is accomplished by **hemoglobin**, the iron-protein molecule carried by the red blood cells. Red blood cells, the major component of blood, have other functions as well. For instance, they contain a large quantity of carbonic anhydrase, which catalyzes the reaction between carbon dioxide and water to facilitate carbon dioxide removal. Hemoglobin also has an additional important role as an acid-base buffer and is responsible for most of the **buffering power** of whole blood (2, 5, 10).

RESPIRATORY ANATOMY AND PHYSIOLOGY

As air passes through the nose, the nasal cavities perform three distinct functions: warming, humidifying, and filtering the air (2, 9).

Air is distributed to the lungs by way of the trachea, bronchi, and bronchioles (Figure 7.6). The **trachea** is called the first-generation respiratory passage, and the right and left main **bronchi** are the second-generation passages; each division thereafter is an additional generation (**bronchioles**). There are between 20 and 25 generations before the air finally reaches the **alveoli** where gases are exchanged in respiration.

Exchange of Air

The amount and movement of air and expired gases in and out of the lungs is accomplished by expansion and contraction of the lungs. The lungs are expanded and contracted in two ways: (1) by downward and upward movement of the diaphragm to lengthen and shorten the chest cavity and (2) by elevation and depression of the ribs to increase and decrease the anteroposterior diameter of the chest cavity (Figure 7.7). Normal, quiet breathing is accomplished almost entirely by movement of the diaphragm. During inspiration, contraction of the diaphragm creates a negative pressure (vacuum) in the chest cavity and air is drawn into the lungs. During expiration the diaphragm simply relaxes; the elastic recoil of the lungs, chest wall, and the abdominal structures compress the lungs and air is expelled. During heavy breathing, the elastic forces are not powerful enough to cause necessary rapid expiration. The extra required force is achieved mainly by contraction of the abdominal muscles, which push the abdomen upward against the bottom of the diaphragm (2, 9).

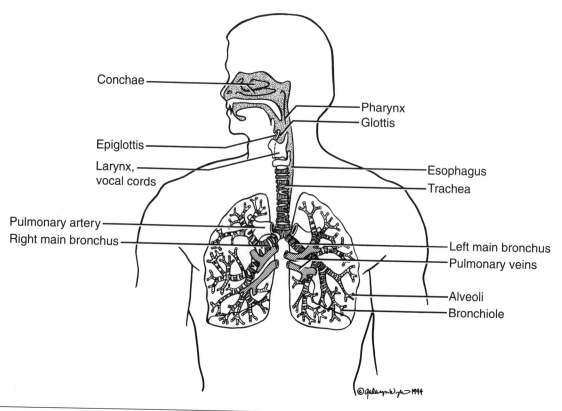

Figure 7.6 Gross anatomy of the human respiratory system.

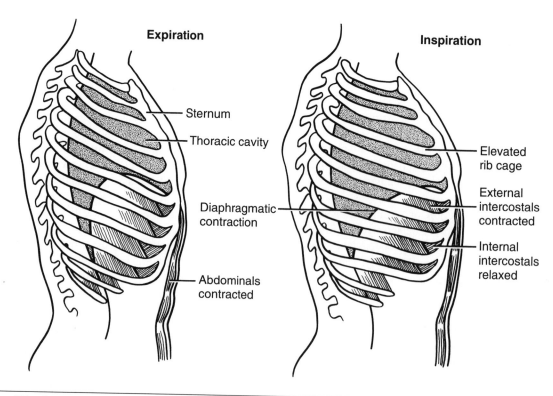

Figure 7.7 Contraction and expansion of the thoracic cage during expiration and inspiration, illustrating diaphragmatic contraction, elevation of the rib cage, and function of the intercostals. The vertical and anteroposterior diameters increase during inspiration.

The second method for expanding the lungs is to raise the rib cage. The chest cavity is small, and in the natural resting position the ribs are slanted downward. Elevating the rib cage allows the ribs to project almost directly forward so that the sternum (breastbone) moves forward, away from the spine, causing the anteroposterior diameter of the chest to be 20% greater during maximum inspiration than during expiration. The muscles that elevate the rib cage are called muscles of inspiration, and the muscles that depress the chest, muscles of expiration.

Pleural pressure is the pressure in the narrow space between the lung pleura and the chest wall **pleura** (membranes enveloping the lungs and lining the chest walls). This pressure is normally slightly negative. Because the lung is an elastic structure, during normal inspiration the expansion of the chest cage is able to pull on the surface of the lungs and creates a more negative pressure, thus enhancing its inspiration. During expiration, the events are essentially reversed.

Alveolar pressure is the pressure inside the lung alveoli when the glottis is open and no air is flowing into or out of the lungs. The pressure in all parts of the respiratory tree all the way to the alveoli is equal to the atmospheric pressure. To cause inward flow of air during inspiration, the pressure in the alveoli must fall to a value slightly below atmospheric pressure. During expiration, alveolar pressure must rise above atmospheric pressure.

During normal, quiet respiration, only 3% to 5% of the total energy expended by the body is required to energize the pulmonary ventilatory process. But during very heavy exercise the amount of energy required can increase to as much as 8% of total body energy expenditure, especially if the person has any degree of increased airway resistance or decreased pulmonary compliance (1, 2, 7, 9).

Exchange of Respiratory Gases

After the alveoli are ventilated with fresh air, the next step in the respiratory process is the diffusion of oxygen from the alveoli into the pulmonary blood and the diffusion of carbon dioxide in the opposite direction. The process of diffusion is a simple random molecular motion of molecules moving in both directions through the capillary wall and alveolar wall. The energy for diffusion is provided by the kinetic motion of the molecules themselves. The rates of diffusion of the two gases are dependent upon their concentrations in the capillaries and alveoli. Net diffusion of the gas will occur from the region of high concentration to the region of low concentration (2, 9).

Control of Respiration

The nervous system adjusts the rate of alveolar ventilation by adjusting the rate and depth of breathing in order to meet the demands of the body. Thus, arterial blood oxygen concentration and carbon dioxide concentration are hardly altered even during strenuous exercise (1, 2, 5, 7, 9, 10).

Respiratory Center. A **respiratory center** composed of several widely dispersed groups of neurons is located bilaterally in the lower portion of the brain stem (the pons and medulla oblongata). It is divided into three major collections of neurons (2, 9) (Figure 7.8):

- The *dorsal respiratory group* plays the fundamental role in the control of respiration. The primary function of the dorsal respiratory group is to cause inspiration; it is also the primary generator of the rhythm of respiration.

- The *ventral respiratory group* of neurons has several important functions. First, respiratory signals from the ventral respiratory group contribute to the respiratory drive for increased pulmonary ventilation, when increased ventilation becomes necessary. Second, stimulation of some of the neurons in the ventral group causes inspiration or expiration depending upon where the stimulus is located. These neurons are especially important in providing the expiratory signals to the powerful abdominal muscles during expiration. Thus, the ventral respiratory group of neurons operates primarily as an overdrive mechanism when high levels of pulmonary ventilation are required.

- The *pneumotaxic center* controls both the rate and pattern of breathing. The primary effect of the center is control of the duration of the filling cycle of the lungs, which tends to limit the volume of inspiration. Secondarily, this increases the rate of breathing because limitation of inspiration shortens expiration and the entire period of respiration.

The ultimate goal of respiration is to maintain the proper concentrations of oxygen, carbon dioxide, and hydrogen ions in the tissues. Excess carbon dioxide or hydrogen ions can cause greatly increased strength of both the inspiratory and expiratory signals to the respiratory muscles. Oxygen, in contrast, does not have a significant direct effect on the respiratory center of the brain, but acts almost entirely on peripheral chemoreceptors (discussed in the next section). It appears that none of the three areas of the respiratory center are affected directly by changes in blood carbon dioxide or hydrogen ion concentrations. Instead, direct chemical control of respiratory center activity is regulated by an additional neuronal area, the chemosensitive area. Located beneath the ventral surface of the medulla, this area is highly sensitive to changes in both blood carbon dioxide and hydrogen ion concentration and in turn excites the other portions of the respiratory center (2, 5, 9, 10).

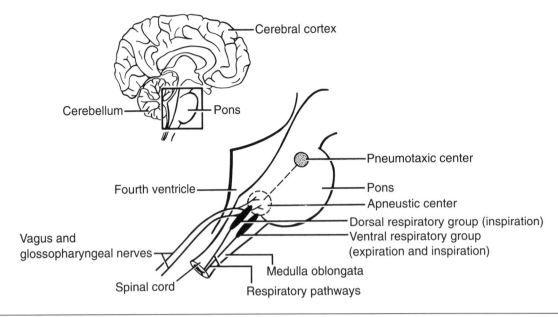

Figure 7.8 The brain's respiratory center.

The chemosensitive area is especially stimulated by hydrogen ions. However, hydrogen ions do not easily cross either the blood-brain barrier or the blood–cerebrospinal fluid barrier. For this reason, changes in hydrogen ion concentration in the blood actually have considerably less effect in stimulating the chemosensitive area than do changes in carbon dioxide, even though carbon dioxide stimulates these neurons only indirectly. However, carbon dioxide and water in tissues form carbonic acid. This in turn dissociates into hydrogen and bicarbonate ions; the hydrogen ions then have a potent direct stimulatory effect (2, 9).

Peripheral Chemoreceptor System. Another accessory mechanism called the **peripheral chemoreceptor system** is also available for controlling respiration (Figure 7.9). Peripheral chemoreceptors are located in several areas outside the brain and are especially important for detecting changes in oxygen concentration in the blood, although they also respond to changes in carbon dioxide and hydrogen ion concentrations. By far the largest number of these chemoreceptors are located in the *carotid bodies*, although a sizable number also exist in the *aortic bodies*. Each of these chemoreceptor-containing bodies receives a special blood supply through a tiny artery directly from the adjacent arterial trunk. Since the flow of blood through the bodies is great—20 times the weight of the bodies themselves each minute—the oxygen concentration in the bodies themselves is approximately equal to that in the arteries. When the oxygen concentration in the arterial blood falls below normal, the chemoreceptors are strongly stimulated and send nervous signals to the respiratory center, which stimulates increased respiration (2, 9).

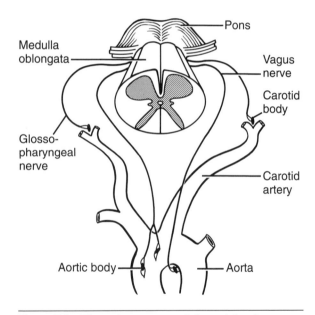

Figure 7.9 The main structures of the peripheral chemoreceptor system.

CARDIOVASCULAR AND RESPIRATORY RESPONSES TO ACUTE EXERCISE

The effects of exercise on cardiovascular and respiratory functions, both acutely and chronically, significantly impact the anatomical and physiological parameters previously described. A basic knowledge of these responses is essential. Beginning with acute responses and followed by the effects of training, these responses are discussed here.

Cardiovascular Responses

The primary function of the cardiovascular system during exercise is to deliver oxygen and other nutrients to the muscles. This section describes systematic mechanisms of these acute responses.

Cardiac Output. The amount of blood pumped by the heart, the **cardiac output**, is determined by the quantity of blood ejected with each contraction (the **stroke volume**), and by the heart's rate of pumping (**heart rate**):

$$\dot{Q} = \text{Stroke volume} \times \text{Heart rate}, \qquad (7.1)$$

where $\dot{Q}$ is the cardiac output. Heart rate is ordinarily measured in beats (contractions) per minute, so cardiac output is usually expressed in units of volume per minute (1-3, 7).

In progressing from rest to steady-state exercise, cardiac output undergoes an initial rapid increase followed by a gradual rise until a plateau is reached. During strenuous exercise, cardiac output increases by about 4 times the resting level of about 5 L/min to an average maximum of 20 to 22 L/min. Stroke volume begins to increase at the onset of exercise and continues to rise until the individual's oxygen consumption is at approximately 50% to 60% of maximal oxygen uptake. At this point, the increase in stroke volume begins to plateau. College-age males have maximal stroke volumes averaging between 100 and 115 ml of blood per min; maximal stroke volumes for college-age females are approximately 25% less, owing to smaller average body size. Heart rate, in contrast, rises in a linear fashion with increasing work load to a maximal per-minute rate equal to approximately 220 less the person's age.

Stroke Volume. Essentially, two physiological mechanisms regulate stroke volume. The first is intrinsic to the myocardium, the muscle tissue of the heart. Primarily as a consequence of increased venous return with exercise, the **end-diastolic volume**—the volume of blood in the left ventricle at the end of the filling phase, or diastole—is significantly increased. The myocardial fibers are thus stretched more than they are when the person is at rest, which results in a more forceful contraction, that is, an increase in force of systolic ejection and greater cardiac emptying. This phenomenon has been termed **Starling's law of the heart**, which, in formal terms, states that the force of contraction is a function of the length of the fibers of the muscle wall. Greater cardiac emptying is characterized by an increase in the **ejection fraction**, the fraction of blood ejected from the end-diastolic volume (1-3, 7).

The second means by which the stroke volume is regulated, in this case increased, is through the action of the sympathetic hormones epinephrine and norepinephrine, which produce augmented ventricular contraction and greater systolic emptying of the heart. There is an increase in sympathetic stimulation with the onset of exercise.

Heart Rate. The inherent rhythmicity and conductivity of the myocardium is influenced by the cardiovascular center of the medulla, which transmits signals to the heart through the sympathetic and parasympathetic components of the autonomic nervous system. The atria are supplied with a large number of both sympathetic and parasympathetic neurons, whereas the ventricles receive sympathetic fibers almost exclusively. Stimulation of the sympathetic cardioaccelerator nerves accelerates depolarization of the SA node, which causes the heart to beat faster. Acetylcholine, a hormone of the parasympathetic nervous system, is released from the vagal nerve endings, retarding the rate of SA node discharge and slowing the heart rate. Vagal stimulation has essentially no effect on myocardial contractility (1-4, 7).

The resting heart rate normally ranges from 60 to 100 beats/min, with fewer than 60 beats/min being described as **bradycardia** and more than 100 beats/min as **tachycardia**. Maximal exercise heart rate was already described. Submaximal heart rate, that is, those rates between resting and maximal levels, relates to a variety of basic metabolic characteristics of the human system as well as to the level of physiological stress. Submaximal heart rate is much less predictable between individuals than resting heart rate and is affected by exercise training.

Oxygen Uptake. The oxygen demand of working muscles is directly related to their mass and metabolic efficiency. Therefore, exercise involving a larger mass of muscle is likely to be associated with a higher total oxygen uptake. **Maximal oxygen uptake** is described as the greatest amount of oxygen that can be utilized at the cellular level for the entire body. It has been found to correlate well with the degree of physical conditioning and has been accepted as an index of total body fitness. The capacity to utilize oxygen is related not only to the lungs' effectiveness, but also to the ability of the heart and circulatory system to transport the oxygen and to the body tissues' ability to utilize it. The maximal oxygen uptake increases and decreases with the degree of physical conditioning. Resting oxygen uptake is estimated at 3.5 ml O_2 per kg of body weight per min (ml $\cdot$ kg^{-1} $\cdot$ min^{-1}); this value is defined as 1 **metabolic equivalent**, or 1 **MET**. Maximal oxygen uptake values may range from 40 to 80 ml $\cdot$ kg^{-1} $\cdot$ min^{-1}, or 11.4 to 22.9 METs, in normal, healthy individuals and depend upon a variety of physiological parameters as well as conditioning level (1, 2, 7).

The oxygen uptake $\dot{V}O_2$ may be calculated as follows:

$$\dot{V}O_2 = \dot{Q} \times \text{a-v}O_2 \text{ difference,} \qquad (7.2)$$

where $\dot{Q}$ is the cardiac output in milliliters per minute and a-vO_2 difference is the arteriovenous oxygen difference (the difference in the oxygen content of arterial and venous blood) in milliliters of oxygen per 100 ml of blood. For example,

$$
\begin{aligned}
\dot{V}O_2 &= (72 \text{ beats/min} \times 65 \text{ ml blood/beat}) \\
&\quad \times 6 \text{ ml } O_2/100 \text{ ml blood} \\
&= 281 \text{ ml } O_2/\text{min.}
\end{aligned}
$$

To get the usual units for oxygen uptake (i.e., ml · kg^{-1} · min^{-1}), we would divide this result by the person's weight in kilograms.

We can manipulate Equation 7.2 to get the following equation (the **Fick equation**) for cardiac output:

$$\dot{Q} = \frac{\dot{V}O_2}{\text{a-v}O_2 \text{ difference}} \cdot \qquad (7.3)$$

For example,

$$
\begin{aligned}
\dot{Q} &= \frac{281 \text{ ml } O_2/\text{min}}{6 \text{ ml } O_2/100 \text{ ml blood}} \\
&= 4{,}680 \text{ ml blood/min} \\
&= 4.68 \text{ L blood/min.}
\end{aligned}
$$

This equation is helpful in understanding the relationship of each parameter to the other and in developing a clearer picture of how exercise may affect each.

Direct measurement of cardiac output is usually limited to animal research because of the difficulty of assessing stroke volume directly, especially with exercise, and thus has little application for use in humans. The indirect Fick method, indicator dilution, and carbon dioxide rebreathing methods for determining cardiac output are commonly used in human measurements. However, cardiac output can be easily computed if the oxygen consumption during a minute has been determined and the arteriovenous oxygen difference is known. Various techniques for measuring cardiac output, oxygen consumption, and the arteriovenous oxygen difference are available in a number of university and hospital exercise laboratories.

Blood Pressure. Systolic blood pressure is used to estimate the strain against the arterial walls during ventricular contraction and, when combined with heart rate, can be used to describe the work of the heart. This estimate of the work of the heart is obtained by multiplying the heart rate and systolic blood pressure and is referred to as the **rate-pressure product**, or double product. Diastolic blood pressure, conversely, provides an indication of peripheral resistance, or the ease with which blood flows from the arterioles into the capillaries. Because the heart pumps blood directly into the aorta, the pressure in the aorta is obviously high, averaging approximately 100 mm Hg (Figure 7.10). Also, because pumping by the heart is pulsatile, arterial pressure fluctuates between a systolic level of 120 mm Hg and a diastolic level of 80 mm Hg (approximate values). As the blood flows through the systemic circulation, its pressure falls progressively to approximately 0 mm Hg by the time it reaches the termination of the vena cava in the right atrium (venous pressure) (2, 3, 8).

The **mean arterial pressure** is the average blood pressure throughout the cardiac cycle. However, it is not the average of systolic and diastolic pressures; rather,

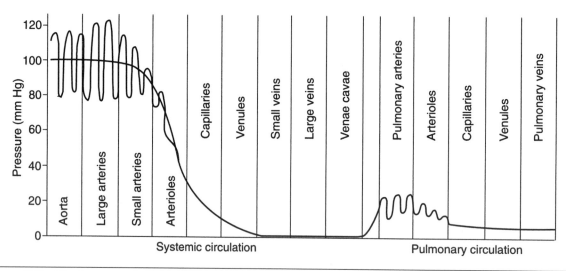

Figure 7.10 Blood pressures in the different portions of the circulatory system.
Reprinted from Guyton (1991).

because the arterial pressure usually remains nearer the diastolic level than the systolic level during a greater portion of the cardiac cycle, the mean arterial pressure is usually slightly less than the average systolic and diastolic pressures. It can be calculated by adding one-third of the difference between systolic and diastolic pressure to the diastolic pressure.

Normal resting blood pressure generally ranges from 110 to 140 mm Hg systolic and 60 to 90 mm Hg diastolic. With exercise, systolic pressure can normally rise up to as much as 220 mm Hg (with heavy exercise in some people), while diastolic pressure will remain at the resting level or decrease slightly (1, 2, 7-9).

Control of Local Circulation.

In the body, blood flow is a function of resistance: as resistance is reduced, blood flow is increased, and as resistance is increased, blood flow is reduced. Resistance is caused by friction between the blood and the internal vascular wall. This resistance is determined by three factors:

- the viscosity of the blood,
- the length of the vessel, and
- the diameter of the vessel (2, 8).

The resistance of the entire systemic circulation is called the **total peripheral resistance**. As blood vessels throughout the body become constricted, total peripheral resistance increases; with dilation, peripheral resistance decreases. A long-term decrease in total peripheral resistance causes a reciprocal increase in cardiac output, whereas a long-term increase in total peripheral resistance causes a corresponding decrease in cardiac output.

In the body, the **viscosity** of the blood (resistance to flow, which is primarily the result of the frictional drag of suspended red blood cells) and the length of the vessel remain relatively constant under most circumstances. The most important factor affecting blood flow is the diameter of the vessel; thus, constriction and dilation of blood vessels (called *vasoconstriction* and *vasodilation*) are the primary mechanisms for regulating regional blood flow.

During exercise, blood flow to active muscles is considerably increased by the dilation of local arterioles, and, at the same time, blood flow to other organ systems is reduced by constriction of the arterioles. For example, renal blood flow at rest is normally about 1,100 ml/min, or approximately 20% of cardiac output. During maximal exercise, however, renal blood flow may be reduced to only 250 ml/min, or about 1% of cardiac output, as blood flow is diverted to the skeletal musculature (1, 7, 8).

Local factors and autonomic nervous control are the two major means for regulating oxygen supply to the tissue with local autoregulatory mechanisms being the primary initial mechanism. Local factors directly influence the smooth muscle bands of the small arterioles to cause vasodilation. A decrease in oxygen supply to skeletal and cardiac muscle produces a potent local stimulus for vasodilation. The response is almost instantaneous and precisely related to the metabolic needs of the tissue. Local increases in temperature, carbon dioxide concentration, acidity, adenosine level, and the levels of magnesium and potassium ions also enhance regional blood flow (2, 8).

Superimposed on vasoregulation caused by local factors is a central vascular control mediated by the autonomic nervous system. Norepinephrine acts as a general vasoconstrictor and is released at certain sympathetic nerve endings. These sympathetic constrictor fibers are called **adrenergic fibers**. Other sympathetic neurons, especially those in skeletal and heart muscle, release acetylcholine; these are the **cholinergic fibers** and their action causes vasodilation. The constrictor nerves are constantly active so that blood vessels are always in a state of constriction. The degree of this constrictor activity is referred to as **vasomotor tone**. Dilation of blood vessels under the influence of adrenergic neurons is due more to a reduction in vasomotor tone than to an increase in the action of either sympathetic (or parasympathetic) dilator nerve fibers. In any case, whatever sympathetic-activated vasoconstriction is present in active tissue is rapidly overridden by the powerful vasodilation induced by metabolism (2, 3, 8).

Some sympathetic nerves terminate in the adrenal medullas. In response to sympathetic activation, these glands secrete large quantities of epinephrine and a smaller amount of norepinephrine into the blood. These hormones bring about a generalized constrictor response, except in the blood vessels of the heart and skeletal muscles. During exercise, this generalized hormonal control of blood flow to specific organs is relatively minor in comparison to the local, rapid, and powerful sympathetic neural drive (1-3, 5, 7, 8, 10).

At the onset of exercise and even before exercise begins, cardiovascular changes are initiated from the nerve centers above the brain's medullary region. These adjustments provide for a significant increase in the rate and pumping action of the heart, as well as predictable alterations in regional blood flow that are proportional to exercise severity. As exercise continues, sympathetic cholinergic outflow and local metabolic factors, which act on chemosensitive nerves and directly on the blood vessels themselves, cause dilation of resistance vessels in active muscles. This reduced resistance permits increased blood flow. As exercise continues, there are also constrictor adjustments in less active tissues; thus, an adequate perfusion pressure can be maintained even with the dilation of the vessels supplying large masses of musculature. This provides appropriate redistribution of blood to meet the metabolic requirements of working muscles (1, 7).

At rest, the systemic veins contain over 50% of all the blood in the circulatory system. For this reason, they are frequently referred to as a blood reservoir for the circulation. Thus, factors affecting venous return are as important as those regulating arterial blood flow. The massaging effect of contracting and relaxing exercising muscles on the veins, as well as the stiffening of the veins themselves, immediately increases the return of blood to the right ventricle. Venous tone increases in both working and nonworking muscles. These adjustments result in maintenance of balance between cardiac output and venous return. Factors affecting blood flow in the venous system are especially important in upright exercise in which the force of gravity tends to counter venous pressures in the extremities (1, 2, 7, 8).

Internal Influences of Cardiorespiratory Responses.

At rest, there are multiple autonomic mechanisms for maintaining appropriate arterial pressure. Almost all these are negative feedback reflex mechanisms. The best known mechanism for arterial pressure control is the baroreceptor reflex. This reflex is initiated by stretch receptors, called baroreceptors or pressoreceptors, located in the walls of the large systemic arteries. A rise in blood pressure stretches the baroreceptors and causes them to transmit signals to the central nervous system. Signals are then sent through the autonomic nervous system to the circulatory system to reduce arterial pressure back toward normal. This is accomplished by two means: (1) vasodilation of the veins and the arterioles throughout the peripheral circulatory system and (2) decreased heart rate and force of heart contraction. Hence, the excitation of the baroreceptors by increasing pressure in the arteries reflexly causes the arterial pressure to decrease because of both a decrease in peripheral resistance and a decrease in cardiac output. Conversely, low pressure has opposite effects, reflexly causing the pressure to rise back toward normal (2, 8).

During exercise, muscles require greatly increased blood flow. Part of this increase results from local vasodilation of the muscle vasculature caused by increased metabolism of the muscle cells. However, additional increases result from simultaneous elevation of arterial pressure. One of the most important functions of nervous control with respect to circulation is its capability to cause very rapid increases in arterial pressure, thus playing a significant role in the perfusion of blood to the working muscles. To accomplish this, the vasoconstrictor and cardioaccelerator portions of the sympathetic nervous system are stimulated as a unit. At the same time, there is inhibition of the normal parasympathetic vagal inhibitory signals to the heart. In consequence, three major changes occur simultaneously, each of which helps to increase the arterial pressure:

- Almost all the arterioles of the body constrict. This greatly enhances the total peripheral resistance, impeding the runoff of blood from the arteries and thereby increasing the arterial pressure.
- The veins are strongly constricted. This displaces blood from the peripheral circulation toward the heart, thus increasing the volume of blood in the heart chambers. This in turn causes the heart to beat with increased force (Starling's law) and therefore to pump increased quantities of blood, raising the arterial pressure.
- Finally, the heart itself is directly stimulated by the autonomic nervous system, which also enhances cardiac output. This obviously contributes to a rise in arterial pressure (1, 2, 7, 8).

An especially important characteristic of the nervous control of arteriole pressure is its rapidity of response, which often begins even before exercise does. Within seconds, arteriole pressure can increase up to twice the normal levels. This increase in pressure plays a significant role in supplying blood to muscles at the onset of exercise.

Respiratory Responses

Physical activity affects oxygen consumption and carbon dioxide production more than any other form of physiological stress. With exercise, large amounts of oxygen diffuse from the capillaries into interstitial fluid and the tissue itself, considerable quantities of carbon dioxide move from the blood into the alveoli, and ventilation increases to maintain the proper alveolar gas concentrations to allow for the increased exchange of oxygen and carbon dioxide (1, 7).

During exercise, significant increases in the **minute ventilation**—the volume of air breathed in 1 min—occur, resulting from increases in the depth of breathing, its rate, or both. During strenuous exercise, the breathing rate of healthy young adults usually increases to 35 to 45 breaths/min, while **tidal volumes** (the amount of air inhaled and exhaled with each breath) of 2 to 2.5 L or greater are common. Consequently, the minute ventilation can easily reach 100 L, or about 17 times the resting value.

During light and moderate steady-state exercise, ventilation (volume of air breathed) increases linearly with oxygen consumption and carbon dioxide production and averages between 20 and 25 L of air per L of oxygen consumed; this is true for exercise levels up to about 55% of maximal oxygen uptake. The ratio of minute ventilation to oxygen consumption is termed the **ventilatory equivalent**. Under these conditions, ventilation is increased primarily by raising the tidal volume. At higher exercise levels breathing frequency takes on a more important role. In more intense submaximal exercise, the minute ventilation takes a sharp upswing and increases disproportionately with increases in oxygen consumption. As a result, the ventilatory equivalent is greater than during steady-state exercise and may increase to 35 or 40 L of air per L of oxygen consumed.

A portion of the air in each breath does not enter the alveoli and is thus not involved in gaseous exchange with the blood. This air, which fills the nose, mouth, trachea, and other nondiffusible conducting portions of the respiratory tract, is contained within the **anatomical dead space**. In healthy subjects this volume averages 150 to 200 ml, or about 30% of the resting tidal volume. Anatomical dead space increases with tidal volume and may actually double during deep breathing owing to some stretching of the respiratory passages with fuller inspiration (Figure 7.11). This increase in dead space, however, is still proportionately less than the increase in tidal volume. Consequently, deeper breathing provides far more effective alveolar ventilation than does similar minute ventilation achieved only through an increase in breathing rate (2, 9).

A portion of the alveoli may not function adequately in gas exchange due to either underperfusion of blood or inadequate ventilation relative to the size of the alveoli. The portion of the alveolar volume with a poor ventilation-perfusion ratio is termed the **physiological dead space**. Physiological dead space in the healthy lung is small and can be considered negligible. In the normal person, the anatomical and physiological dead spaces are nearly equal because all alveoli are functional. However, in persons with partially functional or nonfunctional alveoli, the physiological dead space is sometimes as much as 10 times the anatomical dead space, or as much as 1 to 2 L.

During exercise, alveolar ventilation is maintained through an increase in both the rate and depth of breathing. In moderate exercise, well-trained athletes can adequately achieve alveolar ventilation by increasing tidal volume with increased depth of breathing and only a small increase in breathing rate. Due to this deeper breathing, alveolar ventilation may increase from 70% of the minute ventilation at rest to over 85% of the total exercise ventilation. With more intense exercise, increases in tidal volume begin to plateau, and minute ventilation is further enhanced through an increase in breathing frequency (1, 7).

Gas Responses. At rest, the pressure of oxygen molecules in the alveoli is about 60 mm Hg greater than in the venous blood entering the pulmonary capillaries. Consequently, oxygen diffuses through the alveolar membrane into the blood. Carbon dioxide diffuses in the opposite direction under a slightly greater pressure difference. The process of gas exchange is so rapid in healthy lungs that an equilibrium between blood and alveolar gas occurs in less than 1 s (2, 9).

In the tissues, where oxygen is consumed as part of the metabolic process and an almost equal amount of carbon dioxide is produced, gas pressures can differ considerably from those in arterial blood (Figure 7.12). At rest, the average oxygen pressure in the fluid immediately outside a muscle cell rapidly drops below 40 mm Hg, and the cellular carbon dioxide pressure averages

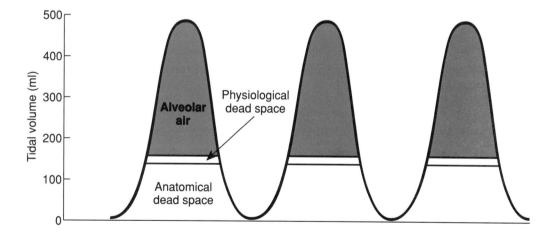

Figure 7.11 Distribution of tidal volume in healthy subject at rest. The tidal volume comprises about 350 ml of ambient air that mixes with alveolar air, about 150 ml of air in the larger passages (anatomical dead space), and a small portion of air distributed to either poorly ventilated or perfuse alveoli (physiological dead space).
Reprinted from McArdle, Katch, and Katch (1986).

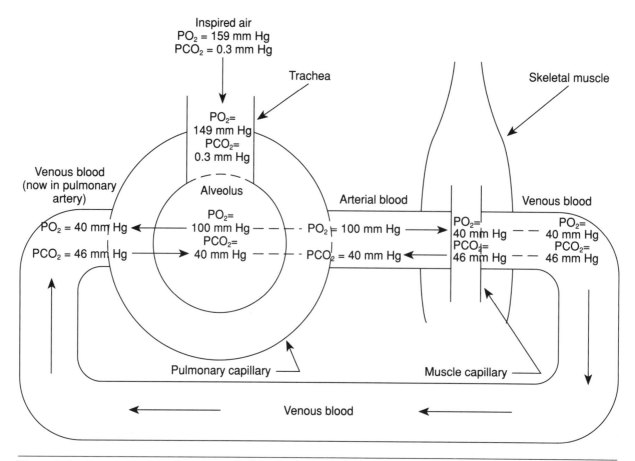

Figure 7.12 Pressure gradients for gas transfer in the body at rest. The pressures of oxygen (PO_2) and carbon dioxide (PCO_2) in ambient air, tracheal air, and alveolar air are shown, as are the gas pressures in venous and arterial blood and muscle tissue.
Reprinted from Fox, Bowers, and Foss (1993).

about 46 mm Hg. During heavy exercise, however, the oxygen pressure in muscle tissue may fall to about 3 mm Hg, whereas the pressure of carbon dioxide approaches 90 mm Hg. Because of these pressure differences, oxygen leaves the blood and diffuses toward the metabolizing cell, and carbon dioxide flows from the cell to the blood (1, 2, 7, 9).

Blood Transport of Gases and Metabolic By-Products. Oxygen is carried in blood in two ways: in solution dissolved in the plasma and combined with hemoglobin. Oxygen is not particularly soluble in fluids. In fact, only about 3 ml of oxygen can be carried per L of plasma, which means that, because the average human being has about 5 L of blood, only 15 ml of oxygen are carried in the fluid portion of the blood. Nevertheless, the small quantity of oxygen transported in the plasma does serve several important functions. The random movement of dissolved oxygen molecules establishes the oxygen pressure of blood and tissue fluids. This pressure of dissolved oxygen plays an im-

portant role in the regulation of breathing and also permits the diffusion of oxygen between alveoli and blood and between blood and tissue (2, 5, 9, 10).

In males there are about 15 to 16 g of hemoglobin and in females about 14 g of hemoglobin per 100 ml of blood. Each gram of hemoglobin can combine loosely with 1.34 ml of oxygen. On the average, approximately 20 ml of oxygen is carried with the hemoglobin in each 100 ml of blood.

Once carbon dioxide is formed in the cell, its only means of transport out of the cell is the process of diffusion and subsequent transport to the lungs. As with oxygen, only a small amount of carbon dioxide—about 5% of that produced during metabolism—is carried in the plasma. Although this quantity is small, it is the random movement of these dissolved carbon dioxide molecules that establishes the carbon dioxide pressure of blood.

Some carbon dioxide is transported in combination with hemoglobin, but most combines with water and is delivered to the lung in the form of bicarbonate (HCO_3^-).

The first step in this process is the combination of carbon dioxide in solution with water in a reversible reaction to form carbonic acid (H_2CO_3). This reaction is slow, and little carbon dioxide would be carried in this form if it were not for the action of the enzyme carbonic anhydrase, which accelerates the interaction of carbon dioxide and water about 5,000 times. Once carbonic acid is formed in the tissues, most of it ionizes to hydrogen ions and bicarbonate ions. The hydrogen ions are then buffered by the protein portion of the hemoglobin to maintain the pH of the blood within relatively narrow limits. Because bicarbonate ions are quite soluble in blood, they diffuse from the red blood cell into the plasma in exchange for chloride ions, which move into the blood cell to maintain ionic equilibrium. Sixty to eighty percent of all carbon dioxide is carried as plasma bicarbonate.

An important by-product of exercise is lactic acid. During moderate steady-state exercise, sufficient oxygen is available to the working muscles. Under these conditions, lactic acid, a major product of metabolism, does not accumulate (i.e., the removal rate equals the production rate). If, however, aerobic metabolism is insufficient to accomplish a given work load, anaerobic metabolism takes over and lactic acid is formed at a rate that exceeds its clearance from the blood. The exercise level or level of oxygen consumption at which blood lactate begins to show a systematic increase above the resting baseline level is termed the onset of blood lactate accumulation (OBLA). Almost all of the lactic acid generated during anaerobic metabolism is buffered in the blood by sodium bicarbonate and results in water and carbon dioxide (1, 7).

CARDIOVASCULAR AND RESPIRATORY RESPONSES TO EXERCISE TRAINING

The effect of exercise training is key to understanding the basis for physical performance or athletic competition. The following section provides a discussion of this subject.

The Heart

The most significant change in central cardiovascular function with long-term aerobic training (6-12 months) is the increase in maximal cardiac output. Because the maximal heart rate may actually even decrease slightly with prolonged exercise training, perhaps as a result of increased vagal tone, the enhanced capacity to increase cardiac output with training results directly from improved stroke volume. The weight and volume of the heart generally increase with prolonged aerobic training.

Cardiac hypertrophy is a normal training adaptation characterized by an increase in the size of the cavity of the left ventricle and a thickening of its walls. In addition, endurance training enhances the contractile state of the myocardium and improves its capability for achieving a larger stroke volume. The increase in stroke volume following aerobic training is usually accompanied by a heart rate reduction during submaximal exercise. Also, the rate of increase in the heart rate with a given work load is much less in the trained athlete than in a sedentary person (1, 7).

Capillary Circulation

Aside from its role in delivering oxygen, nutrients, and hormones, the capillary circulation provides the means for removing heat and metabolic by-products. Increased capillarization in response to the increased density of muscle associated with training has been observed. However, further research is necessary to clarify the role of exercise training and capillary development and to establish the precise physiological role of these adaptations (1, 7).

Blood

Plasma volume and total hemoglobin tend to increase with endurance training, although the amount of hemoglobin per unit volume of blood remains about the same. The increases may enhance circulatory and thermoregulatory dynamics to enhance oxygen delivery capacity during exercise (1, 7).

Ventilation

Aerobic training brings about several changes in pulmonary ventilation during maximal and submaximal exercise. Maximal exercise ventilation increases with improvements in maximal oxygen uptake. This results because the increase in aerobic capacity brings about a larger oxygen requirement and, correspondingly, a larger production of carbon dioxide that must be eliminated through increased alveolar ventilation (1, 7).

Following as few as 4 weeks of training, a considerable reduction in the ventilatory equivalent is observed with submaximal exercise. A smaller amount of air is breathed at a particular rate of submaximal oxygen consumption. In general, the tidal volume becomes larger and breathing frequency is considerably reduced. The exhaled air of trained individuals often contains only 14% to 15% oxygen during submaximal exercise, whereas the expired air of untrained persons may contain 18% oxygen at the same work level.

Ventilatory adaptations appear to be highly specific to the type of exercise used in training, although ventilatory equivalent is generally greater during arm exercise than during leg exercise. Training-induced adaptations in ventilation are observed only during exercise that uses the specifically trained muscle groups. Therefore, it may be that ventilatory adjustment to training results from local, neural, or chemical adaptations in the specific muscles trained through exercise.

Oxygen Extraction

Exercise training produces significant increases in the amount of oxygen extracted from the circulating blood. An increase in the arteriovenous oxygen difference is the result of a more effective distribution of the cardiac output to working muscles as well as of enhanced capacity of the trained muscle cells to extract and utilize oxygen (1, 7).

Lactic Acid

Although the OBLA is reached at about 55% of the healthy, untrained subject's maximal capacity for aerobic metabolism, it occurs at a higher percentage of the athlete's aerobic capacity. This favorable response may be due to the endurance athlete's genetic endowment (type of muscle fiber), specific local adaptations associated with training that favor the production of less lactic acid, and a more rapid rate of removal at any exercise level (1, 7).

Adaptation enhances the cell's capacity to generate ATP aerobically, especially through the breakdown of fatty acids, and may extend the percentage of one's maximal capacity for aerobic metabolism that can be sustained prior to the OBLA. Thus, highly trained endurance athletes may be able to perform at 80% to 90% of their maximal capacity for aerobic metabolism. Additionally, the ability to generate a high lactic acid level in a maximal exercise bout is increased with specific anaerobic training and subsequently reduced with detraining. Studies of well-trained athletes have shown that after they performed strenuous short-term exercise, the blood lactate concentration is 20% to 30% higher than in untrained subjects under similar circumstances. The mechanism for this response is unknown, but may be due to the large difference in the motivation level accompanying the trained state.

EXTERNAL INFLUENCES ON CARDIORESPIRATORY RESPONSE

There are a variety of external influences that will affect both the acute response and the chronic adaptation of the cardiorespiratory system. Some of these are described here.

Altitude

Upon arrival at elevations greater than 2,300 m, physiological adjustments occur to compensate for the thinner air and accompanying reduced alveolar oxygen pressure. Two adjustments are particularly important. First, as a result of the low partial pressure of oxygen, there is a great increase in pulmonary ventilation (hyperventilation). Ventilation may remain elevated for a year or longer if altitude exposure is prolonged. Second, there is an increase in blood flow at rest and during submaximal exercise (Table 7.1) (1, 7).

In the early stages of altitude adaptation, submaximal heart rates and cardiac outputs may increase 50% above sea-level values, whereas stroke volume remains essentially unchanged. Because the oxygen cost of work at high altitudes is essentially no different than at sea level, increases in submaximal blood flow partially compensate for the reduced oxygen in arteriole blood. Hyperventilation and increased submaximal cardiac output provide a rapid and relatively effective counter to the challenge of altitude. Concurrently, other slower-acting physiological and metabolic adjustments occur during a prolonged altitude state. The most important of these are

- the maintenance of the acid-base balance of body fluids altered by hyperventilation,
- increased formation of hemoglobin in red blood cells, and
- changes in local circulation and cellular function.

All these adaptations generally improve tolerance to the relative hypoxia of medium and high altitudes.

Hyperoxic Breathing

It is common to observe athletes breathing oxygen-enriched, or hyperoxic, gas mixtures during rest periods and following strenuous exercise. The belief is that this procedure increases the oxygen-carrying capacity of the blood and thus increases oxygen transport to the exercising muscles. If this were the case, oxygen breathing would certainly improve aerobic capacity and possibly speed up recovery. The fact is, however, that when healthy people breathe ambient air at sea level, the hemoglobin in arteriole blood leaving the lungs is 95% to 98% saturated with oxygen. Thus, breathing high concentrations of oxygen could increase oxygen transport of hemoglobin only to a small extent. However, the positive psychological influence of oxygen breathing should not be discounted, which may justify continuing this practice (1, 7).

There is, however, considerable evidence that breathing hyperoxic gas during submaximal and maximal aerobic exercise enhances physical performance of an aerobic nature. Although the precise mechanism for the

Table 7.1   Adjustments to Altitude Hypoxia

System	Immediate adjustments	Longer-term adjustments
Pulmonary	Hyperventilation	Hyperventilation
Acid-base	Body fluids become more alkaline due to reduction in CO_2 with hyperventilation	Excretion of HCO_3^- by the kidneys and concomitant reduction in alkaline reserve
Cardiovascular	Increase in submaximal heart rate	Submaximal heart rate remains elevated
	Increase in submaximal cardiac output	Submaximal cardiac output falls to sea-level value or below
	Stroke volume remains the same or is slightly lowered	Stroke volume is lowered
	Maximal heart rate remains the same or is slightly lowered	Maximal heart rate is lowered
	Maximal cardiac output remains the same or is slightly lowered	Maximal cardiac output is lowered
Hematologic		Decrease in plasma volume
		Increased hematocrit
		Increased hemoglobin concentration
		Increase in total number of red blood cells
Local		Possible increased capillarization of skeletal muscle
		Increased mitochondria
		Increased aerobic enzymes

beneficial effects of hyperoxia remains unclear, several physiological responses are worthy of consideration. Oxygen breathing during both light and heavy exercise has resulted in reductions in blood lactate, heart rate, and ventilation volume and a significant increase in maximal oxygen consumption. Because the available evidence does not show that hyperoxic gas mixtures increase the maximal cardiac output, the increase in maximal oxygen uptake must be due to an expanded arteriovenous oxygen difference. This may be partially explained by the fact that even a small increase in hemoglobin saturation during hyperoxia, as well as an increase in the oxygen dissolved in the plasma, increases total oxygen availability during strenuous exercise to an efficacious degree. Further, the increase in partial pressure of oxygen in solution caused by breathing hyperoxic gas also facilitates its diffusion across the tissue-capillary membrane to the mitochondria. This may account for its more rapid rate of utilization in the beginning phase of exercise.

In summary, there is no evidence that oxygen breathing during recovery from strenuous exercise will enhance subsequent exercise performance. However, the breathing of hyperoxic mixtures during endurance performance does appear to offer positive ergogenic benefits, although the practical application of this technique during competition is limited.

Smoking

The research relating smoking habits to lung function and exercise performance is meager; most endurance athletes avoid smoking for fear of hindering performance due to a reduction in ventilatory capacity. The chronic smoker does tend to experience the decreased dynamic lung function associated with obstructive lung disorders. Such pathological processes, however, usually take years to develop. In young smokers, chronic alterations in lung function tend to be minimal and insignificant in terms of their effect on physical performance. However, other more acute effects of tobacco smoking may adversely affect exercise capacity. These include the following:

- The effect of nicotine, which constricts the terminal bronchioles of the lungs. This in turn increases the resistance to air flow in and out of the lungs.
- The irritating effects of smoke, which cause increased fluid secretion in the bronchial tree as well as some swelling of the epithelial linings.
- Nicotine paralysis of the cilia on the surfaces of the respiratory epithelial cells. The cilia normally beat continuously to remove excess fluids and foreign particles from the respiratory tract. As a result, debris accumulates in the respiratory passageways and adds to the difficulty of breathing.

Thus, even the light smoker will feel respiratory strain during maximal exercise and a reduction in the level of performance (1, 7).

Carbon monoxide, a component of cigarette smoke, is associated with impaired hemodynamic response to exercise. Compared with oxygen, carbon monoxide more readily combines with hemoglobin, forming carboxyhemoglobin. This results in a reduction of the amount of oxygen that can be carried by hemoglobin and thus a reduction in oxygen that can be provided to the working muscles. Hence, maximal exercise capacity may be lowered and submaximal cardiovascular responses may be increased in an attempt to provide adequate oxygenated blood to the working muscles.

Blood Doping

Red blood cell reinfusion, often called "induced erythrocythemia" or "blood doping," has received attention as a possible ergogenic aid. With this procedure, several units of a person's blood are withdrawn, the plasma is removed and immediately reinfused, and the packed red cells are placed in frozen storage. Following a period of 4 to 6 weeks to allow for natural blood cell replenishment, the stored blood cells are then reinfused 1 to 7 days before an endurance event. As a result, the red blood cell count and hemoglobin level of the blood is elevated 8% to 20%. It is theorized that the added blood volume contributes to a larger maximal cardiac output and that the red blood cell packing increases the blood's oxygen-carrying capacity and thus the quantity of oxygen available to the working muscles. This would certainly be a considerable asset, given that endurance exercise requires a high and sustained level of aerobic metabolism, especially if one's capacity for aerobic metabolism is limited by physiological factors such as oxygen transport. However, although a theoretical basis for blood doping exists, there is limited and conflicting experimental evidence to justify this procedure. It does appear that red blood cell reinfusion results in a 5% to 13% increase in aerobic capacity, a reduced submaximal heart rate and reduced blood lactate for a standard exercise work load, and an augmented endurance performance both at altitude and sea level. However, there is also the potential for increasing hematocrit level (percent of blood volume occupied by cells) too much, leading to increased blood viscosity and decreased aerobic performance (1, 7).

CONCLUSION

Knowledge of cardiovascular and respiratory responses to exercise will help the strength and conditioning professional understand the scientific basis for aerobic conditioning as well as what adaptations to expect and monitor. This information can be of particular value in developing the goals of a conditioning program and can provide a basis for clinical evaluation and the selection parameters that might be included in such an evaluation process.

Key Terms

adrenergic fiber	117	bronchus	111	mean arterial pressure	116
alveolar pressure	113	buffering power	111	metabolic equivalent (MET)	115
alveolus	111	capillary	111	metarteriole	111
anatomical dead space	119	cardiac output	115	minute ventilation	118
aortic valve	108	cholinergic fiber	117	mitral valve	108
arteriole	110	depolarization	110	peripheral chemoreceptor system	114
artery	110	diastole	108	physiological dead space	119
atrioventricular (AV) bundle	109	ejection fraction	115	pleura	113
atrioventricular (AV) node	109	electrocardiogram (ECG)	110	pleural pressure	113
atrioventricular (AV) valve	108	end-diastolic volume	115	pulmonary valve	108
		Fick equation	116	Purkinje fiber	109
atrium	108	heart rate	115	rate-pressure product	116
bradycardia	115	hemoglobin	111	repolarization	110
bronchiole	111	maximal oxygen uptake	115		

Study Questions

1. The contracting left ventricle pushes blood through

   a. the tricuspid valve into the pulmonary circulation
   b. the mitral valve into the peripheral circulation
   c. the aortic valve into the peripheral circulation
   d. the aortic valve into the pulmonary circulation

2. The QRS complex on the ECG represents

   a. electrical stimulus for ventricular contraction
   b. an abnormal heart rhythm
   c. ventricular repolarization
   d. atrial depolarization

3. Normal, quiet breathing during inspiration is accomplished through

   a. relaxation of the diaphragm
   b. contraction of the abdominal muscles
   c. contraction of the diaphragm
   d. positive pressure in the chest cavity

4. Normal responses to exercise include the following *except*

   a. mean arterial pressure rise
   b. stroke volume increase
   c. systolic blood pressure response similar to heart rate
   d. diastolic blood pressure rise

5. Which of the following is not a component of oxygen uptake:

   a. heart rate
   b. systolic blood pressure
   c. stroke volume
   d. arteriovenous oxygen difference

6. Increased blood flow to working muscles is partly accomplished through

   a. dilation of the venous system
   b. decreased carbon dioxide in the blood
   c. decreased acidity of the blood
   d. vasoconstriction of arterioles in other organ systems

7. Which of the following is not an effect of altitude during submaximal exercise:

   a. increased cardiac output
   b. decreased oxygen concentration in arterial blood
   c. hyperventilation
   d. increase of oxygen cost of work

Applying Knowledge of Cardiovascular and Respiratory Anatomy and Physiology

Problem 1

Identify and describe how maximal oxygen uptake is important in a power sport such as football and an endurance sport such as cross-country skiing.

Problem 2

Using the Fick equation as a guide, describe in detail the various physiological adaptations that result from training designed to improve maximal oxygen uptake. Differentiate, where possible, the differences in physiological adaptations resulting from endurance training versus resistance training.

References

1. Fisher, A.G., and C.R. Jensen. *Scientific Basis of Athletic Conditioning*, 3rd ed. Philadelphia: Lea & Febiger. 1989.
2. Guyton, A.C. *Textbook of Medical Physiology*, 8th ed. Philadelphia: Saunders. 1991.
3. Hurst, J.W., R.C. Schlant, C.E. Rackley, E.H. Sonnenblick, and N.K. Wenger. *The Heart*, 8th ed. New York: McGraw-Hill. 1994.
4. Kennedy, H.L. *Ambulatory Electrocardiography and its Technology*, 2nd ed. Philadelphia: Lea & Febiger. 1989.
5. Lee, G.R., ed. *Wintrobe's Clinical Hematology*, 9th ed. Philadelphia: Lea & Febiger. 1989.
6. Marriott, H.J.L., and M.B. Conover. *Advanced Concepts in Arrhythmias*, 2nd ed. St. Louis: Mosby. 1989.
7. McCardle, W.D., F.I Katch, and V.I. Katch. *Exercise Physiology*, 4th ed. Philadelphia: Lea & Febiger. 1994.
8. Milnor, W.R. *Hemodynamics*, 2nd ed. Baltimore: Williams & Wilkins. 1989.
9. Taylor, A.E., K. Rehder, R.E. Hyatt, and J.C. Parker. *Clinical Respiratory Physiology*. Philadelphia: Saunders. 1989.
10. Williams, W.J., E. Beutler, A.J. Erslev, and M.A. Lichtmann, eds. *Hematology*, 4th ed. New York: McGraw-Hill. 1990.

CHAPTER 8

GENERAL ADAPTATIONS TO RESISTANCE AND ENDURANCE TRAINING PROGRAMS

William J. Kraemer

Strength and conditioning training programs attempt to create systematic processes for eliciting physiological adaptations over time (1, 6, 26, 35, 69, 72, 77). The magnitude of change depends on how much adaptational potential exists in the person undergoing training—that is, how much adaptation has already occurred within his or her physiological system. For example, the size of a muscle fiber in a highly trained lifter may increase only 5% in cross-sectional area over a 1-year training cycle, even though the area increased by 40% in the first year of training. The same concept holds true for performance. For example, for a novice weightlifter a 25-kg improvement in the snatch lift in the first 6 to 8 months of training would not be uncommon. In contrast, a highly trained weightlifter might have to train for a year in order to gain just 2.5 kg in the snatch lift. A genetic ceiling exists for every physiological function within each person. Furthermore, performance gains in many sports are typically not related to the change in only one physiological system. The concept of total conditioning addresses this need to train each of the physiological systems related to sport performance (36, 37, 50, 68).

In short, each athlete brings to a strength and conditioning training program his or her own genetic predisposition, potential for improvement, and willingness to put forth the effort required for developing his or her physiological potential through the program. If the athlete has not been involved in any prior training program, positive changes will be observed with almost any training program owing to the athlete's large "adaptational window." However, if continued change is desired for a particular variable once training adaptations have used up a large portion of the adaptational window, the exact nature of the training stimulus becomes all the more important. Adaptational changes to a training program are dynamic and related to the athlete's stage of physical development. Furthermore, training programs can be ineffective owing to their inability to elicit an adequate stimulus for change in a particular physiological system.

I would like to thank Dr. Andrew C. Fry, CSCS, one of my former doctoral students, for his help in writing the section on overtraining. The preparation of this manuscript was supported in part by a grant from the Robert F. and Sandra M. Leitzinger Research Fund in Sports Medicine to the Center for Sports Medicine at The Pennsylvania State University. I would also like to thank Joann Ruble and Carol Glunt for their help in the preparation of the manuscript.

From a physiological point of view, it is much easier to maintain a performance level when training elite athletes than to improve an area that is already using a high proportion of the adaptational window. This is especially true when improvement is desired over short periods of training, such as 8 to 10 weeks (6, 51, 98a).

Elite athletes have to train very hard in order to make small gains in performance. This is achieved by improving the physiological adaptations in the body by small but significant adaptational changes. The smallest differences in performance can make the difference between winning and losing a championship (29, 51). Training for optimal athletic performance is a very demanding task where what you *don't* know as a strength and conditioning professional may hurt the optimal performance of the athlete.

Training must be carefully planned and its effects understood and evaluated. An athlete's body can be overtrained and pushed into physiological states in which adaptation to the training is ineffective or in which risks of injury and illness can produce major setbacks (10, 12, 19, 22, 23, 29). Proper exercise training and recovery can act to maximize the adaptational capacity of each variable trained. Consequently, a number of important concepts need to be understood as one starts to learn more about physiological adaptations to exercise training:

- Each person will respond a little differently to each training program.
- The magnitude of the physiological or performance gain is related to the size of the adaptational window available for change in that athlete.
- The amount of physiological adaptation will depend upon the effectiveness of the exercise prescriptions used in the training programs.
- Training for peak athletic performance is different from training for optimal health and fitness because, in the former, the level of adaptation usually requires considerably higher training intensities and volumes of exercise than would be needed for general health and fitness.

The primary purpose of this chapter is to provide an overview of some of the physiological adaptations that occur with exercise training. This should provide the basis for an understanding of the ultimate result of exercise training, physiological adaptation that leads to enhanced performance.

VARIATIONS IN ENERGY REQUIREMENTS, SOURCES, AND USAGE

An athlete's ability to perform is based on the ability to gain needed energy (4, 5, 8, 9, 99). Energy requirements may be short term or long term, depending on the activity. Long-term performance requires a great deal of energy from aerobic metabolic sources (97). Thus, training that enhances the athlete's ability for various long-term performances at lower power outputs has typically been referred to as **aerobic training**, or **endurance training**. In contrast, short-term performance requires energy from anaerobic sources (although aerobic contributions are greater than might be expected); this type of training has typically been called **anaerobic training**. Anaerobic training has traditionally consisted of many different training modes, from lifting weights to sprint running, in which oxygen delivery is not a limiting factor in performance.

Ultimately, training stimulates adaptations and thus enhances the body's physiological systems for better performance (38, 53-56, 58, 102). Specific programs can focus on a wide range of physical abilities. Preparation of physical abilities can range from an athlete preparing to perform a single lift in weightlifting to performing in an ultra-endurance event (e.g., the marathon or triathlon) (62, 67, 73, 79).

One of the basic aspects of most exercise prescriptions in training programs is related to improving the body's ability to gain energy. Many times we attempt to match the metabolic system of the sport to the training stimulus of the program (63, 64). While this may be an oversimplification of a complex process, from the weight room to the track, training programs are used to enhance energy availability and utilization. A basic understanding of how the body uses energy is fundamental to the development of a proper, goal-specific training program. To date, our understanding of the interaction of the body's different metabolic systems has been simplistic. All energy systems (aerobic and anaerobic) are engaged upon the initiation of physical activity. It is the magnitude and relative proportion of the energy contribution from each source that differ and can dramatically change moment to moment depending upon the demands of the sport. Thus, except for those cases in which a steady-state demand is achieved, activities vary dramatically as to their metabolic profiles during the activity and during periods of rest (18, 95, 105). As a rule of thumb, anaerobic systems predominate in the very early phases (up to 25 s) of continuous activity. Continuous maximal exercise cannot be performed for very long (usually < 3 min); the individual fatigues and has to stop. If exercise continues, the power output is drastically reduced and aerobic metabolism plays the dominant role in continuing the activity. This can be seen in a 200-m sprint, where, at the end of the race, the athlete has no energy left and is unable to maintain the same maximal power output over a greater distance; if the athlete attempts to keep running, the power output has to be drastically reduced (86).

In sports or conditioning activities in which various types of rest intervals (i.e., ceased or reduced activity) are available, recovery starts and continues to various extents based on the amount of time available; during recovery, only the aerobic system is used (126). For example, recovery may mean 25 s in a huddle in football, time-outs in a basketball game, or between periods in a wrestling match. Once the activity starts again, all energy systems are reactivated and performance is dependent upon the available (including recovered) energy supplies (14, 78). **Interval training** (e.g., sprints) and **resistance training** are examples of conditioning activities that use an interplay of activity intervals and rest periods to develop the body's energy systems for repeated and high–power output demands (65). In addition, interval training is a good example of a conditioning method that can enhance the body's ability to perform aerobic or endurance activities as the aerobic system is also dramatically utilized and enhanced (2, 11). Thus, the interplay of energy systems is more dramatic than previously thought. In Figure 8.1 the interplay of different metabolic systems with exercise duration is shown. Understanding the metabolic demands of exercise helps in developing training programs to meet the acute or immediate energy needs of a sport (103, 104, 109, 110).

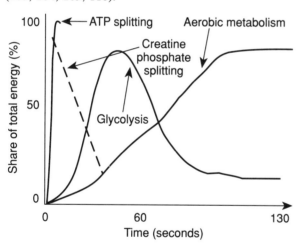

Figure 8.1 Relationship between energy delivery systems and exercise duration.

ANAEROBIC TRAINING

There are two anaerobic energy sources, the phosphagen system and glycolysis (also called anaerobic glycolysis).

Review of Anaerobic Energy Systems

The Phosphagen System. As discussed in chapter 5, the phosphagen system provides the high-energy phosphate compound adenosine triphosphate (ATP). (ATP and creatine phosphate are the major phosphagens.) ATP is immediately available to muscle, so the energy needs of fast and powerful movement are met in the immediate area of the muscle's actin and myosin contractile machinery. In exercising muscles, ATP concentration does not decrease in proportion to the demand for ATP, because the products of ATP hydrolysis— adenosine diphosphate (ADP), inorganic phosphate, and hydrogen ions—all participate in another reaction with creatine phosphate to re-form ATP.

This type of energy availability is vital for sports of very short duration, such as field events and sprints, and burst-like sports, like football, basketball, and wrestling. Training programs enhance the content of phosphagens in the muscle. Increases in ATP and creatine phosphate occur only in muscles being trained, and training activities of higher power output produce larger gains in the muscle's phosphagen content (46).

Glycolysis. Glycolysis is essentially the breakdown of glucose to pyruvic acid and the conversion of this intermediate, in the absence of oxygen, to lactic acid (chapter 5). (Pyruvic acid can also be converted to acetyl CoA and enter the aerobic pathway.) If it is converted into lactic acid, it is then considered anaerobic metabolism. Carbohydrates (e.g., glucose) pass through the glycolytic cycle of reactions and either end up being used in aerobic metabolism or anaerobic metabolism. Thus, the terms ''anaerobic glycolysis'' and ''aerobic glycolysis.''

The series of reactions needed to break down glucose to lactic acid creates a greater time delay in energy production compared with the phosphagen system. In other words, the phosphagen system has a greater potential for supplying energy demands for very quick and powerful muscular actions of short duration. Still, anaerobic glycolysis is instantly initiated with intense exercise; indeed, increases in muscle lactic acid and blood lactate concentrations have been observed after exercise lasting only a few seconds (86).

Lactic acid is produced from glycolytic reactions in the muscle, with carbohydrates providing the only energy substrate. Thus, blood lactate concentrations are lower than muscle concentrations, as lactic acid produced in the muscle can be further broken down and used for energy before it has a chance to pass into the circulation. Many activities that require repeated maximal activity are typically interval in nature. Thus, free radicals, along with other products from glucose degradation, are readily available for energy use (e.g., lactic acid is used for energy production). In addition, these various compounds provide the building blocks for the resynthesis of glucose. Therefore, glycogen stores in the liver and muscle are not typically depleted to the same extent observed consequent to continuous high intensity aerobic exercise.

Physical toleration for intense exercise characterized by anaerobic training has to be developed (122). This is especially true in the case of training protocols and sports that accumulate high concentrations of lactic acid (which, of course, includes hydrogen ions). Lactic acid buildup contributes to a decrease in muscle and blood pH. The acidity of the muscle, moving from a pH of 7.4 to 7.0 after intense exercise (e.g., repeat sprint intervals) or during certain sports (e.g., wrestling and an 800-m race), affects the muscle's ability to maintain force production at high power outputs. Blood pH values as low as 6.9 have been observed in elite anaerobic athletes. The ability to tolerate such demands improves with training as the body adapts to the acidic environment in the muscle. The blood and muscle buffering capacities of the body are increased with anaerobic training as hydrogen ions are neutralized into weak acids. Training gradually exposes the muscle to the lower pH environments and adaptations are important to allow the athlete to compete under such conditions. One can see the effects of this ability to tolerate high lactic acid concentrations as the body buffers a greater amount of the acid associated with its production and the muscle performs more effectively. Thus, a dramatic training effect in athletes is the ability to tolerate acid conditions in the muscle. Additionally, the symptoms of nausea, dizziness, vomiting, and extreme fatigue that occur during the performance of glycolytic-type sports or conditioning activities can be reduced with training.

After 20 to 30 s of intense activity, the aerobic contribution of energy demands increases dramatically to help maintain higher power outputs, with the result that as much as 40% to 45% of the required energy can come from aerobic metabolism. Thus, sports such as wrestling or an 800-m race will have a dramatic aerobic contribution despite the extremely high concentrations of lactic acid found in the muscle and reflected in the blood. In fact, such sports as wrestling and middle-distance sprints can raise blood lactate concentrations 20 to 25 times above resting levels in only a few minutes. Such high concentrations of lactate would not be possible for the athlete to produce unless aerobic metabolic sources allowed anaerobic glycolysis to continue for a longer period of time.

Table 8.1 provides an estimation of the primary contribution from the different energy sources. The table can be used as a guide for exercise prescription, when matching the metabolism of the sport with the training activity is important for enhanced performance potential.

Methods and Modes of Anaerobic Training

Anaerobic training involves a wide range of training methods and modes of exercise. Sprint workouts, stair

Table 8.1 Primary Metabolic Demands of Various Sports

| Sport | Primary metabolic demand from | | |
	Phosphagen system	Anaerobic glycolysis	Aerobic metabolism
Baseball	High	Low	—
Basketball	High	Moderate to high	—
Boxing	High	High	—
Cross-country skiing	—	—	High
Diving	High	Low	—
Downhill skiing	High	Moderate	—
Fencing	High	Moderate	—
Field events	High	—	—
Field hockey	High	Moderate	Moderate
Football	High	Moderate	Low
Gymnastics	High	Moderate	—
Golf	High	—	—
Ice hockey	High	Moderate	Moderate
Lacrosse	High	Moderate	Moderate
Marathon	—	—	High
Soccer	High	Moderate	High
Swimming, short distance	High	Moderate to high	—
Swimming, long distance	High	Moderate to high	—
Tennis	High	—	—
Track, short distance	High	Moderate to high	—
Track, long distance	—	Moderate	High
Ultraendurance events	—	—	High
Volleyball	High	Moderate	—
Wrestling	High	High	—
Weightlifting	High	—	—

Note. All types of metabolism are involved to some extent in all activities. Only the primary or near-primary metabolic systems for each sport are shown in this table.

running, plyometrics (stretch-shortening cycle activities), and wall climbing are just a few of the training activities that can be configured in an anaerobic exercise protocol (61). From the previous discussion it should be clear that in certain anaerobic training programs aerobic metabolism would be highly involved. This would occur more readily with programs that cause large elevations in lactic acid. Anaerobic training programs that concentrate on the phosphagen are typically under 10 s in duration and provide adequate rest (aerobic recovery) so that lactic acid does not accumulate to any large extent (76). Thus, the aerobic system is not as dramatically involved in sustaining the actual training activity, but more involved with recovery. In this style of training the duration of the rest period is a vital factor. If long rest periods are used (1:12), lactic acid concentrations are low, increases in stroke volume are minimal, and improvements in aerobic power are not seen nor are improvements in the body's ability to buffer acid (14, 78). Thus, anaerobic training is actually a continuum from movements that take a fraction of a second to

more metabolically demanding training activities such as sprint intervals with short rest periods.

RESISTANCE TRAINING

One could classify resistance training as an anaerobic form of exercise. Many of these different training programs can be used to enhance the ability of the body to perform at very high force and/or power outputs for a very short period of time to improve the body's ability to perform repeated bouts of maximal activity (43, 57, 66, 74, 92, 125).

Several extensive reviews of the physiological effects of resistance training have been made (71, 73, 74, 116). Table 8.2 gives a summary of the changes reported,

Table 8.2 Comparison of Physiological Adaptations to Resistance Training and Aerobic Training

Variable	Result following resistance training	Result following endurance training
Performance		
Muscle strength	Increases	No change
Muscle endurance	Increases for high power output	Increases for low power output
Aerobic power	No change or increases slightly	Increases
Maximal rate of force production	Increases	No change or decreases
Vertical jump	Ability increases	Ability unchanged
Anaerobic power	Increases	No change
Sprint speed	Improves	No change or improves slightly
Muscle fibers		
Fiber size	Increases	No change or increases slightly
Capillary density	No change or decreases	Increases
Mitochondrial density	Decreases	Increases
Fast heavy-chain myosin	Increases in amount	No change or decreases in amount
Enzyme activity		
Creatine phosphokinase	Increases	Increases
Myokinase	Increases	Increases
Phosphofructokinase	Increases	Variable
Lactate dehydrogenase	No change or variable	Variable
Metabolic energy stores		
Stored ATP	Increases	Increases
Stored creatine phosphate	Increases	Increases
Stored glycogen	Increases	Increases
Stored triglycerides	May increase	Increases
Connective tissue		
Ligament strength	May increase	Increases
Tendon strength	May increase	Increases
Collagen content	May increase	Variable
Bone density	No change or increases	Increases
Body composition		
% body fat	Decreases	Decreases
Fat-free mass	Increases	No change

along with those that occur in aerobic endurance training. Several items in the table are discussed in detail in the following sections.

Changes in Muscle Fibers

Increased muscle size from resistance exercise occurs primarily through muscle fiber hypertrophy. While hyperplasia, the increase in the number of muscle cells, cannot be completely ruled out, it appears not to be a major strategy for muscle tissue adaptations to resistance training and, if it occurs at all, would only involve a small amount of tissue (30). In untrained people a training duration of 4 weeks or more is necessary before significant changes in the size of the muscle fiber are observed (92, 93, 114, 119, 120). Previously trained muscle may be more responsive to heavy resistance exercise and respond in a few weeks with an increase in muscle fiber size. Further study is needed to evaluate the time courses of morphological changes with different initial levels of training. It now appears that heavy chain-myosin proteins in muscle make alterations toward fast types in muscle that is already resistance-trained. Such changes in myosin proteins may contribute to changes in force production capabilities before the enhanced protein accretion that causes hypertrophy occurs. Such basic protein changes in muscle protein structure and function all enhance the functional ability of muscle in response to a heavy resistance training program (118).

The increased cross-sectional area of muscle fibers is caused by the greater number of actin and myosin filaments added to the myofibrils. Heavy resistance training results in increased fiber cross-sectional area of both Type I and Type II muscle fibers; synthesis of contractile proteins appears greatest in Type II fibers (9, 93, 94, 119). Differences among other fiber subgroups are not clear. Powerlifters and Olympic weightlifters have Type II fiber areas almost twice the size of their Type I fiber areas, but bodybuilders do not. Bodybuilders can have a higher percentage of Type I fiber because that sport does not require the same type of strength performance. This suggests that the type of resistance training protocols used may have a significant impact on subsequent muscle fiber adaptations. Fiber areas of lifters are significantly larger than those of runners and other control subjects. Resistance training is a more potent stimulus for muscle fiber hypertrophy than any other form of exercise.

Additional Cellular Adaptations

Heavy resistance training reduces mitochondrial density in the trained muscles, a change that parallels and is thus attributable to increases in muscle size (91, 94). The increase in the amount of contractile protein also indicates decreased capillary density. However, decreases in mitochondrial and capillary densities do not result in reduced ability to perform aerobic exercise. Powerlifters and Olympic weightlifters show significantly lower capillary densities when compared with control subjects, whereas bodybuilders have capillary densities similar to nonathletes. Bodybuilding workouts typically elevate blood lactate concentrations to above 20 mmol/L; this may help get rid of the lactic acid by various mechanisms, making enhanced capillary supply a positive training effect to help in the clearance of lactic acid from the exercising muscle tissue (21, 84, 111). The type of exercise protocols used by bodybuilders may differentially influence cellular adaptations. Such changes may be advantageous for sports such as 800-m races and wrestling that develop large accumulations of lactic acid.

There are many conflicting reports on enzyme changes with resistance training. Further study of enzyme changes with resistance training that use single-fiber analysis schemes to delineate the subtle changes that may occur in specific fiber types are needed.

Heavy resistance training induces increases in energy substrate levels and their availability in muscle (118, 120). After 5 months of training, ATP, creatine phosphate, creatine, and glycogen increased in the triceps brachii (21). Prolonged heavy resistance training may also increase capacity for intramuscular lipid storage. These changes are related to the specific type of resistance training program used, whether it is low-volume, with 5RM (repetition maximum) and long rest periods, or high-volume, with 10RM and short rest periods.

Muscle Strength

Initial gains in muscle strength during the first few weeks of training do not show a concomitant increase in muscle size or muscle cross-sectional area (98a, 107, 108). The quality of the muscle—specifically, the type of muscle proteins that make up the myosin filament—changes, but not enough protein is accumulated in the cells to create increases in muscle fiber size. Within several weeks, however, myofibril proteins start to be added to the muscle fibers, and increases in muscle fiber size are observed at about 8 to 12 weeks of training.

Increases in muscle strength from pretraining values can range from 7% to 45%, the figure for a given person dependent in large part upon the starting level of strength. If a person is untrained, almost any program will bring gains, but the rate of increase declines as training continues. Thus, the design of effective exercise prescriptions becomes increasingly important. The majority of investigations have used untrained subjects and thus a large window of adaptation would be expected and therefore a large increase in strength following just about any training program. If the learning effects are not removed with repeated test familiarization and practice tests, as much as 50% of the strength gain may reflect the acute learning effects (subject improves performance because he or she learns what to do and how to produce force) and not be true physiological gains related to muscle tissue adaptations over the long-term training program. Hoffman et al. (51) found that in highly trained college football players, some protocols demonstrated no significant changes during a 10-week training program. This points to the importance of understanding the training level of athletes when evaluating changes in strength with training. In addition, gender effects also account for the absolute magnitude of strength gains (24, 52, 88, 125).

The effects of training are related to the type of exercise used, its intensity, and its volume (number of sets × number of repetitions). With trained athletes, a higher volume of exercise is typically needed in order for the adaptations to continue to improve (although overtraining is also possible). The use of both eccentric and concentric components in machine stack plate or free-weight resistance exercise may result in optimal improvement in strength and muscle size—an important consideration when examining goals and matching them with resistance training equipment. Multiple sets of an exercise and maximum voluntary contractions are needed when training athletes with progressive resistance training (77). Carefully manipulating intensity and volume is where the "art" of the profession comes in.

An RM Continuum for Training Effects

In a study on the effects of the resistance intensity of the exercise, Anderson and Kearney (3) demonstrated that a repetition continuum exists (Figure 8.2). As the number of repetitions increased, the return on strength gains decreased and local muscular endurance was enhanced. Thus, heavier loads (6-8RM) produced much larger gains in strength than lighter loads (30-40RM). Differences among heavier loads (1-10RM) appeared irrelevant, since they are all typically used in periodized resistance training programs (96). Experimentally, the interaction of volume and intensity can be problematic when trying to compare different RM intensities from 1RM to 10RM. Interpretation may be difficult, and findings may not reflect the long-term efficacy found in different methods of periodized training. Thus, it is apparent that a single optimal program for all people

does not exist. It is rather the appropriate use of basic principles involving proper progression, variation, and individualization of resistance training that are the crucial factors in training success (32, 72, 80).

Neural Adaptations

As noted previously, the correlations between increase in muscle strength and increase in muscle mass are weak within the first few weeks of training (98a, 106, 107). However, factors other than muscle mass contribute to muscle force production, including increased inhibition of antagonistic muscle and better cocontraction of synergistic muscles, increased activation of synergistic muscles, inhibition of neural protective mechanisms, and increased motor neuron excitability.

When starting a training program, a variety of alterations must take place to provide for increased strength, power, and size of the muscles trained. The nervous system and the muscle tissue system are the primary physiological systems involved with the needed adaptations for increased force production. It is thought that they carry on a dramatic and complex interplay. What causes the neural or muscle tissue component to dominate at a given stage of training remains unclear, but could be related to how well trained a person already is or to the configuration of the resistance exercise stimulus used in a program. For example, a very high intensity (5RM and lower) and low-volume multijoint lift training program in a trained athlete may primarily affect neural factors (e.g., recruitment patterns, activation, inhibition, etc.). Muscle fibers may already be at a high percentage of adaptational capacity and, because of the exercise volume, may not be receiving the stimulus needed to further enlarge them. Competitive weightlifters gain much more in strength and power than in number of muscle fibers or muscle hypertrophy. Conversely, when using a program of very high volume and 10RM (moderate) intensity loads with short rest periods, as many bodybuilders do, the focus may shift to the development of muscle mass; such a protocol may enhance the body's natural anabolic hormonal responses to training. Under these circumstances, muscle hypertrophy may be promoted to a larger extent than muscle strength and power. Neural factors play a diminished role in their contribution to the adaptation.

Most training programs will typically focus upon gaining either greater strength and power or muscle

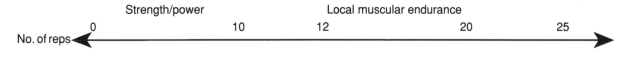

Figure 8.2 Repetition maximum continuum for training effects.

tissue hypertrophy. While typical heavy resistance training programs usually result in increases in all three components, especially in the novice trainee, more advanced programs will attempt to maximize one of the two developmental domains. This interplay between neural and muscle-tissue factors has been observed in competitive lifters and hypothesized to be a tenable mechanism for continued adaptation of the body to resistance training. In Figure 8.3 a theoretical interplay of neural and hypertrophy factors is shown that emphasizes the variety of physiological strategies available for adaptation to training.

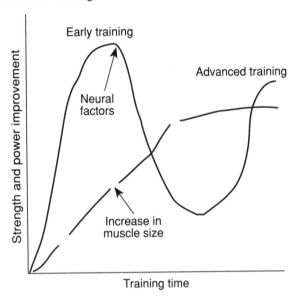

Figure 8.3 Theoretical interplay between neural and muscle tissue factors.

Cardiovascular Responses and Adaptations

Resistance training can benefit the cardiovascular system, but in a manner different from conventional endurance training (7, 41). Improved ability of the heart, lungs, and circulatory system to function under conditions of high pressure and force production demonstrate the positive benefits of heavy resistance exercise in expanding the physiological capacity of the athlete. Since many of the competitive environments involve very similar high-pressor and force production requirements, resistance exercise can help prepare the athlete's body for such extreme competitive demands (26, 45, 49). Although very large increases in acute blood pressure responses to resistance exercise (> 300/ 180 mm Hg) have been observed, especially when a Valsalva movement is performed, no data exist that would indicate resistance training has any negative effects on resting blood pressure (for review see 26). The

ability to tolerate higher blood pressure responses to intense exercise may be viewed as a positive adaptation and a manifestation of the extraordinary plasticity of the lifters' cardiovascular system in response to stress. Male bodybuilders have lower blood pressures than either recreationally trained or sedentary males while performing resistance exercise at the same relative (RM) load.

Cross-sectional echocardiography studies show that highly weight-trained athletes have normal left ventricular, systolic, and diastolic internal dimensions and volumes, in terms of both absolute value and value relative to body surface area (26, 28). Short-term studies on left ventricular cavity changes are inconclusive, suggesting that longer training programs are needed to bring about change (26). The effects of resistance training on cardiac wall thickness are less clear at present because of discrepancies in control subjects, effectiveness of exercise program, and caliber of lifters. Heavy resistance training does appear to increase cardiac wall thickness, but not equally for all people. The increased cardiac wall thickness causes the ratio of septum to free-wall thickness to exceed 1:3. Although this higher-than-normal ratio is usually associated with hypertrophic cardiomyopathy, competitive weightlifters and powerlifters had normal ratios of left ventricular mass to volume and normal wall thickness per body surface area, indicating normal hearts (33, 34). The negative old myth about an "athletic heart" is thus not true and needs to be better understood by both strength and conditioning professionals and clinicians when dealing with young healthy athletes who perform intensive resistance training (59).

One of the more conventional training effects of an endurance training program is to increase an athlete's maximal oxygen consumption (71). Resistance exercise, however, is not very effective in training this variable. Conventional heavy resistance training programs do not increase aerobic power. Exceptions would be relatively untrained people, in whom increases ranging from 5% to 8% in aerobic power result from resistance training. Thus, it is obvious that changes in aerobic metabolism and performance are not optimally affected with resistance exercise. Even increases in maximal oxygen consumption from circuit weight training programs (light loads, short rests, and multiple exercises) are lower than what would be expected from conventional endurance training programs (discussed later in this chapter).

Body Composition

Intense resistance training can cause changes in body composition. Resistance training can increase fat-free mass and decrease the percentage of body fat. Short-term resistance training programs have typically resulted in slight increases in fat-free mass (125). The change in percentage of body fat depends on caloric intake and the metabolic intensity of the resistance training program. Continual, long-term adherence to a heavy resistance training program appears necessary to achieve optimal increases in fat-free mass and decreases in percentage of body fat.

Connective Tissue

At present, little direct evidence exists on the effects of heavy resistance training on changes in connective tissue (17, 115). Stone (115) pointed out that because of the nature of the exercise stimulus, resistance training may have a dramatic effect on the strength of ligaments and tendons. In trained bodybuilders the absolute amounts of connective tissue in the muscle are greater than those in controls, but when corrected for muscle size, the relative amounts of connective tissue remain constant. Resistance exercise may act as a ''growth promoter'' mediated by growth-promoting peptides. Increases in insulinlike growth factor I (IGF-I) have been observed in various heavy resistance exercise protocols (70, 82, 83). A combination of tropic influences could mediate increased connective tissue growth and development resulting from heavy resistance exercise.

Bone Modeling

Elite strength athletes involved in competitive forms of resistance exercise have been shown to possess elevated levels of bone minerals in both the axial and appendicular skeletons, a change that corresponds with the athletes' extremely high levels of leg, hip, back, and upper body strength (16, 17). In order for exercise to be an effective intervention for increasing bone mass in the axial skeleton, the hip and spine must receive direct mechanical loading to produce the functional adaptation of a localized increase in bone mass at these sites. Thus, many investigators have looked to more direct means of loading the axial skeleton in an effort to find a way to control and progressively increase the magnitude of the strain and the rate at which the strain is applied. Resistance exercise typically involves the performance of a selected movement against an external load. This type of training appears to provide an excellent method for controlling the critical aspects of the mechanical strain that are necessary to produce a bone-building response to the activity.

One study (98b), assessing the mineral content of the distal end of the radius in young males, showed that many athletes have greater bone mass than their less active counterparts. The evaluation revealed that top-ranked athletes—specifically, advanced weightlifters and throwers—had a greater bone mineral content than less accomplished athletes. The bone mineral values fell on a continuum, with values higher in athletes who participated in the sports with the greatest degree of lower body loading: weightlifters > throwers > runners > soccer players > swimmers (who were similar to controls).

At the 1983 World Powerlifting Championships a group of competitors was tested for the bone mineral content in the lumbar spine (44). The resulting values were extremely high and correlated well with the aggregate tonnage that each athlete had lifted over the previous year of training. At the time of this study, however, drug testing was not mandatory at international competitions, and it is probable that many of these athletes were involved in exogenous hormone (especially steroid) therapy, which would color the results of the study.

To date, only one longitudinal study has been reported in the literature on the use of traditional resistance exercise training to stimulate bone remodeling. Gleeson et al. (42) recruited premenopausal women (aged 23-46 years) to participate in a 12-month resistance exercise study designed to assess the efficacy of circuit training on the bone mass of the spine and os calcis. The investigators intentionally kept the load, volume, and intensity of exercise low in an effort to improve compliance (although no data exists to say that such a protocol improves exercise adherence). The bone mineral density of the spine increased significantly in the experimental group; however, the gain (0.81%) was small and significant only when compared to the 0.52% decrease experienced by the control group. The bone mass of the os calcis did not change in either group. Two obvious factors may have limited the adaptation of bone to this resistance exercise program. First, the degree of loading on the skeleton was extremely low; resistance exercise programs designed to increase strength typically involve loads greater than 85% of the 1RM or use less than eight repetitions/set. Secondly, the authors reported that none of the exercises directly loaded the spine or heel. The only strain that would have been experienced on the spine consequent to the training would have been that resulting from the involvement of the back musculature in stabilization during the exercises. Thus, the relatively minor changes in bone mass that resulted from the low-intensity resistance exercise program used in this study cannot be generalized to the potential effect that more intense resistance exercise programs may have on bone mass.

Two terms are used to describe the deformation of bone by external loading: *strain magnitude*, which refers to percent of maximal strength and corresponds to the load of the exercise, and *strain rate*, which refers to power output and corresponds to its intensity. The magnitude required to produce an effective stimulus for bone remodeling appears to be a 1RM to 10RM load, or 85% to 100% of 1RM. Multiple (three to six) sets of structural exercises must be performed to achieve the volume of exercise necessary to overload the musculoskeletal system sufficiently to cause hypertrophy and gains in strength. The number of loading cycles (sets and repetitions) seems to be a relatively unimportant factor in bone remodeling, provided that a minimal number of cycles is performed and that other factors dictating the mechanical strain, such as the intensity, load, and exercise selection, are appropriate. To satisfy the need for high strain rates in a dynamic loading program, such weightlifting exercises as cleans, snatches, and jerks should be incorporated into the loading program. Although these exercises require somewhat of a reduction in the magnitude of the exercise load relative to a heavy pressing movement, they dramatically and advantageously increase the rate at which the load is applied to the bone.

To create a continually changing strain distribution pattern, which would itself be viewed as an osteogenic stimulus, the choice of exercises performed needs to be varied on a regular basis, yet still provide a proper exercise stimulus. Possibilities include switching to a related exercise (e.g., snatches to cleans), making minor changes in bar placement or foot stance during squats, and altering hand spacing on the bar during overhead presses, bench presses, and rowing movements. One must keep in mind that, in changing from squats to single-leg extensions, the hip and spine are no longer receiving large compressive forces; thus, the stimulus for bone remodeling at these sites is drastically reduced or even eliminated.

Hormonal Influences

Hormones, and changes in hormone levels consequent to exercise, are vital to adaptations of the body to exercise stress (chapter 6) (39, 40, 70). Anabolic hormones, such as testosterone and growth hormone, influence the development of muscle, bone, and connective tissue. More generally and importantly, hormones are involved with a wide variety of homeostatic mechanisms that are dedicated to keeping the body's functions within a normal range during rest and exercise. If an exercise protocol involves large muscle groups and is intense enough, the exercises will stimulate the neuroendocrine system. Hormonal influences may be involved in adaptations resulting from heavy resistance training. Changes in testosterone and cortisol levels, for example, are directly linked to changes in maximal strength over training periods. Resistance exercise produces significant increases in anabolic hormones (81, 82).

AEROBIC TRAINING

Endurance training and resistance training provide a continuum of modalities that affect various physiological systems (15, 20, 48, 75, 100, 101). The magnitude of change in any program depends on the athlete's pre-training level and the characteristics of the program (89, 90). As with resistance training, endurance training requires proper progression, variation, specificity, and overload if physiological adaptations are to be effected (113). A multitude of adaptations are needed, from the cellular to the organismal level (109).

Over the past 3 decades volumes of information have been produced on endurance exercise and its subsequent training adaptations. As we have noted, aerobic metabolism plays a vital role in human performance and is basic to all sports, if for no other reason than recovery. Metabolically, the Krebs cycle and electron transport chain are the main pathways in energy production. Aerobic metabolism produces far more ATP energy than anaerobic metabolism and uses fats, carbohydrates, and proteins. Many sports involve interactions between the aerobic and anaerobic metabolic systems and thus require appropriate training. For example, soccer, lacrosse, basketball, field hockey, and ice hockey involve continuous movement (and thus constant aerobic demand) intermixed with bursts of sprint and power activities. Proper conditioning of the aerobic system is vital to the ability of the player to sustain such activity and adequately recover. (See Table 8.1, p. 130, for a guide to which energy sources various sports use.)

It appears that every athlete needs to have a basic level of cardiovascular endurance, which can be achieved using a wide variety of training modalities and programs. The traditional modality has been the long, slow distance run. For the strength-and-power athlete, however, this may be irrelevant or even detrimental to power development; adequate gains in aerobic fitness can be accomplished with interval training when appropriate and needed (22, 47). The old concept of an aerobic base for purposes of recovery in anaerobic sports is somewhat misunderstood in that athletes can gain aerobic training adaptations with a variety of training programs (e.g., interval training with short rest periods).

Basic Training Adaptations

One of the most commonly measured adaptations to endurance training is an increase in maximal oxygen uptake associated with an increase in maximal cardiac output (112). As the intensity of exercise increases, the oxygen consumption rises to maximal levels. When the demands increase to where the oxygen consumption can no longer increase, maximal oxygen uptake has been achieved. Endurance training can improve an athlete's aerobic power 5% to 30%, depending on the starting fitness level. Greater improvement can usually be attributed to exceptionally low starting levels. Metabolic changes include increased respiratory capacity, lower blood lactate concentrations at a given submaximal exercise intensity, increased mitochondrial and capillary densities, and improved enzyme activity. Although maximal oxygen uptake may not change with endurance training in athletes year to year, improvement in the oxygen cost of running does improve; several studies have shown a progressive improvement in the economy of running in elite endurance athletes. Long-term endurance training may be more involved with improving the athlete's running economy than with improving the maximal ability to extract and utilize oxygen (i.e., $\dot{V}O_2max$). Runners may not improve their $\dot{V}O_2max$ but performance may be better due to enhanced running economy (73).

The intensity of training is one of the most important factors in improving and maintaining aerobic power. Short, high-intensity bouts of interval sprints can improve maximal oxygen uptake if the interim rest period is also short. Callister et al. (14) showed that long rest periods used with sprints improve sprint speed without significant increases in maximal aerobic power. Therefore, longer training sessions result in lesser degrees of aerobic improvement as less activity is performed per unit of time.

Physiological adaptations vary according to age and gender (20, 123). Maximal aerobic power decreases with age in adults. On the average, age for age, the aerobic power values of women range from 73% to 85% of the values of men. However, the general physiological response to training is similar in men and women. The differences in aerobic power may be caused by several factors, including women's higher percentage of body fat and lower blood hemoglobin values and men's larger heart size and blood volume.

Table 8.3 lists the physiological changes that occur with short-term (3-6 month) endurance training and compares the values with those of elite endurance athletes.

Hormonal Influences

In general, during high-intensity exercise, plasma and serum concentrations of hormones can increase 10 to 20 times over their levels at rest (60, 85). Several mechanisms contribute to these changes, including changes in hepatic and extrahepatic clearance rates, shifts in blood volume, and—our concern here—exercise. High-intensity endurance training augments the absolute secretion rates of many hormones, including epinephrine, in response to maximal exercise, although trained athletes have blunted responses to submaximal exercise. Their hormone concentrations equal those of their untrained counterparts at the same relative exercise intensity. Trained athletes may have more effective mechanisms for receptor-binding interaction in the control and regulation of metabolic function. The greater hormonal

response patterns to maximal exercise appear to augment the athlete's ability to tolerate and sustain prolonged high exercise intensities. When exercise duration is short (from 5-30 s), there are few changes in peripheral blood hormone concentrations.

It appears that the role of hormones in the muscle remodeling process is different in endurance and resistance adaptations. Endurance training, especially running, is often associated with protein sloughing from the muscle, which the body attempts to offset by hormonal anabolic mechanisms. In the case of running, however, catabolic effects predominate and can lead to muscle degradation and reduction in power. It is not uncommon for elite endurance runners who are training with high mileage to be able to jump vertically only several inches. Thus, the use of resistance training to offset the catabolic effects of running may be vital for distance runners; resistance training is the only way to build muscle tissue.

Body Composition

Endurance training is associated with alterations in body composition. Endurance exercise training usually decreases the relative percentage of body fat and has little or no significant effect on fat-free mass. Longer term programs can result in greater decreases in the percentage of body fat (103, 104). When training intensity and volume balance anabolic and catabolic activities in muscle, the optimal prescription depends on the training level of the athletes and the variation in the exercise protocol. Excessive training might lead to a predominance of catabolic activity in the body and cause muscle metabolism not to be able to keep up with the needed amount of protein synthesis.

Neural Adaptations

Adaptations in the nervous system play a role in the early stages of endurance training (107). At the outset, efficiency is increased and fatigue of the contractile mechanisms delayed. The level of motor unit activation in the prime movers needed to maintain a given submaximal force decreases as skill is acquired. Additionally, improved endurance performance may also result in a rotation of neural activity among synergists and among motor units within a muscle. Thus, the athlete produces more efficient locomotion during the activity with lower energy expenditure.

Overview of Exercise Prescriptions

The configuration of the exercise stimulus is vital to the body's adaptational responses. The level of an acute exercise stimulus determines the contributions of various physiological systems in performing the exercise, and the adaptational responses to the training program

Table 8.3 Physiological Variables in Endurance

Variable	Previously untrained subjects[a]		Elite endurance athletes
	Before training	After training	
Heart rate:			
Resting (beats/min)	74	61	45
Maximal	194	190	185
Stroke volume:			
Resting (ml^2)	64	82	127
Maximal	122	142	201
Cardiac output:			
Resting (L/min)	4.5	4.6	4.4
Maximal	22.3	25.8	34.9
Heart volume (ml)	750	823	1,250
Blood volume (L)	4.8	5.2	6.1
Blood pressure:			
Resting (mm Hg)	120/80	124/78	105/65
Maximal	206/85	202/82	209/69
Pulmonary ventilation:			
Resting (L/min)	7	6	6
Maximal, BTPS	123	142	201
Breathing rate, BTPS:			
Resting (breaths/min)	14	12	11
Maximal	42	47	59
TV:			
Resting (L)	0.06	0.6	0.6
Maximal	2.8	3.1	3.1
VC (L)	2.8	3.1	3.1
RV (L)	5.8	6.1	6.4
Arteriovenous oxygen difference:			
Resting (ml/100 ml)	6.1	6.1	6.1
Maximal	14.5	15.2	16.4
Maximal oxygen uptake (ml/kg)	47	55	79
Weight (kg)	75	72	62
% body fat	16.0	14.9	6.7
% Type I fibers	55	55	81
Fiber area:			
Type I (μm^2)	4,730	4,820	4,180
Type IIa	6,860	7,150	4,299
Type IIb	6,167	6,433	3,899
Capillary density:			
Number/mm^2	290	350	460
Number/fiber	1.2	1.4	3.2
Citrate synthetase (activity units)	28	37	78
Hexokinase (activity units)	2.4	2.9	4.2
Lactate dehydrogenase (activity units)	580	654	629
Maximal fiber shortening velocity:			
Type I (fiber lengths/s)	0.86	?	1/10
Type II	4.85	?	1/74

[a]These subjects completed a short-term (3- to 6-month) endurance training program.

depend on the individual's physiological capabilities, which are largely determined by genetic predisposition.

During the past 25 years a great deal of attention has been focused on endurance training. Individualization of training protocols is now widely accepted and implemented for all types of training, for the cardiac patient and the elite endurance athlete. The primary training variables in prescribing endurance exercise are exercise intensity, exercise duration, and training session frequency. In general, as a person becomes fitter, the intensity, duration, and frequency of training sessions must increase to improve physiological function and performance. Elite endurance athletes require careful manipulation of training variables to avoid overuse or overtraining syndromes. Fardy (25) described effective ranges for these variables as the basis of individual fitness levels. Effective ranges for a highly trained athlete might be an intensity of 80% to 90% of maximum heart rate, a duration of 1 to 2 hr, and a frequency of 5 to 7 days/week, whereas corresponding values for a beginner might be 60% to 85%, 15 to 45 min, and 3 to 5 days/week. The training ranges may be modified to vary training and keep the adaptive stimulus high. Few exercise programs use the same protocol every day; scientists need to examine more realistic training protocols that are not as constant. Dynamic, rhythmic large-muscle group exercises (such as cycling or running) are typically used to improve aerobic power. Both intermittent interval and continuous training techniques can improve aerobic fitness.

Compatibility of Resistance and Endurance Training

Combining resistance and endurance activities appears to interfere primarily with strength performances at high velocities of movement (22). When strength and endurance training are done in excess (overtraining), maximal power performance is blunted (23). Possible explanations for this less-than-optimal strength-and-power development include adverse neural changes and the alterations of muscle proteins in the fibers. In contrast, no adverse effects on aerobic power have yet been observed, despite the expected cellular changes caused by heavy resistance exercise (47).

OVERTRAINING

Overtraining has been a topic of great interest over the past decade (12, 13, 87, 117, 124). The concept may be defined as excessive volume or intensity of training, or both, resulting in fatigue (which is due also to a lack of proper rest and recovery). Overtraining itself is simply the stimulus. The *overtraining syndrome* is the condition resulting from overtraining; it is sometimes referred to as ''staleness.'' This syndrome can, but does not always, include a plateau or decrease in performance. (Many alternative terms have been suggested for overtraining, including *burnout*, *chronic overwork*, *physical overstrain*, and *overfatigue*.) Additionally, some authors use the term *overtraining* only when a decline in performance occurs.

Overtraining can occur on a short-term basis, which is termed **overreaching**. Recovery from this condition is easily achieved within a few days; consequently, overreaching is often a planned phase of many training programs. Overreaching can be considered the first stage of the overtraining syndrome, which is itself the final stage of a continuum. The following overtraining continuum illustrates the progression to an overtraining syndrome.

$$\textit{Acute fatigue} \rightarrow \textit{Overload stimulus} \rightarrow \textit{Over-reaching} \rightarrow \textit{Overtraining syndrome}$$

The overtraining syndrome can last as long as 6 months, and recovery may not be immediate. This is especially true for endurance overtraining. In resistance training, however, long-term decrements have not been demonstrated, and many athletes rebound after a period of recovery. Since we now know that such rebounds are possible, it is difficult to determine when overtraining becomes chronically detrimental. In addition, some athletes ''respond'' to overtraining, whereas others do not. (So it is the training professional's responsibility to monitor each athlete's progress.) It appears that overtraining can cause dramatic decreases in performance in previously untrained people.

The overtraining syndrome involves alterations to a number of physiological systems. Two distinct types of overtraining syndromes have been suggested; sympathetic and parasympathetic syndromes. The sympathetic syndrome includes increased sympathetic activity at rest, whereas the parasympathetic syndrome includes increased parasympathetic activity at rest and with exercise. One or both can result from overtraining. Some researchers feel that the sympathetic syndrome develops before the parasympathetic syndrome and is predominant in younger subjects who train for speed or power. All overtraining can eventually result in the parasympathetic syndrome. In actuality, little data exists to support this differentiation. Injury or illness may also result from overtraining.

Overtraining in Aerobic Sports

Differences exist between aerobic and anaerobic overtraining syndromes. Among endurance athletes, physiological responses to increased volume training have been monitored in distance runners, swimmers, cyclists, and rowers. Increased training intensity has also been studied in distance runners and swimmers. Increasing the volume of training often produces performance decrements, but not in all cases. Body weight may or may not decrease, although lowered body fat percentages may result. In addition, muscle size and strength may not be affected. On the other hand, increased training intensity can result in improved physical performance.

Cardiovascular Responses.

Heart rate is affected by greater volumes of training. Resting heart rates may decrease, stay the same, or increase. In at least one instance, the decreased resting heart rates were later followed by increased heart rates. Exercise-induced maximum heart rates decrease from overtraining, as have heart rates at absolute submaximal exercise intensities. Resting blood pressures are generally not affected by increased volumes of training. However, increased training intensity can produce increased resting diastolic blood pressures without affecting resting systolic pressures.

Biochemical Responses.

High training volume results in increased levels of creatine kinase, indicating muscle damage. Lactate concentrations, on the other hand, either decrease or stay the same when training volumes increase. Blood lipids and lipoproteins are not altered by volume overtraining. Muscle glycogen decreases with prolonged periods of overtraining, although this may be largely due to dietary considerations. Decreased glycogen levels may contribute to the lowered lactate responses just noted.

Endocrine Responses.

In general, large increases in training volumes result in a catabolic state for endurance athletes, as is apparent when endocrine levels are monitored. Circulating levels of total testosterone decrease. Concentrations of free testosterone also decrease in some cases. These changes do not appear to be regulated by the pituitary, since luteinizing hormone levels are not affected. The changes in the free testosterone component appear to be independent of protein binding capacity, because concentrations of sex hormone–binding globulin are not altered. Therefore, the decreased ratio of total testosterone to sex hormone–binding globulin that can accompany increased volumes of training seems to be due to altered total testosterone levels.

Cortisol responses to increased volumes of training are variable. Specific responses appear to be dependent on contributing variables, including training protocol, diurnal variations, and whether resting or acute responses were measured. Increased cortisol concentrations have been associated with empirically identified overtraining syndromes and decreased aerobic performance. Pituitary regulation of adrenal cortex activity may be an important factor, in that decreased levels of adrenocorticotropin have resulted from overtraining protocols, although levels of this hormone may eventually increase.

The anabolic-catabolic state of an organism may be quantified by the testosterone-cortisol ratio, which decreases or stays the same with greater training volumes. The free testosterone component may be more influential physiologically. Decreases of 5% to 50% in the ratio of free testosterone to cortisol have also been reported with increased training volumes. A possible marker of an overtraining syndrome is a decrease of 30% or more in this ratio.

Decreased pituitary secretion of growth hormone occurs with overtraining. This and other endocrine responses to an overtraining stimulus appear to be due primarily to impaired hypothalamic function, not pituitary function.

Whether these altered endocrine variables are responsible for performance decrements is open to debate. Levels of testosterone, free testosterone, cortisol, total testosterone, and creatine kinase seem to simply reflect training volumes. Actual physical performance is occasionally related to total testosterone concentrations, but not in all cases.

Catecholamines appear very responsive to an overtraining stimulus. Alterations in basal levels of epinephrine, norepinephrine, and dopamine are reported to be significantly related to the severity of self-reported complaints in overtrained runners. Changes in catecholamine and cortisol concentrations may mirror each other during overtraining, although cortisol is not as sensitive to increased training volume as catecholamines are.

Severely increased volumes of training can result in decreased nocturnal levels of epinephrine, which are indicative of basal levels. Preexercise or resting levels of epinephrine are either unchanged or increased. Exercise performed at an absolute load results in increased epinephrine levels in the presence of overtraining, although maximum levels of epinephrine are unchanged. Nocturnal norepinephrine concentrations decrease with severe volume overtraining, while resting or preexercise levels increase or stay the same. Exercise at an absolute submaximal load will produce increased norepinephrine concentrations, the opposite of a normal resistance training effect. Maximal norepinephrine concentrations are not affected by overtraining.

Basal levels of dopamine decrease with volume overtraining, as do dopamine concentrations at the same absolute work load. With submaximal exercise, dopamine responses vary, but appear to counter norepinephrine patterns.

Although it is often difficult to document, severe volume overtraining of endurance athletes produces characteristics of the parasympathetic overtraining syndrome. This includes reduced sensitivity to catecholamines and may result in advanced cases of severe overtraining syndromes.

Markers of Overtraining. Due to their responsiveness to an overtraining stimulus, many of the previously mentioned physiological variables have been suggested as markers of an overtraining syndrome for endurance athletes. The following is a list of some of these variables (29):

- Decreased performance
- Decreased percentage of body fat
- Decreased maximal oxygen uptake
- Altered blood pressure
- Increased muscle soreness
- Decreased muscle glycogen
- Altered resting heart rate
- Decreased lactate
- Increased creatine kinase
- Altered cortisol concentration
- Decreased total testosterone concentration
- Decreased ratio of total testosterone to cortisol
- Decreased ratio of free testosterone to cortisol
- Decreased ratio of total testosterone to sex hormone–binding globulin
- Increased heart rate
- Decreased sympathetic tone (decreased nocturnal and resting catecholamines)
- Increased sympathetic stress response

Overtraining in Anaerobic Sports

A survey of overtrained athletes found that 77% were involved in sports requiring high levels of strength, speed, or coordination—that is, anaerobically oriented sports. This implies that athletes engaged in anaerobic activities may be more susceptible to an overtraining syndrome, perhaps the previously described sympathetic overtraining syndrome, than are endurance athletes. A theoretical schematic of the development of anaerobic overtraining syndromes is presented in Table 8.4.

Resistance exercise is the most studied anaerobic activity in the overtraining literature; interval sprinting has also been investigated. An important consideration when monitoring resistance exercise is that different exercise protocols produce different endocrine responses. As a result, postexercise observations of circulating hormones may be misleading, with preexercise or basal values preferred. However, when acute responses are properly interpreted, much valuable information is available that is not apparent with resting values. The time of postexercise blood sampling is also very important, since variable endocrine concentrations are observed with different postexercise intervals. In addition, diurnal variations must be accounted for, since acute endocrine responses to a weight training protocol are different during daytime and nightime hours.

Increasing anaerobic training volume or intensity may affect some, but not all, performance variables. It also appears that physical performance may be affected before symptoms of an overtraining syndrome appear. Anaerobic exercise overtraining does not always affect

Table 8.4   Theoretical Development of Anaerobic Overtraining

Stages of overtraining	Anaerobic performance						
	Neural	Skeletal muscle	Metabolic	Cardiovascular	Immune	Endocrine	Psychological
1st (no effect on performance)	Altered neuron function						
2nd (probably no effect on performance)	Altered motor unit recruitment					Altered sympathetic activity and hypothalamic control	
3rd (probably decreased performance)	Decreased motor coordination	Altered excitation-contraction coupling	Decreased muscle glycogen	Increased resting heart rate and blood pressure	Altered immune function	Altered hormonal concentrations	Mood disturbances
4th (decreased performance)		Decreased force production	Decreased glycolytic capacity		Sickness and infection		Emotional and sleep disturbances

From *Physiological Responses to Short-Term High Intensity Resistance Exercise Overtraining* by A. Fry, 1993, unpublished doctoral dissertation, The Pennsylvania State University.

such variables as criteria weightlifting exercises, aerobic power, and vertical jump height. However, decreased body fat, slower sprint speed, and decreased isometric and isokinetic quadricep strength may develop. Increased weight training intensity appears to alter motor patterns before force production capabilities are decreased. Training intensity (a given percent of 1RM) and strength alterations (percent change in 1RM) in resistance exercise are also related to various physical performance tests. Anaerobic overtraining does not ordinarily alter body weight, resting blood pressure, or resting heart rate. Exercise-induced lactate concentrations decrease or are unchanged with anaerobic overtraining.

Endocrine Responses.

Studies of anaerobic overtraining have monitored either resting hormonal concentrations or a combination of resting and acute concentrations. The immediate postexercise responses to weight training vary depending on the exercise protocol. Testosterone concentrations increase after many protocols, depending on exercise intensity and training experience, but not strength levels. In general, acute endocrine responses seem to reflect training stresses and competitive lifting performance. Testosterone may be the hormone most sensitive to the stresses of an anaerobic training program and the one that adapts most readily to increased volumes of training.

Increased volumes of anaerobic exercise result in decreased, increased, or unchanged resting total or free testosterone levels. Exercise-induced testosterone levels either decrease or increase. These seemingly opposing results may be dependent on the training stresses experienced prior to the respective investigations, since increases in exercise-induced testosterone, but not resting levels, have been observed over the course of a year of training. Resting luteinizing hormone levels may increase or stay the same in response to greater training volumes and seem to reflect resting testosterone levels.

Increasing training intensity does not seem to affect resting values of total testosterone, but may produce decreased free testosterone levels. This is accompanied by increased resting luteinizing hormone levels, with intense training affecting the free component of testosterone more. In this manner, luteinizing hormone is most closely associated with free testosterone concentrations following high-intensity training.

Increased volumes of anaerobic exercise usually increase preexercise cortisol concentrations. Normal training for 1 year does not alter resting cortisol levels. Acute cortisol levels, however, will sometimes decrease. Overtraining by increasing exercise intensity will also raise resting levels of cortisol. The relationship between postexercise cortisol and testosterone suggests that cortisol concentrations are not responsible for the resulting testosterone responses.

The resting or exercise-induced anabolic-catabolic status of an athlete, as assessed by the ratio of total testosterone to cortisol, does not change with a year of normal training. Anaerobic volume overtraining lowers or does not affect the ratio of resting total testosterone to cortisol and appears to result in less variability with an exercise stimulus. Increased training intensity also lowers this ratio. Resting levels of sex hormone–binding globulin are not affected by greater training intensities. The ratio of total testosterone to sex hormone–binding globulin, which indicates free testosterone levels, is also unaffected by intensity, although increased training volumes lower this ratio. Acute growth hormone levels decrease after weight training volumes are increased.

Testosterone concentrations are related to performance over a 1-year period, as are ratios of total testosterone to cortisol and total testosterone to sex hormone–binding globulin. In addition, these ratios are related to force production in the quadriceps and competitive lifting performance.

To the author's knowledge, no anaerobic overtraining studies have investigated catecholamine responses. Epinephrine and norepinephrine levels are directly related to exercise intensities. However, the actual time course of epinephrine and norepinephrine secretion differ at various intensities. The acute catecholamine response to anaerobic exercise may also be dependent on the athlete's strength levels and physical characteristics.

Neuromuscular Responses.

As with catecholamines, few data are available on neuromuscular responses to overtraining. Neural adaptations precede contractile tissue adaptations to a resistance exercise program. Neural activity, as indicated by integrated electromyography (IEMG), and force capabilities reflect training volume primarily in elite strength athletes. Diurnal variations are not evident for maximal IEMG activity and isometric force capabilities. Likewise, 1 week of increased volume training did not affect morning or afternoon IEMG activity or force. In addition, increased volumes of anaerobic training did not alter IEMG activity during maximal isometric quadricep force production. Isokinetic quadricep strength may decrease in both volume and intensity overtraining. Increasing training volume, however, does not produce impaired weightlifting performances.

Markers of Overtraining.

The previously mentioned physiological responses to anaerobic overtraining may be markers of an overtraining syndrome. The endocrine responses, however, appear to require longer than 1 week of monitoring to serve as adequate markers. The most effective markers may be those associated with a sympathetic overtraining syndrome, because this may be the first response to anaerobic overtraining.

A recent theory on the mechanisms of overtraining proposes that the central nervous system neurotransmitter serotonin is produced excessively. Serotonin is often associated with sleep and fatiguing conditions. The serotonin precursor, tryptophan, competes with branched-chain amino acids (valine, leucine, and isoleucine) when crossing the blood-brain barrier. It has been theorized that dietary supplementation with branched-chain amino acids would contribute to decreased levels of serotonin in the brain. Overtraining and supplementation studies with weightlifters, however, have not supported this theory.

Psychological Factors in Overtraining

Mood disturbances, as determined from a profile of mood states, have been associated with increased training volumes. Subscales from this profile have been used successfully to identify athletes suffering from an overtraining syndrome, exhibiting the classic ''inverted iceberg profile.'' Heavy training has been accompanied by decreased vigor, motivation, confidence, and concentration and raised levels of tension, depression, anger, fatigue, confusion, anxiety, and irritability. Altered psychological characteristics are also related to changing endocrine profiles. Many athletes may know when they are excessively overtrained, due in part to the concomitant psychological alterations. Many times the psychological factors are observed before changes in physical performance are. Monitoring the mood and mental state of athletes is very important to gaining insights into overtraining (121).

RECOVERY TECHNIQUES

Recovery from exercise has long been a topic of great interest for athletes. However, recovery techniques have been limited to only a relatively small number of studies and are usually discussed more in terms of anecdotal evidence than experimental fact. Efficacy of recovery has thus been attributed to many different modalities—everything from whirlpool baths and massage to electrostimulation, cryotherapy, and heat. Each of these in its own right may be effective in various situations, especially where injury is present. Still, each needs to be examined for each sport for which claims are made.

Warm-up and cool-down activities are typically promoted in sports and can help in preparation and recovery. Warm-up is important to increasing muscle temperature and activating metabolic systems to the level needed at the start of competition. Warm-up is typically followed by flexibility exercises and then more sport-specific warm-up. It is not completely understood how warm-up affects performance and injury prevention, but most athletes feel more comfortable and ready for competition after appropriate warm-up is conducted.

A strong case can be made for cool-down activities. One of the most obvious examples is the importance of proper cool-down in enhancing lactic acid removal from muscle tissue after intense anaerobic activity. The removal of lactic acid is improved when light- to moderate-intensity exercise is performed, as opposed to attempting to recover without any activity in the muscles involved. For example, dramatic elevations in lactic acid levels (20-40 times above resting levels) occur in the muscles after a wrestling match. Rather than allowing the wrestler to come off the mat and slump down on a chair, the wrestler should be encouraged to skip rope or jog around the gym for 5 to 10 min. In a tournament in which another match might be scheduled within the hour, getting rid of the lactic acid, which will inhibit subsequent performance, allows the wrestler to better recover. Regardless of the metabolic nature of the sport, adequate cool-down is needed for the appropriate transition of the body from intense exercise stress to rest.

Nutritional factors probably play the most important role in recovery from exercise training and competition. Within 30 min after a sport activity or exercise training, either of which significantly depletes glycogen stores in the muscles and liver, carbohydrate stores need to be replenished. If carbohydrates are ingested within this acute period of recovery, glycogen repletion is enhanced. Additionally, it is of the utmost importance during and after sport competitions and exercise training sessions that time be taken to drink an adequate amount of fluids to rehydrate the body. Because the thirst mechanism does not indicate perfectly the need for water, athletes often have to be forced to drink adequate amounts of water.

DETRAINING

If inactivity, rather than proper recovery, occurs following exercise, an athlete loses training adaptations—that is, he or she experiences **detraining**. Little is known about detraining following various conditioning protocols. Endurance adaptations are most sensitive to periods of inactivity because of their enzymatic basis. In contrast, strength changes appear more resistant to short periods of inactivity and decay over time at a much slower rate. The exact cellular mechanisms that mediate detraining changes are unknown; further research is needed to clarify the underlying physiological mechanisms; it appears that when detraining occurs, the physiological function goes back to the normal untrained state of the individual.

Periodization of training attempts to provide for adequate recovery while preventing the athlete from becoming detrained. With the use of proper exercise variation, maintenance programs, and active recovery periods, adequate protection against serious detraining effects is possible.

Responses to detraining of various variables are shown in Figure 8.4.

CONCLUSION

Exercise training is related to the configuration of the exercise stimulus to gain specific changes in the body. Exercise programs must adhere to proper specificity, progression, variation, and recovery in order for adaptations to be optimized. Furthermore, different athletes have different adaptational responses to an exercise training program. Optimal training adaptations rest on the process of exercise prescription where the right "tools" are used for the job. In reality, the day-to-day accountability of the athlete to training and the appropriate progression in exercise prescriptions by the strength and conditioning specialist are what make up optimal training programs for athletes.

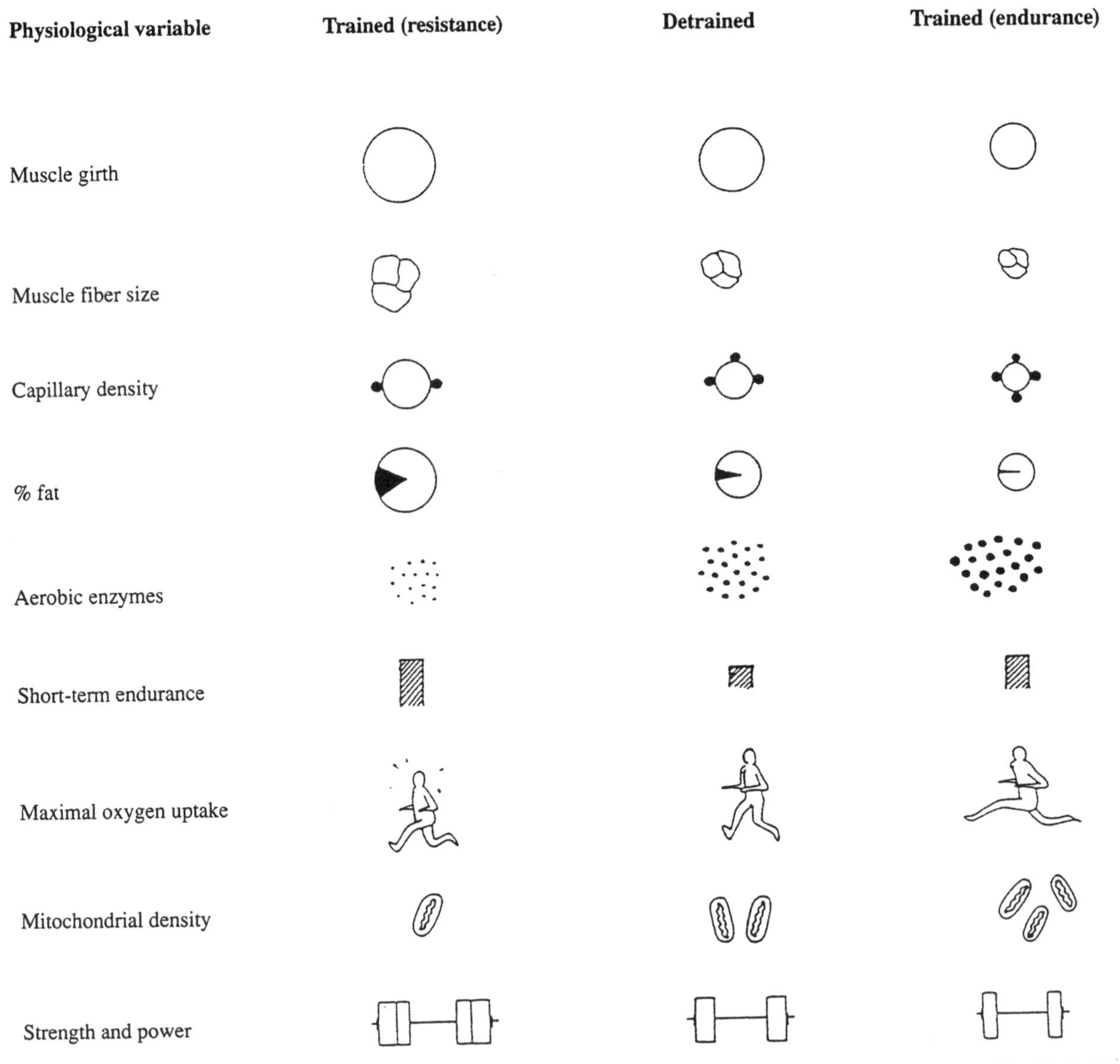

Figure 8.4 Relative responses of physiological variables to training and detraining.
Reprinted from Fleck and Kraemer (1987).

Key Terms

Study Questions

1. The highest lactic acid concentrations in the muscle would be observed after which of the following exercise protocols?

   a. maximal exercise lasting 15 s
   b. maximal exercise lasting 1 to 2 min
   c. two intermittent maximal exercise bouts of 20 s
   d. maximal exercise lasting 30 min

2. Chronic anaerobic training involving glycolysis results in

   a. better blood protein–buffering ability
   b. better hydrogen ion–buffering ability in the muscle and blood
   c. lactate-buffering ability in the blood
   d. hydrogen ion–buffering ability in the muscle only

3. In elite endurance athletes, primary training adaptations are

   I.   increase in maximal oxygen uptake
   II. increase in pulmonary ventilation
   III. increase in running economy
   IV. decrease in muscle fiber size

   a. I and III only
   b. I and II only
   c. I, II, and III only
   d. I, II, III, and IV

4. Many of the primary training adaptations in the aerobic metabolic cycles are related to

   a. increases in enzyme concentrations
   b. decreases in protein metabolism
   c. changes in nerve function
   d. elevations in body core temperature

5. In wrestling or judo what might not change with overtraining?

   a. maximal anaerobic sprint performance
   b. changes in muscle strength at various velocities of movement
   c. resting heart rate
   d. mood states

6. What is the best marker of overtraining in all athletes?

   a. heart rate
   b. blood pressure changes
   c. none at this time
   d. muscle strength changes

7. After an 800-m time trial to get into the finals, an athlete should do which of the following to facilitate removal of lactic acid from the blood?

   a. perform stretching exercises
   b. sit and rest quietly
   c. perform moderate-intensity jogging
   d. drink several glasses of water

8. Long-term recovery is promoted only if

   a. proper nutritional intake is achieved
   b. muscles are immersed in cold water
   c. proper cool-down is performed
   d. muscles are immersed in warm water

9. When endurance athletes detrain, they first observe a decline in

   a. maximal strength
   b. maximal power
   c. maximal oxygen consumption
   d. maximal heart size

10. Detraining results in which of the following?

   a. decreased performance in all cases
   b. a return to exactly the same pretraining values
   c. a decline in all physical functional capacities
   d. a loss of muscle proteins in all cases

Applying Knowledge
of General Adaptations

Problem 1

Set up a three-column table. On the top row list the training goals of strength, power, and local muscular endurance. List the proper RM values below each training goal. Below the RM values list the number of sets to be performed for the untrained athlete and advanced trained athlete. List the reasons for differences in the two training programs and determine the volume of exercise for each training variable.

Problem 2

Characterize the sports of wrestling, soccer, and basketball in terms of the following:

- Which of the sports would have the highest lactic acid response to competition?
- Rank the three sports with regard to their glycolytic component.
- Which of the three sports would have the highest aerobic component?
- Rank the three sports for their aerobic component.
- Since aerobic metabolism starts to play a significant role after about 30 s, explain how the aerobic system interacts with the anaerobic systems in each of the three sports. Give specific examples of the metabolic demands of the various skills used in the three sports.
- Now design a mode-specific resistance training program for each sport that would mimic the metabolic demands of each. Take into consideration the variety of skills performed in each sport.

Problem 3

Describe the differences between aerobic and anaerobic overtraining. Develop a profile for both an aerobic and anaerobic athlete showing overtraining variables. Write down a month-to-month progression of the values for each variable with overtraining being observed at 6 months. Graph the curves. What factors would affect recovery and what might be suggestive of overtraining prior to the 6-month point? Would all athletes on a team respond in the same way to an overtraining situation?

References

1. American College of Sports Medicine. The recommended quantity and quality of exercise for developing and maintaining fitness in healthy adults. *Med. Sci. Sports Exerc.* 10:vii-x. 1978.

2. Andersen, P., and J. Henriksson. Capillary supple of the quadriceps femoris muscle of man: Adaptive response to exercise. *J. Physiol.* 270:677-690. 1977.

3. Anderson, T., and J.T. Kearney. Effects of three resistance training programs on muscular strength and absolute and relative endurance. *Res. Q. Exerc. Sport.* 53:1-7. 1982.

4. Astrand, P.O. Physical performance as a function of age. *JAMA* 205:729-733. 1968.

5. Astrand, P.O., and K. Rodahl. *Textbook of Work Physiology.* 3rd ed. New York: McGraw-Hill. 1986.

6. Atha, J. Strengthening muscle. *Exerc. Sport Sci. Rev.*, D.I. Miller, ed. 9:1-73. 1981.

7. Bevegard, B.S., and J.R. Shepherd. Regulation of the circulation during exercise in man. *Physiol. Rev.* 47:178-213. 1967.

8. Brooks, G.A. Anaerobic threshold: Review of the concept and directions for future research. *Med. Sci. Sports Exerc.* 17:22-34. 1985.

9. Brooks, G.A., and T.D. Fahey. *Exercise Physiology: Human Bioenergetics and Its Applications.* New York: Wiley. 1984.

10. Brown, R.L., E.C. Frederick, H.L. Falsetti, E.R. Burke, and A.J. Ryan. Overtraining of athletes—a round table. *Phys. Sportsmed.* 11(6):93-110. 1983.

11. Brynteson, P., and W.E. Sinning. The effects of training frequencies on the retention of cardiovascular fitness. *Med. Sci. Sports.* 5:20-33. 1973.

12. Budgett, R. Overtraining syndrome. *Br. J. Sports Med.* 24(4):231-236. 1990.

13. Callister, R., R.J. Callister, S.J. Fleck, and G.A. Dudley. Physiological and performance responses to overtraining in elite judo athletes. *Med. Sci. Sports Exerc.* 22(6):816-824. 1990.

14. Callister, R., M.J. Shealy, S.J. Fleck, and G.A. Dudley. Performance adaptations to sprint, endurance and both modes of training. *J. Appl. Sport Sci. Res.* 2:46-51. 1988.

15. Clausen, J.P. Effect of physical training on cardiovascular adjustments to exercise in man. *Physiol. Rev.* 57:779-815. 1977.

16. Colletti, L.A., J. Edwards, L. Gordon, J. Shary, and N.H. Bell. The effects of muscle-building exercise on bone mineral density of the radius, spine, and hip in young men. *Calcif. Tissue Int.* 45:12-14. 1989.

17. Conroy, B.P., W.J. Kraemer, C.M. Maresh, and G.P. Dalsky. Adaptive responses of bone to physical activity. *Med. Exerc. Nutr. Health.* 1(2):64-74. 1992.

18. Costill, D.L. Metabolic responses during distance running. *J. Appl. Physiol.* 28:251-255. 1970.

19. Costill, D.L., M.G. Flynn, J.P. Kirwan, J.A. Houmard, J.B. Mitchell, R. Thomas, and S.H. Park. Effects of repeated days of intensified training on muscle glycogen and swimming performance. *Med. Sci. Sports Exerc.* 20(3):249-254. 1988.

20. Drinkwater, B. Physiological responses of women to exercise. *Exerc. Sport Sci. Rev.* 1:125-153. 1973.

21. Dudley, G.A. Metabolic consequences of resistive-type exercise. *Med. Sci. Sports Exerc.* 20(Suppl.):S158-S161. 1988.

22. Dudley, G.A., and R. Djamil. Incompatibility of endurance- and strength-training modes of exercise. *J. Appl. Physiol.* 59:1446-1451. 1985.

23. Dudley, G.A., and S.J. Fleck. Strength and endurance training: Are they mutually exclusive? *Sports Med.* 4:79-85. 1987.

24. Falkel, J.E., M.N. Sawka, L. Levine, et al. Upper to lower body muscular strength and endurance ratios for women and men. *Ergonomics* 28:1661-1670. 1985.

25. Fardy, P.S. Training for aerobic power. In: *Toward an Understanding of Human Performance*, E.J. Burke, ed. Ithaca, NY: Movement Publications. 1977. pp. 10-14.

26. Fleck, S.J. Cardiovascular adaptations to resistance training. *Med. Sci. Sports Exerc.* 20(Suppl.):S146-S151. 1988.

27. Fleck, S.J., R. Bartels, E.L. Fox, and W.J. Kraemer. Isokinetic total work increases and peak force training cut-off points. *NSCA Journal* 4(2):22-24. 1982.

28. Fleck, S.J., J.B. Bennett, III, W.J. Kraemer, and T.R. Baechle. Left ventricular hypertrophy in highly strength trained males. In: *Proc. 2nd International Conference on Sports Cardiology*, T. Lubich, A. Venerando, and P. Zeppilli, eds. 2:302-311. 1989.

29. Fleck, S.J., and W.J. Kraemer. The overtraining syndrome. *NSCA Journal.* 4(4):50-51. 1982.

30. Fleck, S.J., and W.J. Kraemer. Hyperplasia vs. hypertrophy. *NSCA Journal* 5(1):62-63. 1983.

31. Fleck, S.J., and W.J. Kraemer. *Designing Resistance Training Programs.* Champaign, IL: Human Kinetics. 1987.

32. Fleck, S.J., and W.J. Kraemer. Resistance training: Basic principles. *Phys. Sportsmed.* 16(3):160-171. 1988.

33. Fleck, S.J., and W.J. Kraemer. Resistance training: Physiological responses and adaptations. Part 2. *Phys. Sportsmed.* 16(4):108-124. 1988.

34. Fleck, S.J., and W.J. Kraemer. Resistance training: Physiological responses and adaptations. Part 3. *Phys. Sportsmed.* 16(5):63-73. 1988.

35. Fox, E.L., R.W. Bowers, and M.L. Foss. *The Physiological Basis of Physical Education and Athletics*, 4th ed. Dubuque, IA: Brown. 1988.

36. Fry, A.C., and W.J. Kraemer. Physical performance characteristics of American collegiate football players. *J. Appl. Sport Sci. Res.* 5(3):126-138. 1991.

37. Fry, A.C., W.J. Kraemer, C.A. Weseman, B.P. Conroy, S.E. Gordon, J.R. Hoffman, and C.M. Maresh. The effects of an off-season strength and conditioning program on starters and non starters in women's intercollegiate volleyball. *J. Appl. Sport Sci. Res.* 5(4):174-181. 1991.

38. Gaesser, G.A., and L.A. Wilson. Effects of continuous and interval training on the parameters of the power-endurance time relationship for high-intensity exercise. *Int. J. Sports Med.* 9:417-421. 1988.

39. Galbo, H. Endocrinology and metabolism in exercise. *Int. J. Sports Med.* 2:203-211. 1981.

40. Galbo, H. *Hormonal and Metabolic Adaptation to Exercise.* New York: Thieme-Stratton. 1983.

41. Gettman, L.R., and M.L. Pollock. Circuit weight training: A critical review of its physiological benefits. *Phys. Sportsmed.* 9:44-60. 1981.

42. Gleeson, P.B., E.J. Protas, A.D. LeBlanc, V.S. Schneider, and H.J. Evans. Effects of weight lifting on bone mineral density in premenopausal women. *J. Bone Miner. Res.* 5(2):153-158. 1990.

43. Gollnick, P.D. Relationship of strength and endurance with skeletal muscle structure and metabolic potential. *Int. J. Sports Med.* 3(Suppl. 1):26-32. 1982.

44. Granhed, H., R. Johnson, and T. Hansson. The loads on the lumbar spine during extreme weight lifting. *Spine* 12:146-149. 1987.

45. Harman, E.A., P.M. Frykman, E.R. Clagett, and W.J. Kraemer. Intra-abdominal and intra-thoracic pressure during lifting and jumping. *Med. Sci. Sports Exerc.* 20:195-201. 1988.

46. Harman, E.A., M.T. Rosenstein, P.M. Frykman, R.M. Rosenstein, and W.J. Kraemer. Estimation of human power output from maximal vertical jump and body mass. *J. Appl. Sport Sci. Res.* 5(3):116-120. 1991.

47. Hickson, R.C. Interference of strength development by simultaneously training for strength and endurance. *Eur. J. Appl. Physiol.* 45:255-263. 1980.

48. Hickson, R.C., H.A. Bomze, and J.O. Holloszy. Linear increase in aerobic power induced by a strenuous program of endurance exercise. *J. Appl. Physiol.* 42:372-376. 1977.

49. Hickson, R.C., B.A. Dvorak, E.M. Gorostiaga, T.T. Kurowski, and C. Foster. Potential for strength and endurance training to amplify endurance performance. *J. Appl. Physiol.* 65:2285-2290. 1988.

50. Hoffman, J.R., A.C. Fry, R. Howard, C.M. Maresh, and W.J. Kraemer. Strength, speed, and endurance changes during the course of a Division I basketball season. *J. Appl. Sport Sci. Res.* 5(3):144-149. 1991.

51. Hoffman, J.R., W.J. Kraemer, A.C. Fry, M. Deschenes, and M. Kemp. The effects of self-selection for frequency of training in a winter conditioning program for football. *J. Appl. Sport Sci. Res.* 4(3):76-82. 1990.

52. Hoffman, T., R.W. Stauffer, and A.S. Jackson. Sex differences in strength. *Am. J. Sports Med.* 7:265-267. 1979.

53. Holloszy, J.O. Biochemical adaptations to exercise: Aerobic metabolism. *Exerc. Sport Sci. Rev.* 1:45-71. 1973.

54. Holloszy, J.O. Adaptation of skeletal muscle to endurance exercise. *Med. Sci. Sports.* 7:155-164. 1975.

55. Holloszy, J.O., and F.W. Booth. Biochemical adaptations to endurance exercise in muscle. *Annu. Rev. Physiol.* 38:273-291. 1976.

56. Howald, H. Training-induced morphological and functional changes in skeletal muscle. *Int. J. Sports Med.* 3:1-12. 1982.

57. Jansson, E., B. Sjodin, and P. Tesch. Changes in muscle fibre type distribution in man after physical training: A sign of fibre transformation? *Acta Physiol. Scand.* 104:235-237. 1978.

58. Karvonen, M.J., E. Kentala, and O. Mustala. The effects of training on heart rate: A longitudinal study. *Ann. Med. Exp. Biol. Fenn.* 35:307-315. 1957.

59. Keul, J., H.H. Dickhuth, M. Lehmann, and J. Staiger. The athlete's heart: Haemodynamics and structure. *Int. J. Sports Med.* 3(Suppl. 1):33-43. 1982.

60. Kjaer, M. Epinephrine and some other hormonal responses to exercise in man; with special reference to physical training. *Int. J. Sports Med.* 10:2-15. 1989.

61 Knuttgen, H.G., and W.J. Kraemer. Terminology and measurement in exercise performance. *J. Appl. Sport Sci. Res.* 1:1-10. 1987.

62. Kraemer, W.J. The physiological basis for conditioning in wrestling. *NSCA Journal* 4(3):49. 1982.

63. Kraemer, W.J. Exercise prescription in weight training: A needs analysis. *NSCA Journal* 5(1):64-65. 1983.

64. Kraemer, W.J. Exercise prescription in weight training: Manipulating program variables. *NSCA Journal* 5(3):58-59. 1983.

65. Kraemer, W.J. Exercise recovery. *NSCA Journal* 5(3):35-36, 63. 1983.

66. Kraemer, W.J. Measurement of strength. In: *Proc. White House Symposium on Physical Fitness and Sports Medicine.* A. Weltman and C.G. Spain, eds. Washington, DC: President's Council on Fitness and Sports. 1983. pp. 35-36.

67. Kraemer, W.J. Strength development for collision sports. In: *Proc. White House Symposium on Physical Fitness and Sports Medicine.* A. Weltman and C.G. Spain, eds. Washington, DC: President's Council on Fitness and Sports. 1983. pp. 60-62.

68. Kraemer, W.J. Physiological aspects for conditioning in wrestling. *NSCA Journal* 6(1):40-42. 1984.

69. Kraemer, W.J. Programming: Variables in successful program design. *NSCA Journal* 6(2):54-55. 1984.

70. Kraemer, W.J. Endocrine responses to resistance exercise. *Med. Sci. Sports Exerc.* 20(Suppl.):152-157. 1988.

71. Kraemer, W.J. Physiological and cellular effects of exercise training. In: *Sports-Induced Inflammation*, W.B. Leadbetter, J.A. Buckwalter, and S.L. Gordon, eds. Park Ridge, IL: American Academy of Orthopaedic Surgeons. 1990. pp. 659-676.

72. Kraemer, W.J., and T.R. Baechle. Development of a strength training program. In: *Sports Medicine*, 2nd ed. F.L. Allman and A.J. Ryan, eds. Orlando: Academic Press. 1989. pp. 113-127.

73. Kraemer, W.J., and W.L. Daniels. Physiological effects of training. In: *Sports Physical Therapy*, D.B. Bernhardt, ed. New York: Churchill Livingston. 1986. pp. 29-53.

74. Kraemer, W.J., M.R. Deschenes, and S.J. Fleck. Physiological adaptations to resistance exercise: Implications for athletic conditioning. *Sports Med.* 6:246-256. 1988.

75. Kraemer, W.J., and S.J. Fleck. Aerobic metabolism, training, and evaluation. *NSCA Journal* 5(5):52-54. 1982.

76. Kraemer, W.J., and S.J. Fleck. Anaerobic metabolism and its evaluation. *NSCA Journal* 4(2):20-21. 1982.

77. Kraemer, W.J., and S.J. Fleck. Resistance training: Exercise prescription. Part 4. *Phys. Sportsmed.* 16(6):69-81. 1988.

78. Kraemer, W.J., S.J. Fleck, R. Callister, M. Shealy, G. Dudley, C.M. Maresh, L. Marchitelli, C. Cruthirds, T. Murray, and J.E. Falkel. Training responses of plasma beta-endorphin, adrenocorticotropin and cortisol. *Med. Sci. Sports Exerc.* 21(2):146-153. 1989.

79. Kraemer, W.J., S.J. Fleck, and M.R. Deschenes. A review: Factors in exercise prescription of resistance training. *NSCA Journal* 10(5):36-41. 1988.

80. Kraemer, W.J., A.C. Fry, P.N. Frykman, B. Conroy, and J. Hoffman. Resistance training and youth. *Pediatr. Exerc. Sci.* 1:336-350. 1989.

81. Kraemer, W.J., A.C. Fry, B.J. Warren, M.H. Stone, S.J. Fleck, J.T. Kearney, B.P. Conroy, C.M. Maresh, C.A. Weseman, N.T. Triplett, and S.E. Gordon. Acute hormonal responses in elite junior weightlifters. *Int. J. Sports Med.* 13(2):103-109. 1992.

82. Kraemer, W.J., S.E. Gordon, S.J. Fleck, L.J. Marchitelli, R. Mello, J.E. Dziados, K. Friedl, E. Harman, C. Maresh, and A.C. Fry. Endogenous anabolic hormonal and growth factor responses to heavy resistance exercise in males and females. *Int. J. Sports Med.* 12(2):228-235. 1991.

83. Kraemer, W.J., L. Marchitelli, D. McCurry, R. Mello, J.E. Dziados, E. Harman, P. Frykman, S.E. Gordon, and S.J. Fleck. Hormonal and growth factor responses to heavy resistance exercise. *J. Appl. Physiol.* 69(4):1442-1450. 1990.

84. Kraemer, W.J., B.J. Noble, B.W. Culver, and M.J. Clark. Physiologic responses to heavy-resistance exercise with very short rest periods. *Int. J. Sports Med.* 8:247-252. 1987.

85. Kraemer, W.J., B.J. Noble, B. Culver, and R.V. Lewis. Changes in plasma proenkephalin peptide F and catecholamine levels during graded exercise in men. *Proc. Natl. Acad. Sci. U.S.A.* 82:6349-6351. 1985.

86. Kraemer, W.J., J.F. Patton, H.G. Knuttgen, L.J. Marchitelli, C. Cruthirds, A. Damokosh, E. Harman, P. Frykman, and J.E. Dziados. Hypothalamic-pituitary-adrenal responses to short duration high-intensity cycle exercise. *J. Appl. Physiol.* 66:161-166. 1989.

87. Kuipers, H., and H.A. Keizer. Overtraining in elite athletes: Review and directions for the future. *Sports Med.* 6:79-92. 1988.

88. Laubach, L.L. Comparative muscular strength of men and women: A review of the literature. *Aviat. Space Environ. Med.* 47:534-542. 1976.

89. Lesmes, G.R., E.L. Fox, C. Stevens, and R. Otto. Metabolic responses of females to high-intensity interval training of different frequencies. *Med. Sci. Sports.* 10:229-232. 1978.

90. Lortie, G., J.A. Simoneau, P. Hamel, M.R. Boulag, F. Landry, and C. Bouchard. Responses of maximal aerobic power and capacity to aerobic training. *Int. J. Sports Med.* 5:232-236. 1984.

91. Luthi, J.M., H. Howald, H. Classen, K. Rösler, P. Vock, and H. Hoppeler. Structural changes in skeletal muscle tissue with heavy-resistance exercise. *Int. J. Sports Med.* 7:123-127. 1986.

92. MacDougall, J.D. Adaptations of muscle to strength training; a cellular approach. In: *Biochemistry of Exercise VI: Metabolic Regulation and Its Significance*, B. Saltin, ed. Champaign, IL: Human Kinetics. 1986. pp. 501-513.

93. MacDougall, J.D. Morphological changes in human skeletal muscle following strength training and immobilization. In: *Human Muscle Power*, N.L. Jones, N. McCartney, and A.J. McComas, eds. Champaign, IL: Human Kinetics. 1986. pp. 269-288.

94. MacDougall, J.D., D.G. Sale, J.R. Moroz, G.C.B. Eider, J.R. Sutton, and H. Howald. Mitochondrial volume density in human skeletal muscle following heavy resistance training. *Med. Sci. Sports Exerc.* 11:164-166. 1979.

95. Maresh, C.M., T.G. Allison, B.J. Noble, A. Drash, and W.J. Kraemer. Substrate and endocrine responses to race-intensity exercise following a marathon run. *Int. J. Sports Med.* 10(2):101-106. 1989.

96. Matveyev, L. *Fundamentals of Sports Training.* Moscow: Progress Publishers. 1981.

97. Moody, D.L., J.H. Wilmore, R.N. Girandola, et al. The effects of a jogging program on the body composition of normal and obese high school girls. *Med. Sci. Sports.* 4:210-213. 1972.

98a. Moritani, T., and H.A. De Vries. Neural factors versus hypertrophy in the time course of muscle strength gain. *Am. J. Phys. Med.* 58:115-130. 1979.

98b. Nilsson, B.E., and N.E. Westlin. Bone densities in athletics. *Clin. Orth. Rel. Res.* 77:179-182. 1971.

99. Noble, B.J. *Physiology of Exercise and Sport.* St. Louis: Times Mirror/Mosby. 1986.

100. Patton, J.F., W.L. Daniels, and J.A. Vogel. Aerobic power and body fat of men and women during army basic training. *Aviat. Space Environ. Med.* 51:492-496. 1980.

101. Patton, J.F., W.J. Kraemer, H.G. Knuttgen, and E.A. Harman. Factors in maximal power production and in exercise endurance relative to maximal power. *Eur. J. Appl. Physiol.* 60:222-227. 1990.

102. Pollock, M.L. The qualification of endurance training programs. *Exerc. Sport Sci. Rev.* 1:155-188. 1973.

103. Pollock, M.L., T.K. Cureton, and L. Greninger. Effects of frequency of training on working capacity, cardiovascular function and body composition of adult men. *Med. Sci. Sports Exerc.* 1:70-74. 1969.

104. Pollock, M.L., and A. Jackson. Body composition: Measurement and changes resulting from physical training. In: *Toward an Understanding of Human Performance*, E.J. Burke, ed. Ithaca, NY: Movement Publications. 1977. pp. 21-36.

105. Rowell, L.B. Human cardiovascular adjustments to exercise and thermal stress. *Physiol. Rev.* 54:75-159. 1974.

106. Sale, D.G. Neural adaptation in strength and power training. In: *Human Muscle Power*, N.L. Jones, N. McCartney, and A.J. McComas, eds. Champaign, IL: Human Kinetics. 1986. pp. 289-307.

107. Sale, D.G. Influence of exercise and training on motor unit activation. *Exerc. Sport Sci. Rev.* 15:95-151. 1987.

108. Sale, D.G. Neural adaptation to resistance training. *Med. Sci. Sports Exerc.* 20(Suppl.):S135-S145. 1988.

109. Saltin, B. Physiological effects of physical conditioning. *Med. Sci. Sports Exerc.* 1:50-56. 1969.

110. Saltin, B., and P.O. Astrand. Maximal oxygen uptake in athletes. *J. Appl. Physiol.* 23:252-258. 1967.

111. Schantz, P.G. Plasticity of human skeletal muscle with special reference to effect of physical training on enzyme levels of the NADH shuttles and phenotypic expression of slow and fast myofibrillar proteins. *Acta Physiol. Scand.* 558(Suppl.):1-62. 1986.

112. Scheuer, J., and C.M. Tipton. Cardiovascular adaptations to physical training. *Annu. Rev. Physiol.* 39:221-251. 1977.

113. Sjodin, B., and J. Svedenhag. Applied physiology of marathon running. *Sports Med.* 2:83-99. 1985.

114. Staron, R.S., R.S. Hikida, F.C. Hagerman, G.A. Dudley, and T.F. Murray. Human skeletal muscle fiber type adaptability to various workloads. *J. Histochem. Cytochem.* 32:146-152. 1984.

115. Stone, M.H. Implications for connective tissue and bone alterations resulting from resistance exercise training. *Med. Sci. Sports Exerc.* 20(Suppl.):S162-S168. 1988.

116. Stone, M.H., S.J. Fleck, N.T. Triplett, and W.J. Kraemer. Health- and performance-related potential of resistance training. *Sports Med.* 11(4):210-231. 1991.

117. Stone, M.H., R.E. Keith, J.T. Kearney, S.J. Fleck, G.D. Wilson, and N.T. Triplett. Overtraining: A review of the signs, symptoms and possible causes. *J. Appl. Sports Sci. Res.* 5(1):35-50. 1991.

118. Tesch, P.A. Acute and long-term metabolic changes consequent to heavy-resistance exercise. In: *Muscular Function in Exercise and Training*, P. Marconnet and P.V. Komi, eds. Basel, Switzerland: Karger. 1987. pp. 67-89.

119. Tesch, P.A. Skeletal muscle adaptations consequent to long-term heavy-resistance exercise. *Med. Sci. Sports Exerc.* 20(Suppl.):S124-S132. 1988.

120. Tesch, P.A., P.V. Komi, and K. Häkkinen. Enzymatic adaptations consequent to long-term strength training. *Int. J. Sports Med.* 8(Suppl.1):66-69. 1987.

121. Tharion, W.J., T.M. Rausch, E.A. Harman, and W.J. Kraemer. Effects of different resistance exercise protocols on mood states. *J. Appl. Sport Sci. Res.* 5(2):60-65. 1991.

122. Triplett, N.T., W.J. Kraemer, and M.H. Stone. A brief review: Ammonia and its response to exercise stress. *NSCA Journal* 13(3):61-65. 1991.

123. Vogel, J.A., J.F. Patton, R.P. Mello, and W.L. Daniels. An analysis of aerobic capacity in a large United States population. *J. Appl. Physiol.* 60:494-500. 1986.

124. Warren, B.J., M.H. Stone, J.T. Kearney, S.J. Fleck, R.L. Johnson, G.D. Wilson, and W.J. Kraemer. Performance measures, blood lactate and plasma ammonia as indicators of overwork in elite junior weightlifters. *Int. J. Sports Med.* 13(5):372-376. 1992.

125. Wilmore, J.H. Alterations in strength, body composition, and anthropometric measurements consequent to a 10 week weight training program. *Med. Sci. Sports.* 6:133-138. 1974.

126. Wilt, F. Training for competitive running. In: *Exercise Physiology*, H.B. Falls, ed. New York: Academic Press. 1968. pp. 395-414.

CHAPTER 9

INDIVIDUAL DIFFERENCES AND THEIR IMPLICATIONS FOR RESISTANCE TRAINING

Jean Barrett Holloway

How can a strength and conditioning program be designed so that a person's unique morphology and training background, as well as gender and age, can be considered? Human beings display a wide variety of physiques and habits of physical activity (12), a fact reflected in the abundance of different sports, games, and dance styles that the peoples of the world have developed. In order to respond to the needs of different people, strength and conditioning professionals need to be sensitive to a wide range of possible performance abilities, not just the averaged scores of select groups commonly discussed in the exercise science literature.

There are several general approaches that strength and conditioning professionals can use to improve their ability to respond to a wide variety of people. **Longitudinal studies** of movement behavior, which show the changes in subjects over time, illustrate the development of a person's physical abilities with proper training. Observing the morphology, performances, and training habits of world-record holders in sporting events provides information about human genetic potential in movements such as running, jumping, and lifting. Finally, strength and conditioning professionals can cultivate an interest in the variation of postural habits and typical physical activities of the peoples of different cultures and countries. In the increasingly multicultural society of North America, this information allows more

effective interaction with people of diverse backgrounds. It can also help improve one's perspective on current controversies in the fitness field. Squatting exercises, for example, have been considered by some in the United States to be of questionable safety (19), yet in many Asian countries people of all ages commonly squat in repose, and in Europe the squat is widely used for physical conditioning.

By calling attention to three topics that relate to modifying a training program based upon a person's unique characteristics, this chapter supplements chapters that more generally address the concepts of responses to training, program planning, and exercise techniques. The first section summarizes anatomical and physiological differences in gender with regard to strength and power. The second section deals with the interaction of training stimulus with a person's physical maturity, age, and training background. The last section looks at selected effects of individual morphological and biomechanical differences in the execution of weight training exercises.

GENDER DIFFERENCES IN ANATOMY AND PHYSIOLOGY

The topic of strength training for female athletes and related differences between men and women has been extensively reviewed elsewhere (18,27). The essential point of these papers was that the strength and conditioning professional should use the same approach in constructing a program for a woman as for a man: Each athlete should be assessed as an individual.

Anatomical Differences

The main strength-related anatomical differences between average men and women are in body height, body weight, muscle fiber size, the proportion of hip width to shoulder width, and the proportion of body fat to body weight. These anatomical differences all relate in part to the strength advantage that having a greater amount of muscle tissue affords the average man. There is a good correlation between the amount of cross-sectional area of muscle and the ability to exert force (24,32). A taller, wider skeletal frame can support more muscle tissue than a smaller frame. A body composed of more muscle and less fat has the potential to exert more force. The broader shoulders typical of men can support more muscle tissue and also provide a leverage advantage over the typically narrower shoulders of women in strength expression at the shoulder. The advantages of having more muscle tissue or better leverage can also be used to illuminate strength differences between groups of people or people of the same gender.

Strength and Power Output

On the average, women have roughly two thirds the absolute strength and power output of men. A greater difference is typically found between men and women in absolute upper body strength, as compared with lower body strength. As strength comparisons are made with measures expressing strength relative to body mass and to lean body mass, the gap between men and women narrows (18).

When strength is expressed per unit of muscle cross-sectional area, the potential for force production is the same for men, women, and children of both genders and various ages. This similarity at the cellular level is what strongly supports the use of the same training procedures for men and women (18). Also, strength and muscle hypertrophy responses to training are similar for men and women when measured from the pretraining baseline (see reference 18 for a discussion of recent evidence on female hypertrophy). Again, this supports the use of a similar training methodology for men and women.

The role of hormonal differences in strength responses by individual men and women, between groups of athletes, and between genders is still being researched. Recent evidence indicates that individual testosterone levels may help predict the potential for strength and power development in women, but not in men (16). There may be a threshold level of testosterone that men typically exceed so as to make no appreciable difference in the prediction of their strength development. Women, however, have approximately one tenth the testosterone levels of men, and because individual women vary considerably from one another in testosterone levels, a woman near the testosterone threshold for strength effects may have an advantage over other women.

It is important to remember that there is a considerable range of strength abilities among men and among women and that there is also an overlap of strength abilities, with the result that some women are stronger than some men. The goal of the strength and conditioning specialist is to develop a person toward his or her genetic potential.

HOW TRAINING STIMULUS INTERACTS WITH MATURITY

The theories and concepts contained in this brief discussion are rooted in the field of **motor development**, sometimes termed developmental kinesiology (7). This area of study is concerned with the changes in movement behavior as they occur over a person's lifespan (29,41). Readers interested in further exploration of the field may wish to begin with an overview text such as that cited in reference 13.

Variation in Maturation Rate to Adulthood

"Although development is age-related, it is not age-dependent" (13, p. 69). An appreciation of the differences in the development of motor behavior among individuals can start with the observation of infants and extend throughout life. In infants, the order of the learning of movement skills is the same for all, but the rates at which these skills develop can vary greatly. For example, the sequence of the stability skills that an infant develops is control of the head and neck, control of the trunk, sitting, and standing. One child may stand unsupported at 10 months of age and another at 13 months, but both are quite normal (13).

Variation in the Onset of Puberty. Differences among individuals are very evident during the pubertal growth spurt at the end of childhood, a time when many people have their first exposure to strength training. The onset of puberty can vary from age 8 to 13 years for girls, and from age 9 to 15 years for boys. Girls, however, typically begin puberty about 2 years before boys. After the onset of puberty, the period of rapid growth for boys and girls extends over approximately 4.5 years

(13). Once puberty has begun, changes in such factors as body composition, the reproductive system, and sex characteristics then unfold in a set order. The result is that a group of 14-year-old adolescents can have height differences as great as 9 in (23 cm), and weight differences of up to 40 lb (18 kg) (3).

Maximum Strength Development Follows Maximum Height and Weight Development.

At any given time, the bigger, early-maturing children in such a group will probably have an advantage in absolute strength expression because of their greater amount of muscle tissue as compared with the smaller, later-maturing children (3,23). In boys, maximum strength development typically occurs about 9 months to 1 year after the peak velocity of growth in height and body weight, with body weight being the clearer indicator (2,22). This pattern suggests that during the adolescent growth spurt, muscle increases first in mass and then in ability to express strength (2). This pattern, interestingly, corresponds to the hypertrophy phase followed by the strength phase in the periodization theory of strength training (37,38) discussed in chapter 30.

In girls, maximum strength development also usually occurs after peak velocity of growth in height. There is, however, more individual variation in the relationship of strength to height and body weight for girls than for boys (22,23). This can possibly be explained by the concomitant increase in body fat that occurs during girls' puberty. Unfortunately, sufficient longitudinal data on the dynamic strength and motor performance of girls are lacking (2).

Motor Skills in Early and Late Maturers.

Early maturers often tend to be mesomorphic or endomorphic in general body type. Typical **mesomorphs** are muscular, broad shouldered, thick chested, and narrow waisted. Typical **endomorphs** are rounder and more pear shaped. Late maturers, who keep growing for a longer period of time and so become taller adults, tend to be **ectomorphs** in body type: slender, tall, and more angular (3) (Figure 9.1). In girls, better performance in such motor skills as sprints, the long jump, and the vertical jump, rather than the absolute strength measures just discussed, has been associated with later skeletal and sexual maturation (23). This is in contrast to the typical pattern for boys, which shows early maturers doing better in motor skills. However, boys do seem to reach their best rate of improvement in speed and flexibility tasks before their peak velocity in height occurs (2).

Motor performance is influenced by many interacting biological and environmental factors. There is no strong evidence at this time that regular training either delays or accelerates the process of maturation in either boys or girls (23). Genetic factors strongly dominate adult standing height, limb and trunk lengths, skeletal and sexual maturation, and body type. On the other hand, other physical characteristics related to motor performance, such as body weight, skinfold thickness, and

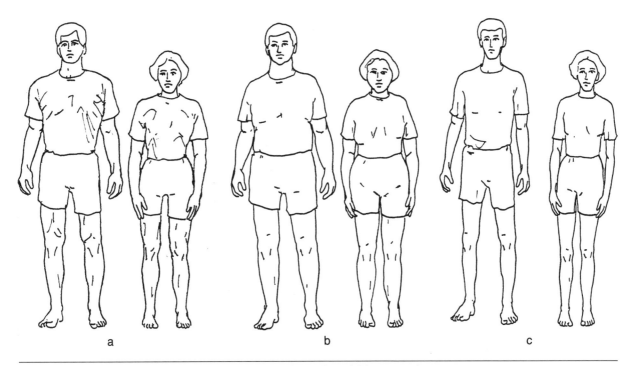

a   b   c

Figure 9.1 General body types. (a) Mesomorph, (b) endomorph, and (c) ectomorph.

body circumference, can be modified considerably by environmental influences, though these influences interact with and are limited by genetic factors (13).

Chronological Age Versus Biological Age. Because of the normal individual variation in rate of development, it is not particularly accurate to define a developmental level in terms of an age in months or years (**chronological age**). Maturity is better gauged with a measure of **biological age**, such as skeletal age, dental age, or sexual age (13), with chronological age ranges used as rough guidelines only. As discussed, degree of maturation is related to a person's ability in strength performance and sports performance. This means that the ideal physical examination prior to participation in sports should include an assessment of physical maturity. Gallahue (13) cites Caine and Broekhoff (5) in a discussion of the inexpensive and noninvasive technique of using the **Tanner stages** of sexual development (40), specifically those associated with the onset of secondary sex characteristics. Problems with embarrassment can be minimized if the potential athlete is asked to rank his or her own maturity level in private, using the drawings of the Tanner stages. In girls, the milestone of **menarche** (the onset of menstruation) is a late event in maturation, occurring approximately 1 year after the time of maximum growth in stature (23). This information might also be useful in a preparticipation examination, because the occurrence of menarche indicates that the rate of growth has slowed.

Sensitivity to individual needs and abilities is especially important for adolescents in the weight room. For example, the strength and conditioning professional may judge that an early-maturing girl is finished with her growth spurt at age 14 and can safely train for a strength and power sport such as competitive weight lifting. A late-maturing boy, on the other hand, may have future potential as a rower or basketball player, but at age 14 may not be ready for heavy resistance training (see reference 26 for training recommendations). The strength and conditioning specialist should frankly explain the reasons for individualized training programs to adolescents, offering special encouragement to late maturers and opportunities for them to develop a variety of motor skills in sports that are less strength dependent.

Successive Movement Ability Phases

Running, jumping, throwing, and balancing skills do not develop automatically in children as they grow older. Human beings develop skill in movements not only because of biologically determined influences of maturation but also because of interacting environmental influences, which include encouragement, instruction,

and opportunity for practice (13). Although the development of movement skills in human beings happens in a seamless, progressive fashion, it is convenient to speak of phases of motor development throughout life. The successful development of each phase is dependent upon the achievement of competence in the foregoing phase; many individual differences in adult motor behavior occur because of incomplete development of various skills at one point or another in childhood.

Motor development specialists theorize that there are **sensitive periods** during a person's life span when the development of a given level of motor skills is optimal (13,42). Thus, the lack of proper opportunity, instruction, or encouragement during a sensitive period can limit a person's ability to fulfill his or her genetic potential in movement skills and in the many aspects of life to which movement skills contribute. According to Wolanski (43), the years from age 8 to 17 (i.e., adolescence) represent an important sensitive period for strength, agility, and explosive movements. During this time there is a high rate of development and a lowered influence of inheritance, with the result that the sensitivity and ability of a person to adapt to a training stimulus, while still within genetically determined individual boundaries, are at their most efficient levels. An example of the application of this principle to coaching methods can be found in how boys have studied gymnastics in Russia. Many of the complex technical moves of the sport are mastered early on, by age 13, so that the remaining adolescent years can largely be used to capitalize on strength development (44).

During all phases of development, movement can be categorized as stabilizing, locomotor, or manipulative in nature. These movement types are often used in combination, but are distinct enough to be categorized separately:

- **Stabilizing movements** "place a premium on gaining and maintaining one's equilibrium in relation to the force of gravity" (13, p. 45). Such movements are required almost all the time in real-life freestanding activities. Examples are body rolling, trunk twisting, and the tight, erect torso required to support a barbell overhead (as for a press, jerk, or snatch) or on the back or chest (as for a back squat, front squat, or clean).

- **Locomotor movements** "involve a change in location of the body relative to a fixed point on the surface" (13, p. 46). Walking, hopping, jumping, and lunging are examples.

- **Manipulative movements** involve motor actions that use an object. Throwing, catching, or kicking an object are examples, as are most weight training exercises in which a bar, dumbbells, or an apparatus is acted upon.

The phases of motor development and their approximate ages of appearance can be summarized as follows (13):

1. **Reflexive movement phase** (in utero to 1 year). Reflexive movements, such as sucking or palmar grasping, are involuntary reactions to an environmental trigger.
2. **Rudimentary movement phase** (birth to 2 years). This phase involves the development of voluntary inhibition of reflex movement and the beginnings of control over movement.
3. **Fundamental movement phase** (2 to 6 or 7 years). Running, jumping (locomotor), throwing and catching (manipulative), and beam walking (stability) are examples of movements that can be developed through the initial, elementary, and mature stages of this phase.
4. **Specialized movement phase** (7 to 14 years and older). Building on the competencies set in the fundamental movement phase, specialized sport, dance, and recreation movements can now be developed. Fundamental movements are combined and refined in transitional, application, and lifelong utilization stages.

Typical Changes in Performance Associated With the Aging Process

Experiences and abilities gained during the aging process are influenced by heredity, previous experiences, and lifestyle choices. There are lifelong opportunities for learning that can improve the quality of life at any point, though they cannot stop the aging process (13).

With age, movements become slower, and more effort and attention may be required to maintain previous levels of coordination. Psychomotor performance measures, such as reaction time, worsen with age, especially as the complexity of the task increases (17).

A decline in many physical performance measures typically occurs with aging. Maximum oxygen uptake, maximum heart rate, strength performance, peak power, and total work performed all gradually decrease from young-adult levels. Muscle mass is also lost with age, and body fat increases (34). There is evidence that muscle fiber size decreases, particularly in fast-twitch fibers, and the total number of muscle fibers also appears to decrease (9). The ratio of the number of fast-twitch fibers to slow-twitch fibers may also change by a selective loss of fast-twitch fibers. Additionally, the rate of protein synthesis is reduced. The loss of muscle mass and the changes in the ratio of fast-twitch to slow-twitch fiber area undoubtedly have an impact on strength and power performance (34).

The mass and structural integrity of bone begin to decline in both average men and women after about the age of 25. The resulting loss of bone strength can become severe in the elderly, with fractures occurring very easily. This disease is called **osteoporosis**, and although it occurs largely in postmenopausal women, there is an increasing rate of incidence among elderly men (25). The maintenance of bone mass is related in part to hormonal and nutritional factors, but it is also related to the level of physical activity of the individual (18). Weight-bearing physical exercise is responsible for the amount of bone mass attained in young adulthood, with men achieving 30% more bone mass than women. This type of exercise can also aid in diminishing the amount of strength and mass that bones lose with aging (25).

The rate at which skeletal muscle can adapt to vigorous chronic exercise is reduced in the elderly (34), but adaptations still take place and improvements in performance levels can occur, though the baseline level may be lower than it would be in a younger person. Pedersen, Puggaard, and Sandager (28) found elderly men and women to be significantly improved in measures of strength, coordination, balance, reaction time, and flexibility after 5 months of gymnastics training. Increases in strength, flexibility, and cardiovascular measures have been observed in elderly women (9) and men (34). The use of resistance training in elderly men has also resulted in muscle hypertrophy similar to that in younger men (4). A similar hypertrophy response has been observed in elderly women (8). Thus, it seems that maintenance of an active lifestyle can encourage more youthful levels of fitness for aging people (1).

Implications of Individual Training History for the Strength and Conditioning Professional

At the college and professional-sport level, the strength and conditioning professional is often involved with training gifted athletes in complex movements. However, not all weight room specialists deal with select, well-developed athletes. Many children and adults in mechanized societies have never properly developed past the fundamental phases of movement (13).

A factor that directly influences a person's development in strength and power, and an important factor in explaining the extremity of gender differences in strength, is culture (27). Western cultures have viewed strength as a masculine characteristic, with the result that girls are typically not encouraged or provided with the means to develop to their genetic potential in physical strength. The strength and conditioning professional who coaches women will very likely have to deal with the low self-expectations and the fear of appearing masculine that this tradition fosters in girls.

Knowledge of the phases of development, especially when considered along with the activity history of a given individual, can help the strength and conditioning professional to assess and (within limits) remedy the quality of movement skill a person can demonstrate. The weight room often provides the first opportunity in many years for a person's fundamental stabilizing movements to be addressed. In a frequently seen example, people with relatively strong hips and legs may nevertheless fail at power cleans or exhibit poor squatting or jerking form because they allow the torso to collapse at key moments. Such trainees need coaching on how to isometrically contract the torso muscles and briefly hold the breath to create sufficient intra-abdominal pressure to help in spinal support. An example of how to remedy the problem of "catching" power cleans is to give the trainee a moderate weight in a slow, basic exercise, such as the front squat, for a few workouts, with instructions to concentrate on keeping an upright, rigid torso. Once the stabilizing skill is mastered in the front squat, it can carry over to the correct moment of receiving the weight in the clean.

The general approach to planning a strength and conditioning program, therefore, varies depending on a person's training history. Two contrasting case histories exemplify this approach:

• Trainee 1. This person was an early maturer and received early and varied motor skills experience, early selection into a sport, and early knowledge of advanced lifting techniques. At age 20, in contrast to someone without such an advantageous background, Trainee 1 needs greater and more frequent training stimulus for progress, though the rate of improvement may be slower because the trainee is functioning close to genetic potential. At age 40, Trainee 1 can still come close to individual personal bests.

• Trainee 2. This person has a poor motor skills background and little knowledge of exercise techniques or personal strength capacity. At age 20, improvement can be more rapid initially compared with someone with better movement experience. However, Trainee 2 has less potential in the long run, cannot withstand as much training stimulus, and needs more and longer rest periods for progress. The strength and conditioning specialist should carefully track training progress and symptoms of overtraining, allowing symptoms to fully subside before assigning the next heavy workout. At age 40, without intervening training, Trainee 2 is far below genetic potential.

INDIVIDUAL BIOMECHANICAL DIFFERENCES: COACHING THE EXECUTION OF EXERCISES

Garhammer (15) has conducted an extensive review of the literature on the biomechanics of weight training and weightlifting; readers are encouraged to consult this. As Cavanagh (6) points out, there is a natural alliance between sport biomechanics and providing better coaching feedback to the athlete. A biomechanist's information, however, still needs to be translated into moment-by-moment coaching in the weight room.

Modest weight rooms may have the basic tools for resistance training but lack the funding for video cameras and other expensive equipment necessary for biomechanical analysis. Under these all-too-common conditions, only the educated eye of the strength and conditioning specialist can determine when to make individual adjustments in exercise execution. That educated eye should also be able to discern when a trainee is lacking in ability to the extent that a particular exercise should not be performed at all. Grossly poor form or pain when a trainee attempts an exercise dictates that another exercise should be substituted.

The author has gleaned many of the following observations from the experience of advanced strength and conditioning specialists.

Posture

Careful observation of an athlete's normal standing and walking posture can provide useful clues to lifting technique and program design. The balance of muscle tensions surrounding joints and the relative tightness or looseness of connective tissue affect the habitual carriage of the body, including posture during weight training.

For example, a posture in which the hips are tucked under the torso (posterior pelvic tilt) and the lordotic curve (the normal inward curve of the lumbar spine) is flattened may indicate tight hamstrings and gluteals, or weak spinal erectors. Such an athlete will find the correct, rigid torso position difficult to maintain in squatting, cleaning, jerking, and snatching. Typically, this error is displayed when the lower back rounds during the pull from the floor, in the bottom position of the squat and clean, and in the initial dip for the jerk. This rounded torso cannot effectively transfer force to the bar, and the amount of weight that can be lifted is reduced. A program that addresses both stretching of the hamstrings and strengthening of spinal erectors is necessary to correct this imbalance.

Similarly, an exaggerated lordotic curve (anterior pelvic tilt) may be the result of tight hip flexors and shortened spinal erectors and weak, lengthened abdominal muscles. This may prevent an athlete from achieving full hip extension in the second pull of the clean or snatch, with the result that heavier attempts are lost in front, unable to be completed. Again, a combination of improvement in hip flexibility and strengthening of the abdominals is needed for the athlete to lift more correctly.

Shoulder posture also gives important clues to lifting problems. A slumping, round-shouldered posture may be the result of both weakness of the upper back and inflexibility of the upper chest and anterior shoulder. In pulling from the floor, the scapulae are too easily pulled away from the spine, the upper back collapses, and the correctly locked torso cannot be maintained. In cleaning and front squatting, the chest cannot be held upright under the weight of the bar and the upper back rounds. The catch in the snatch is severely compromised because of limited range of motion in the shoulder and inability to stabilize the bar overhead. Stretching of the anterior shoulder and the use of a sufficiently light weight to maintain proper torso posture during lifting can correct this weak link.

Although basic multijoint exercises are still a mainstay during a period of posture correction, imbalances of tension and flexibility should be corrected before an athlete begins to lift challenging loads. The use of appropriate assistance exercises can be very important during this corrective period. Once imbalances are corrected, however, assistance work can be minimized, and functional, movement-specific, multijoint weight training will continue the strengthening process in a balanced manner.

Small and Large People

Shorter, more muscular people usually have an advantage over taller, less muscular people in weightlifting and powerlifting movements. This can be explained by considering the definition *work = force × distance*. The distance that a bar of a given weight must travel from the floor to overhead in a snatch or clean and jerk, or from the floor to arms' length in a deadlift, is less in people of shorter stature. Taller people must exert force over a longer distance and must therefore perform more work with the same bar weight. As mentioned earlier, there is a good correlation between the amount of cross-sectional area of muscle and the ability to exert force (24,32), so a muscular individual with a shorter skeletal frame has an advantage of greater strength potential to be exerted through a shorter distance as compared with a taller, less muscular person.

Although larger, well-muscled athletes can often lift impressive absolute amounts of weight compared with smaller athletes, the supporting skeletal extremities of hands or feet may not be much different in size. In large, strong athletes, these extremities, joints, and their connective tissues must withstand training of a heavier absolute load. To minimize overtraining injuries in very large athletes, the total volume of repetitions, the number of training sessions, and the frequency of high-intensity workouts should be less than for very small athletes. More time for recovery may also be necessary. A compromise must be sought, however, so that sufficient repetitions at moderate intensity are done by the large athlete to fulfill muscle hypertrophy requirements. The strength and conditioning professional must be aware of the greater potential for injury at the beginning and end of the exercise movement, when the mass of the athlete and bar must be accelerated and decelerated (37), and must also take care not to overstress the joints of very heavy individuals in jumping and plyometric work, even if they have a good strength base. For example, Stone and O'Bryant (37) recommend that depth jumps not be used for athletes over 230 lb (104 kg).

Machines and Individual Differences

The advantages of free weights over machines have been compiled in three seminal articles (14,35,36); an additional summary is also available in Stone and O'Bryant (37). The major advantages derive from the ability of free-weight exercises to mimic the movement demands of real-life sport and everyday activities and from the numerous possibilities for variation in free-weight exercises. Thus, the strength and conditioning professional can apply the two central principles of **specificity of exercise** (training in a specific manner to produce a specific outcome) and Selye's **general adaptation syndrome** (33) to the use of free weights. The general adaptation syndrome describes the non-specific, three-phase response (alarm, resistance, exhaustion) of the body to any stressor (e.g., the demands of exercise or a virus). Planning a strength training program with sufficient variety and recovery will avoid the ill effects of the exhaustion phase.

In contrast to free weights, most machines create a forced or guided two-dimensional movement pattern for the user. This forced pattern does not allow as much individual variation in movement patterns caused in part by differences in people's limb segment lengths, bone articulations, and muscle attachment sites. Free weights permit three-dimensional movement and do not hinder the individual athlete's movement pattern. Rubber tubing and machines using cables that can move in three dimensions are more adaptable to individual differences. However, cables and rubber tubing typically offer a fast-to-slow movement pattern, with greater resistance and slower speed toward the end of the pattern, which contrasts with the typical slow-to-fast pattern of many sport movements. For example, in throwing and jumping events, the initial speed of motion is relatively slower as the athlete overcomes the resistance of the throwing implement or the body; speed then increases and resistance decreases as the movement progresses.

Another disadvantage of machines is that they typically provide resistance only at a single joint. Thus the part, not the whole, of a motor skill is emphasized and overall coordination is not developed. Also, because most machines support the user, few, if any, demands are made to stabilize and balance the user or the load, which is quite the opposite from the demands of most real-life activities outside the weight room.

As mentioned earlier, assistance exercises (which may involve machines) can be important in the correction of postural imbalances. They can also be useful in the rehabilitation of injuries when the use of the whole body may not be possible, as long as care is taken to suit the exercise to the improvement of the ability required (31). In these cases, the coach can examine a machine for its movement specificity, make sure the load increments on the machine are suitable for the trainee, and have that trainee ''try on'' the machine for comfort. Machine movement tracks, like off-the-rack clothing sizes, are created to fit the average person, but no one is average in all respects. If a particular machine does not fit, try a different brand or substitute a different exercise.

Practical Observations Regarding Specific Free-Weight Exercises

Much has been written about the technique of lifting free weights (21,30,39,42). Readers who require more detail than this chapter offers are urged to turn to these and other references and to view slow-motion videotapes of several current world-class athletes. Sequential still photos can omit critical lifting moments; watching a moving picture (or the real thing) is always desirable and can often deflate the somewhat artificial controversies about technique, such as whether an athlete's heels leave the floor during snatching and cleaning.

Vorobeyev (42) uses body proportions to classify bodies into three types: long arms, long legs, short torso (ectomorph); short arms, short legs, long torso (endomorph); and more proportioned (mesomorph) (see Figure 9.1 on p. 153). Although not every person will clearly fit into a category, some athletes may benefit from the following observations on such body proportion attributes as they relate to the benefits and proper execution of some major free-weight exercises. Be aware that a young athlete may grow and change body proportions over time.

Long Torso. The athlete with a long torso relative to the rest of his or her body has a longer torso length to stabilize during total body and sport movements. Extra torso work, such as good mornings, hyperextensions, and abdominal work, and extra overhead support work, such as overhead squats and jerk recoveries, may be necessary for the athlete to develop control over a

long torso. Front squatting is also very helpful, performed beltless as full squats or to a quarter-squat depth with very heavy weight.

Pulling Off the Floor (Snatch, Clean). In pulling a bar off the floor, foot stance and grip width vary considerably with the individual athlete because of body proportions; they need to be adjusted to permit the hips to be as close to the bar as possible, the shoulders ahead of the bar, and the center of pressure toward the ball of the foot at the moment of liftoff (15,39). It is more difficult for the lifter with long arms, long legs, and a short torso to keep the hips close and the shoulders over the bar at the same time. Additional deadlifting exercises with a snatch grip can develop the strength of the back (especially the latissimus dorsi) to hold a correct position over the bar at liftoff.

Grip and foot stance width may increase slightly with increases in strength and body weight. Large feet give a broader base of support and offer a greater margin for technical error than small feet. If it is possible for the lifter to minimize the turnout of the toes in the liftoff stance, more area of support for front to back balance on the feet can be gained. Very small hands may have trouble with a hook grip or with getting fingers all the way around the bar; straps may be needed.

There is at present little biomechanical data on the powerlifting style of deadlift (15), although it is a core pulling movement for many athletes.

Squat. Advanced athletes who compete and train with squatting movements tend to have legs that are shorter than average relative to height (18). This conception of the ideal squat morphology is supported by research (10,11) that found that the inability of untrained men and women to squat flat-footed was influenced by the relation of femur length, torso length, and height. However, the ability to squat with an erect torso and feet solidly in contact with the floor also depends on ankle and hip flexibility and torso strength. Since body proportions cannot be changed by the coach, the use of weightlifting shoes with a higher heel or standing with heels on a small board or weight plates may help squatting form. Ankle stretches and hip and groin stretches should become part of the regular training program. Finally, marginally acceptable squatting technique may also be improved simply by continuing to perform squats with lighter weights as the coach frequently encourages the squatter to maintain the best technique possible.

Snatch. Snatch grip width can be estimated by measuring the distance between elbows while the athlete is holding the arms straight out to the side (21). Adjustments from this estimate are then made based on comfort and success in lifting. A good initial test for correct grip width is the ability of the athlete to perform over-head squats correctly. Very tall, very long limbed people, such as professional basketball players, may need a wider grip for snatching than the regulation bar length allows; a special bar or clean grip snatches on a regulation bar can be considered.

The ability to overhead squat into the full snatch bottom position is affected by torso strength and by the flexibility of the ankles, hips, shoulders, elbows (which should lock with the humerus fully externally rotated), and wrists. A good stretching program and proper weightlifting shoes can help promote proper form. Wrist discomfort can often be minimized with a tape or Ace elastic bandage wrap. Strength for the hyperextended wrist position can be developed by balancing a small weight plate on the palm of the hand, like a waiter holding a tray, and then flexing the wrist. Also, athletes who teeter on the balls of their feet and lean forward excessively with the torso as they approach the full snatch bottom have to limit themselves to power snatches, catching the bar with their knees partially flexed. As always, the inability to maintain good form limits the amount of weight that can be used in an exercise.

Clean and Jerk.

Many problems in the clean relate to an inability to rack the bar so that it rests correctly on the shoulders and clavicles without shutting off blood flow in the carotid arteries and without resting on the hands alone. The athlete may need to actively shrug up the shoulders to create a shelf for the bar. Ideally, the elbows are high so that the humerus is parallel to the floor in the catch of the clean. Shoulder or wrist inflexibility or injury or an excessive amount of muscle mass in the biceps and other elbow flexors may hamper this ideal high elbow position. Emphasis on the correct rack position while front squatting, stretching the wrists and triceps, and eliminating bicep curls from the program can also encourage correct racking technique.

In the starting position for the jerk, a long humerus can prevent the athlete from lowering the elbows sufficiently to involve the arms in the initial drive (39). An athlete with this disadvantage who needs to use the jerk as a sport training exercise may have to jerk from in back of the neck. Inability of the elbows to lock in the catch of the jerk is a serious disadvantage, because the relatively small elbow extensors must then try to hold a weight that the large hip and leg muscles have driven overhead. Stretching exercises should be used to try to increase elbow range of motion.

An incomplete split in the jerk may be caused by tight hip flexors. Stretching the hips and strengthening the legs with lunges that go through the increased range of motion may help remedy this problem (20).

Bench Press.

Short arms and a large chest cavity are an advantage in bench pressing, since these factors shorten the distance over which the athlete must exert force. Garhammer (15) mentions that a three-dimensional biomechanical analysis of a bench press is needed to illuminate the complex shoulder and shoulder girdle involvement.

CONCLUSION

We have looked at gender differences, physical maturity and aging, and individual biomechanical factors in relation to designing and implementing strength and conditioning programs.

Regarding gender differences, women are smaller than men, have less muscle mass, and can display roughly two-thirds of the absolute overall strength and power of men. Additionally, the traditional upbringing of girls has discouraged them from expressing physical strength. However, women and men respond to strength training in very similar ways from their respective pre-training baselines and have a similar potential for developing force per unit of muscle tissue. Thus, the strength and conditioning professional should use the same basic approach for a man or a woman, which is to assess each athlete as an individual.

The interaction of training stimulus with the maturity of the individual may be studied with reference to motor development theory. Adolescents begin pubertal growth at varying ages. Their gains in height and body weight are related to gains in strength and power performance. A group of teens of the same chronological age may display different degrees of physical maturity, and their training programs need to be adjusted accordingly. Physical maturity can be determined in a preparticipation physical examination by having the young athlete report his or her level of development according to the Tanner scale.

Strength and conditioning professionals should be aware that the general types of body movements (stabilizing, locomotor, and manipulative) do not develop and improve automatically as children grow up. People need encouragement, instruction, and opportunity for practice in order to develop through the successive phases of skill levels. Many adults are incomplete in their development of motor skills because of a lack of these stimuli, especially during the sensitive developmental period of adolescence. Remediation of some skills may need to be included in a training program.

As a person continues to mature, old age causes a decline in most aspects of physical performance, including the strength of muscle and bone. Physical training can be initiated at any age, however, and can benefit a person with improvements over the pretraining baseline.

Previous motor skill experience and lifetime activity habits greatly affect physical capabilities during the aging process, including exercise intensity and frequency.

The strength and conditioning professional needs to take into account the effects of individual biomechanical differences in posture, body size, sport movement pattern, and body proportions when selecting exercises and coaching specific free-weight exercises.

The topics in this chapter are diverse, but all exemplify the attention that the strength and conditioning professional needs to give to the unique characteristics of the trainee in order to design and administer the most effective training program.

Key Terms

biological age	154	longitudinal study	151	rudimentary movement phase	155
chronological age	154	manipulative movement	154	sensitive period	154
ectomorph	153	menarche	154	specialized movement phase	155
endomorph	153	mesomorph	153		
fundamental movement phase	155	motor development	152	specificity of exercise	157
		osteoporosis	155	stabilizing movement	154
general adaptation syndrome	157	reflexive movement phase	155	Tanner stages	154
locomotor movement	154				

Study Questions

1. Many adults have never developed their movement skills past the

   a. reflexive movement phase
   b. rudimentary movement phase
   c. fundamental movement phase
   d. specialized movement phase

2. What is the latest stage of development possible for a 14 year old to have reached?

   a. reflexive movement phase
   b. rudimentary movement phase
   c. fundamental movement phase
   d. specialized movement phase

3. When men and women are compared as to absolute strength performance, which of the following is true, on the average?

   a. Men are stronger.
   b. Women are stronger.
   c. They are the same.

4. When force production per unit of muscle cross-sectional area of men and women is compared, which of the following is true, on the average?

   a. Men have more potential.
   b. Women have more potential.
   c. They are the same.

5. An athlete with a short torso, long arms, and long legs may have difficulty with which two exercises?

   a. the front squat
   b. the jerk
   c. pulling a snatch off the floor
   d. the bench press

6. During adolescence, the period of maximum strength development typically

    a. precedes maximum endurance development
    b. follows maximum endurance development
    c. precedes maximum weight development
    d. follows maximum weight development

Applying Knowledge of Individual Differences

Problem 1

You observe an athlete attempting to back squat to a thighs parallel position, but you see the heels coming up off the floor and the torso leaning forward well before that squat depth can be reached. What factors do you consider in order to explain and remedy this?

Problem 2

On parents' visitation night, you meet 2 ninth-grade boys and their parents. Both boys are highly motivated to get big and strong and want to copy the strength training program you gave to the varsity football team. One boy is short and muscular and brags about his growing moustache; he and his dad are about the same height. The other boy is a little taller than his buddy, slight of build, and it is clear his voice has not yet deepened; both his mom and dad are well above average height. What do you tell these friends about their wanting to train together?

Problem 3

A former national-level gymnast watched the Olympic Games and wants to get in shape to throw the javelin. She is 22, last competed 4 years ago, runs and goes rock climbing often, and does a 20-min machine weight training circuit 3 days a week. What do you tell her to expect from your strength training program regarding frequency of training, intensity of training, choice of weight exercises, and training responses to this style of program?

Problem 4

A 70-year-old man had successful cataract surgery a year ago. He always used to do a lot of yard work, but he could not do that during his recuperation and then got out of the habit. Now he no longer feels strong enough, and he fears that he will hurt himself. He admits to feeling depressed about it and complains that his clothes just hang on him. He wants to know if any of this is correctable. What do you advise?

References

1. American College of Sports Medicine. ACSM position stand: The recommended quantity and quality of exercise for developing and maintaining cardiorespiratory and muscular fitness in healthy adults. *Med. Sci. Sports Exerc.* 22(2):265-274. 1990.
2. Beunen, G., and R.M. Malina. Growth and physical performance relative to the timing of the adolescent growth spurt. In: *Exercise and Sport Sciences Reviews*, vol. 16, K.B. Pandolf, ed. New York: Macmillan. 1988. pp. 503-540.
3. Branta, C. Young athletes: Midgets and giants at the same age. *Motor Dev. Acad. Newslet.* 11(1):2-4. 1990.
4. Brown, A.B., N. McCartney, D. Moroz, D.G. Sale, S.A. Garner, and J.D. MacDougall. Strength training effects in aging (abstract). *Med. Sci. Sports Exerc.* 20(2 [suppl.]):S80. 1988.
5. Caine, D.J., and J. Broekhoff. Maturity assessment: A viable preventive measure against physical and psychological insult to the young athlete? *Phys. Sportsmed.* 12(4):118-124. 1987.
6. Cavanagh, P.R. Biomechanics: A bridge builder among the sport sciences. *Med. Sci. Sports Exerc.* 22(5):546-557. 1990.
7. Clark, J.E., and J. Whitall. What is motor development? The lessons of history. *Quest* 41:183-202. 1989.
8. Cress, M.E., D.P. Thomas, J.C. Agre, R.G. Cassens, and E.L. Smith. Skeletal muscle adaptations to long-term training in elderly women (abstract). *Med. Sci. Sports Exerc.* 21(2 [suppl.]):S64. 1989.
9. Drinkwater, B.L. Exercise and aging: The female masters athlete. In: *Sport Science Perspectives for Women*, J.L. Puhl, C.H. Brown, and R.O. Voy, eds. Champaign, IL: Human Kinetics. 1988. pp. 161-169.

10. Fry, A.C., K.W. Bibi, and T. Eyford. Stature variables as discriminators of foot contact during the squat exercise in untrained females (abstract). *J. Appl. Sport Sci. Res.* 3(3):72-73. 1989.

11. Fry, A.C., T.J. Housh, R.A. Hughes, and T. Eyford. Stature and flexibility variables as discriminators of foot contact during the squat exercise. *J. Appl. Sport Sci. Res.* 2(2):24-26. 1988.

12. Gaisford, J. *Atlas of Man.* New York: St. Martin's Press. 1978.

13. Gallahue, D.L. *Understanding Motor Development: Infants, Children, Adolescents.* Indianapolis: Benchmark Press. 1989.

14. Garhammer, J. Free weight equipment for the development of athletic strength and power, part I. *NSCA Journal* 3(6):24-26, 33. 1981.

15. Garhammer, J. Weight lifting and training. In: *Biomechanics of Sport*, C.L. Vaughan, ed. Boca Raton, FL: CRC Press. 1989. pp. 169-210.

16. Häkkinen, K., A. Pakarinen, H. Kyrolainen, S. Cheng, D.H. Kim, and P.V. Komi. Neuromuscular adaptations and serum hormones in females during prolonged power training. *Int. J. Sports Med.* 11(2):91-98. 1990.

17. Hart, B.A. Psychomotor function and aging. In: *Sport Science Perspectives for Women*, J.L. Puhl, C.H. Brown, and R.O. Voy, eds. Champaign, IL: Human Kinetics. 1988. pp. 171-179.

18. Holloway, J.B., and T.R. Baechle. Strength training for female athletes, a review of selected aspects. *Sports Med.* 9(4):216-228. 1990.

19. IDEA Foundation. Guidelines for training of dance-exercise instructors. (Available from IDEA, 4501 Mission Bay Dr., Suite 3-A, San Diego, CA 92109.) 1986.

20. Jones, L. Problems with the jerk. *Ironsport* 2(3):24-25. 1990.

21. Jones, L. United States Weightlifting Federation Coaching Accreditation Course, Club Coach Manual. (Available from USWF, 1750 E. Boulder St., Colorado Springs, CO 80909.) 1991.

22. Malina, R.M. Growth, strength, and physical performance. In: *Encyclopedia of Physical Education, Fitness, and Sports*, vol. II, G.A. Stull, ed. Salt Lake City: Brighton. 1980. pp. 443-470.

23. Malina, R.M. Growth, performance, activity, and training during adolescence. In: *Women and Exercise: Physiology and Sports Medicine*, M.M. Shangold and G. Mirkin, eds. Philadelphia: Davis. 1988. pp. 120-128.

24. Maughan, R.J. Relationship between muscle strength and muscle cross-sectional area: Implications for training. *Sports Med.* 1:263-269. 1984.

25. Mosekilde, L., and A. Viidik. Age-related changes in bone mass, structure and strength: Pathogenesis and prevention. *Int. J. Sports Med.* 10(suppl.):S90-S92. 1989.

26. National Strength and Conditioning Association. Position paper on prepubescent strength training. (Available from NSCA, P.O. Box 81410, Lincoln, NE 68501.) 1985.

27. National Strength and Conditioning Association. Strength training for female athletes: A position paper. *NSCA Journal* 11(4):43-55; 11(5):29-36. 1989.

28. Pedersen, H.P., L. Puggaard, and E. Sandager. A longitudinal study of muscle function in elderly people: A comparison of different kinds of exercise. *Int. J. Sports Med.* 10(suppl.):S113. 1989.

29. Roberton, M.A. Motor development: Recognizing our roots, charting our future. *Quest* 41:213-223. 1989.

30. Roman, R.A. *The Training of the Weightlifter*, 2nd ed. (A. Charniga, trans.). Livonia, MI: Sportivny Press. 1986.

31. Rutherford, O.M. Muscular coordination and strength training: Implications for injury rehabilitation. *Sports Med.* 5:196-202. 1988.

32. Ryushi, T., K. Häkkinen, H. Kauhanen, and P.V. Komi. Muscle fiber characteristics, muscle cross-sectional area, and force production in strength athletes, physically active males and females. *Scand. J. Sports Sci.* 10(1):7-15. 1988.

33. Selye, H. *The Stress of Life*, rev. ed. New York: McGraw-Hill. 1978.

34. Stamford, B.A. Exercise and the elderly. In: *Exercise and Sport Sciences Reviews*, vol. 16, K.B. Pandolf, ed. New York: Macmillan. 1988. 16:341-379.

35. Stone, M.H. Considerations in gaining a strength-power training effect (machines vs. free weights): Free weights, part II. *NSCA Journal* 4(1):22-24, 54. 1982.

36. Stone, M.H., and J. Garhammer. Some thoughts on strength and power. *NSCA Journal* 3(5):24-25, 47. 1981.

37. Stone, M.H., and H.S. O'Bryant. *Weight Training: A Scientific Approach.* Minneapolis: Burgess International. 1987.

38. Stone, M.H., H.S. O'Bryant, and J. Garhammer. A hypothetical model for strength training. *J. Sports Med. Phys. Fitness* 21:342-351. 1981.

39. Takano, B. Coaching optimal technique in the snatch and clean and jerk. *NSCA Journal* 9(5):50-59; 9(6):52-56. 1987. 10(1):54-59. 1988.

40. Tanner, J.M. Motor development at adolescence. In: *Growth at Adolescence*, 2nd ed., J.M. Tanner, ed. Oxford, UK: Blackwell Scientific. 1962.

41. VanSant, A.F. A life span concept of motor development. *Quest* 41:224-234. 1989.

42. Vorobeyev, A. *Weightlifting.* (W.J. Brice, trans.). Budapest: International Weightlifting Federation. 1978.

43. Wolanski, N. Heredity and psychomotor traits in man. In: *Sport and Human Genetics: The 1984 Olympic Scientific Congress Proceedings*, vol. 4, R.M. Malina and C. Bouchard, eds. Champaign, IL: Human Kinetics. 1986. pp. 123-129.

44. Zatsiorsky, V.M. Biomechanics and training of maximal muscular performance. [Course lectures.] UCLA Dept. of Kinesiology. June–August, 1991.

THE PSYCHOLOGY OF ATHLETIC PREPARATION AND PERFORMANCE: THE MENTAL MANAGEMENT OF PHYSICAL RESOURCES

Bradley D. Hatfield
Evan B. Brody

We believe that excellence in athletic performance is the result of sound skill and physical training accompanied by optimal rest and recovery cycles and appropriate diet. At any particular stage of biological maturity, the phenotypic development of the athlete's genetic potential represents a relatively stable ceiling for performance, but the expression of that skilled performance can vary tremendously from contest to contest and even from moment to moment. We believe that athletes cannot exceed the potential for their stages of physical and skill development, as determined by the factors we have described. The role of sport psychology is to help athletes achieve consistent levels of performance at or near their physical potential by carefully managing their physical resources.

After defining foundational terms, we will address how the mind, or psyche, can influence physical performance and then describe the ideal performance state—the ultimate goal of every athlete. In part, this state is marked by *psychological* and *physiological efficiency* (i.e., employing only the amount of psychic and physical energy required to perform the task). We will discuss two primary psychological influences on sport learning and performance—motivation and anxiety—citing several theories of how these emotional phenomena change athletic performance. Finally, we will discuss techniques including goal setting, relaxation, mental imagery, and psyching strategies that can be employed for mental training, or managing physical resources.

DEFINITION OF KEY CONCEPTS IN SPORT PSYCHOLOGY

The **athlete** is someone who engages in a social comparison (competition) involving psychomotor skill or physical prowess (or both) in an institutionalized setting, typically under public scrutiny or evaluation. The essence of athletic competition involves comparing oneself to others and putting ego and self-esteem on the line in a setting bound by rules and regulations. No wonder athletes get anxious and aroused! The psychologically well-prepared athlete is characterized by efficiency of thought and deed. Efficiency is typically associated with skilled performance, when actions are fluid and graceful. The concept can also be extended to psychological activity; an efficient athlete adopts a task-relevant focus, not wasting attention on task-irrelevant processing like worrying, catastrophizing, and thinking about "other" things, such as a critical audience or coach.

Sport psychology is the subdiscipline of kinesiology (exercise science) that seeks to understand the influence of behavioral processes on skilled movement. Exercise science together with various clinical areas of medicine (physical therapy, orthopedics, cardiology, etc.) comprises the larger field of sports medicine (41), thus sport psychology is classified as a scientific field of study within sports medicine. Within exercise science sport psychology has three major goals:

1. Measuring psychological phenomena
2. Investigating the relationships between psychological variables and performance
3. Applying theoretical knowledge to improve athletic performance

By applying the information gained, athletes can manage their physical resources.

Anxiety: State and Trait

Athletes are frequently concerned about anxiety, arousal, and attention. The first two terms are often used interchangeably to mean stress, but this lack of specificity can cause real confusion and poor communication between athletes, coaches, and sport psychologists.

Anxiety, or more specifically **state anxiety**, is a subjective experience of apprehension and uncertainty accompanied by elevated autonomic and voluntary neural outflow and increased endocrinological activity. State anxiety is a negative experience, but its effects on athletic performance can be positive, negative, or indifferent depending on such factors as the athlete's skill level and personality and the complexity of the task to be performed. State anxiety is distinct from but related to **trait anxiety**, a personality variable or disposition relating to the probability that one will perceive an environment as threatening. In essence, trait anxiety acts as a primer for the athlete's brain to experience state anxiety (64).

Arousal is simply the intensity dimension of behavior and physiology (7). For example, a "psyched-up" athlete may experience tremendous mental activation characterized by positive thoughts and a strong sense of

control (in line with Martens's (45) notion of **psychic energy**). In such a case the athlete would not be described as anxious. Arousal is always present in an individual to some degree as a continuous state ranging from deep sleep, or comatose, to highly excited; it can be indexed by such measures as heart rate, blood pressure, electroencephalography (EEG), electromyography (EMG), and catecholamine levels or with self-report instruments, such as the activation-deactivation checklist (66). The optimal arousal required for efficient performance depends on several factors.

In a nonanxious state, arousal is under the *control* of the athlete; it can be elevated or depressed as needed. The athlete who is psychologically well prepared knows the appropriate zone for optimal performance and can manage it accordingly. In an anxious state arousal is relatively *uncontrolled*. Typically, arousal is too high during state anxiety; the skeletal muscles are tense, the heart is racing, and negative thoughts intrude. This lack of physical and psychological efficiency is typically initiated by uncertainty about a present or anticipated event. At least three important factors are usually present:

- A high degree of ego involvement in which the athlete may perceive a threat to self-esteem
- A perceived *discrepancy* between one's ability and the demands for athletic success
- A fear of the consequences of failure (such as a loss of approval from teammates, coach, family, or peers)

State anxiety, then, typically modifies psychological and physical arousal so that it becomes elevated and uncontrolled. Some investigators have advocated using both cognitive and somatic assessments of arousal because it is a multidimensional, or at least bidimensional, phenomenon (59). **Cognitive anxiety** relates to psychological processes and worrisome thoughts, whereas **somatic anxiety** relates to such physical symptoms as tense muscles, tachycardia, and the butterflies. Because anxiety and arousal are rather vague terms, Table 10.1 includes explanations of more specific terms.

Stress, for our purposes, will be considered as any disruption from homeostasis or mental and physical calm. A stressor is an environmental or cognitive event that precipitates stress (i.e., the stress response). It can be described as a negative (distress) or a positive (eustress) state. Therefore, stress comprises cognitive and somatic anxiety, whereas eustress comprises psychic energy and physiologic arousal.

The cognitive somatic anxiety questionnaire (CSAQ) measures the cognitive and somatic anxiety domains (59). Gould, Petlichkoff, Simons, and Vevera (22) have shown that these two constructs have very different

**Table 10.1 Specific Components
of the Anxiety and Arousal Constructs**

Cognitive anxiety	A psychological state involving task-irrelevant mental processes that are negative in nature, flood attention, and can deter performance proportionally (especially activities requiring high amounts of information processing). That is, the more the athlete experiences cognitive anxiety, the worse the performance, especially when performance depends on complex decision making.
Somatic anxiety	Relatively uncontrolled physiological arousal, which is influenced by cognitive anxiety. Shows an inverted-U relationship to sport performance unless accompanied by significant cognitive anxiety, which causes a sharp decline in performance (i.e., catastrophe theory).
Psychic arousal or energy	A continuum of psychological intensity that is *not* manifested as apprehension and uncertainty, but rather as a sense of activation and focus. It is usually positively related to sport performance unless complex decision-making tasks are involved that require lower levels of psychological arousal.
Physiological arousal	A psychologically neutral intensity dimension of physical arousal. Extreme levels would aid activities requiring heightened energy metabolism, especially those relying primarily upon the ATP-creatine phosphate and glycolytic pathways. Carefully regulated arousal would facilitate endurance and predominantly aerobic activity.

implications for sport performance. Accordingly, a coach should ascertain whether an athlete is predominantly state anxious (experiencing cognitive and somatic anxiety) or predominantly aroused (experiencing psychic energy and physiological arousal), as the mental perspective can have a distinct effect on performance.

The decision branch for the mind to go one way or the other relates to an athlete's perception of the incoming sensory events. Sensation, a first step in the *perceptual process*, is simply the reception of environmental stimuli by the athlete's brain. It is an emotionally neutral process representing an information-gathering phase of psychological activity (58). For example, the athlete's visual cortex in the occipital lobe of the brain registers the sight of a stadium, while the auditory cortex in the temporal lobe receives the roar of the crowd. The brain constantly integrates experiences or memory with these incoming stimuli, perceiving the environment and giving meaning to it. The perceptual process is part of a complex series of neuropsychological events that may ultimately result in interpreting the stadium and crowd noise as either threatening or challenging (i.e., anxiety-provoking or psyched out, vs. psyched-up). Perceiving a challenge promotes the psychic energy condition, and the athlete views competition in an appetitive manner. These two perspectives have important impacts on the athlete's ability to focus on the tasks to be performed and the fluidity, or efficiency, of the coordinated athletic movements.

Attention and Skill

The athlete's ability to focus can be better understood through the construct of attention. Attention is defined as the processing of those environmental cues that come to awareness. The information-processing model views attention as a fixed capacity, like a box, with finite volume (33). This fixed capacity (a scarce commodity) is constantly bombarded by externally (e.g., sights and sounds) and internally (e.g., thoughts and afferent stimuli within the body) generated cues.

Conscious attention is continuously bombarded with a variety of stimuli and thoughts to which it can attend. The ability to inhibit awareness of some stimuli in order to process others is termed *selective attention*, and it suppresses task-irrelevant cues (e.g., people on the sidelines, planes flying over the stadium) in order to process the task-relevant cues in the limited attentional space. For a football quarterback, task-relevant cues might include wind conditions and a receiver's path and speed. Importantly, the ability to focus attention on task-relevant cues and to control distraction is a *skill* that can be learned. Frank Costello (6), formerly a world-class high jump competitor and now a strength and conditioning coach, purposely encouraged people to walk across his approach to the jump during practices while he engaged in mental preparation. The motivation to engage in this attentional training initially stemmed from his experiences with distractions from the media and attendant personnel during a major Madison Square Garden event. He believed if he trained to suppress distraction, the ability would then transfer to competitive situations.

Kandel and Schwartz (39) in a classic treatise described fascinating evidence that emotion can change or alter the neural programming involved in initiating and controlling voluntary movement. In essence, emotion can change the order in which the brain structures and executes commands to the working muscles. Perhaps the frustration incurred by an athlete's inability to block distractions can bring a subcortically controlled movement to a conscious level (i.e., the athlete starts forcing the movement). As the brain changes its programming sequence, the timing and force of the agonistic, antagonistic, and synergistic muscles involved in a particular movement might also be altered. This phenomenon could be relevant particularly to fine motor skills like golf, place-kicking, and high jumping. Richard Demak (11) remarks on this concept in an article entitled ''Mysterious Malady'':

> Mike Stanley, a catcher for the (Texas) Rangers, became so fixated on his throwing percentage (the percentage of base runners a catcher throws out) that he grew terrified of throwing the ball at all. As a result, he sent rainbows to second and third base and little lobs back to the pitcher. Now that Stanley has received some psychological counseling and is making better throws, people are telling him how much stronger his arm is. ''My arm is the same as before,'' Stanley says. ''I'm just not afraid to *let it go* anymore.''
>
> In the (above), it's as if the player suddenly forgot how to throw a baseball, and, in effect, he did. Almost every season there are a few big league players who find themselves unable to perform an act that used to come almost as naturally as breathing. It has happened to infielders who've fired the ball to first more times than they've tied their shoelaces, to catchers who could once gun down the swiftest base runners and to pitchers who have made it to the majors on their pinpoint control. Somehow these players develop a mental block that inhibits the simple act of throwing. (p. 44)

Football coaches often exploit the potential for this psychological neuromotor problem in opponents by calling a time-out just before a field-goal attempt. During the time-out an athlete might flood his attentional capacity with task-irrelevant self-doubt and thoughts of failure. Placekickers can deal with this anxiety and attentional challenge by adopting a ritual or a mental checklist that consciously directs thoughts to task-relevant and controllable concerns (e.g., breathing, checking the turf, and stretching the hamstrings).

The important underlying principle is that thinking about one set of thoughts actively excludes attending to other worrisome thoughts because of the limited capacity of working memory. This human shortcoming can be used to advantage. Prior to a lifting performance, for example, the athlete might use key phrases to focus on the task-relevant cues associated with the lift, such as foot placement, back position, point of visual focus, and knee angle during a squat. This strategy would reduce distractions, which often deter optimal effort. Such focusing strategies can promote mental consistency during the preparatory state, which, in turn, can promote physical consistency—the hallmark of a skilled athlete.

Cue Utilization

At low levels of arousal attentional width is very broad, according to Easterbrook's (1959) **cue utilization** theory (13), and both relevant and irrelevant cues can come to the athlete's awareness. The athlete may not concentrate well at these under-aroused levels. This may explain why some teams commit mental errors when playing against an ''easy'' opponent. As arousal increases, attentional width progressively decreases, enabling more focus (if the athlete has been coached about the proper cues for allocating the narrowed attentional capacity). But a point of diminishing returns may be reached at excessive levels of arousal due to a lack of attentional resources. In other words, too much shrinkage occurs. Figure 10.1 highlights this phenomenon. Consider the case of a young high school basketball player suddenly thrust into a starting role because of injury to a teammate. In her debut the athlete is highly concerned with social evaluation. Suddenly, at an intense moment of play the coach calls a time-out. The athlete is reprimanded for not passing the ball to a teammate who was in an opportunistic position to score. The athlete pleads her case by indicating that she didn't see the open player. In essence, her attentional capacity was flooded with task-irrelevant cognition.

Attentional Style

Nideffer (52) formulated an important concept in sport psychology when he theorized that individuals tend to fall into categories of chronic attentional styles. He developed an instrument to measure these tendencies, the Test of Attentional and Interpersonal Style (TAIS). His studies revealed that attentional style, as a personality trait, tends to be characterized by two dimensions, internal–external and broad–narrow. The first dimension refers to an introspective versus an externally oriented perspective, whereas the second dimension refers to a highly selective versus an integrative (expansive) orientation. Using these dimensions of attention he identified six categories of dispositional styles, which are described in Table 10.2, taken from Iso-Ahola and Hatfield (36).

Understanding this concept can improve coaching effectiveness. For example, a player who tends to become overloaded with external stimuli might be coached to focus on *one* important cue, such as an opponent's footwork. Without such coaching, a player more likely would attend to too many cues, becoming confused and having slowed reaction time.

HOW THE MIND AFFECTS THE ATHLETE'S PHYSICAL PERFORMANCE

The mind-body link was recently illustrated in a study by Hatfield, Spalding, Mahon, Slater, Brody, and

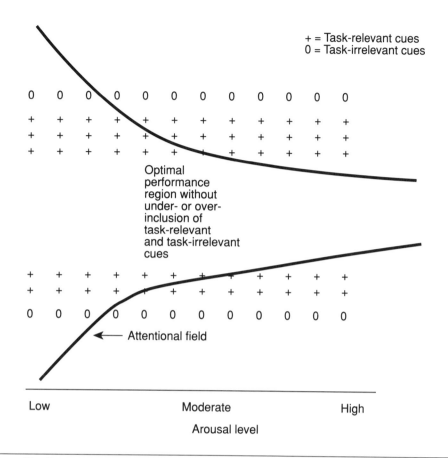

Figure 10.1 Cue utilization.
Reprinted from Landers (1980).

Table 10.2 Attentional Styles

1. Broad external attention focus	Ability to effectively manage many environmental stimuli simultaneously
2. Overloaded by external stimuli	Tendency to be confused because of the intake of too many stimuli
3. Broad internal attentional focus	Ability to effectively manage many internal stimuli (autonomic responses, covert thoughts, etc.)
4. Overloaded by internal stimuli	Tendency to be confused because of the intake of too many internal stimuli
5. Narrow attentional focus	Ability to effectively narrow attention
6. Reduced attentional focus	Tendency to reduce attention so that task-relevant information is lost

Reprinted from Nideffer (1976).

Vaccaro (32) that manipulated cognitive strategies in long-distance runners to examine the effect on physiological efficiency. Some time ago, Morgan and Pollock (49) reported that elite American distance runners tend to carefully monitor their efforts, probably in an attempt to optimize pace, whereas other runners tend to distract themselves more often in an attempt to reduce the perceived pain and fatigue of their efforts. The monitoring strategy was termed *association*, whereas the distracting strategy was called *dissociation*. Because it was unknown whether a strategy of association contributed to superior endurance performance, Hatfield et al. examined the effect of the two strategies on pulmonary activity, oxygen uptake, and muscle tension levels in intercollegiate distance runners during treadmill running (32). During work at anaerobic threshold (i.e., about 75%-80% of aerobic capacity) the associative strategy was manipulated by providing a digital display of minute volume of expired air ($\dot{V}_E$) to the athlete, which was updated every 15 s. Information on the integrated EMG activity of the trapezius and forearm muscles was delivered through a headphone set, a higher pitched tone corresponding to increased tension. The runners completed a continuous 36-min run at steady state, divided into three 12-min segments of association (feedback), dissociation (distraction) and a control condition presented in a random order.

During the feedback attentional state the efficiency of respiratory activity was increased so that oxygen consumption ($\dot{V}O_2$) was maintained at a reduced pulmonary cost relative to the other two conditions. More specifically, $\dot{V}_E$ was reduced during the association analogue, and it showed an increase in tidal volume but a decrease in respiratory rate. On each breath the athletes were unloading more CO_2 and extracting more O_2. They were breathing more *efficiently*. The running pace was constant throughout the 36 min because of the fixed treadmill speed, and, therefore, no conclusions can be reached about the effects of the cognitive strategies on performance. However, in light of Daniels's (8) work on the importance of economy to endurance performance, this study may provide some evidence of how the mind tangibly affects such physical performances.

A series of classic studies relating to the mind-body connection in sport was reviewed by Fenz (16,17). Fenz noted that superior sport parachutists tend to show a more regulated arousal state than their equally experienced but less successful counterparts, their heart rates not rising as high while boarding the aircraft and awaiting exit from the plane (16). Interestingly, he noted a difference in the attentional set of the two groups: The superior performers adopted a task-related focus and monitored external cues, such as wind, clouds, and elevation. The weaker jumpers tended to focus inward, cognitively, and to dwell on possibilities of personal harm and injury. Fenz very creatively related these opposing psychological perspectives to a well-known psychophysiological theory advanced by Lacey and Lacey (40) called the *intake-rejection hypothesis*. This theory holds that externally oriented attention (sensory intake) is associated with a reduced heart rate (i.e., the bradycardia of attention), which increases sensorimotor efficiency. The typical behavioral index of sensorimotor efficiency is reaction time. Lacey and Lacey repeatedly demonstrated that cardiac deceleration, during the warning period of a simple reaction time test, resulted in faster performance. Although the precise mechanism for the cardiac effect on the central nervous system is beyond the scope of this chapter, Fenz's work (16) supported the integrated psychophysiological model for explaining sport performance. He interpreted the mind-set of superior parachutists as analogous to sensory intake, whereas he viewed the inferior performers as falling along the dimension of sensory rejection.

Rejection of the environment, while focusing within, promotes a tachycardia response that Lacey and Lacey said promoted a "stimulus barrier" effect for the CNS. For example, performing mental arithmetic is an intense internally directed cognitive exercise that requires rejection of potentially distracting external cues. Such an exercise is associated with increased heart rate. Of course, the origin of the tachycardia in the inferior parachutists may have been due to the sympathetically mediated fear response, but theoretically Lacey's model would predict an increase in reaction time. With increased reaction time, decision making during descent would be adversely affected.

The task orientation of the superior performers may have controlled heart rate because of attentional capacity. That is, little room would be left for fear-inducing cues. The study, in summary, shows how an athlete's cognitive activity may impact on performance by way of autonomic arousal and its effect on reaction time. With decreased reaction time, the decision-making ability of the superior performers could enable better responsiveness to wind and other task-relevant conditions.

To illustrate another example of the mind-body influence, the cerebral cortex could be in a state of heightened activity if the athlete were in a highly aroused state (whether anxious or psyched-up), which could *facilitate* efferent neural activation to the involved muscles. In essence, there may be increased neural traffic to the muscles because of heightened cortical activation. Such a state might improve gross-motor performance but be debilitating for a fine-motor skill (because of excessive tension in the muscles or a lack of inhibition and relaxation in the antagonistic muscles). In fact, Weinberg provided empirical evidence for such an occurrence (73), finding disruptions in the activation patterns and coordination of the arm muscles (as measured by EMG) in anxious subjects performing an overarm throw for accuracy.

The tonic background level of arousal in any athlete is determined by a diffuse network of cells in the dorsal aspect of the brain stem, arising from the medulla oblongata to the thalamus (see Figure 7.8), called the reticular activating system (RAS). Any increases in physical arousal would increase those afferent signals from the body to the brain and serve as input to this arousal center. The RAS then stimulates or drives the activity of the cortex by way of the appropriate projection fibers. This effect would increase the excitatory connections between the neurons in the athlete's cortex, which, in turn, may increase the neural outflow to the muscles.

Concurrent with the motor outflow to the skeletal muscles, the hypothalamus (a brain stem structure situated just below the thalamus; see Figure 6.1) initiates sympathetic stimulation to the various organs of the body. This increased activation supports striated muscle metabolism. The sympathetic outflow to the viscera emanates from the thoracic and lumbar areas of the spinal column. Finally, the release of norepinephrine, a neurotransmitter, at the ends of the sympathetic neurons causes increased activity in the involved end organs. This sympathetic outflow to the organs extends also to the adrenal medullae, which release adrenaline to the circulation, further prolonging catecholaminergic stimulation. For this reason athletes may suffer pregame jitters for several hours before a contest. Table 10.3 illustrates the connections between the CNS and various organs of the body by way of sympathetic outflow. This is the branch of the autonomic nervous system that mediates the fight or flight response (4).

If sustained, the increased autonomic activity could cause a performance decrement in an endurance sport where efficient energy metabolism is necessary. However, the increased activity could be beneficial—or inconsequential—for other short-duration activities.

Table 10.3 Effects of Autonomic Nerve Stimulation on Various Visceral Effector Organs

Effector organ	Sympathetic effect
Eye	
Iris (radial muscle)	Dilates pupil
Iris (sphincter muscle)	—
Ciliary muscle	Relaxes (for far vision)
Glands	
Lacrimal (tear)	—
Sweat	Stimulates secretion
Salivary	Decreases secretion, saliva becomes thick
Stomach	—
Intestine	—
Adrenal medulla	Stimulates secretion of hormones
Heart	
Rate	Increases
Conduction	Increases rate
Strength	Increases
Blood vessels	Mostly constricts, affects all organs
Lungs	
Bronchioles (tubes)	Dilates
Mucous glands	Inhibits secretion
Gastrointestinal tract	
Motility	Inhibits movement
Sphincters	Stimulates closing
Liver	Stimulates hydrolysis of glycogen
Adipose (fat) cells	Stimulates hydrolysis of fat
Pancreas	Inhibits exocrine secretions
Spleen	Stimulates contraction
Urinary bladder	Helps set muscle tone
Piloerector muscles	Stimulates erection of hair and goose bumps
Uterus	If pregnant, contraction If not pregnant, relaxation
Penis	Erection, ejaculation

Reprinted from Fox (1984).

Afferent stimulation from the heightened visceral activity can present a serious distraction (e.g., perception of butterflies) and further narrow the selective attention available for the task-relevant cues. This distraction may not impact sport performances involving simple decision making, but it could compromise attentionally demanding ones (30).

The mind-body connection is also embodied by the endocrine system. For example, the hypothalamus stimulates the pituitary gland to release adrenocorticotrophic hormone (ACTH), which stimulates the adrenal cortex to release cortisol and other mineralocorticoids. The relevance of cortisol release to athletic conditioning and performance is that it enables the process of gluconeogenesis to occur. This term translates literally to the generation of new glucose. This response is part of the body's attempt to mobilize extra energy resources to meet the demands of any stressor, whether it be physical or psychological.

Either competition or prolonged high intensity training, especially overtraining, can be stressful both physically and mentally (25). Importantly, the substrate for this metabolic process is derived from the breakdown of protein and fat tissues in the body. The carbon, hydrogen, and oxygen derived from catabolic action, as well as the deamination of protein, is reformed to $C_6H_{12}O_6$ (glucose) for energy. This kind of psychoendocrine response is quite adaptive for meeting short-term stressors, but it may be maladaptive with chronic or long-term stressors. The chronic effect could result in loss of weight, lean tissue, and strength, due to muscle atrophy (25). Interestingly, Frankenhauser (20), a prominent researcher who examined the effect of psychological states on endocrine activity, demonstrated that feelings of uncertainty (or lack of control) about future outcomes are a driving force for cortisol secretion.

Tangible physical processes occur in the brain and body as a result of the athlete's thinking processes. These changes in neuromuscular activation, coordination, autonomic arousal, and metabolism can cause changes in motor performance. The changes may be beneficial, detrimental, or neutral, depending on the nature of the task, the athlete's level of skill, and the complexity of the task in terms of decision making.

THE IDEAL PERFORMANCE STATE

The ideal performance state has been studied from a number of measurement perspectives. Williams (79) listed these characteristics that athletes typically report about this state:

- Absence of fear—no fear of failure

- No thinking about or analysis of performance (This would be related to the motor stage of automaticity.)
- A narrow focus of attention concentrated on the activity itself
- A sense of effortlessness—an involuntary experience
- A sense of personal control
- A disorientation of time and space, in which time seems to slow

In a sense, this ideal performance state seems to represent everything that applied sport psychology programs attempt to promote. There is an absence of negative self-talk, a strong feeling of efficacy, and an adaptive focus on the task-relevant cues. Importantly, the athletes trust in their skill and conditioning levels and just "let it happen," without interference from negative associative processes in the cortex.

A good example of this state is reported in the following quote by Walter Payton, one of the premiere running backs of the National Football League (NFL) (1).

I'm Dr. Jekyll and Mr. Hyde when it comes to football. When I'm on the field sometimes I don't know what I am doing out there. People ask me about this move or that move, but I don't know why I did something, I just did it. I am able to focus out the negative things around me and just zero in on what I am doing out there. Off the field I become myself again. (pp. 2-3)

Payton's comments richly reinforce many of the concepts discussed throughout this chapter. It is important to remember that his mental state largely rests on a sound physical training program, as well as on a history of performance success. Payton was a phenomenal physical specimen who, in the off-season, arduously ran wind sprints, trained on hills, and lifted weights. Combined with superior performance on the field, such physical preparatory effort would contribute greatly to the focused, confident psychological state he exuded.

Interestingly, this mind state has been noted by some sport psychologists who have measured regional brain activity in elite athletes during performance (31). Using EEG technology, Hatfield et al. examined left-hemispheric and right-hemispheric activity in world-class competitive marksmen as they prepared for their shots. In essence, researchers showed that the analytical left hemisphere decreased its activation level during the preparatory sighting phase, whereas the right hemisphere (more involved in visual-spatial processing) relaxed too, but not as much. In essence, these highly skilled and focused athletes experienced an overall quieting of the forebrain accompanied by a shift in relative hemispheric dominance. Unfortunately, the dynamics and requirements of rifle marksmanship differ from those of other sports, but marksmen do provide a nice model for studying skilled attentive states, using EEG technology, because they are motionless and yet highly engaged psychologically. It is worthwhile noting the relationship between attentional processes and performance is universal in nature.

It is risky to extrapolate the findings to other athletes, but the statement Payton made when he said, "I don't know why I did something, I just did it," would seem consistent with the hemispheric shift phenomenon. O.J. Simpson, the former running back of the NFL's Buffalo Bills franchise, also reported a kind of "mindless" state. He revealed that even though he thought about "nothing" during a given play, he could recall where each teammate and opponent was situated on the field when he crossed the goal line. Such a contradiction can be resolved by explaining in different terms: Simpson apparently allocated his fixed attentional resources so that he processed spatially oriented cues and could efficiently react to changing conditions on the field. Obviously, being highly skilled, he didn't need to "think" or analyze what he was doing. His high degree of skill probably also minimized engagement in negative self-talk. It may be that such a performance state, as reported by Simpson, would also show relative right-brain dominance if assessed by psychophysiological technology, such as EEG.

Again, this allocation or shift in allocation of attention to process only the cues and cognitive activity that relate to the athlete's performance nicely represents our concept of **mental/psychological efficiency**. We believe that such a state precipitates the fluid, graceful movements of superior performers, which can thematically be described as physically efficient. Thus, such a state exemplifies the optimal mind-body relationship in sport. A practical point for coaches relates to what kind of advice they give an athlete just prior to performance. It would appear counterproductive to engage in much analytical thought about the skill to be performed. An analytical approach may be useful for the novice, but a different approach, allowing the athlete to "just let it happen," should be employed as skill develops.

MOTIVATIONAL PHENOMENA

Intrinsic Motivation

Intrinsic motivation is an important aspect of any athlete. Deci defined this construct as a desire to be competent and self-determining (10). With intrinsic motivation, basically, the athlete is a self-starter because of his or her love of the game. The coach's work of teaching skill and effective strategies with team sports can be much more effective when athletes are *self-motivated*. Surrounded by such players, a coach can concentrate on task-relevant concerns rather than on encouraging effort by cajoling, punishing, or exhorting. Intrinsically motivated athletes are more likely to maintain effort consistently across practice and competition, lessening the coach's responsibilities. How can such a desirable state be maintained or encouraged? The answer lies in Deci's definition, which stresses success (competence) and ''pulling one's own strings'' (self-determination). Appropriate goals, especially ones of a process or performance nature, can increase perceived competence. Additionally, giving the athlete some latitude in decision making would increase perceived self-determination. Effective leaders in business and industry know that placing an appropriate degree of responsibility (i.e., latitude in decision making) with their employees is empowering in terms of increasing commitment, effort, and creativity (67). Authoritarian behavior is sometimes warranted in sport, in that clear directives are needed in a stressful competitive environment, but a total lack of delegated responsibilities could result in a loss of initiative and drive in athletes: Within the team sport setting a diffusion of personal responsibility and leadership behavior might occur.

Another desirable construct is achievement motivation, which relates to the athlete's wish to engage in competition, or social comparison. All things being equal between two athletes, whoever is higher in achievement motivation would be the better athlete because of viewing competition in an appetitive manner.

Achievement Motivation

McClelland, Atkinson, Clark, and Lowell (47) theorized that all people have opposing personality traits within themselves: the *motive to achieve success* (MAS) and the *motive to avoid failure* (MAF). The MAS is self-explanatory, whereas the MAF relates to the desire to protect one's ego and self-esteem. To understand their relevance to the psychology of coaching consider the following.

McClelland et al. (47) showed, by means of an arithmetically stated theory, that MAS-dominated athletes are most intrigued by situations that are either uncertain or challenging, with a 50% probability of success. On the other hand, MAF-dominated players are comfortable in situations where it is either very easy to achieve success *or* extremely difficult (i.e., they would not be expected to win). At a high level of sport involvement it is unlikely that athletes would be dominated by MAF, but they would certainly show degrees or a range of competitiveness. Confronted by a very challenging goal,

such as gaining a significant amount of lean muscle weight during the hypertrophy phase of a periodized cycle, a MAF individual might reduce effort because he fears failure and the threat to self-esteem (he might also claim the goal is unrealistic), whereas a MAS individual might heighten effort in response to the challenge, not perceiving any threat.

During a tense game the coach would want to handle these two players and psychological orientations differently in order to maximize success. Suppose that two defensive backs in a football game—one dominated by MAS and the other by MAF—confronted a situation in which their team, playing defense, has one minute left in the game and leads by only two points. The opposing team's offense has just crossed midfield. The MAS player views this scenario as an opportunity to pursue defensive skills, whereas the MAF player adopts an avoidance behavior. With the first player the coach would not have to issue any motivational instructions because the MAS athlete perceives the outcome as challenging (i.e., 50% probability of success). But with the MAF player, the coach should define the athlete's responsibility to make goal attainment relatively easy. For example, this athlete could be told simply to cover his territory while in a zone defense or simply to execute proper footwork during pass coverage. This kind of coaching instruction removes some of the self-induced pressure, allowing the athlete to focus on task-relevant cues. If success is achieved, the MAF athlete may become more comfortable in highly competitive situations. Likewise, referring to the difficulty a MAF athlete would have with the challenge of weight gain, the strength and conditioning coach should assist the athlete in setting more realistic goals based on the perception of what is realistic.

Positive and Negative Reinforcement in Coaching

Experiences are stored in long-term, or associative, memory where they are powerful determinants of how an athlete interprets a practice or competitive situation (e.g., fear or challenge). Long-term memory may be conceived as the subconscious mind. For it to contribute adaptively to performance, it should be filled with largely positive experience. If one envisions the conscious mind as attentional processing, or working memory, and the subconscious mind as the vast reservoir of stored, or long-term, memory, then the relative magnitude of the latter is overwhelming. And, importantly, long-term memory would largely shape perception and attention. Coaches should be aware, therefore, of the concepts of positive and negative reinforcement as well as positive and negative punishment (43); these kinds of experiences will shape long-term memory.

An important behavioral technology can be used to increase the positive, confident psychological outlook. **Positive reinforcement** is the act of *increasing* the probability of occurrence of a given behavior (a target behavior, like correct footwork in basketball, is termed an operant) by following it with or presenting a given act, object, or event like praise, decals on the helmet, or prizes and awards. **Negative reinforcement** also increases the probability of occurrence of a given operant by *removing* an act, object, or event that is typically aversive (43). For example, if the team particularly hustled in practice (i.e., the operant is enthusiasm and hustle), then the coach could announce that no wind sprints will be required at the session's end. This coaching reinforcement style forces attention on what the athlete is doing *correctly.*

Punishment, on the other hand, is designed to *decrease* the occurrence of a given operant. Such behaviors, by necessity, would be negative things like mistakes or a lack of effort. **Positive punishment** would be the presentation of an act, object, or event following a behavior that could decrease its occurrence. An example is reprimanding a player after a fumble. **Negative punishment**, or *removal* of a contingency, could take the form of revoking privileges or playing time, as in benching. The word *contingency* refers to a conditional consequence, and in the previous sentence it relates to the act of benching. Coaches use both reward and punishment liberally, but arguably reinforcement (i.e., reward) or a *positive approach* is better because it focuses athletes on what they *should do* and what they *did right.* Reinforcement increases a task-relevant focus, as opposed to a worry focus. Secondly, athletes build long-term memories of success and build self-esteem, self-efficacy, and confidence. A task focus usually facilitates reaction time and decision making. Additionally, success-based experiences more likely color the athlete's view of competition or perception as appetitive and as an opportunity to perform.

Of course, coaches should punish unwarranted lack of effort, but it would seem ineffective to punish athletes for making mistakes if they are *trying* to perform correctly. Jimmy Johnson, the head coach of the NFL's Dallas Cowboys franchise, believes strongly in the positive, or reinforcement, style of coaching as seen in this quote from an interview (34):

> I never tell a running back, Don't fumble. I never tell a placekicker, Don't miss. I say to the running back, Protect the ball. I say to the placekicker, Make this. You'd be surprised how few coaches understand the simple psychology I'm using here. But, in my opinion, it is vital psychology. Why? The human mind, upon receiving the message, Don't fumble, will record the word "fumble" and, consciously or not, worry over it. The "don't" doesn't help. If anything, it hurts—because it's a negative. And so the running back who is told, Don't fumble, is more likely to fumble than if the coach had said nothing at all. So I try never to plant a negative seed. I try to make every comment a positive comment.
>
> Some coaches bring their rookies into training camp and—though they might know their first- and second-round picks by name—take the approach with the lower-round picks and free agents that "Oh, I'll learn his name if he makes the team." What they don't understand is that whether a player makes the team might hinge on something as subtle as whether you treat him as an individual that you care about, with talent you believe in. (p. 4-5)

Interestingly, Johnson's use of recognition—addressing each rookie by his first name—a form of positive behavior, may very well allow a player to focus on task or game-relevant cues: The reward of personal recognition by an esteemed figure could both increase arousal and reduce negative or self-deprecating thoughts in the athlete's mind. Johnson's style increases the likelihood that the player will exhibit reduced reaction time, more explosive muscular contractions, and better attention to cues related to defensive reads, "picking up" a receiver's fakes, and so forth. Such a style can indirectly affect the athlete's muscular movements. Furthermore, understanding how the mind functions (i.e., attention) would philosophically guide a coach to feel justified—he understands *why* he would employ such an approach.

INFLUENCE OF AROUSAL ON PERFORMANCE

One of the major tenets of the arousal–performance relationship, derived from the classic work of Yerkes and Dodson (82), is referred to as the **inverted-U theory**.

Inverted-U Theory

Basically, this theory states that arousal facilitates performance up to an optimal level, beyond which further increases in arousal are associated with reduced performance. Figure 10.2 graphically shows this relationship. A number of revisions have been postulated to improve this predictive model, such as Hanin's (26) zone of optimal performance theory, which we shall discuss later. Understanding this inverted-U concept will help coaches and athletes understand *why* arousal affects performance, and it will enable them to gain greater

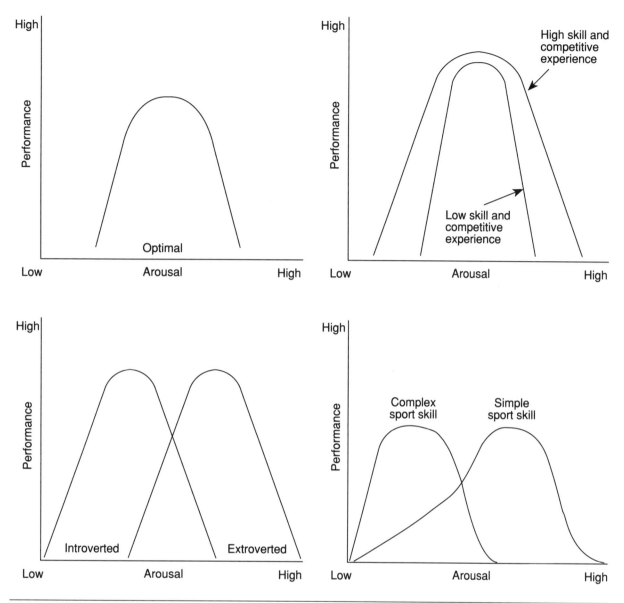

Figure 10.2 Inverted-U theory and its modifications. Reprinted from Hatfield and Walford (1987).

control over what is the appropriate level of arousal for a given athlete within a given sport.

An athlete's skill level can widen, or increase, the latitude of optimal arousal: That is, the more skill an athlete has developed, the more he can tolerate changes in arousal. In the beginning stages of learning a skill the athlete is in a stage of analysis or cognition (18). This means that he or she has to *think* about actions. For example, a novice basketball player has to be conscious of the ball while dribbling and needs to devote some attention to the task. At a given level of arousal, worrisome thoughts compete with an attentional capacity already filled by details of motor performance (i.e., dribbling). If a new situation suddenly develops, the novice's mind is already occupied, and he or she may

not see it. Remember the earlier example of a high school basketball player suddenly thrust into a starting role.

Tucker, Antes, Stenslie, and Barnhardt (68) conducted an ingenious experiment that provides evidence that state anxiety may place a processing load primarily on the left hemisphere. In it they presented high- and low-state anxious subjects with a recognition task both for the left and right brain hemispheres. This recognition task involved split-second decision making about a word presented tachistoscopically in the left visual half-field (the right brain) or the right visual half-field (the left hemisphere). The subject was to determine whether the word was an antonym to a previous display. The two groups of subjects did not differ in their performances (i.e., percent of correct responses) for stimuli presented to the right forebrain, but they showed a marked difference in left forebrain accuracy of detection. The high-state anxious individuals were severely compromised and made more errors. This finding has significant implications for the novice or unskilled athlete, inasmuch as it is believed that analytical processing of motor skill is negotiated by left-brain processing. Attentional capacity would be at a premium in the anxious athlete, who is at the cognitive or analytical stage of skill acquisition. The left forebrain of such a competitor may be so preoccupied that any stimuli arising from the sport situation, such as reacting to a pick in basketball or the signals from a catcher to a pitcher in baseball, would be missed. The functional attention that can be devoted externally is severely limited.

Conversely, Fitts and Posner (18) described the advanced performer as marked by the stage of automaticity. He or she does not need to think about movements, which are initiated subcortically—rather than cortically (as with the novice). Any arousal-inducing thoughts are *not* in competition for attentional space with motoric concerns. That is why advanced performers can call plays, dribble, and coordinate their body movements with the dynamic flow of teammates and opponents more readily than can novices. This does not mean that advanced level athletes necessarily like increased arousal, but they can *tolerate* it to a greater extent.

In coaching, one should *decrease* the decision-making responsibilities of the developing or unseasoned athletes (players who are skilled but lack competitive experience) or have them focus on simple assignments to prevent attentional overload. In coaching Olympic-style lifters during an important meet, instructions to novice competitors should be simple, clear, and direct. When they do experience success, the derived self-confidence may reduce negative self-talk and the sense of further uncertainty that typically characterizes such performers. The optimal arousal point is lower for lesser-skilled athletes compared with more advanced players.

A second factor affecting optimal arousal is the task complexity (53). Most athletic skills are exceedingly complex from a biomechanical perspective, but the complexity that concerns us relates to conscious decision making. For example, sprinting is a very complex phenomenon in terms of motor control and functional anatomy, but, fortunately, athletes do not have to devote much conscious attention to the coordinated action. In fact, the action becomes altered and inefficient if they think about it, because they change the neural sequences for movement initiation. From an attentional perspective, simple skills can tolerate a higher degree of arousal (and attentional narrowing) because they have few task-relevant cues to monitor. Fortunately, physiological arousal, which typically accompanies psychic arousal, may be beneficial. Any increase in neuromuscular activation enables more powerful and explosive movements. However, the situation is dramatically reversed for skills that require tremendous decision-making effort, such as a goalie has in soccer or a catcher has in baseball when facing a critical, bases-loaded pitch. In these instances arousal must be kept relatively low because of the necessity of maintaining attentional width.

Certainly, for athletes to maintain great presence of mind while engaging in physically demanding situations (e.g., a quarterback scanning for secondary receivers while running for his life) is engaging in a very complex task, from an arousal and performance perspective. The physiological-arousal needs of the body are at odds with the lowered psychological-arousal needs of the mind. In short, the more complex the skill, the lower the level of arousal that is required. To illustrate this discussion, Shapiro (60) provided the following quotes about quarterback Joe Montana of the NFL's Kansas City Chiefs after his team's defeat of the Houston Oilers to gain entry to the 1993 AFC championship.

About the only thing Montana can't do is offer detailed explanations of how he's almost always able to find a way to win.

And so, it was left to teammates, past and present, to explain the Montana phenomenon.

On Sunday, all of Montana's receivers talked about his ability to stay calm no matter the situation, no matter the score, no matter how many passes they'd dropped, no matter how many times he'd failed to get them the football.

"Joe is a warrior," said tight end Keith Cash. "He doesn't get ruffled at all. We play with a lot of confidence because he has such confidence. With him, you know he's gonna throw the ball, and if you're open, he's gonna get you the ball."

Added wide receiver Willie Davis, "Every time we're down and Joe is out there, the whole team feels we'll win the game, no matter how far down we are or who we're playing. You never see Joe get rattled. Even if we're wide open and drop a pass on a critical down, he'll never say 'You should have caught it.' All he says is go to the next play, and it's not like he won't throw it to you anymore, either. He tells us, 'Do whatever you want to get open, and I'll find you.' And he does." (p. E7)

It appears that Montana attempts to reduce his teammates' arousal levels by making a stressful, complex task somewhat simple to follow. He reduces the potentially overwhelming information and distracting environmental cues.

A third factor, personality, can also shape the optimal level of arousal. According to Eysenck (14), extroverted individuals differ neurologically from introverts. Extroverts are sensory reducers, whereas introverts are sensory augmenters, or ''increasers.'' Accordingly, because people seek an individual optimal level of arousal, the extrovert ''requires'' heightened stimulation (compared with the introvert) because of tending to reduce or dampen arousing effects. On the other hand, the introvert ''requires'' a lower level of stimulation because of tending to increase arousal. All things being equal between two athletes in terms of physique, height, weight, visual acuity, and muscular strength, the extroverted player can better handle the more arousing, or critical, game situation. In reality, of course, no two athletes are the same physically, so that the extrovert may not be as strong or as skilled as the classic introvert. This is why it is important for coaches to fully understand athletes from both a psychological and physiological perspective.

Trait anxiety also affects the determination of optimal arousal. People with high levels of trait anxiety tend to flood attentional capacity with task-irrelevant cognitions, such as thoughts of failure, catastrophe, or ego-oriented concerns. With a complex decision-making task, these attentionally demanding cues could compromise a player's selective attention. Of course, the athlete with low trait anxiety can handle higher levels of pressure because of the decreased probability of engaging in such personal catastrophizing.

There are probably additional factors that moderate this inverted U, but even the interaction of the few factors described here can add tremendous variation in the optimal level individuals require.

Optimal Functioning

Hanin noted these interactions and developed the zone of optimal functioning theory (26). He basically holds that different people perform with very different levels of arousal. It is unclear whether the factors discussed earlier fully account for such individual differences, but nevertheless some practical determinations can be made. Athletes retrospectively engage in recalling the arousal associated with several performances that differed in quality. The measurement of self-reported arousal can be accomplished by using a standardized psychometric instrument, such as the state anxiety inventory (63), which ranges from a low score of 20 to a maximum of 80. An average score is derived from those associated with the best performances. Hanin argues that a deviation of 4 points around this mean will generate the optimal zone of self-reported arousal. As such, the athlete can monitor his state prior to an important match and make adjustments to ''fall'' into this zone. As discussed

earlier, the athlete should then be able to concentrate, or allocate attention, appropriately as well as ready himself physically.

Catastrophe Theory

According to Fazey and Hardy (15), the assessment of the cognitive and somatic dimensions of arousal can sharpen our ability to predict (and, therefore, control) their impact on performance. Earlier assumptions associated with the inverted-U theory held that increases in arousal beyond the optimal level resulted in gradual, proportionate declines in performance. However, common observation would tell us that this is not always the case—an athlete may suffer a severe dramatic and catastrophic decline rather than a gradual quadratic or curvilinear path, and restoring a degree of calm does not necessarily bring a return to the level of performance exhibited before suffering the decline. In the Fazey and Hardy model, somatic arousal has a curvilinear inverted-U relationship to athletic performance, whereas cognitive anxiety shows a steady negative relationship to performance. When increases in physiological arousal do occur *in the presence of cognitive anxiety*, then a sudden drop—rather than a gradual decline—in performance will occur. The practical implication of catastrophe theory is that the arousal construct needs to be more clearly defined. Arousal is a rather vague term, and it would be more discriminatory to use such terms as psychic energy, cognitive anxiety, physiological arousal, and somatic anxiety.

Self-Efficacy

Of course, the main objective for applied sport psychology is generating a psychological perspective that improves performance, and it has been argued that perceived self-confidence or self-efficacy (2) is a better predictor of task execution than either arousal or anxiety. Self-efficacy is perceived self-confidence toward a given task in a specific situation (2). It is the sense of success that an athlete feels he can control, or that she embodies: Someone who is highly efficacious does not doubt his or her ability to succeed at a given task, even when failure is experienced. Anxiety and arousal would seem to be outcomes then, rather than determinants, of this state. Nevertheless, they still are of significance inasmuch as they represent the state of the mind and body. It may be that psychic energy, cognitive anxiety, physiological arousal, and somatic anxiety interface with self-efficacy and physical performance. Figure 10.3 illustrates how these relationships affect both the confident and the nonconfident athlete.

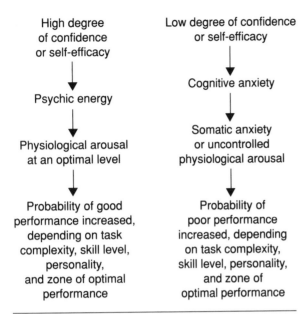

High degree of confidence or self-efficacy	Low degree of confidence or self-efficacy
↓	↓
Psychic energy	Cognitive anxiety
↓	↓
Physiological arousal at an optimal level	Somatic anxiety or uncontrolled physiological arousal
↓	↓
Probability of good performance increased, depending on task complexity, skill level, personality, and zone of optimal performance	Probability of poor performance increased, depending on task complexity, skill level, personality, and zone of optimal performance

Figure 10.3 The relationship between confidence and athletic performance.

MENTAL MANAGEMENT OF PHYSICAL RESOURCES: CONTROLLING PSYCHOLOGICAL PROCESSES

If self-efficacy and a relaxed, confident mind (i.e., the efficient management of an athlete's mental and physical resources) are critical to sport performance, then how can such a state be achieved? We believe the most powerful determinant of confidence and a sense of preparation is quality physical practice in which a number of positive experiences are stored in long-term memory. In essence, the most powerful psychological skills package is quality practice and successful competitive exposure. Gould, Hodge, Peterson, and Giannini provided evidence (23) from their national survey of U.S. coaches that this is a widespread belief and practice. In a sense, coaches act as practicing sport psychologists simply by conditioning and teaching athletes the skills of sport.

Physical training is rich in psychological effect—the two realms cannot really be separated. This is why many athletes develop a strong sense of confidence and psychological preparedness even though they may never have been exposed to formal sport psychology practice in the form of psychological skills techniques, such as mental imagery, hypnosis, and progressive muscle relaxation. Moreover, many athletes have a strong social support system as well, which includes family, friends, coaching personnel, teammates, and others who tend to provide positive feedback and emotional nurturance. Importantly, outstanding coaches at various levels of

play are excellent communicators who provide very specific, focused instructions for their athletes, simultaneously giving ample feedback about the quality of performances in practice and during competition. In fact, athletic coaches tend to assume the role of teachers who often find themselves in a very positively charged emotional environment. That is, their students typically "want to be there" and have high intrinsic motivation. From observational studies of collegiate coaches like John Wooden, former basketball coach at UCLA (65), and Frank Kush, former football coach at Arizona State University and with the NFL's Indianapolis Colts (9), it seems that both leaders tended to be liberal in their use of praise and different styles of interaction with athletes of different temperaments. Granted, Wooden, who won 10 National Collegiate Athletic Association (NCAA) basketball championships in 12 years, was surrounded by extremely talented players who self-selected into the program, but it should also be noted that Wooden also won when he coached teams that varied greatly in terms of physical assets.

Goal Setting

All coaches can probably improve performance quality by directing their athletes' attention to appropriate task-oriented and emotional goals and by instilling a sense of success and self-efficacy through positive and negative reinforcement of desired actions. **Goal setting** can be described as a process whereby progressively challenging standards of performance are pursued with a defined criterion of task performance that increases the likelihood of perceived success (42). For example, a goal for a swimmer may be to execute a technically correct stroke throughout a sanctioned distance, like the 50-m freestyle. In the beginning, the swimmer's level might be so low that such a task would be overwhelming and produce a strong sense of failure and frustration. Yet, the coach may see that the athlete has the physical resources to excel at such an event. That is, there is a high degree of fast-twitch, or Type II, muscle fibers; the swimmer exhibits superior muscular power or speed-strength in the upper and lower body; and he or she also seems to have a high capacity for anaerobic metabolism (according to physiological testing). However, the stroke mechanics are inefficient and therefore the athlete lacks confidence.

Process Goals.
First, the coach and athlete can break the skill and conditioning units down into manageable components (traditionally considered the whole-part-whole method of learning). As each component is mastered, and the athlete focuses on it, a sense of progress and success are nurtured. An important distinction, in terms of setting goals, is the process versus the

outcome (21). Process goals are those over which the athlete has complete control. If the effort is expended, success occurs with a relatively high degree of probability. Examples of process goals within the skill domain would relate to form and technique, although an individually determined time (in the case of the swimmer or track athlete) could also be considered a process goal. An example of a process goal within strength and conditioning is to have the athlete focus on the strategy for weight reduction (e.g., what the athlete must do on a daily basis, such as aerobic activity and weight training), rather than on the actual result (e.g., a loss of weight), thereby increasing a sense of *control* over actions. With process kinds of goals there is a strong contingency between success and effort.

Outcome Goals. On the other hand, outcome goals are ones over which the athlete has little control; typically winning is the primary focus. We believe that winning is a sound goal orientation, but, ironically, that the likelihood of its achievement may be increased by an athlete having both a process and outcome goal orientation, as opposed to a winning-only attitude. Undue emphasis on winning may occupy such a proportion of fixed attentional capacity that it causes narrowing. Task-relevant cues are missed, reaction time is slowed, and coordination is diminished by forcing movements and compromising automaticity, altering the neuromuscular sequencing.

Both process and outcome goals can be applied to the conditioning process as well. For example, emphasizing arm action technique during sprinting illustrates the process orientation, as opposed to focusing only on winning the drill, the outcome. An exception is those instances where an athlete is extremely confident and undermatched in terms of competition and may want to focus solely on outcome and a personal best to maximize motivation.

Short-Term Goals. Beyond the process and outcome distinction, goals can be categorized as short term and long term, or as proximal and distal, respectively. Short-term goals increase the likelihood of success because, although challenging, they are relatively close to the athlete's present ability level. They increase confidence, self-esteem, and self-efficacy. In this regard, short-term process and outcome goals counteract the boredom and frustration that are potential side effects of long, arduous training regimens.

Long-Term Goals. However, the full meaning of the proximal standards of success is framed by an appropriate long-term goal. The athlete may see more relevance in everyday practice goals if it is apparent how they help attain the ultimate level of performance. For example, a young woman who has a long-term goal of winning the floor routine for the NCAA gymnastics championship during her senior year may be much more intense and positive about weight-room conditioning exercises when she perceives their relevance to her dream. An athlete may be more aroused psychologically and physiologically during practice by the perception that today's activity is another brick in the wall of the personal, long-term dream.

Martin and Hrycaiko (46) outlined a very sound program of goal setting in an article discussing the tenets of effective behavioral coaching. In this program a coach specifies the components of a given skill and charts the athlete's success with each part until the whole skill is mastered. Figure 10.4 illustrates this motivational technique for the skill of pass blocking in American football. In behavioral psychology, proximal goals that progressively increase in difficulty are termed *successive approximations*. This is because they increasingly *resemble* the long-term goal. Each targeted goal or behavior is termed an *operant*. **Operants** are clearly defined standards of performance and derive from the term *operationalize*, which means to concretely specify a behavior such that it can be measured.

To understand the effectiveness of such a program, imagine a scenario in which a youth football player attempts to execute the pass-blocking maneuver while simultaneously focusing on the component of proper footwork. Unfortunately, in this scenario he gets knocked down, his helmet is ripped off, his nose is bloodied, *but* his ego is not battered. Why? Because he and his coach observed that he correctly executed his initial footwork and channeled his effort appropriately. Success, in other words, is perceived amidst the apparent catastrophe. The important principle here is that an athlete is more likely to maintain effort with such a perspective. If he has the physical potential to become a skilled football player, then the realization of his potential may increase, instead of his football career being terminated. Perhaps even more important, the athlete continues to build self-esteem, which is a much more important outcome than winning a game.

Process goals and outcome goals, both long term and short term, should always be stated in specific positive terms. It is important to state them positively because of the athlete's fixed attentional capacity. It is more efficient to focus on what is correct than on what is incorrect. What *not* to do requires greater cognitive complexity—too much thinking—and may very well slow reaction time. It is a task-irrelevant cue that needlessly demands attentional resources. Negative goals can paralyze players, because of both increasing fear of failure and the cognitive processing discussed earlier. Athletes who are trying not to look foolish are less

	Date		
Scoring Key I = Needs improvement G = Good N = Excellent			
Arms are crossed at wrist with palms up			
Initial step taken with foot closest to the defender			
Drive out of stance, short initial step(s) toward target			
Arms are brought up and forward on the rotation, aimed at the chest of target			
As rotation of arm starts there is good arch of the back with the head up—forward thrust is from a low position			
On impact, the block is delivered with the forearms, not the head; side view will reveal that both elbows are ahead of the head			
Both fists (closed) are against the chest (not away from the body)			
Elbows at blocker's chest level, not above shoulders			
If fists open, palms should face opponent or rotation not complete			
Blow is delivered from a wide base: Balanced stance avoids easy slip-off and opponent receives full impact of the blow			
Follow through with short, choppy steps (footfire) from a wide stance; take defender in direction he wants to go (control of man essential)			

Figure 10.4 Effective behavioral coaching chart to assess a football player performing the drive block.
Adapted from Martin and Hrycaiko (1983).

likely to be creative and take chances. They think too much and lack mental efficiency. *Positive* goals direct an athlete's attention to task-relevant cues.

The importance of specificity of the goals relates to giving the athlete feedback. Feedback, or the knowledge of success and failure, is more effective in the presence of specific, hopefully quantifiable, goals—as opposed to vague standards of performance. Feedback is a corrective device, much like the operating of a thermostat or cybernetic device. Both success and failure can help the athlete stay on course toward long-term success. For example, a goal of 25 min of continuous running in a heart-rate range of 160 to 170 bpm is a much more engaging task than going "out for a run." The vague statement may be fine for a recreational participant, but it is not helpful for a competitive cross-country runner, especially when the goal is to develop the physiological needs of the individual.

The systematic use of goal setting can increase the psychological development of the athlete while increasing performance. This approach has an abundance of empirical support from research studies where goal setting has been contrasted to relatively vague motivational strategies, such as exhortations to "do your best!"

(74,75). A number of reasons explain why goal setting impacts on performance:

- Goals direct attention by prioritizing an athlete's efforts.
- Goals increase effort because of the contingency between goal attainment and success.
- Goals increase the experience of positive reinforcement through the feedback given to athletes.

It would seem that the informational nature of thoughtfully derived goals, which increase effort because they are challenging yet attainable, is a powerful ingredient for behavioral change.

We would like to note that optimal goal setting requires knowledge of the exercise sciences both in the biophysical and behavioral domains. The efficacy of goals for improving athletic performance lies in their relevance to the physical needs of the athlete. For example, formulating a series of appropriate goals to enable a 400-m runner to decrease his or her time in the event rests on understanding the physical profile, relevant metabolic pathways, and biomechanical technique to be developed.

Of course, some goals may be completely psychological and, therefore, only indirectly performance-based. An example of such a goal is to adopt a positive mood state for an entire practice. Although such goals demand less biophysical knowledge, they may be profoundly useful in increasing performance. That is because they are the goals that an athlete has tremendous control over and they can facilitate inhibiting habitual negative self-talk. However, the most comprehensive goal-setting programs would encompass an integrated knowledge base of several areas of exercise science. We believe this requirement largely defines the uniqueness of sport psychology, or kinesiological psychology, from other behavioral sciences.

Although a scientific and motivationally sound coaching program can greatly help in the development of athletes, several other complementary techniques exist. In reality most athletes probably receive a combination of adaptive and maladaptive experiences during practice and competition, and they may have developed a lack of self-confidence from nonsport experiences. These people need to exert control over their mental and physical states to increase performance and enjoy competition more fully. Therefore, we turn now to some cognitively and somatically based sport psychology techniques athletes can use to better manage their physical resources.

Energizing Techniques

A number of techniques exist with which the athlete can *elevate* his or her level of arousal. The positive effect of such mental preparation or **psyching strategies** on strength performance is well documented in the sport psychology literature (24,50,51,61,69,76,77,78). This relationship has been demonstrated with a static grip strength task (61); by manipulating the subjects' belief in their ability to compete in an arm wrestling match (50); by manipulating expectations on an inclined bench-press strength task (51); and by manipulating preparatory state on a dynamic leg-extension task (69,76,78).

Self-selected forms of mental preparation have been used in many studies to allow subjects to perform at their best (5,61,76). These strategies were later categorized, based on personal interviews and self-report questionnaires. As a result, several forms of mental preparation strategies have been shown to produce greater expressions of force, as compared with nonmental preparation conditions. These include statements of self-efficacy (61,76,78), attentional focus (24,61,76), preparatory arousal (61,76), imagery (61), relaxation (76), and religious beliefs (5).

Studies conducted to examine the effectiveness of mental preparation on strength performance have contrasted mental preparation with other control conditions. These control conditions are not associated with concentration levels that would be conducive to performance enhancement. The comparative conditions include distraction (24,61,69) and a read-only condition (78). Distraction involves a serial-number subtraction task, in which the subject is asked to count aloud backward from 1,000 by sevens (61). The read-only condition involves reading aloud from a selected passage (78). Within this research, a continuum of attentional focus has been examined. Mental preparation facilitates performance by directing the subject's attention toward accomplishing the task. Meanwhile, the distraction conditions seem to direct the subject's attention away from the task.

Weinberg et al. (76) suggest that the mediating mechanism of the *psyching-strength* relationship may be arousal, and Gould et al. (24) obtained self-reported measures of arousal under various types of mental preparation conditions. The results obtained from both the Competitive State Anxiety Inventory (44) and the Activation-Deactivation Checklist (66) revealed that neither score paralleled any changes in performance. The role of self-reported arousal as the major mediator in the psyching strategy–strength performance relationship was not supported.

Wilkes and Summers (78) contrasted several mental preparation strategies, including preparatory arousal, attentional focus, imagery, and statements of self-efficacy, with a control condition to determine effects on a dynamic leg-extension task. All strategies were superior to control. The preparatory arousal strategy, however, distinguished itself from the other techniques. More importantly, the results obtained from self-report measures suggested that attentional narrowing is what all effective mental preparation strategies have in common. Mechanistically, this would seem to provide an explanation for cognitive influence over such tasks.

Many investigators have addressed different mechanisms involved with the expression of greater force. Whether the effect of motivation on endurance (12,56,80), hypnosis on strength (35,48,56), or expectancy on muscular efficiency (12,70,71,72), these studies suggest that maximal performance is limited by psychological inhibitions. Supermaximal performance may be achieved through an active inhibition of these normally protective psychological and neurological inhibitors (35,56,80).

Two mechanisms may allow for greater force expression. The first mechanism, precontraction of antagonistic muscles, has an effect on the expression of force of the agonistic muscle (57). When precontraction of the antagonist occurs prior to a maximal voluntary contraction of the agonist, neural inhibition is overridden and greater activation of the agonist is allowed (57). The second mechanism involves the influence of the Golgi tendon organs. Golgi tendon organs, proprioceptors located in the tendons, monitor tension. Because tendons are attached to muscle, the Golgi tendon organs sense the degree of muscular tension. If the tension is too great, as when damage to the muscle or tendon is sensed, feedback loops from the Golgi apparatus to the CNS enable an inhibition of the contracting muscle and an activation of the antagonistic muscle (3). This occurrence relieves the muscular tension and lessens the risk of injury. Strength training may disrupt Golgi tendon organ inhibition, thus allowing the greater expression of force (19). To illustrate the plasticity of force expression, Ikai and Steinhaus (35) studied the effect of hypnosis, noise, and pharmacological agents on forearm flexor strength performance. Their results suggest that psychologically induced neural inhibition may be overcome by these agents, resulting in heightened performance (i.e., muscular force expression).

Physical Relaxation Techniques

Several physical techniques can help athletes manage their psychological processes. This should not be surprising, in view of the mind-body relationship.

Diaphragmatic Breathing. The first technique to use to reach a higher level of physical and mental relaxation is *diaphragmatic breathing*. Referred to as belly breathing, this form of breathing is a basic stress management technique and a precursor to all other mental-training techniques. It focuses thought on breathing (a controllable aspect of physiology) to clear the mind

and, therefore, attentional capacity. During any mental training exercise, athletes should attempt to engage in deep rhythmic breathing in a relaxed, natural manner. They should avoid hyperventilation and breath holding (Valsalva maneuver). Diaphragmatic breathing is a somatopsychic (muscle-to-mind) technique (27). This means that peripheral (muscular) action is the initiator of central (mental) relaxation. Physiologically, this form of breathing has major influence over heart rate and muscle tension due to feedback mechanisms that link the respiratory and cardiac control centers in the brain stem. The relatively deep inspiration, followed by a controlled expiration, will alter autonomic nervous system (ANS) balance such that an increased expression of vagal tone or parasympathetic activity can occur (54). The parasympathetic branch of the ANS promotes the opposite effect of the sympathetic, mediated fight or flight response. Thus, rhythmic breathing can decrease neural stimulation to both the skeletal muscles and viscera (e.g., heart, lungs, liver) resulting in a sense of deep relaxation.

Diaphragmatic breathing requires that attention be directed away from the chest as the initial origin for the conscious control of breathing, and instead to a conscious focus on the abdominal region as the origin of each full breath. To accomplish this, the abdominal muscles must first relax. Therefore, it is best to start from a standing position, so that breathing is not inhibited. Let the arms hang loosely and concentrate on relaxing, particularly in the neck and shoulder region, by first taking a couple of deep breaths. Next, relax the abdominal muscles so that they appear flaccid. In addition, place your hand on your abdomen. This serves as a form of visible feedback to assist you in ensuring that with the initiation of each breath the abdomen protrudes. The initiation of each breath should occur simultaneously with the protruded, but relaxed, state of the abdominal muscles. You should visibly notice that with each breath the stomach becomes naturally distended. When this portion of the technique is performed properly, the diaphragm (a muscle at the base of the lungs) contracts and drops. This allows a deeper breath to occur. This is the first stage of taking a maximal inhalation. The entire process of inhalation takes place in three different areas and stages: the lower abdominal, the mid-chest, and finally, the upper chest. Diaphragmatic breathing technique can be combined with a more dynamic muscular relaxation technique called progressive muscular relaxation (PMR). Harris and Harris (28) and Williams (79) are excellent sources for learning how to apply both these and other mental training techniques.

Progressive Muscular Relaxation. To achieve an appropriate level of psychic vigor and physiological arousal before performance, many athletes employ progressive muscle relaxation (PMR) (37). PMR is considered a somatic psychological skill, in that it uses the control gained over the body, or soma, in order to effect a state of mental relaxation (as well as obvious physical relaxation). In essence, by going through a series of alternate muscular tensing and relaxation phases, the athlete learns to discriminate, or become *aware* of, somatic tension and thereby learns to *control* it. Therefore, PMR can be defined as a somatic psychological technique by which psychological and physical arousal are self-regulated through the control of skeletal muscle tension. Theoretically, the technique exerts its effect by means of a process termed reciprocal inhibition (81), employing the dualistic mind-body concept and stating that a relaxed body will promote a relaxed mind. Biologically, this probably occurs because of reduced afferent stimulation from the musculature to the reticular-activating system. This reduction in RAS arousal would consequently cause a decline in cortical activity, where thinking and other associative processes occur (i.e., emotional elaboration of cognition by the limbic system). In many cases, a positive side effect of the reduced muscle tension may be an increase in smooth, fluid, or efficient movement as well as an increased range of motion around the joint.

The technique through which one learns to control the somatic input to the central nervous system is a progression of stages leading to achieving complete and total body relaxation voluntarily and instantly, whenever needed. It can be a very effective self-regulation technique for some athletes to use before practice or a competition, or even during an intense moment in a given contest.

First, the athlete will experience alternate tension and relaxation cycles for several small muscle groups throughout the body. Contraction of a given muscle (e.g., the biceps brachii) may occur for 10 to 15 s during which the person generates excessive and uncomfortable levels of tension. Then a similar amount of time follows during which tension release is accompanied by an attempt to achieve deep relaxation (i.e., by trying to feel warmth and heaviness in the limbs). One can save valuable practice time by having athletes use tapes of the PMR instruction at their own convenience. Also, using training tapes at bedtime not only teaches the athlete to relax but may also ensure increased depth of sleep, an essential component to the rest and recovery cycle of hard-training athletes. Ultimately, through diligent mental-relaxation training athletes learn to reduce whole body tension at will.

Autogenic Training.

For athletes who are injured or for some reason find it uncomfortable or impractical to experience sharp tension levels, the PMR cycle described for each muscle group can be replaced with an attentional state that simply focuses on the sense of warmth and heaviness for a particular limb or muscle group. This kind of technique is referred to as autogenic training. Autogenic training can refer to autonomic shifting to parasympathetic dominance. Some older athletes may find this an attractive alternative to PMR.

Mental Imagery

Mental imagery is a form of mental practice that many athletes use. Jack Nicklaus, the famous professional golfer, testified that he visualizes the flight and landing of every shot prior to its actual execution. He believed that this kind of mental preparation promotes better performance. There is countless anecdotal evidence for the efficacy of mental imagery, but is there scientific evidence for this technique?

First, **mental imagery** can be defined as a cognitive psychological skill in which the athlete uses all the senses to create a mental experience of an athletic performance. This means that the athlete simulates reality by mentally rehearsing a movement, imagining visual, auditory, kinesthetic, olfactory, and even exertional cues. During the initial stages of using imagery, the athlete may start with a relatively simple, visual (i.e., unisensory as opposed to a multisensory) perspective. This would help to increase successful practice of the technique. As with learning any skill by proceeding from simple to complex, the person starts with static images, such as imaging a golf ball or mentally examining the visual characteristics of a tennis racquet. The *vividness* or detail of the image should become clearer and clearer with continued practice. Some people have a natural talent for achieving such clarity, but there is no question that everyone can improve with repeated practice.

The perspective of the image can be internal (first person) or external (third person). Although the research literature is unclear as to whether one is superior, it would seem that the more engaging and natural image to the athlete would be appropriate. Of course, the imaginal internal perspective would seem more specific to skill execution inasmuch as actual task performance is accomplished with such an orientation.

If, for example, the athlete successfully visualizes a stationary object with vivid detail, he may then start to move the object or begin to "walk around" it in his mind, viewing it from a number of different perspectives. In the case of an object such as a basketball, the athlete may attempt to bounce it and feel the ball against his fingertips. In this manner he increases complexity by *controlling* the image (e.g., bouncing the ball) or moving it with control as well as bringing a multisensory perspective to bear (i.e., visualization as well as tactile or kinesthetic sensation).

Rehearsing such successful executions during imagined competitive conditions may provide a series of positive memories to be planted in the subconscious mind, thus increasing the athlete's sense of confidence and preparedness for the particular sport. Of course, mental imaging is not as powerful a determinant of self-efficacy as actual success, but it does offer two potentially potent ingredients. First, successful performance is entirely under the control of the athlete during imaging, whereas a degree of uncertainty is inherent about the outcome in reality. In imagery the athlete has a great opportunity to "experience" success. We believe athletes should be realistic in the kinds of success they imagine; that is, the mental images should be personally challenging, yet, realistic. Second, the athlete can "experience" competition repeatedly, fostering a sense of familiarity and preparedness.

It is interesting to think that with some athletes the months of preparation for a season of play—involving off-season, preseason, and in-season conditioning and skill development—may lead to only a few minutes of actual competitive experience. Even for the starters in a given sport, actual competitive experience may be infinitely small relative to physical practice time. Mental imagery, however, allows the athlete to get used to this uncertain environment. Interestingly, it has been reported that Soviet athletes used to visit the venues of Olympic competitions as soon as possible after arriving in the locale or view pictures of the sites in advance of competition so that they could mentally rehearse competing under actual competitive conditions.

Hypnosis

Although hypnosis is misunderstood by many of the general public, it can be an effective tool for psychological arousal and sometimes for behavior or performance change (29). Hypnosis can be defined as an induced state of hypersuggestibility in which positive suggestions relating to an athlete's performance potential can be planted in the subconscious mind. Some athletes may not effectively manage their physical resources because of perceived incompetence or lack of self-efficacy. This is particularly unfortunate when physical tests and a coach's judgment indicate superior potential. The athlete seems to have a mental block in terms of rationally and realistically viewing ability, despite receiving positive performance-based feedback (e.g., they executed a throw well or the coach praised their effort). Such a psychological perspective may inhibit muscular effort or decrease coordination because of forcing the movement, as described earlier. To realize the effect of hypnosis on inhibitory processes, consider the case described years ago by Johnson and Kramer (38) in which an athlete, under hypnotic suggestion, was able to dramatically increase the number of repetitions for a bench-press exercise. Did such a psychological technique result in improved chronic strength and muscular endurance? Obviously not, but it did result in the increased expression of the athlete's strength and endurance potential. In this case, there may have been an actual neurological disinhibitory process occurring at the spinal motor neuron level. The realization and discovery that he or she can perform at such a high level may profoundly alter an athlete's self-concept and, indirectly, future performance.

Certainly, not all athletes operate so far below potential that hypnosis would effect such dramatic change. Only a small portion of the population can achieve an effective hypnotic trance, which may be due to a fear of losing control to an external other, the hypnotherapist. However, hypnosis is an invaluable technique whereby the athlete actively learns to *take control* of the mind in an attempt to engage in more adaptive behavior.

Systematic Desensitization

Sometimes fears are learned by association of previously neutral stimuli with a stressful event. For example, an adult nonswimmer, who experienced a threatening event in the water as a child, may avoid activities around water because of a learned association. This individual may become fearful and, therefore, tense doing basic resistance or stretching exercises in a pool, even ones that require no swimming skill. Understanding exercise science is crucial in an example like this. For example, the aquatic environment is a great aid in enhancing flexibility. To benefit maximally from a stretching program, however, one must learn to fully relax. If one purpose of the pool session is to enhance flexibility, the inability of a nonswimmer to relax in that environment could easily negate the gains in flexibility.

One technique that helps an athlete initially confront or reduce their fear is systematic desensitization (SD) (81). SD is a hybrid of cognitive and somatic techniques that allows an athlete to replace a fear response to various cues with a relaxation response. This adaptive, learned replacement process, the principle behind SD, is called *counterconditioning*.

To practice the technique an athlete should be reasonably skilled at both PMR and mental imagery. He or she should construct a hierarchy, or progression, of fearful events and situations that are specific to the person's perception. For example, a competitive gymnast who suffered a serious injury on the balance beam may list a series of fearful scenes proceeding from warming up prior to her event to the actual movement that precipitated her injury. The hierarchy might consist of approximately 10 to 12 intervening scenarios, or whatever number is appropriate.

In a relaxed setting the athlete images the first scene and experiences a *mild* degree of anxiety. At the same time, PMR is instituted and, theoretically, a strong relaxation response should overcome the relatively weak fight or flight syndrome. This technique is practiced until the athlete can hold the image clearly while maintaining a relaxed state. The athlete progresses through the hierarchy, receiving conditioned fear in small manageable doses that are overcome with the relaxation achieved with PMR and rhythmic breathing. Such a procedure prevents cognitive avoidance and counterconditions a new response (relaxation) to the formerly fear-inducing stimuli.

Cognitive-Affective Stress Management

Smith (62) discusses a program for stress management entitled cognitive-affective stress management training, or SMT. This stress reduction technique consists of these five phases:

1. Pretreatment assessment
2. Education
3. Skill acquisition, in which an integrated coping response is learned
4. Skill rehearsal, in which the coping technique is applied
5. Post-treatment evaluation

The principle underlying SMT effectiveness is termed overload because the program's goal is for the athlete to experience supernormal levels of fear or affect, which he or she learns to "turn off" by means of the coping response. In a sense, the psychological overload principle is analogous to the overload concept in resistance training, where an athlete efficiently executes movements in the athletic context because of having trained with weights and resistances greater than those forces encountered in competition. Theoretically, controlling such high fear levels during the practice of SMT should increase the athlete's confidence to cope with real stressors.

CONCLUSION

The coach and athlete can increase performance outcomes and the enjoyment of competition by attending to the psychological aspects of performance. We believe that a positive, goal-oriented coaching approach is one of the most powerful contributors to psychological preparation for sport. The physical and nutritional preparation of the athlete is also a powerful contributor. An adequate understanding of the mind and body relationship can facilitate communication and aid the athlete to control and manage emotion and arousal. Using appropriate psychological techniques can further help this self-management process. We believe that the experience of success in sport may be important in and of itself, but the greatest outcome may be the enhanced self-esteem and confidence that the athlete achieves, thus positively altering the self-concept.

Key Terms

arousal	164	mental/psychological efficiency	170	psychic energy	164
athlete	163			psyching strategy	179
cognitive anxiety	164	operant	177	somatic anxiety	164
cue utilization	166	positive/negative punishment	172	sport psychology	164
goal setting	176			state anxiety	164
inverted-U theory	172	positive/negative reinforcement	172	trait anxiety	164
mental imagery	181				

Study Questions

1. According to the inverted-U theory of arousal
   a. stress is defined as an emotional reaction to objective danger
   b. higher goals will be set if former goals are successfully completed
   c. simple tasks require low levels of arousal
   d. high levels of arousal may be detrimental to the performance of complex decision-making tasks

2. All anxiety states really *begin* with

   a. the athlete's objective sport situation
   b. the athlete's mental perception of the situation
   c. the limbic system arousal
   d. sensory processing

3. In a critical and arousing game situation a coach would probably throw in the ___ athlete if personality was the only concern regarding performance and game execution.

   a. introverted
   b. extroverted

4. An effective quarterback who looks over the defensive team's alignment and sets up to pass while scanning downfield for both primary and secondary receivers would probably fall into which of the following attentional categories of the TAIS (Nideffer's test of attentional and interpersonal style)?

   a. OIT (overloaded internal)
   b. BIT (broad internal)
   c. BET (broad external)
   d. NAR (narrow)

5. When Walter Payton was interviewed after a game, he stated he really did not have to think about what he was doing during the game—it just happened and was second nature. In sport psychology terms he was in a state of

   a. automaticity
   b. fixation
   c. cognition

6. Which of the following best explains the principle of reciprocal inhibition and how it promotes a reduction in psychological stress?

   a. Muscle relaxation reduces somatic tension.
   b. Attention focused on the muscles reduces distracting thoughts.
   c. A relaxed body promotes a relaxed mind.
   d. A sense of control over the body builds confidence.

7. If a coach tries to increase a player's motivation to play hard on Sunday, he could let him off a practice on Tuesday and Wednesday. This would be an example of

   a. positive reinforcement
   b. negative reinforcement
   c. positive punishment
   d. negative punishment

8. When arousal increases up to a high or stressful level, the width of the athlete's attentional field that can be devoted to the task, or the athlete's functional attention, is

   a. decreased
   b. increased
   c. stays the same

9. Elite athletes tend to engage predominantly in left-brain (analytical) thinking while they perform.

   a. true
   b. false

10. If an athlete is having trouble improving performance, then he or she might concentrate on form or technique, rather than on winning or losing. Such a goal is referred to as

    a. an external goal
    b. an internal goal
    c. an outcome goal
    d. a process goal

Applying Knowledge of the Psychology of Athletic Preparation and Performance

Problem 1

The head coach of one of your most successful sports wants to incorporate sport psychology into her team's strength and conditioning program. She has given you 1 hour a week for the next 5 weeks to talk with and teach the team about mental conditioning. Briefly describe the format and content of each session.

Problem 2

A few days prior to a big game you notice the freshman quarterback under your charge is somewhat distant and seems to be constantly out of breath. After talking with him, you realize he simply needs to learn to regulate his arousal level. He asks if you know of any skills that he can learn before the game to maintain some calm. Briefly describe to him how you can control arousal through breathing.

Problem 3

As strength and conditioning coach, you have several athletes this season with chronic injuries. As you interview each one, several common themes present themselves. First, you notice that each of these athletes always focuses on lifting as much weight as possible. Second, they seem impatient with conducting their training sessions in a proper fashion, including proper warm-up exercises (i.e., 5-min bike ride with a proper amount of flexibility work). Third, they always seem to be impatient with the process of strength and conditioning. What can you teach these athletes about proper and realistic goal setting to avoid injury and to structure success?

Problem 4

You have been responsible for the strength and conditioning program for a world-class athlete for the past 6 months in preparation for the world championships. The athlete arrives at the event a few days before you, and she proceeds to call you on the phone to tell you about the qualifying times of other competitors. The athlete is quite upset, wondering how in the world she can be competing against athletes of such calibre, having had only 6 months training. What do you tell this athlete, who is genetically gifted and as maximally prepared as possible, when she doubts her abilities in comparison with others'?

References

1. Attner, P. Payton vs. Harris vs. Brown. *Sporting News*, (Oct. 1) pp. 2-3. 1984.
2. Bandura, A. Self-efficacy: Toward a unifying theory of behavior change. *Psychol. Rev.* 84(2):191-215. 1977.
3. Basmajian, J.V. and C.J. De Luca. *Muscles Alive: Their Functions Revealed by Electromyography* (5th ed.). Baltimore: Williams & Wilkins. 1985.
4. Cannon, W.B. *The Wisdom of the Body*. New York: Norton. 1932.
5. Caudill, D., R. Weinberg, and A. Jackson. Psyching-up and track athletes: A preliminary investigation. *J. Sport Psychol.* 5:231-235. 1980.
6. Costello, F. Personal communication. 1993.
7. Cox, R.H. *Sport Psychology: Concepts and Applications*. Dubuque, IA: Brown & Benchmark. 1994.
8. Daniels, J.T. A physiologist's view of running economy. *Med. and Sci. Sports Exerc.* 17:332-338. 1985.
9. Darst, P.W., E. Langsdorf, D.E. Richardson, and G.S. Krahenbuhl. Analyzing coaching behavior and practice time. *Motor Skills: Theory Into Practice.* 5(1):13-22. 1981.
10. Deci, E.L. Intrinsic motivation: Theory and application. In *Psychology of Motor Behavior and Sport 1977*. D.M. Landers and R.W. Christina, eds. Champaign, IL: Human Kinetics Publishers. 1978.
11. Demak, R. Mysterious malady. *Sports Illustrated*. 74(13):44-49. 1991.
12. Eason, R.G. Electromyographic study of local and generalized muscular impairment. *J. Appl. Physiol.* 15(3):479-482. 1960.
13. Easterbrook, J.A. The effect of emotion on cue utilization and the organization of behavior. *Psychol. Rev.* 66:183-201. 1959.

14. Eysenck, H.J. *The Biological Basis of Personality*. Springfield, IL: Thomas. 1967.

15. Fazey, J. and L. Hardy. *The Inverted-U Hypothesis: A Catastrophe for Sport Psychology?* [British Association of Sport Sciences Monograph No. I.] Leeds: National Coaching Foundation. 1988.

16. Fenz, W.D. Coping mechanisms and performance under stress. In: *Psychology of Sport and Motor Behavior II, Penn State HPER Series, No. 10*. D.M. Landers, ed. University Park: Pennsylvania State University Press. 1975.

17. Fenz, W.D. Learning to anticipate stressful events. *J. Sport Exerc. Psychol.* 10:223-228. 1988.

18. Fitts, D.M. and M.I. Posner. *Human Performance*. Blemont, CA: Brooks/Cole. 1967.

19. Fleck, S.J. and W.J. Kraemer. *Designing Resistance Training Programs*. Champaign, IL: Human Kinetics. 1987.

20. Frankenhauser, M. Psychoneuroendocrine approaches to the study of stressful person-environment transactions. In: *Nebraska Symposium on Motivation 1978*. Howe and Dienstbier, eds. Lincoln, NE: University of Nebraska Press. 1979.

21. Gould, D. Goal setting for peak performance. In: *Applied Sport Psychology: Personal Growth to Peak Performance*. J.M. Williams, ed. Mountain View, CA: Mayfield. 1993.

22. Gould, D., L. Petlichkoff, H. Simons, and M. Vevera. The relationship between competitive state anxiety inventory-z subscale scores and pistol shooting performance. *J. Sport Exerc. Psychol.* 9:33-42. 1987.

23. Gould, D., K. Hodge, K. Peterson, and J. Giannini. An exploratory examination of strategies used by elite coaches to enhance self-efficacy in athletes. *J. Sport Exerc. Psychol.* 11(2):128-140. 1989.

24. Gould, D., R. Weinberg, and A. Jackson. Mental preparation strategies, cognition, and strength performance. *J. Sport Psychol.* 2:329-339. 1980.

25. Hackney, A.C., S.N. Pearman, III, and J.M. Nowacki. Physiological profiles of overtrained and stale athletes: A review. *J. Appl. Sport Psychol.* 2:21-33. 1990.

26. Hanin, Y.L. Interpersonal and intragroup anxiety in sports. In: *Anxiety in Sports: An International Perspective*. D. Hackfort and C.D. Spielberger, eds. New York: Hemisphere, 1989. pp. 19-28.

27. Harris, D.V. *Involvement in Sport: A Somatopsychic Rationale for Physical Activity*. Philadelphia: Lea & Febiger. 1973.

28. Harris, D.V. and B.L. Harris. *The Athlete's Guide to Sports Psychology: Mental Skills for Physical People*. New York: Leisure Press. 1984.

29. Hatfield, B.D. and F.S. Daniels. The use of hypnosis as a stress management technique. *Motor skills: Theory Into Practice*, 5(1):62-68. 1981.

30. Hatfield, B.D. and D.M. Landers. Psychophysiology in exercise and sport research: An overview. *Exer. Sport Sci. Rev.* 15:351-388. 1987.

31. Hatfield, B.D., D.M. Landers, and W.J. Ray. Cognitive processes during self-paced motor performance: An electroencephalographic profile of skilled marksmen. *J. Sport Psychol.* 6:42. 1984.

32. Hatfield, B.D., T.W. Spalding, A.D. Mahon, B.A. Slater, E.B. Brody, and P. Vaccaro. The effect of psychological strategies upon cardiorespiratory and muscular activity during treadmill running. *Med. Sci. Sports Exerc.* 24(2):218-225. 1992.

33. Hillyard, S.A. and T.W. Picton. Event-related brain potentials and selective information processing in man. In: *Progress in Clinical Neurophysiology* (Vol. 6. Cognitive Components in Cerebral Event-Related Potentials and Selective Attention). J. Desmedt, ed. Basel: Karger. 1979.

34. Hinton, E. Treat them as winners and they will win. *Parade Mag.* (August 15), pp. 4-5. 1993.

35. Ikai, M. and A.H. Steinhaus. Some factors modifying the expression of human strength. *J. Appl. Physiol.* 16(1):157-163. 1961.

36. Iso-Ahola, S.E. and B.D. Hatfield. *Psychology of Sports: A Social Psychological Approach*. Dubuque, IA: W.C. Brown. 1986.

37. Jacobson, E. *Progressive Relaxation* (1st ed.). Chicago: University of Chicago Press. 1929.

38. Johnson, W.R. and G.F. Kramer. Effects of different types of hypnotic suggestions upon physical performance. *Res. Q.* 31:469-473. 1960.

39. Kandel, E.R. and J.H. Schwartz. *Principles of Neural Science*. New York: Elsevier. 1985.

40. Lacey, J.I. and B.C. Lacey. Studies of heart rate and other bodily processes in sensorimotor behavior. In: *Cardiovascular Psychophysiology*. P.A. Obrist, A.H. Black, J. Brener, and L.V. Cara, eds. Chicago: Aldine. 1974.

41. Lamb, D.R. The sports medicine umbrella. *Sport Med. Bull.* 19(4):8-9. 1984.

42. Locke, E.A. and G.P. Latham. The application of goal setting to sports. *J. Sport Psychol.* 7:205-222. 1985.

43. Martens, R. *Social Psychology and Physical Activity*. New York: Harper & Row. 1975.

44. Martens, R. *Sport Competition Anxiety Test*. Champaign, IL: Human Kinetics. 1977.

45. Martens, R. *Coaches Guide to Sport Psychology*. Champaign, IL: Human Kinetics. 1987.

46. Martin, G. and D. Hrycaiko. Effective behavioral coaching: What's it all about? *J. Sport Psychol.* 5(1):8-20. 1983.

47. McClelland, D.C., J.W. Atkinson, R.W. Clark, and E.L. Lowell. *The Achievement Motive*. New York: Appleton-Century-Crofts. 1953.

48. Morgan, W.P., R.H. Needle, and L.L. Coyne. Psychophysiologic phenomena and muscular performance [Abstract]. *AAHPER Abst.* 71. 1966.

49. Morgan, W.P. and M.L. Pollock. Psychologic characterization of the elite distance runner. *Ann. NY Acad. Sci.* 301:482-503. 1977.

50. Nelson, L.R. and M.D. Furst. An objective study of the effects of expectation on competitive performance. *J. Psychol.* 81:69-72. 1972.

51. Ness, R.G. and R.W. Patton. The effect of beliefs on maximum weight-lifting performance. *Cog. Ther. Res.* 3(2):205-211. 1979.

52. Nideffer, R. Test of attentional and interpersonal style. *J. Pers. Soc. Psychol.* 34:394-404. 1976.

53. Oxendine, J.B. Emotional arousal and motor performance. *Quest* 13:23-30. 1970.

54. Porges, S.W., P.M. McCabe, and B.C. Yongue. Respiratory-heart rate interaction: Psychophysiological implications for pathophysiology and behavior. In: *Perspectives in Cardiovascular Psychophysiology.* J.T. Caccioppo and R.E. Petty, eds. New York: Guilford. 1982.

55. Porter, K. and J. Foster. *Visual Athletics: Visualization for Peak Sport Performance.* Dubuque, IA: W.C. Brown. 1990.

56. Roush, E.S. Strength and endurance in the waking and hypnotic states. *J. Appl. Physiol.* 3(7):404-410. 1951.

57. Sale, D. Neural adaptation in strength and power training. In: *Human Muscle Power.* N.L. Jones, N. McCartney, and A. McComas, eds. Champaign, IL: Human Kinetics. 1986. pp. 289-307.

58. Schiffman, H.R. *Sensation and Perception: An Integrated Approach.* New York: Wiley. 1976.

59. Schwartz, G.E., R.J. Davidson, and D.J. Goleman. Patterning of cognitive and somatic processes in the self-regulation of anxiety: Effects of meditation versus exercise. *Psychosom. Med.* 40:321-328. 1978.

60. Shapiro, L. Montana plays for it again. *Washington Post* (Jan. 18), p. E7. 1994.

61. Shelton, T.O. and M.J. Mahoney. The content and effect of "psyching-up" strategies in weight lifters. *Cogn. Ther. Res.* 2(3):275-284. 1978.

62. Smith, R.E. A cognitive-affective approach to stress management training for athletes. In: *Psychology of Motor Behavior and Sport - 1979.* C.H. Nadeau, W.R. Halliwell, K.M. Newell, and G.C. Roberts, eds. Champaign, IL: Human Kinetics. 1980.

63. Speilberger, C.D. *Understanding Stress and Anxiety.* London: Harper & Row. 1979.

64. Speilberger, C.D., R.L. Gorsuch, and R.F. Lushene. *Manual for the State-Trait Anxiety Inventory.* Palo Alto, CA: Consulting Psychologists Press. 1970.

65. Tharp, R.G. and R. Gallimore. What a coach can teach a teacher. *Psychol. Today* (Jan.) 9:74-78. 1976.

66. Thayer, R.E. Measurement through self-report. *Psycholo. Rep.* 20:663-678. 1967.

67. Tichy, N.M. and S. Stratford. *Control Your Destiny or Someone Else Will.* New York: Doubleday. 1993.

68. Tucker, D.M., J.R. Antes, C.E. Stenslie, and T.M. Barnhardt. Anxiety and lateral cerebral function. *J. Abnorm. Psychol.* 87(3):380-383. 1978.

69. Tynes, L.L. and R.M. McFatter. The efficacy of "psyching" strategies on a weight-lifting task. *Cogn. Ther. Res.* 11(3):327-336. 1987.

70. Vidacek, S. and J. Wishner. Influence of expectation of task duration on efficiency of muscular activity. *J. Appl. Psychol.* 55(6):564-569. 1971.

71. Vidacek, S. and J. Wishner. Task difficulty and the efficiency of muscular activity. *J. Appl. Psychol.* 56:510-512. 1972.

72. Voor, J.H., A.J. Lloyd, and R.J. Cole. The influence of competition on the efficiency of an isometric muscle contraction. *J. Motor Beh.* 1(3):210-219. 1969.

73. Weinberg, R.S. The effects of success and failure on the patterning of neuromuscular energy. *J. Motor Beh.* 10:53-61. 1978.

74. Weinberg, R.S., L.D. Bruya, H. Garland, and A. Jackson. Effect of goal difficulty and positive reinforcement on endurance performance. *J. Sport Exerc. Psychol.* 12:144-156. 1990.

75. Weinberg, R.S., C. Fowler, A. Jackson, J. Bagnall, and L. Bruya. Effect of goal difficulty on motor performance: A replication across tasks and subjects. *J. Sport Exerc. Psychol.* 13:160-173. 1991.

76. Weinberg, R.S., D. Gould, and A. Jackson. Cognition and motor performance: Effect of psyching-up strategies on three motor tasks. *Cogn. Ther. Res.* 4(2):239-245. 1980.

77. Weinberg, R.S., D. Gould, and A. Jackson. Relationship between the duration of the psych-up interval and strength performance. *J. Sport Psychol.* 3:166-170. 1981.

78. Wilkes, R.L. and J.J. Summers. Cognition, mediating variables and strength performance. *J. Sport Psychol.* 6:351-359. 1984.

79. Williams, J.M. Psychological characteristics of peak performance. In: *Applied Sport Psychology: Personal Growth to Peak Performance.* J.M. Williams, ed. Mountain View, CA: Mayfield. 1993.

80. Wilmore, J.H. Influence of motivation on physical work capacity and performance. *J. Appl. Physiol.* 24(4):459-463. 1968.

81. Wolpe, J. *Psychotherapy by Reciprocal Inhibition.* Stanford, CA: Stanford University Press. 1958.

82. Yerkes, R.M. and J.D. Dodson. The relationship of strength of stimulus to rapidity of habit formation. *J. Comp. Neurol. Psychol.* 18:459-482. 1908.

CHAPTER 11

PERFORMANCE-ENHANCING SUBSTANCES: EFFECTS, RISKS, AND APPROPRIATE ALTERNATIVES

Karl E. Friedl

Ergogenic substances—performance-enhancing drugs and dietary supplements—have been around for almost as long as athletes have competed:

> Doping follows just one step behind discoveries of herbs and drugs. Centuries ago, Incas chewed coca leaves to sustain strenuous work, and Berserkers ate mushrooms containing muscarine before battle. Now sport is faced with drugs developed with recombinant-DNA technology (27).

Today there is a long list of chemicals that are banned from national and international competition because they are reputed to give unfair advantage to the user. Other chemicals that can be obtained through ingestion of dietary supplements and that are not classified as drugs are big business for manufacturers who market to athletes. The majority of these substances are promoted on the basis of unfounded claims. When a substance is proven to be effective, or at least a consensus is reached by athletic administrators that it is, it too is added to the list of banned substances. Thus, most substances that have a sound basis in performance enhancement are banned to athletes at the upper levels of competition.

Some athletes try to gain advantage by using supplements that are reputed to be ergogenic but are not banned; other competitors use banned substances with the belief that they can stay ahead of the drug testers. The consequence of this is that athletes who would normally not use any of these substances may feel pressured to use them just to stay abreast of their

The opinions or assertions contained herein are the private views of the author and are not to be construed as official or as reflecting the views of the Department of the Army or the Department of Defense.

I am grateful to Ms. Sherryl Kubel for her dedication and effort in obtaining copies of the references used in this paper. I wish to acknowledge the courtesy extended to me by Dr. Debbie Drechsler-Parks in providing facilities to complete this chapter at the Environmental Stress Laboratory at the University of California, Santa Barbara. Dr. Everett Harman, CSCS, provided careful and valuable editing of this manuscript.

competitors. Athletes who are well informed can confidently ignore useless and possibly harmful products, even if their fellow athletes claim otherwise. It may also be possible to steer athletes away from the use of banned drugs if the athletes can be made aware that any competitors who cheat run a high risk of being detected.

Any ergogenic substance has some benefit-risk trade-off. Steroid abuse is a prime example of an emotional issue in which opposing forces exaggerate the risks and the benefits. Promoters tend to exaggerate the benefits, while some coaches or athletic administrators who would rather not see the substances used have a tendency to overstate the risks. Many substances carry some medium- or long-term health risks; others carry the risk of serious penalties and public humiliation. At a minimum, ergogenic substances distract the athlete from full attention to proven training techniques; and even effective substances may produce side effects that may emerge at just the wrong time and hinder peak performance.

It is important for the strength and conditioning professional to be able to discuss the risks and benefits of the main ergogenic substances that athletes are likely to encounter. The strength and conditioning professional is likely to be the first authoritative source whom the athlete approaches for reliable information. It is also important for the advancement of the profession that proper training and nutrition be distinguished from a pharmacological approach, which detracts from sport by providing unfair advantage. The strength and conditioning professional must be able to draw this dividing line. At higher levels of administration, the strength and conditioning professional may also become involved in decisions about which substances may provide unfair advantage in a specific event and what kind of surveillance might prevent such use.

TYPES OF PERFORMANCE-ENHANCING SUBSTANCES

The two principal categories of performance-enhancing substances considered in this chapter are (a) naturally occurring hormones and the drugs that mimic their effects and (b) dietary supplements. Other important substances that are used by some athletes but that do not fall directly into the category of ergogenic aids (e.g., cocaine and alcohol) will not be discussed here.

The distinction between a drug and a dietary supplement is not intuitively obvious; it is an important one, however, because it determines whether or not a product must meet Food and Drug Administration (FDA) approval for safety and effectiveness. If it is not classified as a drug or advertised as having therapeutic value, the FDA generally does not regulate the sale of a product. This means that any manufacturer can introduce a new dietary supplement to the market without any special approval and that the FDA will not investigate its safety or effectiveness unless a health risk is brought to the agency's attention (83). For example, amino acid supplements were largely unregulated until the outbreak several years ago of eosinophilia-myalgia syndrome. This disease was traced to a tryptophan product after the outbreak of nearly 1,600 cases of severe illness and 33 deaths suggested a problem (61). Athletes who use dietary supplements are often human guinea pigs for substances that have not been tested even on real guinea pigs.

Part of the FDA definition of a drug is a substance that changes the body's structure or function. This includes substances that stimulate hormone secretion. Also, if a substance looks like a medicine or is administered differently from the way in which foods would be (e.g., intranasally or by injection), it may be classified as a drug.

Dietary supplement is a catch-all term that includes substances that the FDA does not consider drugs and that also do not fall into the categories of normal foods or food additives. Generally, dietary supplements are highly refined products that would not be confused with a food. These may not have any positive nutritional value; hence, they are not referred to as nutritional supplements. Carbohydrate loading to bolster glycogen stores before an athletic competition is "sports nutrition," but a tablet of a single purified amino acid not promoted for medicinal properties is a "dietary supplement." Examples of dietary supplements are trace minerals such as chromium, single amino acids such as ornithine, plant sterols such as β-sitosterol, and most vitamins.

Ergogenic substances are usually banned from athletic competition when a consensus is reached that they may provide a competitive edge. This does not require conclusive proof that a substance does anything advantageous; it simply represents an agreement among administrators that it might. A few substances have been banned for other reasons, such as medical safety (e.g., narcotics) and social unacceptability (e.g., marijuana) (27). The following are examples of substances currently banned by the International Olympic Committee (28):

Psychomotor stimulants—Amphetamine, Cocaine, Methylphenidate
Sympathomimetic amines—Ephedrine, Isoprenaline
Other central nervous system stimulants—Caffeine, Doxapram, Strychnine
Anabolic (male sex) steroids—Testosterone, Stanozolol, Nandrolone, Norethandrolone, Methandienone

Other hormones—Growth hormone, Erythropoietin
Narcotic analgesics—Codeine, Heroin, Hydromorphone, Methadone, Morphine
Beta-blockers
Masking agents and diuretics—Probenecid, Furosemide

Some of the substances are illegal under governmental statute as well: Anabolic steroids are prohibited by most athletic organizations, with the risk of sanctions against the athlete and possibly against the athlete's team or school, and recent federal law makes their possession for other than medical use a misdemeanor, punishable by up to 1 year in jail and a $1,000 fine.

Performance-enhancing substances tend to be sport specific, providing competitive advantages that may not be useful to all athletes. It is incorrect to assume that athletes in all sports face the same problems of unfair ergogenic substance use by their competitors. Beta-adrenergic agonists and anabolic steroids may be popular with strength athletes because they increase lean mass, whereas substances that enhance aerobic and endurance performance, such as caffeine and erythropoietin, are more likely to be used by marathoners and cyclists. Athletes who require precise control of heart rate, such as biathletes during marksmanship events, benefit from beta-blockers, whereas beta-adrenergic agonists would be likely to impair their performance.

ANABOLIC STEROIDS AND OTHER HORMONES

Various hormones that are naturally produced in the body produce ergogenic effects. Table 11.1 summarizes these hormones, synthetic analogues used by athletes, and related information. Of the principal hormones made by the body, only the male sex steroids, erythropoietin, and epinephrine are likely to produce substantial ergogenic advantages in healthy adults. Because of their widespread use by athletes, the synthetic derivatives of male sex steroids are the most important ergogenic substances for the strength and conditioning professional to be knowledgeable about. These substances can be referred to as androgens, androgenic steroids, or **anabolic steroids** interchangeably (although some authors attempt to make a distinction between these terms on the basis of differential "masculinizing" and "muscle-building" properties).

Anabolic Steroids

Steroids encompass a wide variety of different useful chemicals and hormones, including the estrogens and progestogens used in birth control pills; the glucocorticoids, such as cortisone and prednisone, used as anti-inflammatory drugs in muscle injury or asthma; and the anabolic steroids, such as testosterone enanthate, which are used in a very limited number of therapeutic applications, including hormone replacement for men with low circulating levels. Thus, an athlete may use steroids in the form of asthma medication or female oral contraceptives; these should not be confused with the anabolic steroids.

Actions of Androgens. The primary androgen is testosterone, most of which is synthesized in the testes

Table 11.1   Naturally Occurring Hormones and Their Synthetic Analogues

Hormone (origin)	Synthetic analogues used by athletes	Ergogenic effects of the analogues	Substances purported to promote the hormone's effects
Growth hormone (pituitary)	Recombinant human growth hormone	Increased muscle mass and decreased body fat in growth hormone–deficient men	Arginine and other amino acids
Luteinizing hormone (pituitary)	Human chorionic gonadotropin	Claimed effect: fat reduction	Clomid
Anabolic (male sex) steroids (testes, adrenal cortex, ovaries)	Methyltestosterone, oxandrolone, oxymetholone, methandrostenolone	Increased muscle mass and other actions	So-called steroid replacers: boron, sterols, animal testes
Erythropoietin (kidneys)	Recombinant human erythropoietin	Increased red blood cell production in patients with anemia	Transfusions, B vitamins
Thyroxine (thyroid gland)	Synthroid	Decreased body fat, but also sacrifices lean mass (muscle, bone)	—
Epinephrine (adrenal medulla)	Clenbuterol and other beta-agonists	Increased muscle mass and decreased body fat	—

from cholesterol. Androgens are the primary determinants of male physical characteristics; the default condition, so to speak, in humans is the female form. Thus, when receptors (the cell proteins through which a hormone produces biological actions) for testosterone are deficient, such as in a rare condition called complete testicular feminization syndrome, a genetic male develops into a person who is by all external appearances female.

For most hormones there are well-described diseases produced by excessive secretion, such as hyperthyroidism and acromegaly from excess thyroid and growth-hormone production, respectively; there is no such disease of androgen overproduction for mature men. Although there are a number of disorders for which reducing the androgen levels helps treatment (e.g., prostate disease and some sexually deviant behaviors), androgens appear to play permissive or potentiating roles rather than causative roles in these disorders. Male-pattern balding is a more innocuous example of the same phenomenon; castration would prevent balding, but balding will not necessarily occur in men without a genetic predisposition, even with high testosterone exposure (67).

Results of Unnatural Use of Anabolic Steroids.

Phenotypes are reversed when anabolic steroids are administered to a woman; she will adopt male physical characteristics, including increased upper body muscularity; decreased body fat, especially from the breasts and hips; deepening of the voice; and increased facial hair. Thus, the primary known risk to a woman using anabolic steroids, besides the risks that are also known for men, is masculinization (137). Some of these changes may not be reversible, including the deeper voice, male-pattern balding, and enlargement of the clitoris.

For an adolescent boy using synthetic anabolic steroids, the primary risk is accelerated puberty, which would encompass a rapid growth in size and precocious display of secondary sexual characteristics. Higher doses can also produce early closure of the ends of the long bones, thus terminating bone growth and potentially resulting in short stature for the boy.

Exposure of a fetus to elevated levels of testosterone produces permanent effects on brain development, with dramatic effects on the number and structure of sex-specific neurons. Fetal exposure to testosterone is also thought to be associated with an increased incidence of left-handedness, such language disorders as dyslexia, autoimmune disease, and migraine headaches (99, 100). It has also been suggested that anabolic steroids naturally exert a permanent organizing influence on the brain in boys around the time of puberty, enhancing, for example, the development of spatial ability (75).

Whether or not other, more subtle effects on personality and emotional development occur in children exposed to high doses of anabolic steroids is currently unknown.

Types of Anabolic Steroids.

All anabolic steroids appear to work through the same receptors in the body, although their effects can differ in various tissues because of differences in the metabolites they form and how well they attach to certain proteins. The term *anabolic steroid* was originally coined in the 1930s to describe the nitrogen-retaining action of androgenic steroids, as a marker of muscle- or protein-building effect. This effect on nitrogen balance is temporary and lasts only for a few weeks when an androgen is given continuously at the same dose (87). In the past, androgens have been referred to as having a high "anabolic index" if they produce less effect on reproductive tissues than on growth of the levator ani muscle in the rat, compared with the relative effects of various testosterone compounds (72). Only recently have more direct effects on skeletal muscle been demonstrated, and no studies have yet compared the effects of different steroids on muscular hypertrophy or compared unwanted side effects. Thus, the anabolic potency of an androgen is an elusive property. In practical terms, this means that there is no highly "anabolic" steroid that is known to help an athlete more than other anabolic steroids, even though there is much anecdotal gym lore on this subject. A high dose of nearly any anabolic steroid is likely to achieve a muscle-building effect in most people. As a rule, injectable steroids are more potent than oral steroids because of their route of delivery and perhaps also because they do not require additional modification to protect them from immediate metabolism by the liver.

Table 11.2 summarizes the principal oral and injectable anabolic steroids that have been reported in various surveys of athlete use. Athletes typically use higher doses of the substances than men who take them medicinally to "replace" their own low testosterone levels. Methandrostenolone (Dianabol), for example, maintains normal secondary sexual characteristics in hypogonadal men at a replacement dose of approximately 15 mg/day; athletes have reported using up to 300 mg/day (53, 93). Although this drug has not been available for medical use in the United States for over a decade, it is readily obtained through black-market sources and remains one of the most used oral androgens. Testosterone enanthate, a testosterone ester and the main injectable steroid used by athletes, is readily available in the United States and is used clinically for some rare diseases and for replacement treatment. A replacement dose is approximately 75 to 100 mg/week administered every 1-2 weeks. Injectable steroids are administered intramuscularly, typically by deep gluteal injections. Higher doses (250 mg/week) may be administered for up to 6 months to treat men with low sperm

**Table 11.2   Principal Anabolic Steroids
Used by Athletes**

Generic name or category	Example trade names
Orally active steroids	
Methandrostenolone	Dianabol
Oxandrolone	Anavar
Stanozolol	Winstrol
Oxymetholone	Anadrol
Fluoxymesterone	Halotestin
Methyltestosterone	Oreton-M
Mesterolone	Proviron
Injectable steroids	
Testosterone esters[a]	Delatestryl, Sustanon
Nandrolone esters[a]	Deca-durabolin
Stanozolol	Strombaject
Methenolone enanthate	Primobolan-Depot
Boldenone undecylenate	Parenabol
Trenbolone acetate	Parabolan

[a]These are general categories of substances; many different preparations of each are available.

counts (the drug suppresses sperm production but, when it is withdrawn, sperm production usually surges past pretreatment levels and in some men may remain elevated for years). Athletes have reported using this drug in doses of 1,000 mg or more per week.

The injectable compounds have a wide range of half-lives. Among the testosterone esters, testosterone propionate remains in the circulation for approximately 1.5 days, whereas testosterone buciclate lasts for 3 months after a single injection (16).

Oral Anabolic Steroids.   Anabolic steroids that can be taken orally have some undesirable pharmacological effects unlike those of the natural male sex hormones and some of the injected steroids. These substances are commonly made by modification of the basic androgen structure in what is referred to as a 17-alkyl substitution, a process that enhances the longevity of the compound in circulation and slows its removal or conversion by the liver. (This is why these steroids can be taken orally; even though they are delivered directly to the liver upon absorption, they remain relatively intact.)

The most consistent health risks that have been observed with 17-alkylated anabolic steroids are all related to the liver, either by directly affecting it or altering something regulated by it. Adverse effects include decreased high-density lipoprotein (HDL) cholesterol levels (which increases the risk for coronary artery disease), increased risk of liver tumors, and possible liver

damage. The very predictable reduction in HDL cholesterol is an early indication of the negative effect of oral anabolic steroids on liver function. This reduction is a consequence of the stimulated activity of a liver enzyme that regulates cholesterol metabolism. It is unusual to see persistent elevation of other biochemical markers of liver damage with steroid use; reports of this effect are most likely due to transient elevation similar to the occurrence following very intense exercise bouts (113, 122).

The liver tumors that result from oral anabolic steroid use are generally benign, so the true rate of occurrence may be substantially underreported; athletes may not know they have them. Although the tumors can sometimes regress with simple cessation of steroid use, at least one athlete has died from the rupture of such a tumor (37a).

Testosterone Esters.   Even the testosterone esters, pharmacological compounds that duplicate the circulating testosterone originating in the testes (81), act on the body differently from anything that the body produces because of the way in which very high doses of the synthetic testosterones can be delivered continuously instead of in daily cycles. With repeated cycles of high-dose steroid use and withdrawal, the athlete is essentially putting himself through repeated pubertal cycles and sustaining unknown consequences of readaptation to the drug with each cycle. The doses also greatly exceed what is found in nature, with athletes injecting as much as 1,000 mg/week, approximately 10 times the dose that would maintain normal male levels. With doses at this level, new health risks may arise that result from stimulation of receptors other than androgen receptors (e.g., glucocorticoid and estrogen receptors) or from abnormally high levels of some of the androgen metabolites. For example, estrogen, one of the main metabolites of testosterone, can cause stroke in men (32); three cases of stroke, all associated with gynecomastia (male development of breasts), have been reported in athletes using high-dose steroids (54).

At lower (but much higher than natural) doses, 200 to 250 mg/week, testosterone esters have been administered to healthy men for over a year in male contraceptive trials (152). Nearly all oral and injectable anabolic steroids reduce the secretion of follicle stimulating hormone and luteinizing hormone, which are responsible for sperm development and testicular production of testosterone; however, their use does not guarantee a sperm count of zero in all men (152). If a large dose of an anabolic steroid is administered, the production of testosterone by the testes is reduced because the body "senses" adequate androgen levels. The reduction in sperm production is accompanied by reduced testicular size. When the steroid use is discontinued, sperm count and testicular size return to normal (sperm count may rebound to higher than normal) over a period of 4 to 6 months. There is no evidence that for normal men the reduction in sperm count is irreversible.

Other risks associated with injectable anabolic steroids include those associated with needle use by people without medical training. Several cases of AIDS, hepatitis, and gluteal abcess have been recorded. Other risks can be anticipated for athletes who inject black-market products, because there is no way of knowing what is actually in a vial or how the substance has been handled. The FDA has warned consumers that there are products available that carry counterfeit labels—that is, labels duplicated from a genuine steroid manufacturer's label and put on a vial of substance not made by a legitimate drug company. Tests of such black-market "anabolic steroid" products have demonstrated that the contents can range from nothing other than the liquid base to caffeine, a cheaper steroid, or a lower concentration of steroid (147).

Who Uses Anabolic Steroids? Strength athletes are not the only users of anabolic steroids. Athletes in many sports have tested positive for anabolic steroids, although clearly the strength sports, including football and weightlifting, are high-risk sports for steroid abuse (153). People outside of organized sports also use steroids to enhance appearance rather than performance. A national survey of American high school senior males found that 7% were using or had used anabolic steroids (23). One third of the admitted steroid users were not involved in school-sponsored sports, and more than a quarter of users stated that their main reason for using steroids was for appearance, not to improve athletic performance. Recently, H.G. Pope and his colleagues (personal communication, 1992) described a subset of bodybuilders with an altered self-image, who believe that they look small and weak even though they are large and muscular and who expend inordinate effort to increase their body size through weight training and the use of ergogenic substances. Pope calls this condition "reverse anorexia nervosa." These bodybuilders appear to be substantially different from competitive athletes in terms of their objectives, the greater health risks that some are willing to take, and their dosing with extremely large quantities of steroids. This phenomenon suggests reasons why the most serious illnesses associated with steroid use have occurred almost exclusively in bodybuilders and not in other steroid-using athletes (54).

Ergogenic Benefits. The known and suspected risks of steroid use are not as extreme as some writers would lead athletes and coaches to believe. However, the benefits are also less well defined than is generally acknowledged (12). Without question, testosterone is responsible for much of the increases in muscle mass and strength that occur in boys as they go through puberty. The absence of this testosterone effect results in a distinctive smaller and weaker upper body (seen in men with Kleinfelter's syndrome, for example). Once established, many of the naturally induced masculinization effects are apparently not readily reversed. The established example of this phenomenon is the castration of horses; if castration is performed too late, the gelding retains much of his muscular appearance and aggressive personality. The question relevant to male athletes is, Does anabolic steroid supplementation to normally masculinized men *further* increase muscle mass or enhance performance in some other way?

Androgens do clearly increase body mass, including the nonfat component in normal men not engaged in intensive resistance training (52, 55, 148, 152) and in weight-trained men (53). For a period of time this was postulated to be from an increase in body water (73). More recent studies have demonstrated the presence of androgen receptors in skeletal muscle (65, 103), as well as increases in muscle protein synthesis and muscle RNA content in men (64) and in muscle tropomyosin in guinea pigs (96, 110) during testosterone treatment. Only a few people demonstrate large responses to moderately high doses of anabolic steroids; for most people to achieve substantial increases, much higher doses must be used (51). This relationship may reflect the differential sensitivity of genes that determine the appearance of androgen-dependent characteristics in an individual (10, 11). The increase in fat-free mass and possible reduction in fat mass last for several months after cessation of use (52) (Figure 11.1). Thus athletes may derive a benefit from steroid use even if they stop using the drugs far enough in advance of competition to obtain a negative drug test. This is why unannounced year-round drug testing of some elite athletes is important to preventing unfair drug use.

Despite the benefit of increased muscle mass, no enhancement of athletic performance by anabolic steroids has ever been rigorously demonstrated. Most studies have generally involved low doses close to those used for replacement therapy in hypogonadal men. Furthermore, the typical end point measured has been a 1RM (repetition maximum) lift of some kind, frequently one for which the athlete was not training (69). It is not surprising, then, that these studies showed either mild strength improvements or no effect. In none of the studies has anaerobic power been examined (even though the public has generally credited Ben Johnson's Pyrrhic victory in the sprint in the 1988 Olympics to his anabolic steroid use). No studies have addressed the question of whether anabolic steroids help or actually hinder endurance athletes, even though many claims

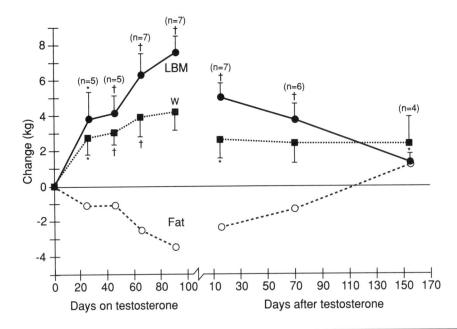

Figure 11.1 Changes in body composition with anabolic steroid administration (200 mg/wk testosterone enanthate for 12 wk) and following drug cessation in normal healthy men. LBM (●) = lean body mass; W (■) = body weight; Fat (○) = fat mass; * = p < 0.05; † = p < 0.01.
Reprinted from Forbes, Porta, Herr, and Griggs (1992).

have been made for performance-limiting mechanisms that might be overcome by such drug use (e.g., the ability to increase training volume without injury and fatigue, enhanced motivation, and a glycogen-sparing effect). Although "everyone knows that anabolic steroids work," nobody has yet demonstrated what kind of physical performance enhancement they might provide.

Athletes claim that steroids are useful in a wide variety of other areas, including replacement treatment of reduced testosterone levels caused by intensive workouts, counteracting the catabolic influences of naturally secreted corticosteroids, increasing the oxygen-carrying capacity of the blood, increasing aggressiveness, and enhancing strength through neuromuscular or other changes separate from muscle hypertrophy. Some of these purported benefits can be dismissed on the basis of available data, although others, such as increased aggressiveness and neuromuscular changes (92, 95, 108), may have some basis.

There is no evidence that there exists a training-induced androgen deficiency in athletes that requires replacement treatment with synthetic anabolic steroids. The data used to support this notion is from starved and sleep-deprived soldiers, in whom testosterone levels can be restored to normal with adequate sleep and food. Other studies have reported chronically low testosterone levels in male distance runners compared with controls (8, 149). However, these are small differences with no clear physiological significance, even if they are statistically significant. In other words, there is no apparent male response parallel to the female "athletic amenorrhea" associated with high training volume.

During intense exercise, and even during intensely stressful military field training, corticosteroids do not generally increase to the range that would be observed with corticosteroid drug administration, and only at much higher levels is testosterone production likely to be suppressed by these hormones. Thus, there is also little evidence of the corticosteroid-related breakdown of muscle tissue that occurs with pharmacological administration of corticosteroids.

Although anabolic steroids can improve hematocrit in patients with anemia, there is little evidence that the commonly used anabolic steroids increase hematocrit or the oxygen-carrying capacity of the blood in normal men.

One of the potentially most potent, and possibly most hazardous, effects of high-dose anabolic steroid use is increased aggressiveness. The East Germans reportedly used anabolic steroids for this effect, delivering high doses to the central nervous system by taking steroids through the nose. This has not been well studied, but anecdotal reports suggest that this practice markedly increased aggressiveness and enhanced performance among their athletes (40). The effect of anabolic steroids on aggressiveness is strongly suspected from case reports (116, 117), even though this effect has only been clearly demonstrated in animals (138). Studies in humans usually have demonstrated improved motivation and improved feelings of well-being in androgen-deficient men treated with anabolic steroids, but even the early studies failed to confirm an increased work capacity in normal men (127). Men subjectively report greater motivation and increased self-confidence with high-dose anabolic steroid use. However, the case reports collected by Pope and Katz (116, 117) and the anecdotal findings of other researchers suggest that in some people, these psychological changes can emerge as reckless behavior and loss of judgment. Psychosis may occur in some susceptible individuals or perhaps at doses that also activate corticosteroid-specific responses (corticosteroids have been known to produce psychosis).

Potential Risks to Performance.
Effects of anabolic steroids that are not readily controllable by the user and that can ruin performance may include uncontrolled emotional responses directed at a teammate when teamwork is critical, an unanticipated decline in performance when steroid use is suddenly stopped, and an undesirable increase in body weight in a marathoner who uses steroids in hopes of extending training capacity. One aspect of steroid use that is virtually unstudied is the effects on performance after an athlete stops using anabolic steroids.

Signs of Anabolic Steroid Use.
Other than a positive drug test or direct observation of use, there is no way of being certain that an athlete is using anabolic steroids. However, there are symptoms that might warrant discussion of steroid abuse with an athlete. The most reliable sign of use is an unexpectedly large increase in body size, possibly accompanied by substantial gains in strength. A jump in size along with a new acne problem, gynecomastia, or a sudden change in behavior might suggest the possibility of anabolic steroid use in an athlete. In a medical screening by a physician, a subnormal HDL cholesterol level (<25 mg/dl) and soft and inappropriately small testes may be a consequence of anabolic steroid use. An unannounced urinalysis would provide certain evidence of recent anabolic steroid use (28).

Other Hormones

Human Chorionic Gonadotropin.
Human chorionic gonadotropin is a hormone obtained from the urine of pregnant women and is very closely related in structure and function to luteinizing hormone. Injected into men, it can increase testicular testosterone production; testosterone levels can be nearly doubled within 4 days after a large intramuscular injection (31). However, this rise cannot be readily sustained, owing to feedback mechanisms in the body. One of the primary risks of the hormone is receptor desensitization in the testes owing to excessive stimulation by the hormone followed by a period in which additional hormone artificially administered or luteinizing hormone naturally secreted from the pituitary does not produce a normal testosterone secretory response (60). The other primary risk in athletes is the stimulation of excess estrogen production by the testes, leading to gynecomastia in some cases (58). Although some athletes claim human chorionic gonadotropin is useful in reducing body fat, there is no sound reason for an athlete to use it as a performance enhancer.

Growth Hormone.
Because growth hormone is much less frequently abused than steroids and because many good reviews of growth hormone use by athletes exist (97, 120, 144), our discussion here will not be exhaustive. Growth hormone is a protein secreted from the pituitary; it is named for one of its best known actions, the stimulation of physical growth of the body. It also has important metabolic actions, such as maintaining blood glucose levels, increasing the uptake of glucose and amino acids into muscle cells (74), and stimulating release of fatty acids from the fat cells.

The main source of pharmacological growth hormones is laboratory synthesis of the relatively complicated molecule using recombinant DNA technology. Until 1986, the only source of the hormone was the pituitaries of human cadavers; this made the hormone exceedingly expensive. Growth hormone from animals cannot be used because human growth hormone receptors accept only the human variety. High cost before 1986 did not prevent athletes from using growth hormone but it did substantially restrict its use. The FDA hastened its approval of recombinant growth hormones after 3 men with growth hormone deficiency were infected from using cadaveric hormone and died from Creutzfeld-Jakob disease, a slow infectious disease affecting the brain somewhat like Alzheimer's disease (88). Recombinant growth hormone does not carry this risk. Because of increased availability and decreasing cost, recombinant human growth hormone now presents society with ethical issues about using the drug to increase stature in normal children and alter body composition in normal adults.

Many effects of growth hormone actually occur through the actions of other hormones produced and secreted from the liver in response to growth hormone stimulation, such as insulinlike growth factors (IGFs). IGFs are now being synthesized using recombinant DNA technology and tested in the treatment of patients with catabolic diseases (151). It can be reasonably expected that within a short period of time athletes will also obtain and abuse these hormones. IGFs appear to be required in very large doses to promote protein anabolism; risks are associated with insulinlike effects and reduction in blood glucose levels (101, 139).

Excessive natural secretion of growth hormone produces well-known clinical syndromes for which people seek medical treatment. Excessive secretion during childhood causes *gigantism*, a condition in which a person becomes abnormally tall. After puberty, once linear growth has stopped, excess secretion of growth hormone causes *acromegaly*, a disfiguring disease characterized by a widening of the bones, arthritis, organ enlargement, and metabolic abnormalities. Acromegalics suffer from a diabeticlike condition that can include glucose intolerance and damage to small blood vessels leading to blindness and kidney failure. Acromegalics also experience increases in muscle mass but tend to complain of muscle weakness; thus, there is apparently something abnormal about the excess muscle produced by growth hormone, although the nature of this effect has not been explained. Dr. Charles Kochakian (personal communication, 1989), a pioneer in anabolic drugs, has described this difference using a comparison of two rats, one treated with rat growth hormone, the other with an anabolic steroid. Both had increased body weight, but the underside of the growth hormone–treated rat felt soft and mushy, whereas the steroid-treated rat had a hard, muscular feel.

Several recent studies have demonstrated moderate effects on body composition and other benefits when growth hormone is used in replacement therapy (30). For example, when men with established growth hormone deficiencies were treated with nightly injections of recombinant human growth hormone for 6 months, their lean body mass increased an average of 12 lb (5.4 kg), and they lost approximately the same amount of fat (126). Side effects included fluid retention and joint pain. Another study tested recombinant human growth hormone in elderly men who had reduced circulating levels of insulinlike growth factor I (IGF-I). Similar results were obtained: an increase in lean body mass and decreased body fat, as well as a thickening of the skin; all occurred without adverse effects (123). One further study indicated changes in the opposite direction. Young men followed for the first year after they stopped using growth hormone to increase stature experienced a decline in muscle fiber size and strength and an increase in the proportion of body fat (124).

It is important to note that the changes in body composition in these studies were produced in subjects deficient in their own production of growth hormone or IGF-I. There is no evidence that supplemental growth hormone produces effects of the same magnitude (it may not even produce normal muscle) or enhances athletic performance in a normal man or woman. One study with seven trained adults given growth hormone 3 days per week for 6 weeks demonstrated modest changes

in body composition but no strength assessment was performed (37b). Growth hormone treatment is also extremely expensive; a 1-year supply for growth hormone–deficient patients, such as those in the studies just described, costs about $13,000. The results produced in these studies were unimpressive compared with what an athlete could do with sound training. Finally, if an athlete can achieve a very long term increase in growth hormone levels through nightly injections of recombinant human growth hormone, then he or she will presumably face all the metabolic and health consequences of acromegalics, who tend to die young from heart disease. Apparently, few athletes are actually using this hormone, which suggests that they may well be aware that the substance probably does little to enhance performance, carries risks, and is very expensive.

Erythropoietin. Erythropoietin is another protein hormone that can be produced by new recombinant DNA techniques and which is reportedly being abused by athletes (1). Erythropoietin is naturally produced primarily in the kidneys and stimulates production of new red blood cells. Its level increases in response to such endurance exercise as marathon running (129). In certain types of anemia, especially in kidney patients with inadequate erythropoietin production, the recent availability of recombinant human erythropoietin has improved the quality of life (46). In normal men administered the recombinant hormone there is also a substantial increase in hematocrit and hemoglobin; after 6 weeks of treatment, hematocrit increased in healthy men from 44.5% to 50% (18). There is a sound basis for an ergogenic effect—enhanced oxygen-carrying capacity of the blood when hematocrit is increased—allowing athletes to work at a higher level of oxygen consumption. This benefit has been demonstrated in numerous studies on blood doping, in which athletes are reinfused with their own red blood cells after a period of collection and storage (19, 24, 44). It might even be argued that endurance athletes are actually ''deficient'' in red cells, with a ''sports anemia'' that occurs when hematocrit does not increase appropriately in response to hemodilution because the oxygen delivery capacity of the circulatory system has also improved (66).

On the other hand, there is a high risk that the additional red blood cells will impede performance as the blood becomes more viscous and thermoregulatory ability becomes compromised. Even in a controlled laboratory setting, one of the few studies using recombinant human erythropoietin administered to normal men demonstrated a large rise in systolic blood pressure during submaximal exercise (18). During endurance events the additional problem of dehydration could compound cardiovascular risks, by eliminating any safety margin in the balance between performance advantages from artificially increased hematocrit and decrements from increased blood viscosity. Reports of multiple deaths of Belgian and Dutch cyclists suspected of having abused erythropoietin suggest a potentially fatal outcome; in this case it is speculated that sudden heart failure occurred when the athletes' hematocrit suddenly rose to 50% to 60% (50). Consequently, endurance athletes should stay away from this drug because of the real danger of sudden death.

Other actions of erythropoietin on the body, in addition to those effects which would be produced with blood doping, may also exist and remain to be investigated. For example, in normal men treated with recombinant human erythropoietin, the lymphocyte count decreased (18), suggesting that erythropoietin may have regulatory effects on cells other than red blood cells, including cells involved in immune function.

Thyroid Hormone. The side effects of thyroid hormone use are significant enough to have curtailed its use among athletes. The most significant problem is that thyroid hormones tend to catabolize muscle, even if they also burn fat (112). Recent animal studies have demonstrated that thyroid hormones cause a shift from slow-twitch to fast-twitch muscle (20, 86), but the relevance to normal men and women is unknown. Thyroid hormones can weaken bones by causing demineralization every time the hormones are readministered (119). The only use for pharmacological thyroid hormones is replacement therapy in thyroid disease.

Beta-Adrenergic Agonists. Synthetic beta-adrenergic agonists (or simply beta-agonists) are substances chemically related to epinephrine, a hormone produced in the adrenal medulla that regulates lipolysis (the breakdown of fat) (4), thermogenesis (increased energy expenditure for heat production), and other aspects of sympathetic activity. Beta-agonists were originally developed for the treatment of asthma and other life-threatening medical conditions. Recently, some of these compounds have been found to have specific effects on body composition, such as increases in lean mass and decreases in stored fat; this effect has resulted in the name *nutrient-partitioning agents* for these drugs (17).

The implicit proof of the effectiveness of beta-agonists is their increasing use in livestock raising. Without question these drugs work in the species for which they are intended, increasing protein synthesis and muscle mass and decreasing fat mass by enhanced lipolysis and lowered lipogenesis (fat synthesis and storage) (15, 71). The main drugs used in animals are ractopamine (pigs), cimaterol (sheep), and clenbuterol (chickens and cattle).

Athletes have begun using these agents, primarily clenbuterol, which is available in Europe as an over-the-counter asthma medication. It is taken orally; athletes typically administer it in doses ranging from 20 to 60 µg/day in 2-week cycles. They claim that the cycling is necessary because of a reported receptor desensitization that results in diminished anabolic responsiveness to the drug (41, 114). At present, there is no available human data establishing the effects on body composition of these drugs. Athletes are using them solely on the basis of anecdotes and self-experimentation. Doses appropriate to livestock may produce quite different effects in humans because of differences in receptor distribution and sensitivity. Other related compounds appear to be more specific to a special class of beta-receptor associated with the actions on body composition but with relatively little of the other epinephrinelike effects, such as increased heart rate and tremors (2); these are currently being tested in human clinical trials as anti-obesity agents (29, 76).

The risks associated with beta-agonists are not well established. Based on reports on an epidemic poisoning that was linked to the consumption of beef liver contaminated with clenbuterol, side effects include sleeplessness, nervousness, and increased heart rate (98). It has been argued that because these agents have been long used in the treatment of asthma in doses comparable to those being used by athletes, they have a proven record of safety (41). However, the safety of asthma medications themselves is currently the topic of intense debate, with the possibility that a higher mortality in asthma patients is due not to the severity of their disease but the frequent use of their beta-agonist medications (25). The risks associated with unlimited dosing when athletes self-administer drugs without medical guidance may be reasonably expected to produce cardiac abnormalities and other effects related to sympathetic stimulation.

It is well known that beta-adrenergic stimulation may impair certain types of athletic performance. Tremor and increased heart rate induced by high levels of epinephrine secreted in response to the stress of competition is detrimental to marksmanship performance and other athletic skills requiring fine motor control, such as ski jumping and diving. In these latter cases, drugs that block beta-receptors have been used by athletes for competitive advantage (91).

Drug Testing

Drug testing for banned substances can be a reliable and effective means of maintaining a "level playing field." Many of the difficulties with drug detection that existed more than a decade ago (9) have been resolved. Drug testing cannot catch every user, but it can be effective in keeping most athletes honest. Athletes who think they can beat the testing can never really be certain, because drug testers are continually developing and improving testing methods. The list of well-known athletes who have been publicly disgraced for errors in judgment is growing.

The key elements of an effective drug program include year-round, randomized, and unannounced testing. The collection procedure has to be meticulously correct to ensure that the urine sample produced is the athlete's own and that there are no mix-ups in the subsequent handling of the sample. The tests must be performed by a competent laboratory certified in this type of work. The remainder of the potential problems with drug testing concern technological aspects of detecting the various substances.

Tests can usually be developed for any substance that does not occur naturally in the body (28, 130). Very sensitive methods, such as mass spectroscopy, can be readily applied to many different types of substances; the appearance of previously ignored substances (e.g., clenbuterol and cimaterol) now triggers quick chemical characterization and identification (34). Most sports organizations have already outlawed "related substances" in their lists of banned substances. Thus, there is no such thing as a "designer" ergogenic substance—one that has minor alterations in chemical composition and that can be used with impunity by athletic competitors (28, 82).

Naturally occurring ergogenic substances, such as caffeine, are assigned a threshold value so that several cups of coffee do not cause the athlete to fail a drug test but the use of high-dose caffeine tablets would. Some substances, such as recombinant human growth hormone and erythropoietin and synthetic testosterone are more difficult to test for because they are indistinguishable from the naturally occurring hormones. Establishing a "normal" range of concentrations is problematic, especially for athletes who may naturally produce higher-than-average levels of these substances. The testing strategy has been to identify associated biochemical changes or by-products associated with natural-hormone production by the body. For example, the use of testosterone will produce several telltale alterations, including suppression of some pituitary hormones, abnormally low levels of steroid metabolites, and an abnormally high level of circulating testosterone (68). A testicular tumor or other abnormality might produce a similar result, but such a diagnosis would clear the athlete of any wrongdoing. The only currently available test for growth hormone and erythropoietin is a direct measure of blood levels. Concentrations above the normal range of these hormones, whose levels are tightly regulated by the body, may be adequate proof of drug use. With erythropoietin, for example, a high hematocrit

and a high level of circulating erythropoietin concentration may be used as the criterion for a positive drug test.

Substances used to mask illicit ergogenic substances are now themselves banned and can be detected. Most of these "masking agents" are diuretics, which dilute the urine specimen and make it harder to obtain a positive test. Most testing labs are able not only to detect diuretics; they can concentrate urine specimens and adjust pH so that a proper drug screen can be performed. Another "masking agent," probenecid, is a weak diuretic that used to be prescribed to prevent urinary excretion of penicillin and was coincidentally found to reduce excretion of androgenic steroids (59). Probenecid is banned and can be detected in drug screens.

The most recent problem in drug testing emerged following the public release of secret East German records of athlete drug use (40). A steroid nasal spray that produced an almost immediate response through its effects on the brain was used, reportedly enhancing aggressiveness and performance. The effectiveness of the nasal approach remains to be scientifically demonstrated. In any case, if such effects actually result, then a new drug test and perhaps a different timing sequence in the testing procedure will have to be developed.

Drug testing has been considerably refined over the past several decades and is now technologically sophisticated enough to detect most banned substances. This should give athletes some assurance of fairness, at least at the higher levels of competition, where testing is likely to be performed in an effective manner. This should also convince athletes that they are putting themselves and their teams at great risk if they choose to use banned substances. Athletes with questions about banned substances and preparations that might contain banned substances may call the U.S. Olympic Committee Drug Hotline at (719) 578-4574.

DIETARY SUPPLEMENTS

Dietary supplements are useful primarily to athletes who have a specific nutritional deficiency. Many advertised supplements do not serve any useful purpose. There are no established nutritional deficiencies associated with sport training that would necessitate supplementation over normal ingestion of food and drink. Doses of dietary supplements exceeding minimum requirements have not generally been demonstrated to produce ergogenic effects. The examples that follow demonstrate how athletes are taken advantage of in their search for performance enhancers. (Caffeine may be one of the few naturally occurring substances that is not banned at low doses of use and that may bring about a performance-enhancing effect for certain sports.)

The claims of the manufacturers of dietary supplements are usually so flimsy that they can be dismissed as having no credible basis without the need for conducting expensive experiments. On the chance that a substance works through some mechanism previously unknown to science, evaluative studies are sometimes performed, particularly when the manufacturer is willing to support the work and athletes are claiming efficacy. An example of this is a very careful and detailed study performed on the effects of γ-oryzanol, a sterol extracted from rice bran; unfortunately for the manufacturer, the study demonstrated no effect on any physiological measures in a group of strength athletes (80).

It is more typically the case that products have simply not been tested for efficacy or for safety, despite the claims on the container or in accompanying literature. It is not practical for anyone to be performing the expensive and elaborate tests necessary to screen all of these substances. Safety tests are usually performed only after a question of health risk arises. For example, there was concern on the basis of one case that Siberian ginseng tablets used by a pregnant woman might cause masculinization of the baby. To determine if this presented a public-health risk, a detailed rat bioassay was conducted on the substance. Not only were the tablets found to be devoid of androgenic activity (and therefore probably not the cause of the problem), but it also turned out that they were prepared from a plant species other than ginseng (7, 145).

Vitamins

A reduction in physical performance is observed in chronic vitamin deficiencies, especially deficiencies in some of the B vitamins (13, 21, 142). However, this does not lead to the conclusion that greater-than-normal intake of certain vitamins enhances performance (85, 141, 146, 150). Furthermore, arguments that athletes on normal diets become vitamin deficient during intensive training are not well supported by the data (121, 128, 141, 146).

Fifty years ago, Keys and Henschel (84) examined the benefits of vitamin supplementation in army rations in reducing fatigue and increasing the work capacity of soldiers during prolonged severe exercise and during semistarvation. When the soldiers were given supplements of vitamins B_1, B_2, and C in amounts greater than 100% of current Recommended Daily Allowances (RDAs), the researchers found no benefit in strength, endurance, resistance to fatigue, or recovery from exertion. Recent studies have still not shown a performance benefit (133). New data suggest that some vitamins are important in disease prevention and may be more effective in this role in higher-than-normal levels of intake, but there is no basis for the use of vitamins as

performance enhancers in an athlete who is not vitamin deficient (105). In fact, excess vitamin use can produce health problems, especially with overuse of vitamin B_6 and fat-soluble vitamins, such as vitamins A and D. For example, doses exceeding 10 times the RDA for vitamin D can produce excessive calcium deposition and weight loss; intake of more than 600 mg/day of vitamin B_6 can produce loss of sensation in peripheral nerves (146).

One claim about vitamin supplementation of athletes merits further investigation. Vitamins C and E are antioxidants, which reduce tissue damage caused by certain chemicals generated in the body during trauma and high levels of stress. It has been proposed that the use of these vitamins in doses higher than their RDAs may hasten physiological recovery or minimize illness and injury following intensive workouts. (Vitamin B_{12} has been promoted to athletes for this effect as well.) To date there is no convincing evidence to support this contention.

"Steroid Replacers"

There is a long list of substances that have been promoted to athletes as "steroid replacers," substances that may increase testosterone levels either through stimulation of testosterone production by the body or by acting as precursors for steroid production. All these claims are completely unfounded, but, couched in scientific terms, the advertisements for these products can be very convincing (57).

Testosterone in the body is manufactured from cholesterol. Thus, pure butter, which is high in cholesterol, could be justifiably sold as a steroid precursor, although putting more cholesterol into a normal person does not increase testosterone levels, because the body already makes far more cholesterol than it needs for the small amount used in steroid production. Plant sterols such as β-sitosterol are sold as "steroid replacers" solely on the basis of their relationship to cholesterol, but are no more likely than butter to influence testosterone levels.

Another class of steroid precursors is the group of substances known as sapogenins (e.g., diosgenin and smilogenin or the plant products advertised as Mexican yam, Diascorea, and Smilax), which have been used to produce steroids in chemical laboratories. From a single precursor substance (e.g., diosgenin), testosterone, estrogens, and corticosteroids can all be synthesized in the laboratory, but no synthesis occurs in the human body because it lacks the necessary enzymes.

Some manufacturers sell preparations of desiccated organs, such as testes, from other species, under the pretext that they will provide some significant amount of natural steroid; they do not. A product known as Yohimbe bark was doctored by one manufacturer with methyltestosterone, a banned anabolic steroid, until it was pulled from the market by the FDA (36).

Boron is another "steroid alternative" that manufacturers claim will increase testosterone levels in the body by 300% within 14 days of use. However, boron may actually cause a decrease in testosterone levels (57). The manufacturers' claim for boron originated with their misinterpretation of a scientific study on postmenopausal women.

"Growth Hormone Releasers"

The intravenous infusion of the amino acid arginine produces a relatively consistent increase in growth hormone secretion in normal subjects (102) and is used by endocrinologists to test a patient for a normal growth hormone response. This is the basis of the marketing of "growth hormone releasers." However, it has never been demonstrated that oral administration of arginine produces a similar rise in growth hormone or that any such rise would be adequate to produce any performance-enhancing effect.

Another amino acid, ornithine, is reportedly 3 times more potent than arginine in the stimulation of growth hormone in the intravenous test. The effects of oral administration of ornithine on growth hormone release in bodybuilders were investigated in one study, with various dose levels up to about 12 g. Although all doses used produced measurable increases in circulating ornithine levels, only the highest dose produced a significant rise in growth hormone 90 min later (22). This increase was less than the typical rise observed during sleep in normal people, which led the authors to question the significance of this brief elevation (Figure 11.2). The greatest problem was that at the dose that produced the growth hormone response, all subjects complained of stomach cramping and diarrhea. It was not clear whether these symptoms or the ingested ornithine actually produced the growth hormone response.

It is questionable whether amino acids can promote a growth hormone response at tolerated oral doses and whether a rise in growth hormone will be meaningful in terms of body composition or performance enhancement in normal subjects (70). Based on the ornithine experiment, the doses of the amino acids typically sold in health food stores (e.g., 250-mg tablets of arginine and ornithine) would not be expected to produce any change in growth hormone levels.

One of the best growth hormone "releasers" is resistance exercise, or perhaps any exercise that produces a large rise in lactic acid (49, 89). The rise in growth hormone levels that can be produced in men and women with high-intensity resistance workouts combined with short rest periods is as large (90) as the rise obtained with intravenous arginine infusion (see Figure 11.2). The reasonable conclusion from the available data is

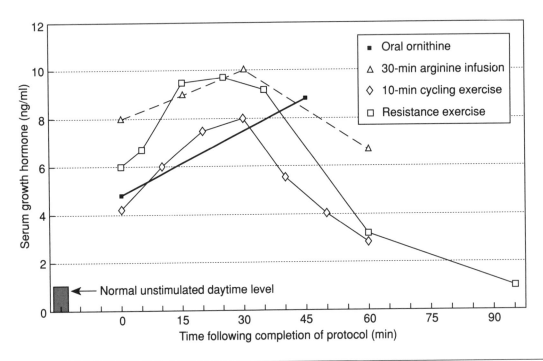

Figure 11.2 Growth hormone response following four protocols (22, 49, 89). The normal nocturnal rise that occurs during rapid–eye movement sleep is as high as or higher than peak levels achieved for each of these stressors or challenges. Oral ornithine is timed from the point at which it appeared in the blood (45 min after ingestion).

that athletes should not waste any money on "growth hormone releasers."

L-Carnitine

L-Carnitine is a dietary supplement with a theoretical basis sufficient to justify testing it for performance-enhancing effects. L-Carnitine is essential for the transport of certain types of fats into the mitochondria for energy production. It is synthesized in the body and is stored primarily in skeletal and cardiac muscle. During intense exercise, carnitine levels appear to decline in muscle because most of it is tied up as acetylcarnitine (125). However, very little change in muscle total carnitine occurs, even after several weeks of intensive training, in sprinters and in distance runners (3). There is therefore no basis for a deficiency condition.

The theory is that if muscle carnitine levels can be increased, there will be a greater utilization of fat during exercise and a saving of glycogen. There are, however, several problems with this line of reasoning (56). The first relates to providing carnitine to the muscle from an oral source. The intestine cannot absorb more than a 2-g dose of L-carnitine, a dosage estimated to increase muscle levels by only 1% to 2% (77). In one study, supplementation with 1 g/day for 4 months produced only small changes in muscle levels in athletes (3). The second problem is that even if muscle carnitine levels could be increased through diet, there are sufficient feedback regulators, such as malonyl-CoA, a product of metabolism, that prevent the transport of additional fats into the mitochondria through the carnitine system. The most serious problem is that there may be good reasons to reduce fatty acid transport into the mitochondria at certain times, such as when oxygen availability is reduced and when the mitochondria may already be flooded with energy substrates (125). Numerous studies have examined the performance-enhancing effect of carnitine (63, 109, 136, 143), but only one (143) has reported a benefit. Animal studies also indicate no benefit during endurance exercise (5, 132).

The use of carnitine by healthy athletes carries potential risks. Several animal studies and one human study have produced muscle carnitine deficiency with administration of D-carnitine or a mixture of D- and L-carnitine (14, 106). In the human study (14) neuromuscular abnormalities were produced in several patients with kidney disease.

Chromium and Vanadium

Chromium is another substance that has been promoted to athletes as a performance enhancer. Chromium is considered a trace essential element and may be involved in glucose regulation (131). The basis of its ergogenic use is a claim that it enhances insulin action and improves muscle glycogen stores, although there is no evidence for this from animal studies (26). Data that have been well circulated by chromium distributors but that have never appeared in a scientific report demonstrate increased lean mass and decreased body fat in men in a weightlifting class and members of a college football team who were fed chromium picolinate (47). Even considering these data, there is no good evidence that chromium does anything to enhance athletic performance (104).

Similarly, vanadium (sold as vanadyl sulfate) has no clear benefit to anyone except a diabetic rat. Several researchers have argued that vanadium has high potential for toxicity, because the dose range in which it helps diabetic rats overlaps with the range in which the rats begin to die from the treatment (43).

Bicarbonate and Other Buffering Agents

A key limiter of intense physical exercise may be an increase in hydrogen ions, which results in such effects as decreased glycolytic enzyme activity and reduced muscle contractile function. Thus, if the decline in intramuscular pH could be slowed by buffers such as sodium bicarbonate, fatigue might be delayed and anaerobic performance enhanced (107). Early studies reported that fruit juices (because of their high citrate levels) and bicarbonate enhanced swimming and running performance (39). Numerous studies have examined the possible performance enhancement of buffers, and some, but not all, report small benefits. Most of the studies that found a performance benefit used at least 300 mg of sodium bicarbonate per kg body weight, given 1 to 3 hr before a competitive event (94). The greatest drawback is that this dose of sodium bicarbonate produces diarrhea, cramps, and bloating in many of the users. Physical training improves the buffering capacity of muscle (111), and proper diet and training may be the surest way to delay fatigue and avoid detrimental side effects (78).

Caffeine and Other Stimulants

Before drug testing of athletes became routine at major competitions, stimulants such as amphetamines, cocaine, caffeine, and strychnine were among the most commonly used doping agents (27). There is little question about the usefulness of stimulants to many types of athletic endeavors; their effects include reduced fatigue, increased alertness, increased confidence, and even euphoria. The benefits produced by amphetamines, for example, were established over 40 years ago in studies of competitive runners and swimmers (134, 135) and of soldiers during prolonged marches (38, 140). There are also risks to performance and health. By delaying fatigue and producing euphoric effects, stimulants carry the risk that an athlete will be pushed beyond safe physiological limits and could suffer serious consequences; soldiers on amphetamines were more likely to continue marching and ignore injuries (38, 140). An additional risk associated with many stimulants is the development of drug dependence.

Because stimulants have to be used at the time of competition to gain an ergogenic advantage, drug testing has substantially curbed this type of cheating. However, a gray area exists for the few stimulants (e.g., caffeine) that are also available in food items and those such as ephedrine that may be accidentally encountered in over-the-counter decongestants and other medications.

Caffeine is present in such foods as chocolate and, of course, in coffee and tea. A typical cup of freshly brewed coffee contains approximately 120 mg of caffeine. More than three cups of coffee drunk shortly before competition would be required to exceed the urinary caffeine limits of 12 µg/ml. The ergogenic potential of caffeine has been the subject of many studies and extensive reviews (33, 42, 45, 48, 62, 79, 118). The primary benefit is a glycogen-sparing effect through increased availability of fatty acids; at least part of this effect may be the result of stimulation of adrenaline release. Caffeine also has stimulant effects of its own that delay fatigue and increase alertness. Caffeine has well-known direct effects in the enhancement and prolongation of cyclic adenosine monophosphate (cAMP) stimulation; thus, in combination with exercise or a beta-agonist such as ephedrine, the effects may be more than just additive (6, 115). The principal drawback to caffeine use is its diuretic effect, which occurs most prominently in nonhabitual users and whose results can range from inconvenience to performance-threatening dehydration. Nervousness and irritability may also result from caffeine ingestion.

Athletes have taken banned substances by mistake, as part of dietary supplements. In some cases, the ingredients have been accurately labeled as "all natural," even though one of the natural ingredients was caffeine in a dose high enough to produce a positive drug test (35). Other preparations labeled as "vitamins" have reportedly contained banned substances that yielded positive drug tests for athletes (35). Ma Huang, a component of many products sold in nutritional supplement stores, is a Chinese herb that contains ephedrine, another banned substance. Athletes should be wary of dietary supplements, both for the dubious benefits of the supplements themselves and for their possible "hidden" pharmacological ingredients.

CONCLUSION

How athletes approach the use of performance-enhancing substances depends in part on information received from strength and conditioning professionals. Ignorance and exaggeration serve no one, and accurate information should be given about the risks and benefits of substances that an athlete may contemplate using. Armed with the best facts available, an athlete should reach the conclusion that the substances that work to enhance performance are banned and/or illegal (e.g., anabolic steroids), that some pose a real health risk (e.g., erythropoietin), that most dietary supplements do not work at all, and that no ergogenic aids are worth the risk to an athlete's reputation and health. Every substance with a potential ergogenic benefit carries some disadvantages, including adverse health consequences or the potential for directly impairing performance when used at the wrong dose, by an individual who responds differently, or in a particular competitive circumstance. This jeopardizes all the hard work that has gone into an athlete's performance.

In addition to these reasons for an athlete to avoid the lure of ergogenic substances, there is the ethical issue expressed by Drs. Catlin and Hatton (27): "The goodness of sport includes mediating the learning of essential values: discipline, endeavor, seeking to triumph but surviving loss, and trust in others, coach or teammates. Doping issues force a higher level of learning more important than trust: personal responsibility."

Key Terms

anabolic steroid	190	dietary supplement	189	ergogenic substance	188

Study Questions

1. Which one of the following is true about dietary supplements?
   a. a product must be safe to use or it can't be sold
   b. a product must be effective or there won't be a market for it
   c. government agencies must approve any supplements sold for human use
   d. there are no guarantees about safety or effectiveness

2. An athlete can be put in jail just for using

   a. erythropoietin
   b. growth hormone
   c. anabolic steroids
   d. clenbuterol

3. A healthy male adult using orally active (17-alkylated) anabolic steroids faces increased health risks including

   a. permanent sterility and brittle bones
   b. liver tumors and reduced blood HDL cholesterol
   c. stroke and permanent sterility
   d. none, except for risks associated with injection of any substance

4. In addition to the health risks faced by an adult, an adolescent boy using anabolic steroids may risk

   a. reduced adult stature and possible behavioral problems
   b. nothing, other than accelerated maturation
   c. deformed facial characteristics and large ears
   d. weak muscles and poor weight-gain

5. Which one of the following potential effects of anabolic steroids is best supported by scientific evidence?

   a. counteracting the effects of training stress
   b. more rapid recovery from injury
   c. increased muscle mass
   d. reduced interest in sex

6. Which one of the following is effective in increasing steroid hormone levels or steroid action in the body?

   a. sterols such as γ-oryzanol
   b. boron
   c. human chorionic gonadotropin
   d. beta-agonists such as clenbuterol
   e. Yohimbe bark extract

7. There are several good reasons that a healthy adult athlete should not use growth hormone. Which one of the following is *not* one of the reasons?

   a. high cost
   b. potential health risks
   c. ergogenic benefits are uncertain
   d. adults will become excessively tall

8. Which one of the following is not known to increase circulating growth hormone levels?

   a. ornithine
   b. sleep
   c. high-intensity exercise
   d. boron

9. Which one of the following is the best reason for endurance athletes to stay away from erythropoietin use?

   a. several bicyclist deaths may have been caused by erythropoietin use
   b. it is well known to cause heart failure
   c. it is well known to reduce resistance to infectious disease
   d. it may reduce the ability of blood to carry oxygen

10. Which three of the following substances are known to produce an anabolic effect (increase lean body mass)?

    a. testosterone
    b. chromium
    c. clenbuterol
    d. growth hormone
    e. L-carnitine
    f. thyroid hormones

Applying Knowledge of Performance-Enhancing Substances

Problem 1

Some have suggested that athletes are "dying in the locker room" from the use of anabolic steroids. Others counter that athletes should be allowed to use steroids if they want to because they either "don't work anyway" or they are at least as safe as many over-the-counter drugs. What do you think about these opinions, and how do you think strength and conditioning training would be affected if anabolic steroid use was openly permitted?

Problem 2

The athletes you train have worked hard to achieve their goals. One of the athletes is looking forward to the ultimate contest of his career, and he wants any competitive edge that he can legitimately get. He's heard about a product called Masterblaster 2000 that he can buy in a health foods store for $75 for a month's supply. That sounds like a bargain for all its ingredients: lots of amino acids (including arginine), chromium picolinate, boron, L-carnitine, and various natural herbs, including ephedra, ginseng, and smilax. The label even has a graph that shows a positive relationship between something called "anabolic effect" and months of product use. The athlete is convinced that this product must have some benefit or the superstar on the label wouldn't endorse it and the store wouldn't be allowed to sell it. Now he has come to you for advice about how much he should take. What would you tell him?

Problem 3

One of your athletes gains 10 lb (4.5 kg) of what looks like mostly lean mass in just over a month, his performance has suddenly shot up, and he seems to have a new acne problem that you never noticed before. You overheard him recently telling some other athletes that competitors are using anabolic steroids and getting away with it because of a new product called Maskall, which is guaranteed by the distributor to hide steroid use in a urinalysis. You guess that he is probably the one who recently left the syringe and empty steroid vial in the locker room trash can. You like the improved performance of this athlete. He stands to gain great fame and fortune if he does well in next month's competition. But you also know that drug testing will be mandatory for the winners. You care about your team and this athlete. What do you do?

References

1. Adamson, J.W., and D. Vapnek. Recombinant erythropoietin to improve athletic performance. *N. Engl. J. Med.* 324:698-699. 1991.
2. Arch, J.R.S., A.T. Ainsworth, M.A. Cawthorne, V. Piercy, M.V. Sennitt, V.E. Thody, C. Wilson, and S. Wilson. Atypical β-adrenoceptor on brown adipocytes as target for anti-obesity drugs. *Nature* 309:163-165. 1984.
3. Arenas, J., J.R. Ricoy, A.R. Encinas, P. Pola, S. D'Iddio, M. Zeviani, S. Didonato, and M. Corsi. Carnitine in muscle, serum, and urine of nonprofessional athletes: Effects of physical exercise, training, and L-carnitine administration. *Muscle Nerve* 14:598-604. 1991.

4. Arner, P., E. Kriegholm, P. Engfeldt, and J. Bolinder. Adrenergic regulation of lipolysis in situ at rest and during exercise. *J. Clin. Invest.* 85:893-898. 1990.

5. Askew, E.W., G.L. Dohm, P.C. Weiser, R.L. Huston, and W.H. Doub Jr. Supplemental dietary carnitine and lipid metabolism in exercising rats. *Nutr. Metab.* 24:32-42. 1980.

6. Astrup, A., S. Toubro, S. Cannon, P. Hein, and J. Madsen. Thermogenic synergism between ephedrine and caffeine in healthy volunteers: A double-blind, placebo-controlled study. *Metabolism* 40:323-329. 1991.

7. Awang, D.V.C. Maternal use of ginseng and neonatal androgenization. *JAMA* 266:363. 1991.

8. Bagatell, C.J., and W.J. Bremner. Sperm counts and reproductive hormones in male marathoners and lean controls. *Fertil. Steril.* 53:688-692. 1990.

9. Bannister, R. Anabolic steroids in sport: Discussion. *Br. J. Sports Med.* 9:100-109. 1975.

10. Bardin, C.W., and J.F. Caterall. Testosterone: A major determinant of extragenital sexual dimorphism. *Science* 211:1285-1294. 1981.

11. Bardin, C.W., J.F. Caterall, and O.A. Janne. The androgen-induced phenotype. In: *Anabolic Steroid Abuse*, research monograph 102, G.C. Lin and L. Erinoff, eds. Washington: National Institute on Drug Abuse, 1990. pp. 131-141.

12. Bardin, C.W., R.S. Swerdloff, and R.J. Santen. Androgens: Risks and benefits. *J. Clin. Endocrinol. Metab.* 73:4-7. 1991.

13. Bates, C.J., H.J. Powers, and D.I. Thurnham. Vitamins, iron, and physical work. *Lancet* 2:313-314. 1989.

14. Bazzato, G., C. Mezzina, M. Ciman, and G. Guarnieri. Myasthenic like syndrome associated with carnitine in patients on long term haemodialysis. *Lancet* 1:1041-1042. 1979.

15. Beermann, D.H., D.E. Hogue, V.K. Fishell, R.H. Dalrymple, and C.A. Ricks. Effects of cimaterol and fishmeal on performance, carcass characteristics and skeletal muscle growth in lambs. *J. Anim. Sci.* 62:370-380. 1986.

16. Behre, H.M., and E. Nieschlag. Testosterone buciclate (20 Aet-1) in hypogonadal men: Pharmacokinetics and pharmacodynamics of the new long-acting androgen ester. *J. Clin. Endocrinol. Metab.* 75:1204-1210. 1992.

17. Bergen, W.G., and R.A. Merkel. Body composition of animals treated with partitioning agents: Implications for human health. *FASEB J.* 5:2951-2957. 1991.

18. Berglund, B., and B. Ekblom. Effect of recombinant human erythropoietin treatment on blood pressure and some haematological parameters in healthy men. *J. Intern. Med.* 229:125-130. 1991.

19. Brien, A.J., and T.L. Simon. The effects of red blood cell infusion on 10-km race time. *JAMA* 257:2761-2765. 1987.

20. Brik, H., and A. Shainberg. Thyroxine induces transition of red toward white muscle in cultured heart cells. *Basic Res. Cardiol.* 85:237-246. 1990.

21. Brouns, F., and W. Saris. How vitamins affect performance. *J. Sports Med. Phys. Fitness* 29:400-403. 1989.

22. Bucci, L., J.F. Hickson, J.M. Pivarnik, I. Wolinsky, J.C. McMahon, and S.D. Turner. Ornithine ingestion and growth hormone release in bodybuilders. *Nutr. Res.* 10:239-245. 1990.

23. Buckley, W.E., C.E. Yesalis, K.E. Friedl, W.A. Anderson, A.L. Streit, and J.E. Wright. Estimated prevalence of anabolic steroid use among male high school seniors. *JAMA* 260:3441-3445. 1988.

24. Buick, F.J., N. Gledhill, A.B. Froese, L. Spriet, and E.C. Meyers. Effect of induced erythrocythemia on aerobic work capacity. *J. Appl. Physiol.* 48:636-642. 1980.

25. Burrows, B., and M.D. Lebowitz. The β-agonist dilemma. *N. Engl. J. Med.* 326:560-561. 1992.

26. Campbell, W.W., M.M. Polansky, N.A. Bryden, J.H. Soares Jr., and R.A. Anderson. Exercise training and dietary chromium effects on glycogen, glycogen synthase, phosphorylase and total protein in rats. *J. Nutr.* 119:653-660. 1988.

27. Catlin, D.H., and C.K. Hatton. Use and abuse of anabolic and other drugs for athletic enhancement. *Adv. Int. Med.* 36:399-424. 1991.

28. Catlin, D.H., R.C. Kammerer, C.K. Hatton, M.H. Sekera, and J.L. Merdink. Analytical chemistry at the games of the XXIIIrd Olympiad in Los Angeles, 1984. *Clin. Chem.* 33:319-327. 1987.

29. Cawthorne, M.A., M.V. Sennitt, J.R.S. Arch, and S.A. Smith. BRL 35135, a potent and selective atypical β-adrenoceptor agonist. *Am. J. Clin. Nutr.* 55:252S-257S. 1992.

30. Christiansen, J.S., and J.O.L. Jorgensen. Beneficial effects of GH replacement therapy in adults. *Acta Endocrinol.* 125:7-13. 1991.

31. Cooke, R.R., R.P. McIntosh, J.G.A. McIntosh, and J.W. Delahunt. Serum forms of testosterone in men after an hCG stimulation: Relative increase in non-protein bound forms. *Clin. Endocrinol.* 32:165-175. 1990.

32. Coronary Drug Project Research Group. The coronary drug project: Findings leading to discontinuation of the 2.5 mg/day estrogen group. *JAMA* 226:652-657. 1973.

33. Costill, D.L., G.P. Dalsky, and W.J. Fink. Effects of caffeine ingestion on metabolism and exercise performance. *Med. Sci. Sports* 10:155-158. 1978.

34. Courtheyn, D., C. Desaever, and R. Verhe. High-performance liquid chromatographic determination of clenbuterol and cimaterol using post-column derivatization. *J. Chromatog.* 564:537-549. 1991.

35. Cowart, V. State-of-art drug identification laboratories play increasing role in major athletic events. *JAMA* 256:3068-3074. 1986.

36. Cowart, V.S. Dietary supplements: Alternatives to anabolic steroids? *Phys. Sportsmed.* 20:189-198. 1992.

37a. Creagh, T.M., A. Rubin, and D.J. Evans. Hepatic tumours induced by anabolic steroids in an athlete. *J. Clin. Pathol.* 41:441-443. 1988.

37b. Crist, D.M., G.T. Peake, R.B. Loftfield, J.C. Kroner, and P.A. Egan. Supplemental growth hormone alters body composition, muscle protein metabolism and serum lipids in fit adults: Characterization of dose-dependent and response-recovery effects. *Mech. Age. Dev.* 58:191-205. 1991.

38. Cuthbertson, D.P., and J.A.C. Know. The effects of analeptics on the fatigued subject. *J. Physiol.* 106:42-58. 1947.

39. Dennig, H., J.H. Talbott, H.T. Edwards, and D.B. Dill. Effect of acidosis and alkalosis upon capacity for work. *J. Clin. Invest.* 9:601-613. 1931.

40. Dickman, S. East Germany: Science in the disservice of the State. *Science* 254:26-27. 1991.

41. Di Pasquali, M. Clenbuterol: A new anabolic drug. *Drugs in Sport* 1:8-11. 1992.

42. Dodd, S.L., E. Brooks, S.K. Powers, and R. Tulley. The effects of caffeine on graded exercise performance in caffeine naive versus habituated subjects. *Eur. J. Appl. Physiol.* 62:424-429. 1991.

43. Domingo, J.L., M. Gomez, J.M. Llobet, and J. Corbella. Oral vanadium administration to streptozotocin-diabetic rats has marked negative side-effects which are independent of the form of vanadium used. *Toxicology* 66:279-287. 1991.

44. Ekblom, B., A.N. Goldbarg, and B. Gullbring. Response to exercise after blood loss and reinfusion. *J. Appl. Physiol.* 33:175-180. 1972.

45. Erickson, M.A., R.J. Schwarzkopf, and R.D. McKenzie. Effects of caffeine, fructose, and glucose ingestion on muscle glycogen utilization during exercise. *Med. Sci. Sports Exer.* 19:579-583. 1987.

46. Erslev, A.J. Erythropoietin. *N. Engl. J. Med.* 324:1339-1344. 1991.

47. Evans, G.W. The effect of chromium picolinate on insulin controlled parameters in humans. *Int. J. Biosoc. Med. Res.* 11:163-180. 1989.

48. Falk, B., B. Burstein, I. Ashkenazi, O. Spilberg, J. Alter, E. Zylber-Katz, A. Rubinstein, N. Bashan, and Y. Shapiro. The effect of caffeine ingestion on physical performance after prolonged exercise. *Eur. J. Appl. Physiol.* 59:168-173. 1989.

49. Felsing, N.E., J.A. Brasel, and D.M. Cooper. Effect of low and high intensity exercise on circulating growth hormone in men. *J. Clin. Endocrinol. Metab.* 75:157-162. 1992.

50. Fisher, L.M. (1991, May 19) Stamina-building drug linked to athletes' deaths. *New York Times*, p. 14.

51. Forbes, G.B. The effect of anabolic steroids on lean body mass: The dose-response curve. *Metabolism* 34:571-573. 1985.

52. Forbes, G.B., C.R. Porta, B.E. Herr, and R.C. Griggs. Sequence of changes in body composition induced by testosterone and reversal of changes after drug is stopped. *JAMA* 267:397-399. 1992.

53. Freed, D.J.L., A.J. Banks, D. Longson, and D.M. Burley. Anabolic steroids in athletics: Crossover double-blind trial on weightlifters. *Br. Med. J.* 2:471-473. 1975.

54. Friedl, K.E. Effects of anabolic steroids on physical health. In: *Anabolic Steroids in Sport and Exercise*, C.E. Yesalis, ed. Champaign, IL: Human Kinetics. 1992. pp. 109-150.

55. Friedl, K.E., J.R. Dettori, C.J. Hannan Jr., T.H. Patience, and S.R. Plymate. Comparison of the effects of high dose testosterone and 19-nortestosterone to a replacement dose of testosterone on strength and body composition in normal men. *J. Steroid Biochem. Molec. Biol.* 40:607-612. 1991.

56. Friedl, K.E., and R.J. Moore. Ergogenic aids: Clenbuterol, Ma Huang, caffeine, L-carnitine and growth hormone releasers. *NSCA Journal* 14(4):35-44. 1992.

57. Friedl, K.E., R.J. Moore, and L.J. Marchitelli. Steroid replacers: Let the athlete beware. *NSCA Journal* 14(1):14-19. 1992.

58. Friedl, K.E., and C.E. Yesalis. Self-treatment of gynecomastia in bodybuilders who use anabolic steroids. *Phys. Sportsmed.* 17:67-79. 1989.

59. Gardner, L.I., J.F. Crigler, and C.J. Migeon. Inhibition of urinary 17-ketosteroid excretion produced by "Benemid." *Proc. Soc. Exp. Biol. Med.* 78:460-463. 1951.

60. Glass, A.R., and R.A. Vigersky. Resensitization of testosterone production in men after human chorionic gonadotropin–induced desensitization. *J. Clin. Endocrinol. Metab.* 51:1395-1400. 1980.

61. Glickstein, S.L., E. Gertner, S.A. Smith, R.I. Roelofs, D.E. Hathaway, P.A. Schlesinger, and E.S. Schned. Eosinophilia-myalgia syndrome associated with L-tryptophan use. *J. Rheumatol.* 17:1534-1543. 1990.

62. Graham, T.E., and L.L. Spriet. Performance and metabolic responses to a high caffeine dose during prolonged exercise. *J. Appl. Physiol.* 71:2292-2298. 1991.

63. Greig, C., K.M. Finch, D.A. Jones, M. Coopers, A.J. Sargeant, and C.A. Forte. The effect of oral supplementation with L-carnitine on maximum and submaximum exercise capacity. *Eur. J. Appl. Physiol.* 56:457-460. 1987.

64. Griggs, R.C., W. Kingston, R.F. Jozefowicz, B.E. Herr, G. Forbes, and D. Halliday. Effect of testosterone on muscle mass and muscle protein synthesis. *J. Appl. Physiol.* 66:498-503. 1989.

65. Gustafsson, J.A., T. Saartok, E. Dahlberg, M. Snochowski, T. Haggmark, and E. Eriksson. Studies on steroid receptors in human and rabbit skeletal muscle: Clues to the understanding of the mechanism of action of anabolic steroids. *Prog. Clin. Biol. Res.* 142:261-290. 1984.

66. Hallberg, L., and B. Magnusson. The etiology of "sports anemia." *Acta Med. Scand.* 216:145-148. 1984.

67. Hamilton, J.B. The role of testicular secretions as indicated by the effects of castration in man and by studies of pathological conditions and the short lifespan associated with maleness. *Recent Prog. Horm. Res.* 3:257-322. 1948.

68. Hatton, C.K., and D.H. Catlin. Detection of androgenic anabolic steroids in urine. *Clin. Lab. Med.* 7:655-668. 1987.

69. Haupt, H.A., and G.D. Rovere. Anabolic steroids: A review of the literature. *Am. J. Sports Med.* 12:469-484. 1984.

70. Hawkins, C.E., and J. Walberg-Rankin. Oral arginine does not affect body composition or muscle function in male weight lifters. *Med. Sci. Sports Exer.* 23:S15. 1991.

71. Helferich, W.G., D.B. Jump, D.B. Anderson, D.M. Skjaerlund, R.A. Merkel, and W.G. Bergen. Skeletal muscle alpha-actin synthesis is increased pretranslationally in pigs fed the phenethanolamine ractopamine. *Endocrinology* 126:3096-3100. 1990.

72. Hershberger, L.G., E.G. Shipley, and R.K. Meyer. Myotrophic activity of 19-nortestosterone and other steroids determined by modified levator ani muscle method. *Proc. Soc. Exp. Biol. Med.* 83:175-180. 1953.

73. Hervey, G.R., A.V. Knibbs, L. Burkinshaw, D.B. Morgan, P.R. Jones, D.R. Chettle, and D. Vartsky. Effects of methandienone on the performance and body composition of men undergoing athletic training. *Clin. Sci.* 60:457-461. 1981.

74. Hesse, D.G., D.E. Matthews, R.L. Leibel, J.M. Gertner, D.A. Fischman, and S.F. Lowry. Recombinant growth hormone enhances muscle myosin heavy-chain mRNA accumulation and amino acid accrual in humans. *Proc. Natl. Acad. Sci. U.S.A.* 86:3371-3374. 1989.

75. Hier, D.B., and W.F. Crowley. Spatial ability in androgen-deficient men. *N. Engl. J. Med.* 306:1202-1205. 1982.

76. Halloway, B.R., R. Howe, B.S. Rao, and D. Stribling. ICI D7114: A novel selective adrenoceptor agonist of brown fat and thermogenesis. *Am. J. Clin. Nutr.* 55:262S-264S. 1992.

77. Hultman, E., G. Cederblad, and P. Harper. Carnitine administration as a tool to modify energy metabolism during exercise. *Eur. J. Appl. Physiol.* 62:450. 1991.

78. Hunter, G., and M. Bamman. Blood buffering. *NSCA Journal* 13:61-65. 1991.

79. Ivy, J.L., D.L. Costill, W.J. Fink, and R.W. Lower. Influence of caffeine and carbohydrate feedings on endurance performance. *Med. Sci. Sports.* 11:6-11. 1979.

80. Johnson, R.L., R.E. Keith, B. Bonner, R.D. Lewis, M.H. Stone, W.J. Kraemer, and B. Warren. The physiological effects of gamma oryzanol on weight-trained young men. *J. Appl. Sports Sci. Res.* 5:170. 1991.

81. Junkmann, K., and H. Witzel. The chemistry and pharmacology of steroid hormone esters. *Monographs on Therapy* 3(Suppl.):1-57. 1958.

82. Kammerer, R.C. Drug testing and anabolic steroids. In: *Anabolic Steroids in Sport and Exercise*, C.E. Yesalis, ed. Champaign, IL: Human Kinetics. 1992. pp. 283-308.

83. Kessler, D.A. The Food and Drug Administration and its problems [letter reply]. *N. Engl. J. Med.* 326:70-71. 1992.

84. Keys, A., and A.F. Henschel. Vitamin supplementation of U.S. Army rations in relation to fatigue and the ability to do muscular work. *J. Nutr.* 23:259-269. 1942.

85. Keys, A., A.F. Henschel, H.L. Taylor, O. Mickelsen, and J. Brozek. Absence of rapid deterioration in men doing hard physical work on a restricted intake of vitamins of the B complex. *J. Nutr.* 27:485-496. 1944.

86. Kirschbaum, B.J., H.B. Kucher, A. Termin, A.M. Kelly, and D. Pette. Antagonistic effects of chronic low frequency stimulation and thyroid hormone on myosin expression in rat fast-twitch muscle. *J. Biol. Chem.* 265:13974-13980. 1990.

87. Kochakian, C.D. Anabolic-androgenic steroids: A historical perspective and definition. In: *Anabolic Steroids in Sport and Exercise*, C.E. Yesalis, ed. Champaign, IL: Human Kinetics. 1993. pp. 3-33.

88. Kolata, G. New growth industry in human growth hormone? *Science* 234:22-24. 1986.

89. Kraemer, R.R., J.L. Kilgore, G.R. Kraemer, and V.D. Castracane. Growth hormone, IGF-1, and testosterone responses to resistive exercise. *Med. Sci. Sports Exerc.* 24:1346-1352. 1992.

90. Kraemer, W.J., S.E. Gordon, S.J. Fleck, L.J. Marchitelli, R. Mello, J.E. Dziados, K.E. Friedl, E. Harman, C. Maresh, and A.C. Fry. Endogenous anabolic hormonal and growth factor responses to heavy resistance exercise in males and females. *Int. J. Sports Med.* 12:228-235. 1991.

91. Kruse, P., J. Ladefoged, U. Nielsen, P.E. Paulev, and J.P. Sorensen. Beta blockade used in precision sports: Effect on pistol shooting performance. *J. Appl. Physiol.* 61:417-420. 1986.

92. Kurz, E.M., D.R. Sengelaub, and A.P. Arnold. Androgens regulate the dendritic length of mammalian motoneurons in adulthood. *Science* 232:395-398. 1986.

93. Liddle, G.W., and H.A. Burke. Anabolic steroids in clinical medicine. *Helv. Medical Acta* 27:504-513. 1960.

94. Linderman, J., and T.D. Fahey. Sodium bicarbonate ingestion and exercise performance: An update. *Sports Med.* 11:71-77. 1991.

95. Luine, V., F. Nottebohm, C. Harding, and B.S. McEwen. Androgen affects cholinergic enzymes in syringeal motor neurons and muscle. *Brain Res.* 192:89-107. 1980.

96. Lyons, G.E., A.M. Kelly, and N.A. Rubinstein. Testosterone-induced changes in contractile protein isoforms in the sexually dimorphic temporalis muscle of the guinea pig. *J. Biol. Chem.* 261:13278-13284. 1986.

97. MacIntyre, J.G. Growth hormone and athletes. *Sports Med.* 4:129-142. 1987.

98. Martinez-Navarro, J.F. Food poisoning related to consumption of illicit β-agonist in liver. *Lancet* 336:1311. 1990.

99. Marx, J.L. Autoimmunity in left-handers. *Science* 217:141-144. 1982.

100. Marx, J.L. The two sides of the brain. *Science* 220:488-490. 1983.

101. Mauras, N., F.F. Horber, and M.W. Haymond. Low dose recombinant human insulin-like growth factor-I fails to affect protein anabolism but inhibits islet cell secretion in humans. *J. Clin. Endocrinol. Metab.* 75:1192-1197. 1992.

102. Merimee, T.J., D. Rabinowitz, and S.E. Fineberg. Arginine-initiated release of human growth hormone: Factors modifying the response in normal man. *N. Engl. J. Med.* 280:1434-1438. 1969.

103. Michel, G., and E.E. Baulieu. Androgen receptor in rat skeletal muscle: Characterization and physiological variations. *Endocrinology* 107:2088-2098. 1980.

104. Moore, R.J., and K.E. Friedl. Physiology of nutritional supplements: Chromium picolinate and vanadyl sulfate. *NSCA Journal* 14(3):47-51. 1992.

105. National Research Council, Subcommittee on the Tenth Edition of RDAs. *Recommended Dietary Allowances*. Washington: National Academy Press. 1989. 283 pp.

106. Negrao, C.E., L.L. Ji, J.E. Schauer, F.J. Nagle, and H.A. Lardy. Carnitine supplementation and depletion: Tissue carnitines and enzymes in fatty acid oxidation. *J. Appl. Physiol.* 63:315-321. 1987.

107. Newsholme, E.A., E. Blomstrand, P. Hassmen, and B. Ekblom. Physical and mental fatigue: Do changes in plasma amino acids play a role? *Biochem. Soc. Trans.* 19:358-362. 1991.

108. Nordeen, E.J., K.W. Nordeen, D.R. Sengelaub, and A.P. Arnold. Androgens prevent normally occurring cell death in a sexually dimorphic spinal nucleus. *Science* 229:671-673. 1985.

109. Oyono-Enguelle, S., H. Freund, C. Ott, M. Gartner, A. Heitz, J. Marbach, F. Maccari, A. Frey, H. Bigot, and A.C. Bach. Prolonged submaximal exercise and L-carnitine in humans. *Eur. J. Appl. Physiol.* 58:53-61. 1988.

110. Papanicolaou, G.N., and E.A. Falk. General muscular hypertrophy induced by androgenic hormone. *Science* 87:238-239. 1938.

111. Parkhouse, W.S., and D.C. McKenzie. Possible contribution of skeletal muscle buffers to enhanced anaerobic performance: A brief review. *Med. Sci. Sports Exerc.* 16:328-338. 1984.

112. Pasquali, R., G. Baraldi, P. Biso, D. Piazzi, M. Capelli, and N. Melchionda. Effect of "physiological" doses of triiodothyronine replacement on the hormonal and metabolic adaption to short-term semistarvation and to low-calorie diet in obese patients. *Clin. Endocrinol.* 21:357-367. 1984.

113. Petera, V., K. Bobek, and V. Lahn. Serum transaminase (GOT, GPT) and lactic dehydrogenase activity during treatment with methyltestosterone. *Clin. Chim. Acta* 7:604-606. 1962.

114. Phillips, W.N. Clenbuterol use climbing. *Anabolic Reference Update #22.* Golden, CO: Mile High. 1990. pp. 1-2.

115. Poehlman, E.T., P. LaChance, A. Tremblay, A. Nadeau, J. Dussault, G. Theriault, J.P. Despres, and C. Bouchard. The effect of prior exercise and caffeine ingestion on metabolic rate and hormones in young adult males. *Can. J. Physiol. Pharmacol.* 67:10-16. 1989.

116. Pope Jr., H.G., and D.L. Katz. Affective and psychotic symptoms associated with anabolic steroid use. *Am. J. Psychiatry* 145:487-490. 1988.

117. Pope Jr., H.G., and D.L. Katz. Homicide and near-homicide by anabolic steroid users. *J. Clin. Psychiatry* 51:28-31. 1990.

118. Powers, S.K., and S. Dodd. Caffeine and endurance performance. *Sports Med.* 2:165-174. 1985.

119. Ribot, C., F. Tremollieres, J.M. Pouilles, and J.P. Louvet. Bone mineral density and thyroid hormone therapy. *Clin. Endocrinol.* 33:143-153. 1990.

120. Rogol, A.D. Growth hormone: Physiology, therapeutic use, and potential for abuse. *Exerc. Sport Sci. Rev.* 17:353-357. 1989.

121. Rokitzki, L., A. Berg, and J. Keul. Blood and serum status of water- and fat-soluble vitamins in athletes and non-athletes. *Int. J. Vitam. Nutr. Res.* [suppl.] 30:192-197. 1989.

122. Ross, J.H., E.C. Attwood, G.E. Atkin, and R.N. Villar. A study of the effects of severe repetitive exercise on serum myoglobin, creatine kinase, transaminases and lactate dehydrogenase. *Q. J. Med.* 206:268-279. 1983.

123. Rudman, D., A.G. Feller, H.S. Nagraj, G.A. Gergans, P.Y. Lalitha, A.F. Goldberg, R.A. Schlenker, L. Cohn, I.W. Rudman, and D.E. Mattson. Effects of human growth hormone in men over 60 years old. *N. Engl. J. Med.* 323:1-6. 1990.

124. Rutherford, O.M., D.A. Jones, J.M. Round, C.R. Buchanan, and M.A. Preece. Changes in skeletal muscle and body composition after discontinuation of growth hormone treatment in growth hormone deficient young adults. *Clin. Endocrinol.* 34:469-475. 1991.

125. Sahlin, K. Muscle carnitine metabolism during incremental dynamic exercise in humans. *Acta Physiol. Scand.* 138:259-262. 1990.

126. Salomon, F., R.C. Cuneo, R. Hesp, and P.H. Sonksen. The effects of treatment with recombinant human growth hormone on body composition and metabolism in adults with growth hormone deficiency. *N. Engl. J. Med.* 321:1797-1803. 1989.

127. Samuels, L.T., A.F. Henschel, and A. Keys. Influence of methyl testosterone on muscular work and creatine metabolism in normal young men. *J. Clin. Endocrinol.* 2:649-654. 1942.

128. Saris, W.H.M., J. Schrijver, M.A. von Erp Baart, and F. Brouns. Adequacy of vitamin supply under maximal sustained workloads: The Tour de France. In: *Elevated Dosages of Vitamins: Benefits and Hazards*, P. Walter, G. Brubacher, and H.B. Stachlin, eds. Lewiston, NY: Hans Huber. 1989. pp. 205-212.

129. Schwandt, H.J., B. Heyduck, H.C. Gunga, and L. Rocker. Influence of prolonged physical exercise on the erythropoietin concentration in the blood. *Eur. J. Appl. Physiol.* 63:463-466. 1991.

130. Schwartz, R.H. Urine testing in the detection of drugs of abuse. *Arch. Intern. Med.* 148:2407-2412. 1988.

131. Schwarz, K., and W. Mertz. Chromium (III) and the glucose tolerance factor. *Arch. Biochem. Biophys.* 85:292-295. 1959.

132. Simi, B., M.H. Mayet, B. Sempore, and R.J. Favier. Large variations in skeletal muscle carnitine level fail to modify energy metabolism in exercising rats. *Comp. Biochem. Physiol.* 97A:543-549. 1990.

133. Singh, A., F.M. Moses, and P.A. Deuster. Chronic multivitamin-mineral supplementation does not enhance physical performance. *Med. Sci. Sports Exer.* 24:726-732. 1992.

134. Smith, G.M., and H.K. Beecher. Amphetamine sulfate and athletic performance. *JAMA* 170:542-557. 1959.

135. Smith, G.M., and H.K. Beecher. Amphetamine, secobarbital, and athletic performance. *JAMA* 172:1502-1514. 1960.

136. Soop, M., O. Bjorkman, G. Cederblad, L. Hagenfeldt, and J. Wharen. Influence of carnitine supplementation on muscle substrate and carnitine metabolism during exercise. *J. Appl. Physiol.* 64:2394-2399. 1988.

137. Strauss, R.H., M.T. Liggett, and R.R. Lanese. Anabolic steroid use and perceived effects in ten weight-trained women athletes. *JAMA* 253:2871-2873. 1985.

138. Svare, B.B. Anabolic steroids and behavior: A preclinical research prospectus. In: *Anabolic Steroid Abuse*, research monograph 102, G.C. Lin and L. Erinoff, eds. Washington: National Institute on Drug Abuse. 1990. pp. 224-241.

139. Turkalj, I., U. Keller, R. Ninnis, S. Vosmeer, and W. Stauffacher. Effect of increasing doses of recombinant human insulin-like growth factor-I on glucose, lipid, and leucine metabolism in man. *J. Clin. Endocrinol. Metab.* 75:1186-1191. 1992.

140. Tyler, D.B. The effect of amphetamine sulfate and some barbiturates on the fatigue produced by prolonged wakefulness. *Am. J. Physiol.* 150:253-262. 1947.

141. van Dale, D., J. Schrijver, and W.H.M. Saris. Changes in vitamin status in plasma during dieting and exercise. *Int. J. Vitam. Nutr. Res.* 60:67-74. 1990.

142. van der Beek, E.J. *Marginal Deficiencies of Thiamin, Riboflavin, Vitamin B-6 and Vitamin C: Prevalence and Functional Consequences in Man.* The Hague: CIP-Gegevens Koninklijke Bibliotheek. 1992.

143. Vecchiet, L., F. Di Lisa, G. Pieralisi, P. Ripari, R. Menabo, M.A. Giamberardino, and N. Siliprandi. Influence of L-carnitine administration on maximal physical exercise. *Eur. J. Appl. Physiol.* 61:486-490. 1990.

144. Wadler, G.I., and B. Hainline. Human growth hormone. In: *Drugs and the Athlete.* Philadelphia: Davis. 1989. pp. 70-74.

145. Waller, D.P., A.M. Martin, N.R. Farnsworth, and D.V.C. Awang. Lack of androgenicity of Siberian Ginseng. *JAMA* 267:2329. 1992.

146. Walter, P. Supraphysiological dosages of vitamins and their implications in man. *Experientia* 47:178-181. 1991.

147. Walters, M.J., R.J. Ayers, and D.J. Brown. Analysis of illegally distributed anabolic steroid products by liquid chromatography with identity confirmation by mass spectrometry or infrared spectrophotometry. *J. Asso. Off. Anal. Chem.* 73:924-926. 1990.

148. Welle, S., R. Jozefowicz, G. Forbes, and R.C. Griggs. Effect of testosterone on metabolic rate and body composition in normal men and men with muscular dystrophy. *J. Clin. Endocrinol. Metab.* 74:332-335. 1992.

149. Wheeler, G.D., S.R. Wall, A.N. Belcastro, and D.C. Cumming. Reduced serum testosterone and prolactin levels in male distance runners. *JAMA* 252:514-516. 1984.

150. Williams, M.H. Vitamin supplementation and athletic performance. *Beiheft Int. Z. Vitamin Ern Arhungsforshung* 30:163-191. 1989.

151. Wilmore, D.W. Catabolic illness: Strategies for enhancing recovery. *N. Engl. J. Med.* 325:695-702. 1991.

152. World Health Organization Task Force on Methods for the Regulation of Male Fertility. Contraceptive efficacy of testosterone-induced azoospermia in normal men. *Lancet* 336:955-959. 1990.

153. Yesalis, C.E., W.A. Anderson, W.E. Buckley, and J.E. Wright. Incidence of the nonmedical use of anabolic-androgenic steroids. In: *Anabolic Steroid Abuse*, research monograph 102, G.C. Lin and L. Erinoff, eds. Washington: National Institute on Drug Abuse. 1990. pp. 97-112.

CHAPTER 12

NUTRITIONAL FACTORS IN PERFORMANCE AND HEALTH

Michael H. Stone

It has only been within the last century that a real understanding of some of the details of nutritional effects on aging, general health, and athletic performance has emerged. Sports nutrition is now one of the most studied areas of nutrition, and many long-held concepts of good nutrition, particularly those relevant to athletes, are being challenged.

Recent information from studies of carbohydrate and protein needs for exercise and training has brought about a reevaluation of previous concepts of athletic nutrition and has led to a restructuring of the diets of athletes. Clearly, carbohydrates may be thought of as an ergogenic aid; they contribute to liver and muscle glycogen content, which in turn contributes to long-term endurance, as well as to maintaining the intensity of repeated bouts of anaerobic exercise. Periodic feedings of carbohydrates during long-term exercise may maintain blood glucose and reduce dependence on liver and muscle glycogen, thus prolonging exercise or allowing for higher intensity exercise. Only a few years ago most sports scientists and nutritionists recommended that the recommended daily allowance (RDA) for protein was sufficient for athletic endeavors. Several sports scientists are now recommending increases in dietary protein for both endurance and strength-and-power athletes (15). Certain vitamins and minerals are also receiving new emphasis for their importance in training and long-term health. Poor nutrition, on the other other hand, may contribute to certain types of overtraining (122).

In short, what is eaten, how it is eaten, and when it is eaten may have marked effects on health and performance. The purpose of this chapter is to summarize current knowledge of nutritional and dietary factors, especially those that affect performance.

PROTEIN

Athletes and strength and conditioning professionals, particularly those involved in strength-and-power sports, have an interest in the role of protein in the diet and in the usefulness of protein supplementation. There is still confusion and controversy today regarding the protein requirements for athletes in training. Many athletes and coaches believe, based on personal experience and anecdotal evidence, that additional protein consumption is necessary for optimal or maximal performance or muscle gain. Even scientists disagree on the exact protein requirements of athletes, particularly those engaged in high-intensity or high-volume physical training. Part of the confusion derives from inadequacies in the experimental design of scientific studies—in particular, the use of short-term studies and poorly designed training programs. A lack of understanding of all aspects of protein metabolism also contributes to the problem. This section reviews the major features of protein metabolism and discusses the effects of physical training on protein requirements.

Protein Metabolism and Function

Approximately 9% to 15% of the total caloric intake of most people in the United States consists of protein (56,106). **Proteins** are relatively complex molecules that have enzymatic and structural functions and are important in a variety of biosynthetic and bioenergetic reactions related to body growth, maintenance and repair, and energy production. Because energy requirements take priority over tissue anabolic reactions (tissue building), protein can also be used as an energy source if carbohydrates and fat in the diet are inadequate (62). An important function of skeletal muscle is to serve as a reservoir for protein, which can be broken down for energy when normal dietary intake is low, as in the extreme case of starvation (119).

Muscle protein is in a constant state of turnover. The amount of protein in muscle is determined largely by the balance between protein anabolism and catabolism (14). If dietary protein above requirement is ingested, it can be oxidized for energy or converted to fat (56,126,127). Thus, eating an excessive amount of protein (or carbohydrates and fat) can increase body fat deposition.

Composition of Proteins

The basic units of protein structure are **amino acids**. All amino acids contain nitrogen. The nitrogen is necessary for the formation of peptide bonds. Proteins are essentially long chains of amino acids linked together by peptide bonds. Thus, protein requirements are related to the requirement for amino acids. Free amino acids are normally found only in small quantities in the foods we eat. Proteins found in food contain mixtures of amino acids that must be digested before the amino acids can be made available.

Synthesis of proteins in humans requires approximately 22 distinct amino acids. Nine of these are **essential amino acids** in adults (Table 12.1): the body cannot synthesize them but must obtain them from plant or animal proteins ingested in the diet. The remaining *nonessential amino acids* can, of course, be obtained from ingested proteins, but can also be synthesized from other substances (such as carbohydrates), as long as there is an adequate source of nitrogen in the body (such as other amino acids). Dietary proteins that contain very low amounts of one or more of the essential amino acids are known as *incomplete proteins* (94). Incomplete proteins are generally of plant origin—nuts, grains, legumes, and seeds. However, the quantity of protein available in some of these products, such as beans, is relatively high and can partially offset the lower biological value. Dietary proteins that contain all the amino acids needed (essential and nonessential) for the synthesis of human tissue protein have a high biological value

Table 12.1 Nonessential and Essential Amino Acids

Nonessential	Essential
Glycine	Leucine
Alanine	Isoleucine
Aspartic acid	Valine
Glutamic acid	Threonine
Serine	Lysine
Cystine, cysteine	Methionine
Tyrosine	Phenylalanine
Arginine	Tryptophan
Proline	Histidine[a]
Hydroxyproline	
Glutamine	
Asparagine	

[a]Some adults can synthesize histidine on their own. For other adults and for infants, histidine is an essential amino acid.

and are known as *complete proteins* (106). These proteins are generally found in animal sources and products: meat, dairy products, eggs, and fish.

Very low dietary intake of an essential amino acid reduces the rate of protein synthesis and impairs the use of other amino acids for protein synthesis. Impaired protein synthesis allows protein catabolic effects to predominate, resulting in increased excretion of nitrogen. Measuring the **nitrogen balance** (nitrogen intake vs. nitrogen loss) provides an estimate of a person's protein balance. A negative nitrogen balance occurs when nitrogen loss is greater than intake, indicating a loss of body protein. A positive nitrogen balance exists when nitrogen intake is greater than loss, which indicates an increased state of protein anabolism. A negative nitrogen balance can occur even if only one of the essential amino acids is limiting as a result of inadequate amounts from the diet (106). A negative nitrogen balance can also occur if the proportions of essential amino acids in the diet are unbalanced and overall protein intake is not sufficient to offset the lack of nitrogen balance.

Two incomplete proteins that are each limiting because of deficiencies in different essential amino acids can provide complete protein when both are eaten together, a practice called *mutual supplementation*. It is important for vegetarians to eat foods that contain such *complementary proteins*, which together will provide all the essential amino acids. The following are combinations of plant groups (along with some common examples) that can provide complementary proteins:

- Traditional combinations
    —Soybeans + rice
    —Peas + wheat
    —Beans + corn

- Lentils + wheat or rice
- Cereals + legumes
- Whole grains + sunflower seeds

The timing of meals also is important for optimum protein synthesis. Mutual supplementation is less effective if all of the essential amino acids are not ingested within a 2-hr period (3). Eating two different incomplete proteins at different meals greatly separated in time does not result in effective mutual supplementation. Additionally, physical exercise and other vigorous physical activities immediately after a meal tend to reduce the absorption of amino acids (and some other nutrients) from the intestinal tract.

Protein quality is an important factor in establishing the daily intake requirement for protein. Many food products claim to have a high protein content; however, the quality of the protein may be poor because of deficiencies in essential amino acids. Dietary variety increases the potential for ingesting high-quality protein foods and increases the potential for easily meeting protein requirements, along with the requirements for other essential nutrients.

Digestion of Proteins

Mechanical breakdown in the form of mastication (chewing) of large food particles begins the process of digestion of dietary proteins. Hydrochloric acid and pepsin released from the stomach wall act to further break down smaller particles in the stomach. No amino acids are absorbed through the stomach of adults. Various digestive enzymes in inactive form, including trypsin, chymotrypsin, and carboxypeptidase, are released from the pancreas into the small intestine, where they are activated. These enzymes catalyze the cleavage of the peptide bonds between amino acids to form small peptides and amino acids. Amino acids can be absorbed by the mucosal cells in the intestinal wall, but are typically absorbed as peptides (dipeptides or tripeptides) then broken down into individual amino acids and released into the blood. Approximately 95% to 97% of all amino acids are absorbed in the small intestine; under normal, nonpathological conditions only small amounts of protein are found in the large intestine.

Amino acid absorption in the small intestine is rapid and dependent upon specific active transport systems. Amino acids can be grouped into several structurally related groups; each group has its own transport system to facilitate absorption along the small intestine (56,106). There is competition among amino acids of the same group for transport sites (10); absorption occurs on a first-come-first-served basis. For example, the amino acids lysine, arginine, cystine, and ornithine share the same transport systems. An excessive amount of one of these amino acids can impair the absorption of the other three. Therefore, ingesting a food or protein supplement containing an excess of one or more amino acids could result in decreased absorption of other amino acids.

Amino acid competition for shared transport systems occurs on a first-come-first-served basis (106). Protein obtained from the typical food we eat apparently has the optimum amino acid combinations. The time involved in the digestive process allows for gradual absorption of amino acids and small peptides. Because of the mechanism and timing of the digestion of normal food protein, a steady, but not overwhelming, supply of amino acids is available to the body. It is possible that predigested proteins, which contain free amino acids, can overwhelm available transport systems, reducing total amino acid absorption.

Almost all proteins that enter the stomach and small intestines will be digested. Most enzymes or peptide hormones taken orally are rendered ineffective by digestion and absorption. Glandular products and other protein-containing substances, which are touted as anabolic steroid substitutes, will not be effective, because they are broken down just like other proteins before entering the blood. Once absorbed from the small intestine, amino acids travel to the liver via the portal circulation. From the blood, amino acids can be taken up by various tissues and, depending upon specific needs, enter various biochemical pathways.

Protein Metabolism and Control

The RDA for protein in adults is 0.8 g of protein per kg of body weight per day (94). A margin of safety is included in the RDA in an attempt to account for individual differences in protein metabolism; variations in the biological value of protein; nitrogen loss via urine, feces, and sweat; and degree of physical activity. Apparently there is no need for additional protein in the diet, above the RDA, to compensate for physical activity due to the built-in margin of safety.

It has been assumed that the RDA is unaffected by caloric consumption. However, caloric intake must be adequate, or total protein requirements can increase. Typically, as caloric expenditure increases with the demands of training, food consumption and caloric intake also increase. Protein intake would then need to increase in proportion to the greater caloric consumption, and the increased protein intake would then maintain normal nitrogen balance. However, this increased protein intake does not always occur. For example, when an athlete switches from one phase of a training program to another, at least 2 to 4 weeks is required to readjust energy and protein intake and output; longer adjustment periods may be necessary if body mass is lost or gained (4,106). Thus, changes in the volume or intensity of physical training could result in changes in body mass and protein status (body protein content), at least for the period of adjustment.

Proteins are degraded by the liver into their constituent amino acids. All amino acids undergo reactions that ultimately result in the donation of their amine groups ($-NH_2$) to α-ketoglutarate to form glutamic acid. In mammalian liver cells the final degradation and disposal of amino acid nitrogen is linked to the deamination of glutamic acid and the subsequent production of ammonia. Ammonia is highly toxic and must be quickly removed. Most of it is converted to urea, a nontoxic substance that is excreted in the urine. Exercise can markedly increase ammonia and urea concentrations as a result of increased protein catabolism and degradation.

Protein metabolism is affected by various hormones (49,128). Testosterone, insulin, and growth hormone are anabolic hormones that enhance protein synthesis or inhibit catabolism. Cortisol has catabolic properties that increase the rate of protein degradation. These hormones have wide-reaching metabolic and physiological effects. They affect not only protein metabolism, but also carbohydrate and lipid (fat) metabolism, mineral and water balance, growth, behavior, and numerous other functions related to protein status. Changes in resting blood hormone concentrations and concentration changes resulting from exercise can affect protein metabolism, both synthesis and degradation.

Effects of Exercise

During exercise, protein synthesis is depressed and protein degradation is unchanged or increased (31). This increases the availability of amino acids for catabolism. Training may increase the need for protein in the diet (86,110). Some studies have suggested that intensive aerobic (44,51,52) and anaerobic (weightlifting) training (21,81) can produce a negative nitrogen balance, which, depending upon its degree and duration, can produce losses in lean body mass that could include structural and enzymatic proteins, antibodies, and other necessary proteins. This could increase the chances of developing injury or disease (122,140).

Related to the observation of a negative nitrogen balance with intensive training are studies and reviews suggesting that intensive or high-volume aerobic training increases the need for specific amino acids, especially branched-chain amino acids (BCAAs) (31,39,61). Studies with animals (47) have demonstrated that BCAAs can donate nitrogen to pyruvate, which can be formed from glucose and amino acids. Pyruvate and BCAAs can be combined as follows:

$$\text{Pyruvate} + \text{BCAA} \rightarrow \text{Alanine} + \alpha\text{-Ketoacid}$$

Alanine, as a nontoxic carrier of nitrogen, transports amino groups to the liver for gluconeogenesis, a process by which lactate and amino acids are converted into glucose. Aerobic exercise can greatly enhance this process (41). The oxidation of the resulting α-ketoacid can provide additional fuel to meet metabolic demands in the muscle or liver. Both liver and muscle can catabolize significant amounts of protein and release amino acids (30,32,85,143). Such exercise-induced changes in protein metabolism may be physiologically significant in three ways (31):

- Amino acid conversion to Krebs cycle intermediates can enhance the rate of oxidation of acetyl-CoA generated from glucose and fatty acid oxidation.
- Increased conversion of amino acids to glucose helps to prevent hypoglycemia.
- Oxidation of certain amino acids may provide energy for muscular contraction.

The net effect is related to accelerated gluconeogenesis; the faster gluconeogenesis proceeds, the more protein is catabolized.

Recent studies of urinary 3-methylhistidine excretion lend further support to the concept of accelerated protein catabolism as a result of exercise. This amino acid is formed primarily as a result of actin and myosin breakdown and is not reused in the synthesis of new protein (14). Intense endurance exercise in the rat (34) and weight training in humans (34,40,107) have been shown to increase 3-methylhistidine excretion following exercise, which suggests an increase in protein catabolism. The exact nature of the increase in protein catabolism as a result of exercise is unknown but probably depends on multiple factors, including the volume, intensity, and type of exercise.

An important factor influencing the rate of protein use may be initial muscle glycogen concentrations (85,110). A greater reliance on protein for energy may occur if skeletal muscle glycogen stores are low. Perhaps 10% or more of total energy demands can be derived from protein during aerobic work if muscle glycogen is not adequate (85). The probability of lean tissue loss is compounded when exercise is coupled with chronic overwork and inadequate diet (120,122,140). Consequently, dietary protein should represent approximately 12% to 15% of the calories consumed by athletes in hard training or physical laborers performing very hard work. Carbohydrates should represent 55% to 60% of the dietary calories to insure adequate glycogen concentrations in muscle and liver, thus reducing potential protein catabolism (110,122).

Loss of body mass and adverse changes in body composition as a result of chronic overwork may also be related to psychological changes, such as loss of appetite (5,122,141). These changes would probably lead to a performance decrement, especially in activities requiring high levels of strength or power. It is also probable that various hormones play important roles in this process.

Protein Intake

Several recent reviews have suggested that athletes need protein intakes above the RDA (15,19,33,84,137,138). A given athlete's specific need is dependent upon several factors, including exercise type, intensity, and volume; length of training period; carbohydrate intake; environmental conditions; quality of protein ingested; and gender (84). Both endurance training and resistance training may increase the protein need (84,126,127), although the exact mechanisms are unclear and may be different. Among endurance athletes, the underlying mechanisms could include tissue repair and use of the BCAAs for auxilliary fuel, while for strength-and-power athletes it is likely tissue repair and maintenance of a positive nitrogen balance so that the hypertrophic stimulus is maximized (84).

Daily protein requirements for endurance athletes range from 1.2 to 2.2 g per kg of body weight (19,44, 84,126,127). Much of the increase in protein requirement for endurance athletes is due to the oxidation of BCAAs (44,84). Supplementation with BCAAs could thus theoretically prolong endurance performance (11). Tryptophan, an amino acid that causes feelings of sleepiness, lethargy, and fatigue—likely as a result of its conversion to the neurotransmitter serotonin—has recently been implicated in fatigue and in the etiology of the overtrained state (1,88,97,98). Tryptophan and the BCAAs compete with each other for entry through the blood-brain barrier (97,98,142). Serum concentrations of tryptophan and brain concentrations of tryptophan are highly correlated in rats (1,142). During exercise, when the blood BCAA concentration decreases as a result of increased amino acid catabolism, the relative concentration of tryptophan increases (1), which may in turn raise the concentration of tryptophan in the brain, leading to an increase in the concentration of serotonin, resulting in increased feelings of fatigue (97,98). While experimental evidence confirms the increase in serotonin within the brains of untrained rats as a result of endurance exercise (1) there are as yet no data confirming that this results in the same type of fatigue as that experienced with short-term or chronic overwork. However, BCAA supplementation in humans has produced both increases (93) and decreases (105,130) in endurance performance. Decreased performance could occur as a result of increased ammonia concentrations that have been shown to occur with BCAA supplementation (90,132) or due to a decrease in Krebs cycle intermediates as a result of increasing the BCAA aminotransferase

reaction (which requires Krebs cycle intermediates) (131). Increased ammonia concentrations have been associated with decreased endurance performance in animals (2). Carbohydrate supplementation appears to attenuate or reduce reliance on BCAA metabolism during exercise (131). Additional study is necessary to establish the role of amino acid supplementation, especially as it relates to fatigue and overwork.

Tarnopolsky et al. (126) present evidence suggesting that the protein requirement for strength-and-power athletes is about 1.76 g · kg^{-1} · day^{-1}. Some evidence suggests that dietary increases in protein may enhance increases in strength and muscle mass among strength athletes, even though initial protein intake values were already above the RDA. Increasing the protein intake among elite Romanian weightlifters from 225% to 438% of the RDA (approximately 3.5 g · kg^{-1} · day^{-1} to 4.0 g · kg^{-1} · day^{-1}) resulted in gains in muscle mass of 6% and maximum strength of 5% (35). Additionally, increased protein intake may be essential when an athlete attempts to lose weight with a hypocaloric diet (for example, when trying to make weight in sports with weight classes), in order to partially offset the accompanying negative nitrogen balance and loss of lean tissue (133). However, untrained subjects who undertook weight training and ingested amounts of protein equivalent to 3.67 times the RDA did not show alterations in lean body mass compared with controls (134). Supplementation with amino acids had no effect on performance or endocrine status in elite junior weightlifters over a 1-week period (46).

Initiation of training or raising training volume or intensity can cause a decreased or negative nitrogen balance even when energy requirements are adequately met by the diet (51,52,84). Return of the nitrogen balance toward positive values as training proceeds may be partially explained because of changes in exercise intensity. It is known that the intensity and relative intensity (percent of maximal intensity) of exercise affects protein use during exercise and training (19,84). As training proceeds and adaptation takes place, the relative intensity may decrease and reduce dependence upon protein (84). Increases in training volume and intensity may be accompanied by a decrease in resting testosterone concentrations (55,92), which can reduce the "anabolic state" of the organism. Among well-trained cyclists, 8 weeks of increased training volume reduced resting testosterone concentrations, but protein supplementation reduced the fall in testosterone concentrations and increased growth hormone concentrations. Carbohydrate supplementation had no effect (54).

During periods of increased volume or intensity of training, when negative nitrogen balances are likely to occur, protein intakes as high as 2 g · kg^{-1} · day^{-1} may not be sufficient to maintain a positive nitrogen balance

(19), perhaps even larger intakes of protein may not produce a positive nitrogen balance. It is possible that too little protein, especially when coupled with a hypocaloric diet, may potentiate or worsen overtraining resulting from overwork. In any case, the protein intake for athletes should be higher than the RDA, particularly during periods of increased volume or intensity of training and should represent at least 12% to 15% of the caloric intake, assuming that caloric intake increases in proportion to the increased energy requirements of training. If there is a decrease in caloric intake, the percentage of caloric intake represented by protein should be raised above 15%.

CARBOHYDRATES

Carbohydrates are compounds composed of carbon, hydrogen, and oxygen in the ratio of approximately 1:2:1, with at least three carbon atoms. Carbohydrates can be classified into three primary groups:

- *Monosaccharides*, or simple sugars, typically contain three to seven carbon atoms. Biologically important monosaccharides include glucose and fructose (fruit sugar).

- *Oligosaccharides* are carbohydrates made up of 2 to 10 monosaccharides chemically bonded together. For example, sucrose (table sugar), a *disaccharide*, is a combination of glucose and fructose.

- *Polysaccharides* contain more than 10 monosaccharides bonded together, in linear or complex branching chains. *Homopolysaccharides* contain only one type of monosaccharide. **Glycogen**, for example, contains only glucose units, arranged in a highly branched structure. A storage form of carbohydrate, glycogen is the only important homopolysaccharide in animal metabolism. Plant starch is a mixture of two glucose homopolysaccharides: amylose (a linear polymer) and amylopectin (a branching polymer). These two substances are the most common polysaccharides in the American diet. *Heteropolysaccharides* contain two or more monosaccharides in their structure. Examples are mucopolysaccharides, which form the ground substance of connective tissue.

Carbohydrates are the preferred metabolic fuel. They are especially important in the performance of aerobic endurance activities and in anaerobic activities that involve high volumes (e.g., repeated anaerobic bouts). Because carbohydrates can be synthesized from amino acids, they are required for growth only to a small extent. Carbohydrates are found in almost all foods except pure fats (106). Low-carbohydrate diets are often associated with symptoms of fatigue, and adaptation to such diets is difficult (17,77,106,122).

Carbohydrates function in physiological phenomena other than energy supply, including

- avoiding ketosis (formation of ketones as a result of excessive fat metabolism),
- reducing the loss of cations (positive ions),
- formation of the cell coat,
- formation of the ground substance of cartilage and bone, and
- formation of heparin, a naturally occurring blood anticoagulant (82,106).

Both liver and muscle glycogen act as stores of carbohydrates. Of the total caloric intake in the typical American diet, approximately 45% to 55% consists of carbohydrates. Excess carbohydrates are converted to body fat.

Digestion of Carbohydrates

Nondigestible plant polysaccharides include pectin, hemicellulose, and cellulose. Other polysaccharides found primarily in fruits and vegetables, such as galactogens, inulin, and raffinose, are partially digestible. Starches and most oligosaccharides are completely digestible.

Digestion of complex carbohydrates begins with mastication. In the mouth, the enzyme salivary amylase begins to catalyze the breakdown of starch to maltose, a disaccharide of two molecules of glucose; this stage of digestion occurs only if there is sufficient time between chewing and swallowing. The optimum stomach pH range for amylase activity is 6.6 to 6.8; the enzyme acts until the pH is further decreased by stomach acid. Although some additional digestion of carbohydrates may occur in the stomach as a result of acid hydrolysis, most digestion of carbohydrates normally occurs after the stomach contents move into the duodenum of the small intestine, into which amylase is secreted from the pancreas. Pancreatic amylase further breaks down carbohydrates into maltose, maltotriose (a trisaccharide), and a mixture of dextrins (oligosaccharides). Enzymes found on the surface of the wall of the small intestine are responsible for the final hydrolysis of these molecules into glucose (106).

Disaccharides (either from starch breakdown or ingested as is) are broken down into their constituent monosaccharides through the action of *disaccharidases* in the intestinal mucosa—for example, sucrase (for sucrose) and lactase (for lactose). A disaccharidase deficiency results in incomplete hydrolysis of a disaccharide before absorption (25,106). One of these disaccharidases, lactase, breaks down lactose into glucose and galactose prior to absorption. Lactase insufficiency is a common disaccharidase deficiency that creates a condition known as lactose intolerance. Lactose remains unabsorbed in the digestive tract and is fermented in the large intestine, causing flatulence, abdominal bloating, and sometimes cramps (25,102,106). People with lactose intolerance usually must abstain from or greatly reduce intake of foods containing lactose, such as milk and some milk products.

Absorption of the products of digestion occurs primarily in the duodenum of the small intestine. Monosaccharides are absorbed and appear in the blood within a few minutes (102). More complex carbohydrate foods such as starches are absorbed within 30 to 60 min after initiation of mastication (102).

Galactose and glucose are absorbed by a selective sodium-dependent active transport system. Because of this selectivity in the active transport system, glucose and galactose are absorbed faster than other hexoses, which are absorbed by diffusion (106). Fructose is absorbed by facilitated diffusion and enters faster than mannose, xylose, or arabinose (104). After absorption, monosaccharides enter the bloodstream and can be taken up by the liver or other tissues (17,106). Most absorbed fructose is transported to the liver, where it is converted to glucose, which can be released into the blood or stored as liver glycogen.

Carbohydrate Metabolism

The entry of glucose into muscle fibers is regulated by a family of small proteins known as **glucose transporters (GLUTs)**. Under normal basal conditions, glucose transport is regulated by GLUT-1, which is located along plasma membranes and capillary endothelial cells. GLUT-4 is likely a more important glucose transporter in skeletal muscle because it is more efficient than the others. GLUT-4 is normally stored in an intracellular pool. Insulin stimulation or exercise causes a translocation of GLUT-4 from the intracellular pool to the plasma membrane and T-tubules; this results in an acceleration of cellular glucose uptake (7,8,45,63,115). Once the glucose has entered the cell it may be stored or used for energy depending upon the needs of the cell. Storage and breakdown of carbohydrate are important considerations in understanding how muscles maintain and supply adequate energy substrate for contraction.

Glycogen is stored in muscle and the liver bound to two enzymes: glycogen synthetase, responsible for glycogen buildup, and phosphorylase, responsible for glycogen breakdown (17,45,77,83). Two other important enzymes are hexokinase (found in muscle, liver, and other cells) and glucokinase (found only in the liver). These enzymes are responsible for phosphorylating (adding a phosphate group to) the sixth carbon of glucose, as seen in the following reaction (17,77,83):

$$\text{ATP} + \text{Glucose} \xrightarrow{\text{Hexokinase or glucokinase}} \text{ADP} + \text{Glucose-6-phosphate}$$

In most cells, including liver and muscle, conversion of glucose into glycogen requires this reaction; it is also a necessary first step for entry of glucose into glycolysis (17,77,83).

Glucokinase becomes more active as blood glucose concentrations increase, so that the liver can take up more glucose and convert it to glycogen. The increased activity of glucokinase results from an induction effect of insulin, which causes increases in the synthesis and concentration of glucokinase. Insulin can increase in blood concentration in response to increasing blood glucose concentration. When blood glucose falls, the activity of glucokinase falls and less glycogen will be stored in the liver (17,77,83).

Hormones have profound effects on carbohydrate storage and breakdown. Blood glucose concentrations can be elevated by epinephrine, cortisol, glucagon, and, indirectly, by growth hormone; they can be decreased by insulin. Glycogen synthesis and storage in the liver and muscle can be enhanced by insulin and testosterone. Glycogen stores are mobilized by epinephrine and glucagon. As with proteins and fats, the regulation of carbohydrate energy substrates depends on neural and hormonal factors that can be modified by such factors as nutritional status, physical exercise, and training (15,16).

Carbohydrate Intake

The importance of carbohydrates in the diets of athletes and physical laborers was recognized as early as 1901 (135). In 1939, diets high in carbohydrate content were found to enhance subjects' ability to perform prolonged heavy physical activity (22). Numerous studies have documented a strong relationship between a high-carbohydrate diet, preexercise muscle glycogen concentration, and work performance and endurance (9,73,103,118). Additionally, muscle glycogen concentration may be related to muscle strength and short-term, high-intensity (anaerobic) exercise (42,67).

Because of the relationship of dietary carbohydrate to muscle and liver glycogen stores (114,135) and to the protein-sparing effect of high concentrations of muscle glycogen (84), dietary carbohydrate is an important factor to consider in physical training. In some cases, carbohydrate-poor diets or training programs that chronically deplete glycogen stores may be a strong contributing factor to overwork and reduced performance (122). Most carbohydrate intake should be complex carbohydrates rather than simple sugars. Daily carbohydrate intake should range from 6 to 11 g/kg of body mass. Carbohydrate intake beyond this range does not appear to provide additional benefit. The proportion of dietary calories derived from carbohydrates should be about 55% to 60% for athletes who are in hard training and eating sufficient calories (125).

LIPIDS

Lipids are substances that can be extracted from biological material with such organic solvents as ether, chloroform, and acetone and that are relatively insoluble in water. Lipids include both solid fats and liquid oils (102). Lipids are important for many metabolic processes; they are also associated with several diseases, including cardiovascular diseases and some types of cancer (13). Lipids function

- as sources of energy,
- as structural components of cell membranes and the myelin sheath of neurons,
- as transporters of lipid-soluble vitamins, and
- in the synthesis of cholesterol and production of associated steroid hormones.

Lipids are found in all cells. Adipose cells, which are filled almost entirely with fat, and vacuoles in muscle fibers are the primary sites of lipid storage (17,83,106). Lipids constitute about 40% of the total dietary calories consumed in the typical American diet (102). Excessive fat intake results in increased stored fat.

Lipids can be classified into three groups: simple lipids, compound lipids, and derived lipids. *Simple lipids* include fatty acids and triglycerides. *Fatty acids*, the simplest lipids, are monocarboxylic acids with long-chain hydrocarbon side groups. Fatty acids may be saturated or unsaturated. *Unsaturated* fatty acids contain one (monounsaturated) or more (polyunsaturated) double bonds between carbon atoms; *saturated* fatty acids have all single bonds between carbons. Most fatty acids found in commonly eaten foods are straight-chain saturated or unsaturated acids containing an even number of carbons. Linoleic, oleic, palmitic, and stearic acids account for 90% of the fatty acids found in typical American diets. Linoleic, linolenic, and arachidonic acids are synthesized in only very small amounts in the human body; they are thus *essential fatty acids* that must be eaten in the diet (102,106). Essential fatty acids are found in a variety of foods, so deficiencies are not common among Americans. These substances are the precursors of *prostaglandins*, lipids that have hormonelike activity. The actions of prostaglandins include (a) relaxation and contraction of smooth muscle, (b) blood pressure reduction, and (c) inhibition of gastric secretions (106).

Triglycerides are composed of the three-carbon molecule glycerol and three fatty acids, one attached to each of the glycerol carbons. Triglycerides make up 95% of the fats found in foods (102), and most fatty acids are ingested as triglycerides.

Triglycerides with long-chain ($\geq$ eight carbon atoms) saturated fatty acids are solids at room temperature; those with short-chain saturated fatty acids or unsaturated fatty acids (or a combination) are generally liquids. Some exceptions occur; for example, coconut oil is saturated but exists as a liquid (102). Triglycerides are a storage form of lipids in animals.

Compound lipids are lipids combined with another moiety; they include lipoproteins, glycolipids, and phospholipids. *Lipoproteins* are a transport vehicle for various lipids traveling between tissues in the blood. *Glycolipids* are carbohydrate-containing lipids that constitute part of the structure of cellular membranes and the myelin sheath of nerves (106). *Phospholipids* are components of all cells; they are found primarily in the cell membrane itself and in subcellular membranes. The structure of phospholipids is similar to that of triglycerides. Phospholipids' basic structure consists of a phosphatidic acid core which contains only two fatty acids and a phosphate group attached to the third glycerol carbon. Phospholipids differ primarily in the type of compound attached to the phosphate group. Because phospholipids have a fat-soluble portion (the fatty acid end) and a water-soluble portion (the glycerol and organic base portion) they function as liaisons between fat-soluble and water-soluble substances that must pass through the cell membrane. The role of phospholipids in the structure of cell membranes ordinarily precludes their use as energy sources (106).

Derived lipids (lipids derived from other lipids or precursor molecules) include alcohols, sterols, steroids, and hydrocarbons. These lipids serve a variety of functions, including functions in the cell membrane, formation of vitamin D, and formation of steroid hormones. *Cholesterol*, a sterol, is likely the most familiar derived lipid. Cholesterol is synthesized from acetate in all animal tissues; it is the most common sterol found in animal tissue and is found in its free form or bound to fatty acids as cholesterol esters. Cholesterol is a precursor of cholic acid (one of the bile acids), vitamin D, and the steroid hormones, including estradiol, progesterone, testosterone, and adrenal steroids.

Digestion of Lipids

Lipid digestion begins with mastication. Although virtually no hydrolysis of triglycerides occurs in the mouth, the presence of triglycerides and other lipids stimulates the release of lingual lipase from serous glands at the base of the tongue (106). Lingual lipase becomes active in the stomach, with optimum hydrolysis of lipids occurring at a pH range of 4.5 to 5.4 (57). Less than 10% of the total digestion of triglycerides occurs in the stomach.

After the first lipids enter the duodenum, gastric emptying slows, possibly due to the effects of the hormone enterogastrone. The slowing of gastric emptying produces a rate of lipid entrance into the duodenum that correlates with the ability of lipases released from the pancreas to hydrolyze the lipids. The lipase glycerol ester hydrolase breaks down triglycerides into fatty acids, glycerol, and monoglycerides (102,106). Cholesterol esterase breaks down cholesterol esters into cholesterol and fatty acids. The hydrolysis of triglycerides is dependent on the presence of bile salts from the gall bladder, which, along with cholesterol and fatty acids, acts as a detergent and aids in the emulsification of triglyceride particles (106).

The breakdown products of lipid hydrolysis aggregate into aggregates called *micelles*, which interact with the mucosal (wall) cells of the intestine. In this manner, the contents of the micelle are transported into the body. Short- and medium-chain fatty acids are absorbed through the mucosal cells into the portal vein and transported directly to the liver. Long-chain fatty acids and glycerol are resynthesized into triglycerides, bound with protein and other lipids, and formed into chylomicrons and a small amount of very low density lipoproteins (VLDL). The chylomicrons and VLDL enter the lymphatic system and eventually enter the blood through the thoracic duct (106).

Lipid Transport and Cellular Uptake

Chylomicrons and VLDL containing dietary lipids can be broken down by body tissue; remnants are taken up by the liver, where they are converted into other lipids and bile salts. Certain lipoproteins are created in the liver and released into the blood (106). Lipoprotein molecules contain various combinations of triglycerides, phospholipids, and cholesterol surrounded by phosphotydyl choline and a protein coat. The coat surrounding each type of lipoprotein contains a specific protein, which represents one of several different classes of protein that impart different properties to specific lipoproteins. The protein portion of a lipoprotein, in part, serves to make the lipids more water soluble and protects them from being hydrolized when they are transported in the blood (87,106).

Lipoproteins released from the liver and from chylomicrons contain triglycerides. In order to enter the cell the triglyceride must first be broken down into glycerol and free fatty acids. This process is catalyzed by the enzyme lipoprotein lipase, which is bound to capillary endothelial cells (18). In fat cells, free fatty acids and glycerol are converted and stored as triglycerides; this process also occurs to a lesser degree in muscle and other

tissues (17,37,64,71). Within adipose tissue, hormone-sensitive lipase breaks down triglycerides to free fatty acids and glycerol. Hormone-sensitive lipase activity is enhanced by fasting and by several different hormones, including catacholamines and glucagon (106). The reaction controlled by hormone-sensitive lipase is the rate-limiting step for lypolysis (60). The free fatty acids from fat cells are released into the blood and can be taken up by other body tissues and used for energy, stored as triglycerides, or incorporated into cell membranes (106). Muscle hormone-sensitive lipase breaks down stored triglycerides and makes them available for oxidation in the mitochondria (17,64,83).

The liver releases VLDL, some low-density lipoproteins (LDL), and high-density lipoprotein (HDL) precursors into the blood. As these lipoproteins pass through various tissues, particularly muscle, lipoprotein lipase removes the triglycerides. As with chylomicrons and VLDL absorbed from the intestine, the removal of triglyceride results in breaking triglyceride down into glycerol and free fatty acids. The glycerol and free fatty acids enter the cell and can be reformed into triglyceride and stored, or they can be oxidized.

The removal of triglyceride from VLDL leaves a remnant in the blood—the intermediate-density lipoprotein (IDL). Most of the IDL is degraded in the liver and the cholesterol removed and converted to bile salts (37,50). Some of the IDL has additional triglyceride removed and is converted to LDL (37,50). LDL is a major cholesterol carrier (17,37,106) that binds to receptors in various tissues, including liver, muscle, and arteries (17,37,50). Cholesterol can be deposited in these tissues by this mechanism (17,37,50) and can then be used in the structure of cell membranes or in the production of vitamin D or steroid hormones. Uncontrolled or excessive binding of LDL to arterial wall receptors is likely a major step in the formation of atherosclerotic plaques (37,50).

As a result of certain disease states or the ingestion of excessive amounts of dietary cholesterol, liver cholesterol concentrations can increase. Increased liver cholesterol causes a decrease in the number of receptors for IDL and LDL. The result is a greater conversion of IDL to LDL. The increase in LDL concentration can result in a greater deposition of cholesterol into arterial walls.

HDL can remove cholesterol from arterial walls or accept cholesterol from VLDL. The transfer of cholesterol from arterial walls or VLDL is accomplished via the enzyme lecithin cholesterol acetyl transferase (50). HDL is degraded in the liver by the enzyme hepatic lipase. The activity of hepatic lipase is negatively correlated with blood HDL concentrations (139).

Because of the mechanisms controlling lipoprotein production and degradation, these blood lipids are associated with risk for cardiovascular disease. Total cholesterol, VLDL, and especially LDL in the blood are generally associated with increased risk for cardiovascular disease. Low LDL:HDL ratios or low total cholesterol:HDL cholesterol ratios (TC:HDL-C) are generally associated with a reduced risk for cardiovascular disease (27,95,102). Values for total cholesterol and the TC:HDL-C ratio for Americans are shown in Tables 12.2a and 12.2b (95,102). Reductions in total cholesterol and the TC:HDL-C ratio have been associated with reduced incidence and mortality from cardiovascular disease. However, low total cholesterol or reductions in total cholesterol may not be associated with an overall reduction in mortality (20,75,96). Recent reviews suggest that low total cholesterol (<160 mg%) may be related to an increased incidence of intra-cranial hemorrhage and a variety of noncardiovascular diseases including liver and pancreatic cancer, digestive diseases, and cirrohsis of the liver, as well as behavioral disorders such as alcohol dependence syndrome and suicide (76,96). Although a cause-and-effect relationship between low total cholesterol and these diseases is unclear (96), caution should be taken in suggesting reductions of total cholesterol below 160 mg%.

Table 12.2a Blood Cholesterol Levels and Risk Classification for Cardiovascular Disease in Americans

Level (mg%)		
Children and adolescents	Adults	Classification
< 170	< 200	Desirable
170-199	200-239	Borderline
≥ 200	≥ 240	High

Table 12.2b Risk for Cardiovascular Disease in Americans Associated With Ratios of Total Cholesterol to High-Density Lipoprotein Cholesterol

Age	Sex	Level of potential risk for ratio shown		
		Low	Average	High
5-19	M	2.3-2.5	2.8-3.4	3.8-4.6
	F	2.3-2.4	3.0-3.1	4.0-4.2
20-39	M	2.5-3.3	3.5-4.7	5.3-6.9
	F	2.3-2.4	3.0-3.4	4.5-5.3
40-59	M	2.4-2.8	3.5-4.9	6.6-6.1
	F	2.4-2.8	3.5-3.8	5.2-6.7
≥ 60	M	2.9-3.0	4.3-4.4	6.1-6.8
	F	2.6-2.8	3.8-4.0	5.8-7.4

Lipid Metabolism

Lipids have a wide range of physiological functions. They are crucial to biological structures and are a prime source of energy. As with proteins and carbohydrates, hormones can have profound effects on lipid metabolism. In general, lipid synthesis is promoted by insulin, and lipolysis (lipid breakdown) is promoted by growth hormone, thyroxine, catecholamines, and cortisol (92, 106).

Mobilization of free fatty acids is important during aerobic exercise (17,77) and is a consequence of anaerobic exercise, with considerable mobilization of free fatty acids occurring after exercise. This suggests that fatty acid oxidation can occur during aerobic exercise and as a result of anaerobic exercise. Fatty acid oxidation is related to body fat losses as a result of exercise. Thus both aerobic and anaerobic exercises of sufficient volume and intensity can alter body fat (92).

As noted previously, abnormal blood lipid levels are related to cardiovascular disease. Both endurance and resistance training can beneficially alter lipid profiles (65,120,121,124), although the mechanisms are unclear. These alterations are apparently related to the volume and intensity of training (120,121).

Lipid Intake. The American diet consists of approximately 42% fat, in terms of calories consumed—16% saturated, 19% monounsaturated, and 7% polyunsaturated fats—with cholesterol making up less than 1% of caloric intake (129). Diets relatively high in saturated fats and cholesterol have been shown to increase blood cholesterol. The general recommendation is that fat compose 30% or less of the total calories eaten (100-102). Most of these calories (20%) should be from monounsaturated or polyunsaturated sources and only 10% from saturated fat sources. Cholesterol intake should be approximately 100 mg/1,000 kcal consumed and usually should not exceed 300 mg/day (102). (This recommendation is given primarily to reduce the incidence of cardiovascular disease.)

Recent evidence suggests that unsaturated fats in large amounts may promote the production of free radicals through lipid peroxidation (68,72,106). Free radicals are unstable molecules or fragments of molecules that have unpaired electrons in their outer orbits (113). They are very reactive, have short half-lives and interfere with normal reactions occurring in biochemical pathways within cells (113). Free radicals have been associated with aging and various types of degenerative diseases, including cancer (68,72). Perhaps simply eating less total fat (approximately 20% to 25% of total calories) would reduce both the potential for cardiovascular disease and free-radical production.

VITAMINS AND MINERALS

Vitamins are organic substances that are essential in minute amounts for normal metabolic functioning in a given organism but that usually cannot be synthesized by the organism; they must therefore be ingested in the diet. Most water-soluble vitamins act as *coenzymes*, which are organic molecules, loosely bound to enzymes, that are required for enzymatic reactions to occur. Fat-soluble vitamins have antioxidant or hormonelike activity. **Minerals** (salt ions) act as *cofactors* or are part of a structure such as bone; the term *cofactor* has the same functional definition as that of coenzyme and encompasses both coenzymes and minerals used in this function (Table 12.3). Vitamins and minerals are needed in a number of synthetic and energy-producing reactions and are important for optimum and maximum physical performance. The adult RDAs for vitamins and minerals are shown in Table 12.4 (102,106).

There are at least two ways in which vitamins and minerals can be the cause of subnormal physical performance. First, the RDAs for vitamins and minerals—or the person's individual requirements—are not being met. It is known that diets deficient in vitamins and minerals produce decrements in physical performance (77,125). However, athletes who eat a diet that contains enough calories and that is nutritionally sound should get amounts of most vitamins and minerals at RDA levels or above.

Table 12.3 **Vitamins: Functions, Sources, and Effects of Deficiencies**

Vitamin	Function	Food source	Effects of deficiency
Water-soluble vitamins			
Thiamin (B$_1$)	Coenzyme for carbohydrate metabolism	Grains, nuts, eggs, liver, green leafy vegetables	Beriberi, neural pathologies
Riboflavin (B$_2$)	Coenzyme for protein, fat, and carbohydrate metabolism	Beans, root crops, fish, meat, dairy products, eggs, green leafy vegetables	Dermatitis, blurred vision, nausea
Niacin	Krebs cycle coenzyme	Red meat, grains, nuts, legumes	Pellegra
Pyridoxine (B$_6$)	Coenzyme for lipid and amino acid metabolism	Red meat, tomatoes, corn, spinach, grains, legumes	Dermatitis, nausea
Cobolamin (B$_{12}$)	Red blood cell formation, amino acid metabolism	Red meat, dairy products, eggs	Pernicious anemia, neural pathology
Pantothenic acid	Coenzyme for steroid synthesis; coenzyme for Krebs cycle	Grains, liver, green vegetables	Adrenal deficiency, neuromuscular degeneration
Folic acid	Coenzyme in nucleic acid and red blood cell production	Green vegetables, liver	Anemia, red blood cell formation, pathology
Biotin	Coenzyme in lipid synthesis; coenzyme in conversion of pyruvate to glucose	Liver, eggs	Fatigue, depression, dermatitis
Ascorbic acid (C)	Collagen formation; acts in various metabolic reactions; acts as an antioxidant	Citrus, tomatoes, green vegetables	Scurvy
Fat-soluble vitamins			
Retinol (A)	Formation of rhodopsin, regulation of bone and tooth growth	Fish liver oils, green and yellow vegetables, liver	Epithelial and neural disorders, night blindness
Calciferol (D)	Calcium and phosphorus absorption	Fish liver oils, egg yolk, liver	Rickets in children
α-Tocopherol (E)	Antioxidant; DNA, RNA, and red blood cell formation	Nuts, wheat germ, vegetable oils, liver, eggs, fish	Abnormal membrane function
Vitamin K	Coenzyme for prothrombin and clotting factor synthesis	Green leafy vegetables, liver	Delayed clotting

Table 12.4   Recommended Daily Allowances (RDAs) for Adults

	RDA	
	Males	Females
Vitamin		
Thiamin (B$_1$)	1.5 mg	1.1 mg
Riboflavin (B$_2$)	1.7 mg	1.3 mg
Niacin	19 mg	15 mg
Pyridoxine (B$_6$)	2.0 mg	1.6 mg
Pantothenic acid	NA	NA
Folic acid	200 μg	180 μg
Biotin	NA	NA
Cobolamin (B$_{12}$)	2.0 μg	2.0 μg
Ascorbic acid (C)	60 mg	60 mg
Retinol (A)	1,000 μg	800 μg
Calciferol (D)	10 μg	10 μg
α-Tocopherol	10 mg	8 mg
Vitamin K	80 mg	65 mg
Mineral		
Calcium	800 mg	800 mg
Phosphorus	1,200 mg	1,200 mg
Iron	12 mg	10 mg
Zinc	15 mg	12 mg
Iodine	150 μg	150 μg
Selenium	30 μg	65 μg

Note. Data from references 102, 106.

Second is the possibility that training may alter vitamin and mineral status (tissue concentrations of vitamins and minerals) even though the RDA is being met. The requirements for some vitamins, such as vitamins B$_1$ and B$_2$ and niacin, are approximately proportionate to the metabolic demands of physical exercise and the cumulative energy expense of training (12). It has been assumed that, as metabolic demands increase and the amount of food eaten increases to compensate for the increased caloric expenditure, the extra food will contain adequate amounts of vitamins and minerals; however, this may not always occur. It is possible that very intense or very high volume training may produce subnormal tissue concentrations of some vitamins or minerals, which would result in impaired performance or contribute to symptoms of chronic overwork. It is also possible that both factors could contribute; training coupled with low energy consumption or diets deficient in certain vitamins and minerals could cause performance decrements.

Although a few studies suggest that performance can be increased by vitamin or mineral supplementation (28,125), most have found no performance enhancement (61,91,136). Unfortunately, there are very few data concerning vitamin or mineral intake or serum concentra-

tions in subjects or athletes in hard (high-intensity or high-volume) training.

Zalessky (144) has presented evidence suggesting that multivitamin therapy enhances the performance and "general well-being" of athletes with a low work tolerance. A summary of Soviet research on nutrition (28) suggested that stressful situations, including environmental stresses, sports activities, and military tasks, increased the need for vitamins and minerals, especially water-soluble vitamins and vitamins A and E.

Low dietary intake of vitamins A and B$_1$ (relative to caloric intake) has been noted in football players and wrestlers, and low potassium intake noted in wrestlers (112). One study evaluated the blood concentrations of 55 20-year-old male trained subjects (cross-country runners, wrestlers, and handball players) and 20 sedentary controls (53). Both groups had lower-than-normal concentrations of vitamins B$_1$, B$_6$, and E. The frequency of vitamin deficiency and, in many cases, the severity of the deficiency were higher in the athletic group, even though their vitamin and caloric intake was higher. A 1-month supplementation improved the vitamin status of the control group but did not completely restore vitamin status in those of the athletic group (53). This suggests that training can alter the vitamin status of athletes.

Subnormal serum concentrations of potassium and magnesium have been reported in male and especially in female athletes participating in a variety of sports (125). Anemia and low serum iron and ferritin concentrations have been detected in both female and male distance runners (23,24,29,99,109). Ferritin is a protein that binds iron and is stored in the liver, spleen, and bones (106). Thus, ferritin represents a storage form of iron. It should also be noted that a vegetarian diet may produce changes in ferritin status. Female distance runners who consumed less than 100 g of red meat per week had significantly lower serum ferritin and total iron-binding capacity than a control group eating substantially more red meat per week (117). This suggests that the form in which dietary iron is consumed can play an important role in iron status.

Among endurance athletes, iron deficiency may be associated with decreased maximal oxygen uptake and particularly reduced performance if hemoglobin is reduced (26). Supplementation appears to return maximal oxygen uptake to normal values faster than it does endurance performance. Iron uptake usually increases during periods of iron deficiency; however, low iron values may not be responsive to diet in some athletes (109). Some research has shown that athletes may absorb less than half the dietary iron of anemic sedentary individuals (38). This reduced absorption of iron, as well as increased hemolysis (breakdown of red blood cells) as a result of various athletic endeavors, can contribute to anemia.

Calcium and phosphorus are major constituents of teeth and bones. Bones act as storage depots for both minerals and, under the influence of the endocrine system, can play an important role in maintaining blood calcium concentrations. Both calcium and phosphorus have a relatively high rate of turnover and must be continuously replaced through the diet.

Osteoporosis is a condition in which there is a loss of bone mass; it can result in considerable structural weakness of the affected bone. Two types of osteoporosis are recognized. Type 1 osteoporosis normally occurs in people 50 to 60 years of age and is associated with distal radius and vertebral fractures. Type 1 is 8 times more prevalent in women than in men. Type 2 osteoporosis is associated with hip, pelvic, and distal humerus fractures and usually occurs after age 70; it is twice as prevalent in women as in men (70). Because of the greater prevalence in women, osteoporosis may be associated with menopause and subsequent reductions in estrogen concentrations. Estrogen supplements after menopause may decrease the rate of bone loss, but will not result in replacement of lost bone (89). Dietary calcium may be important in preventing and perhaps in treating osteoporosis. The calcium RDA for children aged 1 to 10 years and for adults over 24 years old is 800 mg/day; the RDA for people 11 to 24 years of age is 1,200 mg/day. However, the actual requirements for premenopausal and postmenopausal women may be considerably higher (1,500 mg/day). Many women take in less than the RDA (59). Increasing the calcium content of the diet may be essential, especially for women, in order to reduce the potential for developing osteoporosis.

Physical training may also help prevent and reverse osteoporosis. Studies and recent reviews of the literature suggest that training, particularly using weight-bearing and weight-training exercise, may increase the density and tensile strength of bone and connective tissue in general (80,108,116,120). It is also possible that diet and exercise may reduce the potential for developing osteoporosis better than either diet or exercise alone. In postmenopausal women the combination of estrogen replacement and physical training may reduce bone loss better than either alone (6). However, caution should be used in selecting the volume and intensity of exercise. Some evidence suggests that high-volume or low-intensity exercise carried out for relatively long periods may reduce bone density; this is especially apparent among both men and women distance runners. Women athletes who become amenorrheic as a result of high training loads may be particularly susceptible to training-induced reductions in bone mineral content (36,90). Because of the susceptibility of women athletes, especially distance runners, to developing low bone densities, increased dietary calcium may be of particular benefit for them.

EFFECTS OF DEPRESSED APPETITE

Loss of appetite that often accompanies overwork may result in less consumption of energy-containing and other nutrients (69). This could potentiate symptoms of overtraining and result in reduced performance. Alterations in dietary intake among junior elite weightlifters as a result of a 1-week camp have been observed (122,123). Although the subjects ate a greater proportion of calories in carbohydrates during the week, their total energy consumption decreased 350 kcal as a result of lower fat intake and simply eating less. Many of the athletes reported depressed appetites. Intake of B vitamins decreased over time. If this trend had continued over several weeks, it would likely have contributed to an overtrained condition. It is probable that decreased vitamin and mineral intake and low serum concentrations for these nutrients are associated with or contribute to an overtraining process (122).

CALORIC DENSITY AND NUTRIENT DENSITY

Because of differences in molecular structure, the number of kilocalories liberated metabolically is different for the same weight of the food substances protein, carbohydrate, and fat. Carbohydrates and protein yield approximately 4 kcal/g, while fat yields approximately 9 kcal/g. The caloric values of these foods are termed *physiological fuel values* (106).

Using these values, the energy intake of a diet can be calculated. This can be accomplished by adding up the grams of proteins, carbohydrates, or fats consumed and then multiplying by the appropriate physiological fuel value. Additionally, if the total caloric consumption is known and the percentage of the total represented by proteins, carbohydrates, and fats is also known, then the kilocalories represented by the individual food substances can be calculated. An example is shown on page 223.

Nutrient density refers to the amount of nutrient per calorie (102). For example, table sugar (sucrose) is not nutrient dense; it contains almost no vitamins and minerals. Many vegetables and meats contain high densities of various vitamins and minerals. Although nutrient density is not usually a problem for large athletes who eat very large amounts of food, smaller athletes who eat low-calorie diets should pay attention to the vitamin

Calculating Energy Intake

A 100-kg athlete has a daily intake of 75 g of protein, 700 g of carbohydrate, and 150 g of fat. What is (a) the percentage intake of each food type by weight, (b) the total energy intake, and (c) the percentage energy intake of each food type?

(a) Protein: $\dfrac{75 \text{ g}}{75 \text{ g} + 700 \text{ g} + 150 \text{ g}} \times 100\% = 8.1\%$

Carbohydrate: $\dfrac{700 \text{ g}}{925 \text{ g}} \times 100\% = 75.7\%$

Fat: $\dfrac{150 \text{ g}}{925 \text{ g}} \times 100\% = 16.2\%$

(b) Kilocalories of protein: 75 g × 4 kcal/g = 300 kcal

Kilocalories of carbohydrate: 700 g × 4 kcal/g = 2,800 kcal

Kilocalories of fat: 150 g × 9 kcal/g = 1,350 kcal

300 kcal + 2,800 kcal + 1,350 kcal = 4,450 kcal

(c) Protein: $\dfrac{300 \text{ kcal}}{4,450 \text{ kcal}} \times 100\% = 6.7\%$

Carbohydrate: $\dfrac{2,800 \text{ kcal}}{4,450 \text{ kcal}} \times 100\% = 62.9\%$

Fat: $\dfrac{1,350 \text{ kcal}}{4,450 \text{ kcal}} \times 100\% = 30.3\%$

Note that because of the difference in the per-gram amount of energy in fats versus proteins and carbohydrates, the percent compositions by weight and by energy differ from each other.

In certain cases, such as carbohydrate loading (see Carbohydrate Loading section), an athlete may want to adjust the percentage caloric intake of the three food types (keeping total caloric intake constant). He or she then needs to know the mass of each food type that should be eaten. The following calculation is then used:

A 100-kg athlete has a total energy consumption of 6,000 kcal/day and desires an energy breakdown of 15% protein, 60% carbohydrate, and 25% fat. How many grams of each food type should the athlete eat?

Protein: 6,000 kcal × 0.15 × 1 g/4 kcal = 225 g

Carbohydrate: 6,000 kcal × 0.60 × 1 g/4 kcal = 900 g

Fat: 6,000 kcal × 0.25 × 1 g/9 kcal = 167 g

---

and mineral content of the food they eat, that is, the food's nutrient density.

CARBOHYDRATE LOADING

Carbohydrate loading is a technique used to enhance muscle glycogen prior to long-term endurance exercise (101,102). Traditionally, carbohydrate loading has been performed in two stages. Stage 1 consists of glycogen depletion; the athlete eats a low-carbohydrate diet (<40% of total caloric intake) for 3 days and engages in 2 or 3 prolonged exercise sessions at 80% to 90% of maximal oxygen uptake. Stage 2 consists of 3 days of rest or very low intensity exercise immediately before competition and a high-carbohydrate diet (85% to 90% of total caloric intake). Stage 2 can cause an increase in muscle glycogen to levels above normal (supercompensation effect). Stage 1, however, can cause several undesirable side effects, including physical and mental fatigue, depression, and irritability, which often lead to poorer-than-expected performance. Because of these side effects, a modified carbohydrate-loading program is recommended. For example, during Stage 1, a 50% (by calories) carbohydrate diet can be used along with a 6-day training taper. During the last 3 days of the training taper a 70% carbohydrate diet is used (101,102). Some endurance athletes simply eat a high-carbohydrate diet all the time and use a training taper before competition with excellent success.

PRE-EVENT AND POSTEVENT MEALS

The nutritional balance of a meal can have physiological and psychological consequences (100,102). A pre-event meal high in protein may be of little benefit (except psychologically); a meal high in fat may reduce performance by slowing gastric emptying. Carbohydrate is an important consideration in the pre-event meal because of its relationship to performance. Ingesting relatively large amounts of glucose or sucrose 30 to 60 min before exercise can result in a rebound depression of blood glucose as a result of increased insulin (43). However, other studies suggest that a rebound effect will not occur even with simple sugars and that a glucose meal 30 to 60 min before exercise may make more glucose available to the muscle during exercise (48,58). In one study, ingestion of 150 g of carbohydrate (84% of which was maltodextrin, a glucose polymer) 5 min prior to a cycle ride to exhaustion at 62% of maximal oxygen uptake resulted in increased plasma insulin, increased glucose, and prolonged time to exhaustion (112). Nieman (100) suggests a 500- to 800-kcal (125- to 200-g) carbohydrate diet 3 to 5 hr before exercise with an additional 150 to 200 g ingested 5 min prior to long-term endurance events. Large amounts of carbohydrates consumed in short time periods should be ingested as carbohydrate drinks; otherwise, the amount of food that would have to be eaten might cause considerable discomfort.

During prolonged exercise (78) and *perhaps* during repeated bouts of anaerobic exercise (79), beverages containing glucose or glucose polymers may minimize disturbances in temperature regulation and cardiovascular function better than water alone. The solutions should be 4% to 20% carbohydrate and be consumed every 15 to 20 min, especially during the last stages of long-term endurance events when blood glucose may be dropping. However, solutions above 10% may be unsuitable for some types of exercise, such as long (>3-hr) endurance events, because of gastric upset and decreased gastric emptying.

Although increasing the concentration of carbohydrate in solution will increase absorption, this is offset by decreased gastric emptying. Carbohydrate solutions greater than 20% should not be used, because they slow gastric emptying to the point that increased absorption will not compensate for the increased carbohydrate concentration. Fructose should be avoided during exercise because it tends to cause gastric upset.

The postevent meal should contain a high carbohydrate content to help replenish glycogen stores. Some research suggests that a solution containing 500 to 800 kcal (125-200 g) of carbohydrates ingested within 2 hr after an event causes a more rapid restoration of glycogen stores than lower carbohydrate intakes (66). Glycogen repletion may be maximized by consuming 0.7 to 3.0 g of carbohydrate per kg body weight every 2 hr following exercise (45,111). Simple carbohydrates ingested during the first 6 hr following exercise elicit greater glycogen repletion than do complex carbohydrates (74). Additionally, evidence suggests that glucose may more readily increase muscle glycogen, and fructose may more adequately restore liver glycogen (45).

CONCLUSION

Athletes may need dietary protein in excess of the RDA, particularly during periods of heavy loading. Protein intake should be 12% to 15% of the total calories consumed. However, most athletes appear to ingest considerably more than the RDA, usually as a result of increased caloric intake resulting from training; it is not unusual for athletes, especially strength-and-power athletes, to eat as much as 2 to 3 g · kg^{-1} · day^{-1}. Because of this high protein intake, protein supplements are not generally warranted. Carbohydrate ingestion is related to liver and muscle glycogen stores and to both aerobic and anaerobic endurance. In addition to its endurance effects, a high-carbohydrate diet can be beneficial in sparing protein, which may otherwise be catabolized as a result of training.

Some research has indicated that vitamin and mineral deficiencies can occur in athletes as a result of training or poor diets. Iron status is particularly important among female athletes and can be affected markedly by diet or training. The calcium content of the diet is also especially important, in that it relates to the potential for the development of osteoporosis. A broad-based vitamin and mineral supplement, containing nutrients at about 100% of RDA, may be useful in lowering the potential for reduced vitamin and mineral status in some athletes and athletic situations.

Key Terms

amino acid	211	glycogen	215	nutrient density	222
carbohydrate	215	lipid	217	protein	211
essential amino acid	211	mineral	220	vitamin	220
glucose transporter (GLUT)	216	nitrogen balance	211		

Study Questions

1. According to Tarnopolsky et al. 1992, what is the RDA for strength athletes in $g \cdot kg^{-1} \cdot day^{-1}$?

   a. 1.54
   b. 1.23
   c. 0.82
   d. 1.76

2. Which simple sugar is best for liver glycogen replenishment?

   a. glucose
   b. lactose
   c. maltose
   d. fructose

3. Urea production is responsible for the removal of the toxic substance

   a. *N*-methylhistidine
   b. branched-chain amino acids
   c. estradiol
   d. ammonia

4. Retinol is the chemical name for vitamin

   a. K
   b. D
   c. E
   d. A

5. Retinol is a ___ vitamin.

   a. water-soluble
   b. fat-soluble

6. The current RDA for calcium for adult males older than 24 years of age is ___ mg/day.

   a. 1,000
   b. 1,500
   c. 1,200
   d. 800

Applying Knowledge of Nutritional Factors

Problem 1

A 62-kg long-distance runner complains that during a marathon he fatigues very quickly after 18 to 19 miles (29-31 km). Analysis reveals that his daily diet of 3,000 kcal is made up of

12% (by calories) protein, 60% carbohydrate, and 28% fat. He says that his pre-event meal is a candy bar eaten about 2 hr before the race and that he only drinks water during the race. How might adjusting his nutritional intake increase his stamina?

Problem 2

An elite 48-kg weightlifter in a preparation period of training is having difficulty in recovering from her training sessions. She is training 2 to 3 times/day, 4 to 5 days/week. Although the training program is difficult, it does not appear to be excessive. Analysis shows that her daily diet of 2,500 kcal is made up of 15% (by calories) protein, 45% carbohydrate, and 40% fat. How might adjusting the weightlifter's diet increase her ability to recover?

Problem 3

The best-laid plans often go wrong. In Problem 2 the weightlifter tried to rigorously adhere to the prescribed diet. However, as she increased the percentage of carbohydrate calories and decreased the percentage of fat calories her total calories dropped. Because of this her body mass began to drop and her body fat decreased from 11% to 8% and she became amenorrheic. What should she do?

References

1. Acworth, I., J. Nicholass, B. Morgan, and E.A. Newsholme. Effect of sustained exercise on concentrations of plasma aromatic and branched-chain amino acids and brain amine. *Biochem. Biophys. Res. Commun.* 137(1):149-153. 1986.

2. Alborn, E.N., J.M. Davis, and S.P. Baily. Effects of ammonia on endurance performance in the rat. *Med. Sci. Sports Exerc.* 24(5[Suppl.]):S50. 1992.

3. Alfin-Slater, R. *Nutrition for Today.* Dubuque, IA: Brown. 1973.

4. Astrand, P.O., and K. Rodahl. *Textbook of Work Physiology*, 2nd ed. New York: McGraw-Hill. 1970.

5. Ayers, J.W.T., Y. Komesu, R.A. Romani, and R. Ansbacher. Anthropometric, hormonal, and psychological correlates of semen quality in endurance-trained male athletes. *Fertil. Steril.* 43:917-921. 1985.

6. Ballard, J., J. Holtz, B. McKeown, and S. Zinkgraf. Effect of exercise and estrogen upon postmenopausal bone mass. *Med. Sci. Sports. Exerc.* 20(Suppl.):S51. 1988.

7. Banks, E.A., J.T. Brozinick, B.B. Yespelkis, H.Y. Kang, and J.L. Ivy. Muscle glucose transport, GLUT-4 content and degree of exercise training in obese Zucker rats. *Amer. J. Physiol.* 263(5, part 1):E1010-E1015. 1992.

8. Barnard, R.J., and J.F. Youngren. Regulation of glucose transport in skeletal muscle. *FASEB J.* 6(14):3238-3244. 1992.

9. Bergstrom, J., and E. Hultman. Muscle glycogen synthesis after exercise: An enhancing factor to the muscle cells in man. *Nature* 210:309. 1966.

10. Bleich, H.L., E.S. Boro, M.H. Sleisenger, and Y.S. Kim. Protein digestion and absorption. *N. Engl. J. Med.* 300(12):659-663. 1971.

11. Blomstrand, E., F. Celsing, and E.A. Newsholme. Changes in plasma concentrations of aromatic and branched chain amino acids during sustained exercise in man and their possible role in fatigue. *Acta Physiol. Scand.* 133:115-123. 1988.

12. Bobb, A., D. Pringle, and A.J. Ryan. A brief study of the diet of athletes. *J. Sports Med.* 9:255-262. 1969.

13. Boissoneault, G.A., C.E. Elson, and M.W. Pariza. Net energy effects of dietary fat on chemically induced mammary carcinogenesis in F344 rats. *J. Natl. Cancer Inst.* 76:335-338. 1986.

14. Booth, F.W., W.F. Nicholson, and P.A. Watson. Influence of muscle use on protein synthesis and degradation. *Exerc. Sports Sci. Rev.* 10:27-48. 1982.

15. Brooks, G.A. Amino acid incorporation and protein metabolism during exercise and recovery. *Med. Sci. Sports Exerc.* 19(Suppl.):S150-S156. 1987.

16. Brooks, G.A., K.E. Brauner, and R.G. Cassens. Glycogen synthesis and metabolism of lactic acid after exercise. *Amer. J. Physiol.* 224:1162-1186. 1973.

17. Brooks, G.A., and T.D. Fahey. *Exercise Physiology: Human Bioenergetics and its Applications.* New York: Wiley. 1984.

18. Brown, M.S., P.T. Kovanen, and J.L. Golstein. Regulation of plasma cholesterol by lipoprotein receptors. *Science* 212:628-635. 1981.

19. Butterfield, G.E. Whole-body protein utilization in humans. *Med. Sci. Sports Exerc.* 19(Suppl.):S157-S165. 1987.

20. Capurso, A. Lipid metabolism and cardiovascular risk: Should hypercholesterolemia be treated in the elderly? *J. Hypertens.*[Suppl.]10(2):S65-S68. 1992.

21. Celajowa, I., and M. Homa. Food intake, nitrogen, and energy balance in Polish weightlifters during training camp. *Nutr. Metab.* 12:259-274. 1970.

22. Christensen, E., and O. Hansen. Arbeits fahigheit und ernahrung. *Scand. Arch. Physiol.* 81:169. 1939.

23. Clement, D.B., and R.C. Asmundsun. Nutritional intake and hematological parameters in endurance runners. *Phys. Sports Med.* 10:37-43. 1982.

24. Clement, D.B., and L.L. Sanchuk. Iron status and sports performance. *Sports Med.* 1:65-74. 1984.

25. Dahlqvist, A. The intestinal disaccharidases and disaccharide intolerance. *Gastroenterology* 43:694-696. 1962.

26. Davies, K.J.A., C.M. Donavan, C.J. Refino, G.A. Brooks, L. Parker, and P.R. Dallman. Distinguishing effects of anemic and muscle iron deficiency on exercise bioenergetics in the rat. *Am. J. Physiol.* 246:E535-E543. 1984.

27. Davies, K.J.A., J.J. Maguire, and G.A. Brooks. Muscle mitochondrial bioenergetics, oxygen supply and work capacity during dietary iron deficiency and repletion. *Am. J. Physiol.* 242:E418-E427. 1982.

28. Dibbern, V. Nutrition Research - USSR. (U) Dst-18105-144. U.S. Army Document. 1981.

29. Diehl, D.M., T.G. Lohman, S.C. Smith, and R. Kertaer. Effects of physical training and competition on the iron status of female hockey players. *Int. J. Sports Med.* 7(5):264-270. 1986.

30. Dohm, G.L., A.L. Hecker, W.E. Brown, G.J. Klain, F.R. Puente, E.W. Askew, and G.R. Beecher. Adaptation of protein metabolism to endurance training: Increased amino acid oxidation in response to training. *Biochem. J.* 164:705-708. 1977.

31. Dohm, G.L., G.J. Kasperek, E.G. Tapscott, and H. Barakat. Protein metabolism during endurance exercise. *Fed. Proc.* 44:348-352. 1985.

32. Dohm, G.L., F.R. Puente, C.P. Smith, and A. Edge. Changes in tissue protein levels as a result of endurance exercise. *Life Sci.* 23:845-849. 1978.

33. Dohm, G.L., E.B. Tapscott, and G.J. Kasperek. Protein degradation during endurance exercise and recovery. *Med. Sci. Sports Exerc.* 19(Suppl.):S166-S171. 1978.

34. Dohm, G.L., R.T. Williams, G.J. Kasperek, and A.M. Van Rij. Increased excretion of urea and *N*-methylhistidine by rats and humans after a bout of exercise. *J. Appl. Physiol.* 52:27-33. 1982.

35. Dragon, G.I., A. Vasilu, and E. Georgescu. Effect of increased supply of protein on elite weight-lifters. In: *Milk Proteins*, T.E. Galesloot and B.J. Tinbergen, eds. Wageningen, The Netherlands: Poduc. 1985. pp. 99-103.

36. Drinkwater, B.L., K. Nilson, C.H. Chesnut, W.J. Bremer, S. Shainholtz, and M.B. Southworth. Bone mineral content of amenorrheic and eumenorrheic athletes. *N. Engl. J. Med.* 311:277-282. 1984.

37. DuFax, B., G. Assmann, and W. Hollman. Plasma lipoproteins and physical activity: A review. *Int. J. Sports Med.* 3:123-136. 1982.

38. Ehn, L., B. Carlwark, and S. Hoglund. Iron status in athletes involved in intense physical activity. *Med. Sci. Sports Exerc.* 12:61-64. 1980.

39. Evans, W.J., E.C. Fisher, R.A. Hoerr, and V.R. Young. Protein metabolism and endurance exercise. *Phys. Sports Med.* 11:63-72. 1983.

40. Evans, W.J., C.N. Meredith, J.G. Cannon, C.A. Dinarello, W.R. Frontera, V.A. Hughes, B.H. Jones, and H.G. Knuttson. Metabolic changes following eccentric exercise in trained and untrained men. *J. Appl. Physiol.* 61:1864-1868. 1986.

41. Felig, P., and J. Wahren. Amino acid metabolism in exercising man. *J. Clin. Invest.* 50:2703-2714. 1971.

42. Forsberg, A., P. Tesch, and J. Karlsson. Effects of prolonged exercise on muscle strength performance. In *Biomechanics* VI-A, E. Asmussen and K. Jorgensen, eds. Baltimore: University Park Press. 1978.

43. Foster, C., D.L. Costill, and W.J. Fink. Effect of preexercise feedings on endurance performance. *J. Appl. Physiol.* 11:1-15. 1979.

44. Freidman, J.E., and P.W.R. Lemon. Effect of protein intake and endurance exercise on daily protein requirements. *Med. Sci. Sports Exerc.* 17(Suppl.):S231. 1985.

45. Friedman, J.E., P.D. Neufer, and G.L. Dohm. Regulation of glycogen resynthesis following exercise. *Sports Med.* 11(4):232-243. 1991.

46. Fry, A.C., W.J. Kraemer, M.H. Stone, B.J. Warren, J.T. Kearney, C.M. Maresh, C.A. Weseman, and S.J. Fleck. Endocrine and performance responses to high volume training and amino acid supplementation in elite junior weightlifters. *Int. J. Sports Nutr.* 3(3):306-322. 1993.

47. Galim, E.B., K. Hruska, and D.M. Bier. Branched chain amino acid nitrogen transfer to alanine in vivo in dogs: Direct isotopic demonstration with [^{15}N]leucine. *J. Clin. Invest.* 66:1295-1304. 1980.

48. Gleeson, M., R.J. Maughan, and P.L. Greenhaff. Comparison of the effects of pre-exercise feeding of glucose, glycerol and placebo on endurance and fuel homeostasis in man. *Eur. J. Appl. Physiol.* 55:645-653. 1986.

49. Goldberg, R.L. Hormonal regulation of protein degradation and synthesis in skeletal muscle. *Fed. Proc.* 39:31-36. 1980.

50. Goldstein, J., T. Kita, and M. Brown. Defective lipoprotein receptors and atherosclerosis. *N. Engl. J. Med.* 309:288-292. 1983.

51. Gontzea, I., P. Sutzescu, and S. Dumitrache. The influence of muscular activity on nitrogen balance and on the need for protein. *Nutr. Rep. Int.* 10:35-43. 1974.

52. Gontzea, I., P. Sutzescu, and S. Dumitrache. The influence of adaptation to physical effort on nitrogen balance in man. *Nutr. Rep. Int.* 11:231-236. 1975.

53. Guilland, J-C., T. Penaranda, C. Gallet, W. Boggio, F. Fuchs, and J. Keppling. Vitamin status of young athletes including the effects of supplementation. *Med. Sci. Sports Exerc.* 21:441-449. 1989.

54. Hackney, A.C., R.L. Sharp, W.S. Runyan, and R.J. Ness. Resting hormonal changes during intensive training: Effects of a dietary protein supplement. Conference Abstracts, Southeast Chapter of the American College of Sports Medicine meeting. January 1989.

55. Häkkinen, K., A. Pakarinen, M. Alen, H. Kauhanen, and P.V. Komi. Relationship between training volume, physical performance capacity, and serum hormone concentrations during prolonged training in elite weightlifters. *Int. J. Sports Med.* 8:61-65. 1985.

56. Hamilton, E.M.H., E.N. Whitney, and F.S. Sizer. *Nutrition: Concepts and Controversies.* St. Paul: West. 1985.

57. Hamosh, M., and R.O. Scow. Lingual lipase and its role in the digestion of dietary lipid. *J. Clin. Invest.* 52:88-95. 1973.

58. Hargreaves, M., D.L. Costill, W.J. Fink, D.S. King, and R.A. Fielding. Effects of pre-exercise carbohydrate feedings on endurance cycling performance. *Med. Sci. Sports Exerc.* 19:33-36. 1987.

59. Heaney, R.P. The role of calcium in prevention and treatment of osteoporosis. *Phys. Sportsmed.* 15(11):83-88. 1987.

60. Hollet, C.R., and J.V. Auditore. Localization and characterization of a lipase in rat adipose tissue. *Arch. Biochem. Biophys.* 121:423-430. 1967.

61. Hood, D.A., and R.L. Terjung. Amino acid metabolism during exercise and following endurance training. *Sports Med.* 9(1):23-35. 1990.

62. Horton, E.S. Effects of low-energy diets on work performance. *Am. J. Clin. Nutr.* 35:1228-1233. 1982.

63. Houmard, J.A., P.C. Egan, P.D. Neufer, J.E. Friedman, W.S. Wheeler, R.G. Israel, and G.L. Dohm. Elevated skeletal muscle glucose transporter levels in exercise-trained middle-aged men. *Am. J. Physiol.* 261(4, part 1):E437-E443. 1991.

64. Hultsmann, W.C. On the regulation of the supply of substrates for muscular activity. *Bibl. Nutr. Dieta* 27:11-15. 1979.

65. Hurley, B.F., D.R. Seals, J.M. Hagberg, A.C. Goldberg, S.M. Ostrove, J.O. Hollozsy, W.G. Weist, and A.P. Goldberg. Strength training and lipoprotein lipid profiles: Increased HDL cholesterol in body builders vs. power-lifters and effects of androgen use. *JAMA* 252:507-513. 1984.

66. Ivy, J.L., A.L. Katz, C.L. Cutler, W.M. Sherman, and E.F. Coyle. Muscle glycogen synthesis after exercise: Effect of time of carbohydrate ingestion. *J. Appl. Physiol.* 64:1480-1485. 1988.

67. Jacobs, I., P. Kaiser and P. Tesch. The effects of glycogen exhaustion on maximal short-term performance. In: *Exercise and Sport Biology. International Series on Sport Sciences*, vol. 12, P. Komi, ed. Champaign, IL: Human Kinetics. 1982. pp. 103-108.

68. Jenkins, R.R. Free radical chemistry: Relationship to exercise. *Sports Med.* 5:156-170. 1988.

69. Jequier, E. Energy, obesity and body weight standards. *Am. J. Clin. Nutr.* 45:1035-1047. 1987.

70. Johnston, C.C., and C. Slemeda. Osteoporosis: An overview. *Phys. Sportsmed.* 15(11):65-68. 1987.

71. Jones, N.L., J.F. Heigenhauser, and A. Kuksis. Fat metabolism in heavy exercise. *Clin. Sci.* 59469-59478. 1980.

72. Kagan, V.E., V.B. Spirichev, and A.N. Erin. Vitamin E, physical exercise and sport. In: *Nutrition in Exercise and Sport*, J.F. Hickson and I. Wolinsky, eds. Boca Raton, FL: CRC Press. 1989. pp. 255-278.

73. Karlsson, J., and B. Saltin. Diet, muscle glycogen, and endurance performance. *J. Appl. Physiol.* 31:203-206. 1971.

74. Kiens, B., A.B. Raben, A.K. Valeus, and E.A. Richter. Benefit of dietary simple carbohydrates on the early postexercise muscle glycogen repletion in male athletes (abstract). *Med. Sci. Sports Exerc.* 22(Suppl.):S88. 1990.

75. Klepzig, H., and M. Kaltenbach. Cholesterol lowering and life expectancy: A critical review (English abstract). *Z-Kardiol.* 81(7):347-353. 1992.

76. Kritchevsky, S.B., and D. Kritchevsky. Serum cholesterol and cancer risk: An epidemiologic perspective. *Annu. Rev. Nutr.* 12:391-416. 1992.

77. Lamb, D. *Physiology of Exercise.* New York: Macmillan. 1984.

78. Lamb, D.R., and G.R. Brodowicz. Optimal use of fluids of varying formulations to minimize exercise-induced disturbances in homeostasis. *Sports Med.* 3:247-274. 1986.

79. Lambert, C.P., M.G. Flynn, J.B. Boone, T.J. Michaud, and J. Rodriguez-Zayas. Effects of carbohydrate feeding on multiple-bout resistance exercise. *J. Appl. Sports Sci. Res.* 5(4):192-197. 1991.

80. Lane, N., W. Bevier, M. Bouxsein, R. Wiswell, R. Careter, and D.R. Marcus. Effect of exercise intensity on bone mineral. *Med. Sci. Sports. Exerc.* 20(Suppl.):S51. 1988.

81. Laritcheva, K.A., N.I. Valovarya, V.I. Shybin, and S.A. Smirnov. Study of energy expenditure and protein needs of top weightlifters. In: *Nutrition, Physical Fitness, and Health. International Series on Sport Sciences*, vol. 7, J. Pavizkova and V.A. Rogozkin, eds. Baltimore: University Park Press. 1978. pp. 53-61.

82. Lehninger, A.L. *Bioenergetics.* New York: Benjamin. 1973.

83. Lehninger, A.L. *Biochemistry*, 2nd ed. New York: Worth. 1975.

84. Lemon, P.W.R. Protein and exercise: Update 1987. *Med. Sci. Sports Exerc.* 19(Suppl.):S179-S190. 1987.

85. Lemon, P.W.R., and J.P. Mullin. Effect of initial muscle glycogen levels on protein catabolism during exercise. *J. Appl. Physiol.* 48:624-629. 1980.

86. Lemon, P.W.R., and F.J. Nagle. Effects of exercise on protein and amino acid metabolism. *Med. Sci. Sports Exerc.* 13:141-149. 1981.

87. Leon, A.S. Physical activity levels and coronary heart disease. *Med. Clin. North Am.* 69:3-20. 1985.

88. Liberman, H.R., S. Corkin, and B.J. Spring. Mood, performance and pain sensitivity: Changes induced by food constituents. *J. Psychiatr. Res.* 17:135-146. 1983.

89. Lindsay, R. Estrogen and osteoporosis. *Phys. Sportsmed.* 15(11):105-108. 1987.

90. MacLean, D.A., and T.E. Graham. Branched-chain amino acid supplementation augments ammonia responses during prolonged exercise in humans. *Med. Sci. Sports Exerc.* 24(5[Suppl.]):S150. 1992.

91. McMillan, J., R.E. Keith, and M.H. Stone. The effects of vitamin B_6 and exercise on the contractile properties of rat muscle. *Nutr. Res.* 8:73-80. 1988.

92. McMillan, J., M.H. Stone, J. Sartain, D. Marple, R.E. Keith, D. Lewis, and C. Brown. The 20-hr hormonal response to a single session of weight-training. *J. Strength Cond. Res.* 7(1):9-21. 1993.

93. Mitchell, R., R. Kreider, R. Miller, C. Cortes, and V. Mirieal. Effects of amino acid supplementation on metabolic responses to ultraendurance training on performance. *Med. Sci. Sports Exerc.* 23(4[Suppl.]):S15. 1991.

94. National Academy of Sciences. *Recommended Dietary Allowances*, 10th ed. 1989.

95. National Cholesterol Education Program (NCEP), National Heart, Lung and Blood Institute, U.S. Department of Health and Human Services, Public Health Service, National Institutes of Health. NIH Publication No. 88-2925. 1988.

96. Neaton, J.D., H. Blackburn, D. Jacobs, L. Kuller, D.J. Lee, R. Sherwin, J. Shih, J. Stamler, and D. Wentworth. Serum cholesterol level and mortality findings for men screened in the Multiple Risk Factor Intervention Trial. Multiple Risk Factor Intervention Trial Research Group. *Arch. Intern. Med.* 152(7):1490-1500. 1992.

97. Newsholme, E. The metabolic causes of fatigue/overtraining. Keynote address at the Southeast Chapter of the American College of Sports Medicine meeting, Charleston, SC. February 1990.

98. Newsholme, E.A., I.N. Acworth, and E. Blomstrand. Amino acids, brain neurotransmitters and a functional link between muscle and brain that is important in sustained exercise. *Adv. Biochem.* 1:127-133. 1985.

99. Nickerson, H.J., and A.D. Trip. Iron deficiency in adolescent cross-country runners. *Phys. Sportsmed.* 11:60-66. 1983.

100. Nieman, D.C. *Fitness and Sports Medicine*. Palo Alto, CA: Bull. 1987.

101. Nieman, D.C. *Fitness and Your Health*. Palo Alto, CA: Bull. 1993.

102. Nieman, D.C., D.E. Butterworth, and C.E. Nieman. *Nutrition*. Dubuque, IA: Brown. 1992.

103. O'Keeffe, K., R.E. Keith, D.L. Blessing, G.D. Wilson, and K.L. Young. Dietary carbohydrate and endurance performance. *Med. Sci. Sports Exerc.* 19:S538. 1987.

104. Opie, L.J., and E.A. Newsholme. The activities of fructose 1,6-diphosphate, phosphofructokinase, and phosphoenol-pyruvate carboxykinase in white and red muscle. *Biochem. J.* 103:391-399. 1967.

105. Petrozello, S.J., D.M. Landers, J. Pie, and J. Billie. Effect of branched-chain amino acid supplements on exercise-related mood and performance. *Med. Sci. Sports Exerc.* 24(5[Suppl.]):S2. 1992.

106. Pike, R.L. and M. Brown. *Nutrition: An Integrated Approach*, 3rd ed. New York: Macmillan. 1984.

107. Pivarnik, J.M., J.F. Hickson, and I. Wolinsky. Urinary 3-methylhistidine excretion increases with repeated weight training exercise. *Med. Sci. Sports Exerc.* 21:283-287. 1989.

108. Rifkind, B.M., and P. Segal. Lipid Research Clinics program reference values for hyperlipidemia and hypolipidemia. *JAMA* 250:1869-1872. 1984.

109. Risser, W.L., E. Lee, H.B.W. Poindexter, M.S. West, J.M. Pivarnik, J.M.H. Risser, and J.F. Hickson. Iron deficiency in female athletes: Its prevalence and impact on performance. *Med. Sci. Sports Exerc.* 20:116-121. 1988.

110. Rozenek, R., and M.H. Stone. Protein metabolism related to athletes. *NSCA Journal* 6(2):42-62. 1984.

111. Sherman, W.M., and G.S. Wimer. Insufficient carbohydrate during training: Does it impair performance? *Sport Nutr.* 1(1):28-44. 1991.

112. Short, S.H., and W.R. Short. Four-year study of university athletes' dietary intake. *J. Am. Diet. Assoc.* 82:632-645. 1983.

113. Sjodin, B., Y.H. Westing, and F.S. Apple. Biochemical mechanisms for oxygen free radical formation during exercise. *Sports Med.* 10(4):236-254. 1990.

114. Simonses, J.C., W.M. Sherman, D.R. Lamb, A.R. Dernbach, J.A. Doyle, and R. Strauss. Dietary carbohydrate, muscle glycogen and power output during rowing training. *J. Appl. Physiol.* 70(4):1500-1505. 1991.

115. Slentz, C.A., E.A. Gulve, K.J. Rodnick, E.J. Henriksen, J.H. Youn, and J.O. Hollozsy. Glucose transporters and maximal transport are increased in endurance trained rat soleus. *J. Appl. Physiol.* 73(2):486-492. 1992.

116. Smith, E.L., and C. Gilligan. Effects of inactivity and exercise on bone. *Phys. Sportsmed.* 15(11):91-94. 1987.

117. Snyder, A.C., L.L. Dvorak, and J.B. Roepke. Influence of dietary iron source on measures of iron status among female runners. *Med. Sci. Sports Exerc.* 21:7-10. 1989.

118. Snyder, A.C., D.R. Lamb, T. Baur, D. Conners, and G. Brodowicz. Maltodextrin feeding immediately before prolonged cycling at 62% VO₂max increases time to exhaustion. *Med. Sci. Sports Exerc.* 15:126. 1983.

119. Sparge, E. Metabolic functions of skeletal muscles of man, mammals, birds, and fishes: A review. *J. R. Soc. Med.* 72:921-925. 1979.

120. Stone, M.H. Muscle conditioning and muscle injuries. *Med. Sci. Sports Exerc.* 22(4):457-462. 1990.

121. Stone, M.H., S.J. Fleck, W.J. Kraemer, and N.T. Triplett. Health- and performance-related potential of resistance training. *Sports Med.* 11(4):210-231. 1991.

122. Stone, M.H., R. Keith, J.T. Kearney, G.D. Wilson, and S.J. Fleck. Overtraining: A review of the signs and symptoms of overtraining. *J. Appl. Sports Sci. Res.* 5(1):35-50. 1991.

123. Stone, M.H., R.E. Keith, D. Marple, S.J. Fleck, and J.T. Kearney. Physiological adaptations during a one-week junior elite weightlifting training camp. Conference Abstracts, Southeast Chapter of the American College of Sports Medicine meeting. January 1989.

124. Stone, M.H., and G.D. Wilson. Resistive training and selected effects. In: *Medical Clinics of North America*, L. Goldberg and D. Elliot, eds. Philadelphia: Saunders. 1985. pp. 109-122.

125. Strauzenberg, S.E., F. Schneider, R. Donath, H. Zerbes, and E. Kohler. The problem of dieting in training and athletic performance. *Bibl. Nutr. Dieta* 27(27):133-142. 1979.

126. Tarnopolsky, M.A., S.A. Atkinson, J.D. MacDougall, A. Chesley, S. Phillips, and H.P. Schwarcz. Evaluation of protein requirements for trained strength athletes. *J. Appl. Physiol.* 73(5):1986-1995. 1992.

127. Tarnopolsky, M.A., J.D. MacDougall, and S.A. Atkinson. Influence of protein intake and training status on nitrogen balance and lean body mass. *J. Appl. Physiol.* 64(1):187-193. 1988.

128. Tischler, M.E. Hormonal regulation of protein degradation in skeletal and cardiac muscle. *Life Sci.* 28:2569-2576. 1981.

129. U.S. Department of Agriculture, Human Nutrition Information Service. *Nationwide Food Consumption Survey.* Continuing Survey of Food Intakes by Individuals: Women 19-50 Years Old and their Children 1-5 Years, 1 Day, 1985, USDA rept. 85-1. Men 19-50 Years, 1 Day, 1985. USDA rept. 85-3. 1985.

130. Vandewalle, L., A.J.M. Wagenmakers, K. Smets, F. Brouns, and W.H.M. Saris. Effect of branched-chain amino acid supplementation on exercise performance in glycogen depleted subjects. *Med. Sci. Sports Exerc.* 23(4[Suppl.]): S116. 1991.

131. Wagenmakers, A.J., E.J. Beckers, F. Brouns, H. Kuipers, P.B. Soeters, G.J. Van der Vusse, and W.H.M. Saris. Carbohydrate supplementation, glycogen depletion and amino acid metabolism during exercise. *Am. J. Physiol.* 260(6, #1): E883-E890. 1991.

132. Wagenmakers, A.J.M., K. Smets, L. Vandewalle, F. Brouns, and W.H.M. Saris. Deamination of branch-chain amino acids: A potential source of ammonia production during exercise. *Med. Sci. Sports Exerc.* 23(4[Suppl.]):S116. 1991.

133. Walberg, J.L., M.K. Leidy, D.J. Sturgill, D.E. Hinkle, S.J. Ritchey, and D.R. Sebolt. Macronutrient needs in weight lifters during caloric restriction. *Med. Sci. Sports Exerc.* 19(2):S70. 1987.

134. Weideman, C.A., M.G. Flynn, F.X. Pizza, R. Coombs, J.B. Boone, E.R. Kubitz, and W.F. Simpson. Effects of increased protein intake on muscle hypertrophy and strength following 13 weeks of resistance training. *Med. Sci. Sport Exerc.* 22(2):S37. 1990.

135. Williams, M.H. *Nutritional Aspects of Human Physical and Athletic Performance.* Springfield, IL: Charles C Thomas. 1976.

136. Williams, M.H. *Nutrition for Fitness and Sport.* Dubuque, IA: Brown. 1983.

137. Wilmore, J.H., and B.J. Freund. Nutritional enhancement of athletic performance. *Nutr. Abstr. Rev.* A54:1-6. 1984.

138. Wolfe, R.R. Does exercise stimulate protein breakdown in humans? Isotopic approaches to the problem. *Med. Sci. Sports Exerc.* 19(Suppl.):S172-S178. 1987.

139. Wood, P.D., and M.L. Stefanick. Exercise, fitness, and atherosclerosis. In: *Exercise, Fitness, and Health,* C. Bouchard, R.J. Shepard, T. Stephens, J.R. Sutton, and B.D. McPherson, eds. Champaign, IL: Human Kinetics. 1990.

140. Wright, J.E., and M.H. Stone. NSCA statement on anabolic drug use. *NSCA Journal* 7(5):45-59. 1985.

141. Yates, A., K. Leehey, and C.M. Shisslak. Running: An analogue of anorexia? *N. Engl. J. Med.* 308:251-253. 1983.

142. Yokogoshi, H., T. Iwata, K. Ishida, and A. Yoshida. Effect of amino acid supplementation to low-protein diet on brain and plasma levels of tryptophan and brain 5-hydroxyindoles in rats. *J. Nutr.* 117:42-47. 1987.

143. Young, V.R., and H.N. Munro. *N*-methylhistidine (3-methylhistidine) and muscle protein turnover: An overview. *Fed. Proc.* 37:2291-2300. 1978.

144. Zalessky, M. Coaching, medico-biological, and psychological means of recovery. *Legkaya Athletika* 7:20-22. 1977.

CHAPTER 13

WEIGHT GAIN AND WEIGHT LOSS

Michael H. Stone

Knowledge of weight gain and weight loss principles is essential if strength and conditioning professionals are to prescribe training programs that bring about desired results. This chapter begins by discussing the energy cost of exercise, an understanding of which is important in regulating body mass and body composition, improving health-related parameters, and reducing the potential for overtraining. Next, the effects of exercise on water and electrolyte levels in the body are discussed. Finally, this chapter provides information important for gaining and losing weight for competitive purposes so that one's safety, health, and competitive edge are not compromised.

ENERGY COST OF EXERCISE

Energy is commonly measured in kilocalories (kcal). A **kilocalorie** is the work or energy required to raise the temperature of one kilogram of water one degree celsius. A person's rate of energy expenditure is related to body mass, intensity of exercise, and work efficiency. Thus, as intensity of exercise increases, the rate of caloric expenditure increases, and the more total work accomplished, the more energy is used—energy cost. Additionally, the total energy expenditure of training is directly or indirectly related to several physical and physiological parameters, including body mass and body composition, substrate mobilization, alterations in serum lipids, and cardiovascular function. Considering these relationships, a reasonable estimate of the **energy**

cost (the total energy used) of various exercises is valuable in planning training programs. Typical rates of energy consumption for various activities are listed in Table 13.1 (2,30,33). As the table indicates, some activities have a wide range of energy costs. This is the result of the numerous determining variables just noted as well as of practical aspects of the sport. The energy

Table 13.1 Energy Cost of Sports Activities

Activity	Energy cost (kcal/min)
Lying supine	1
Sitting	1-1.5
Standing	1-1.5
Basketball (mean values for a game)	1-15
Cycling at 4 km/hr (2.5 mph)	7
Football (while active)	6-14
Jogging at 160 m/min (6 mph)	7-9
Sprinting	18-22
Volleyball (mean values for a game)	3-6
Weight training (mean values)	
Circuit	9-10
Priority	5-10
Small muscle mass	3-7
Large muscle mass	6-18
Combination (emphasizing large muscle mass)	9-10

Note. Data from references 2, 30, 33.

cost of playing basketball, for example, can result in widely varying energy expenditures depending on which position is being played and the size of the player.

The energy cost of exercise and training can be important from the standpoints of health and performance. It has been suggested that in terms of health, especially as it concerns reducing the risk for cardiovascular disease, energy-cost volume and intensity thresholds should be met (25). The intensity threshold is approximately 7.5 kcal/min, and the volume threshold begins at approximately 500 kcal/week above resting levels. The benefits increase up to about 2,000 extra kcal/week. Training programs that cost more than 2,000 kcal/week above baseline may improve performance but are unlikely to produce additional health benefits. Considering the rate of energy expenditure of various activities, it is apparent that several different activities, including weight training, can meet these intensity and volume thresholds, provided the activity selected is performed in a vigorous manner and the volume is high. It has been suggested that there may be a graded relationship between energy expenditure and health benefits, especially decreased risk for cardiovascular disease (9,10). Thus, to a point, the greater the energy expenditure, the greater the health benefits.

Many athletes train several times a day, several days a week. Because of this, considerable total work is performed with a concomitantly large total energy expenditure. In order to reduce the potential for non-beneficial adaptations, such as chronic overwork and loss of weight or lean body mass, adequate calories must be consumed to balance the caloric expenditure. Typical daily caloric expenditure and caloric consumption for various sports are listed in Table 13.2 (3,23,35). As with the activities shown in Table 13.1, it is important to note that some sports may have a wide range of

Table 13.2 Caloric Expenditure and Consumption of Sports Activities

Activity	Expenditure (kcal · kg⁻¹ · day⁻¹)	Consumption (kcal/day)
Untrained	< 40	2,000-3,000
Marathon	50-80	2,500-6,000
Basketball	55-70	5,000-6,000
Sprinting	55-65	4,300-6,000
Judo	55-65	3,000-6,200
Throwing (field events)	60-65	6,000-8,000
Weightlifting	56-75	3,000-10,000

Note. Energy expenditure values are those of male athletes during training and event performance. Data from references 3, 23, 35.

energy expenditure and caloric consumption. This is largely due to differences in the body masses of participating athletes and in training intensities and volumes. For example, a superheavy weightlifter (140 kg) expends considerably more energy performing the same training exercises at the same relative intensity (percent 1RM) than a 60-kg athlete does; the superheavy lifter also requires a much greater caloric consumption. Additionally, the size of the muscle mass involved also affects the rate of energy use and the total energy used. Large–muscle mass weight training exercises require a greater rate of energy use (higher exercise intensity) than small–muscle mass exercises. The rest periods between sets during resistance training can also influence the energy used during a training session. Shorter rest periods can increase the average energy consumption of a training session.

Priority weight training is a method of resistance training in which the most important exercises relative to goal accomplishment (usually large–muscle mass exercises) are placed first and the less important exercises are performed after the more important ones. With a priority program, all of the sets and repetitions for each exercise are performed before proceeding to the next exercise and sufficient rest is taken between sets so that each set can be completed (36). In circuit weight training, upper- and lower-body exercises are typically alternated with each set, and short (<1-min) rest periods are used. Completion of one set of each exercise constitutes one circuit. Several circuits, typically using 6 to 12 exercises, may be accomplished. Circuit weight training usually emphasizes smaller muscle mass exercises compared with priority training. Because of the short rest periods and the use of many small–muscle mass exercises, the exercise intensity of circuit weight training is typically lower than that of priority training (36). As can be seen in Table 13.1, priority weight training that emphasizes large–muscle mass exercises produces energy expenditures similar to those of circuit weight training that emphasizes short rest periods (but uses many small–muscle mass exercises). (See chapter 12.)

Considering the possible energy expenditures as a result of high-level (high-load) training, it is not unreasonable to expect the strength and conditioning professional and athlete to put considerable thought into the selection of exercises, the length of workouts, and the number of workouts per day.

WATER AND ELECTROLYTES

Water is the most plentiful component of the human body. By weight, water makes up about 60% of a man's body and 50% of a woman's body. About 55% of the body's water is found in the cells, about 39% in the interstitial fluid (between cells), and about 6% in the plasma and lymph. Functions of **intracellular water** (the water in the cells) include providing form and structure, as well as a medium for biochemical reactions. **Extracellular water** (the water in the interstitial fluid, plasma, and lymph) provides a medium for transport and exchange of nutrients, metabolic by-products, gases, and heat (20). Small changes in intracellular or extracellular water content may cause functional changes—any biochemical reaction dependent on water, electrolyte balance, thermo-regulation, etc.

Dehydration resulting in the loss of as little as 2% of body mass can adversely affect a variety of physiological functions and lead to performance decrements (26,29). Of particular importance is the association of dehydration with inadequate thermal regulation, which could in turn result in heat exhaustion or heat stroke. Thus, dehydration during exercise should be avoided.

Although sweating rates are affected by various factors, including temperature, humidity, and clothing worn, it is not uncommon to lose 2% to 3% of body mass, most of it water, during typical exercise regimens. During very long term exercise, such as running a marathon, or repeated high-intensity exercise, such as fall football training, losses of up to 8% of body mass can occur when fluid replacement is inadequate (12,26,28). Of great importance is the observation that the sensation of thirst lags behind the need for water replacement (15,26). The recommendation for water replacement is 500 ml every 30 min during long-term exercise such as a marathon (26); this level of water replacement is also reasonable for repeated high-intensity exercise, especially in the heat, such as football training. Less water replacement is probably needed during exercise sessions in which smaller amounts of body water are lost.

Electrolytes are minerals that have a positive or negative charge, are soluble in body fluids, and are associated with cell membrane electrical potentials (20,26,27). Marked loss of electrolytes can interfere with cellular active transport systems, upset fluid balance, and indirectly affect thermoregulation and various metabolic functions. The most important electrolytes are sodium, potassium, and chloride. Sodium and potassium carry positive charges; chloride is negatively charged. All three electrolytes are easily obtained in ordinary foods.

Sodium and potassium are related to hypertension (high blood pressure). A high sodium intake tends to increase blood pressure; when the potassium intake is 40% higher than sodium intake, blood pressure may decrease. Thus, the sodium-potassium ratio is of primary concern in reducing hypertension, especially among sodium sensitive people (21). A sodium-potassium ratio of 0.6 is generally recommended to help reduce the incidence of hypertension (27).

Electrolytes are usually available in sports drinks that also contain carbohydrates (27). Sports drinks are used to prevent dehydration, counter any losses of electrolytes through sweating, and replace carbohydrates (26). There is some question as to the usefulness of adding electrolytes to sports drink. Although various electrolytes and vitamins are lost in sweat, these losses are not usually significant, particularly in acclimatized individuals (20,26). Furthermore, athletic training results in adaptations that further minimize electrolyte losses through sweating. Under certain conditions, however, the ingestion of electrolytes may be beneficial. During exercise lasting more than 4 hr, such as ultramarathons, low blood sodium levels may occur (26). Physical activity in very hot environments may also (although rarely) result in low blood sodium concentrations, especially in unacclimatized or partially acclimatized people; this condition usually takes 3 to 5 days of activity to develop (22,32).

WEIGHT GAIN

In many sports, such as football, throwing events, and the heavier classes in weightlifting, it is not unusual for athletes to weigh 100 to 150 kg. In attempting to achieve these large body masses, considerable thought should be placed into proper nutrition and physical training programs that can enhance gains in lean body mass, reduce gains in body fat, and allow an achievement of optimal or maximum performance. Athletes trying to gain body mass should consider the following points:

1. The goals of weight gain should be to maximize gains in lean body mass (muscle and connective tissue) and to minimize gains in body fat. Athletes *already in training* should keep in mind that their weight gains will almost always be accompanied by fat gain (17-19) and that substantial increases in body mass will likely be accompanied by an increase in percent body fat. The increase in percent body fat can be minimized by appropriate training and dietary practices. (See the Energy Cost of Exercise section at the beginning of this chapter.)

2. An increase in body mass is best accomplished through specific training programs, particularly weight training (36), associated with an increased caloric consumption. Increased dietary calories should be made up of appropriate percentages of protein, carbohydrate, and fat, as described in chapter 12.

3. Even when **isocaloric diets** (diets with the same number of kcals) are eaten, more fat weight is gained on the diets higher in fat content

(11,13,38). When gaining body mass, care should be taken to keep the fat content of the diet under 30% of consumed calories. Admittedly, this can be difficult, especially when one is consuming a substantial diet (> 5,000 kcal/day); plan meals carefully. Individual differences can be marked. People eating different amounts of calories and proportions of protein, carbohydrates, and fat can maintain similar proportions of body fat even though caloric expenditure is similar (24).

4. Commercial weight gain products are usually not warranted. Some of these products are relatively high in fat content (30% or more). You can usually add extra energy to your diet by simply ingesting extra food. If factors such as training, work, or school schedules; cost; and individual characteristics and tastes preclude the ingestion of additional food, a supplement may be useful. One useful source of protein, carbohydrates, and extra calories is skim milk, which can be flavored to taste. The use of anabolic steroids to gain weight is unwarranted and potentially dangerous (41).

5. Body mass gains should be relatively slow, about 0.5 to 1.0 kg/week; this rate tends to reduce fat gains (8). Prolonged weight gain (> 6 months), in which a relatively large gain in body mass is the goal, should occur at an even slower rate, 0.25 to 0.5 kg/week, to insure that most of the gain is in lean body mass.

6. Monitor body composition closely and often (every 1-2 weeks) by skinfold or hydrostatic weighing. If the percentage of body fat begins to rise markedly, consider changing your diet or training protocol. Observation suggests that high-level athletes in training and attempting to gain body mass usually gain 1% to 3% in body fat for each 10 kg of body mass gained.

After an athlete's career has ended, considerable thought should be given to weight reduction, particularly if the athlete is heavy; examples are linemen, throwers, and heavy classes in weightlifting and wrestling. Reduction in body mass and beneficial alterations in body composition can reduce the potential for cardiovascular and other degenerative diseases. In the college and professional athletic setting, it would not be unreasonable to make counseling on nutrition and proper training available through a certified strength and conditioning specialist. The specialist should have access to a nutritionist or registered dietitian and make every effort to keep up-to-date in sports nutrition.

WEIGHT LOSS

In sports that have stringent body weight limitations, such as weightlifting, wrestling, boxing, and lightweight crew, care must be taken in maintaining proper body mass. It is often necessary to lose body mass in order to compete in a lower weight class. Even in sports in which there are no weight classes, such as gymnastics, one needs a low body fat to be competitive. Achieving a new, lower weight class or low body fat often requires considerable body mass reduction. Athletes attempting to lose body mass should consider the following points:

1. The ideal weight is not the lowest body mass an athlete can maintain. Starved (or markedly dehydrated) athletes do not perform at maximum or optimal levels. Caloric restriction can potentiate overtraining and thus reduce performance (34). Some evidence suggests that caloric restriction in adolescents can result in shorter adult stature (4,31).

2. Previously untrained subjects can lose body fat and gain lean body mass as a result of caloric restriction and training (5,6); however, it is unlikely that athletes already possessing a relatively low body fat content can achieve body mass reduction without losing some lean body mass. Substantial amounts of body mass cannot be lost without losing marked amounts of lean body mass, particularly in association with caloric restriction (7,40). The loss of lean body mass can be minimized through training, particularly weight training (7,14), and by a high-protein diet during caloric restriction (40). The use of fad diets, such as total-liquid diets, should be discouraged.

3. The maximum rate of acceptable body mass loss appears to be approximately 1% of body mass per week. Based on studies of wrestlers (16), this would amount to approximately 0.5 to 1.0 kg/week and would represent a daily caloric deficit of 500 to 1,000 kcals/day. Faster rates (> 1.0 kg/week) can potentiate the loss of lean body mass and glycogen stores, increase the possibility of dehydration, and decrease vitamin and mineral status (4,5,16,28). Additionally, loss of body mass carried out longer than 4 weeks or a total body mass loss of more than 5% may potentiate a change in vitamin and mineral status that would reduce performance (16). It should be noted that the weight loss needs of very small or very large athletes have not been adequately addressed. For example, a female weightlifter with a body mass of 50 kg and who is trying to reduce body mass to 48 kg probably should not lose more than 0.50 kg/week, a value that represents 1% of her body mass. In contrast, a defensive lineman with a body mass of 150 kg may safely lose 1.5 kg/week, which amounts to 1% of his body mass.

4. In males, low body fat is associated with a low testosterone concentration and increased incidence of injury (37,39). Body composition should be checked to make sure that the male athlete does not decrease body fat below 5% to 6% of total body weight. In females, body fat should probably not drop to less than 10% (4,28).

5. Rapid reductions in body mass can be accomplished by short-term fluid restriction resulting in some degree of dehydration. However, this practice has been discouraged by the American College of Sports Medicine because of the following potentially harmful side effects:

- Reduced muscular strength and power
- Decreased low- and high-intensity exercise endurance
- Lower blood and plasma volumes
- Reduced cardiac function
- Reduced maximal oxygen uptake
- Impairment of thermal regulation
- Decreased renal function
- Decreased glycogen concentration
- Loss of electrolytes

Rehydration and reestablishment of electrolyte homeostasis may take more than 5 hr to accomplish (4). It may be noted that very rapid body mass losses, of up to 2% of total body mass, on the day of competition can be achieved with little effect on cardiovascular function (1) or strength performance (39). However, the necessity of rapid body mass loss as a result of dehydration should be avoided, if possible. Vorobeyev (39) suggests that the cumulative effects of several rapid dehydrations per year, even though small, may have harmful consequences. It would also be reasonable when trying to make weight to avoid foods that cause water retention, such as very salty foods (28).

CONCLUSION

The total energy cost of exercise can depend on a number of factors, including body mass and the volume and intensity of exercise. Knowledge of the energy cost of exercise is important in helping to regulate body mass and body composition, improve health-related parameters, and reduce the potential for overtraining. Dehydration and subsequent body mass loss can harm performance and health. Care should be used in proper hydration before, during, and after physical activity.

Weight gain can be accomplished most successfully by a combination of training, especially weight training, and an increase in caloric intake. The fat content of the diet should be kept relatively low and the rate of gain should be less than 1.0 kg/week; this will reduce fat gains.

Weight loss can be successfully accomplished as a result of training and reduced caloric intake. A high-protein diet, weight training, and a rate of body mass reduction of less than 1.0 kg/week can minimize the loss of lean body mass. Weight loss typically should not exceed 5% of body mass or be prolonged (> 4 weeks). Rapid weight loss through dehydration should be discouraged because of the possibility of both short-term and long-term nonbeneficial effects. Heavy athletes should reduce body mass after retiring from competition.

Key Terms

electrolyte	233	extracellular water	233	isocaloric diet	233
energy cost	231	intracellular water	233	kilocalorie	231

Study Questions

1. Athletes attempting to gain weight should

   I. maximize gains in lean body mass
   II. minimize fat gains
   III. gain weight as fast as possible
   IV. gain weight as slowly as possible

   a. I and II
   b. I and III
   c. I and IV
   d. I only

2. Weight loss should proceed slowly in order to

   I.   conserve lean body mass
   II. conserve vitamin status
   III. conserve fat stores

   a. I and II
   b. I and III
   c. I only
   d. II only

3. Compared with a priority weight-training session that emphasizes large–muscle mass exercises, jogging at 6 mph (9.7 km/hr) has a(n) ___ rate of energy expenditure.

   a. slightly lower
   b. slightly higher
   c. equal
   d. much higher

4. In males, body fat usually should not drop below ___ in order to reduce injury potential.

   a. 5% to 6%
   b. 3% to 4%
   c. 6% to 7%
   d. 7% to 8%

5. When a football player attempts to lose weight through caloric restriction, loss of lean body mass can be minimized by

   a. increasing protein intake and engaging in weight training
   b. increasing fat intake and engaging in weight training
   c. decreasing fat intake and engaging in high-volume aerobic training
   d. increasing protein intake and engaging in high-volume aerobic training

Applying Knowledge
of Weight Gain and Weight Loss

Problem 1

A basketball forward reports to fall training at a university. His height is 189 cm (6 ft 2 in), and his body mass is 120 kg (264 lb). He and his coach believe he needs to lose weight. How should this be done?

Problem 2

A lineman has been injured during the first game of the season. His injury requires that he miss six games and the practice sessions for them. The school's certified strength and conditioning specialist is concerned that the lineman will decondition—this would include body mass and body composition changes—during the 6 weeks of recovery from the injury. What should be done?

References

1. Adolph, E.F. *Physiology of Man in the Desert*. New York: Interscience. 1947.

2. American Alliance for Health, Physical Education, Recreation and Dance. *Nutrition for the Athlete*. Washington: Author. 1971.

3. American College of Sports Medicine. *Encyclopedia of Sports Sciences and Medicine*. New York: Macmillan. 1971.

4. American College of Sports Medicine. Weight loss in wrestlers. *Med. Sci. Sports Exerc.* 8:xi-xiii. 1976.

5. American College of Sports Medicine. Proper and improper weight loss programs. *Med. Sci. Sports Exerc.* 15:534-539. 1983.

6. American College of Sports Medicine. The recommended quantity and quality of exercise for developing and maintaining cardiorespiratory and muscular fitness in healthy adults. *Med. Sci. Sports Exerc.* 22:265-274. 1990.

7. Ballor, D.L., V.L. Katch, M.D. Beque, and C.R. Marks. Resistance weight training during caloric restriction enhances lean body weight maintenance. *Am. J. Clin. Nutr.* 47:19-25. 1988.

8. Birrer, R.B. *Sports Medicine for the Primary Care Physician.* Norfolk, CT: Appleton-Century-Crofts. 1984.

9. Blair, S.N. Exercise and chronic disease: Emerging evidence for a protective effect. Keynote address, Southeast Chapter of the American College of Sports Medicine meeting, Norfolk, Virginia. January 1993.

10. Blair, S.N., H.W. Kohl III, R.S. Paffenbarger, D.G. Clark, K.H. Cooper, and L.W. Gibbons. Physical fitness and all-cause mortality. *JAMA* 262(17):2395-2401. 1989.

11. Boissoneault, G.A., C.E. Elson, and M.W. Pariza. Net energy effects of dietary fat on chemically induced mammary carcinogenesis in F344 rats. *J. Natl. Cancer Inst.* 76:335-338. 1986.

12. Bowers, R.W., and E.L. Fox. *Sports Physiology*, 3rd ed. New York: Saunders. 1992.

13. Donato, K., and D.M. Hegsted. Efficiency of utilization of various sources of energy for growth. *Proc. Natl. Acad. Sci. U.S.A.* 82:4866-4870. 1985.

14. Donnelly, J.E., and D.J. Jacobson. Body composition changes with very low calorie diets and exercise. *Med. Sci. Sports Exerc.* 19(suppl.):S69. 1987.

15. Engell, D.B., O. Maller, M.N. Sawka, R.P. Francesesconi, L. Drolet, and A.J. Young. Thirst and fluid intake following graded hypohydration levels in humans. *Physiol. Behav.* 40:226-236. 1987.

16. Fogleholm, G.M., R. Koskinen, J. Laasko, T. Rankinen, and I. Ruokonen. Gradual and rapid weight loss: Effects on nutrition and performance in male athletes. *Med. Sci. Sports Exerc.* 25(3):371-377. 1993.

17. Forbes, G.B. Some influences on lean body mass: Exercise, androgens, pregnancy and food. In: *Diet and Exercise: Synergism in Health Maintenance*, P.L. White and T. Mondeika, eds. Chicago: American Medical Association. 1983.

18. Forbes, G.B. Body composition as affected by physical activity and nutrition. *Fed. Proc.* 4:343-347. 1985.

19. Forsberg, A., P. Tesh, and J. Karlsson. Effects of prolonged exercise on muscle strength performance. In: *Biomechanics VI-A*, E. Asmussen and K. Jorgensen, eds. Baltimore: University Park Press. 1978.

20. Herbert, W.G. Water and electrolytes. In: *Ergogenic Aids in Sport*, M.H. Williams, ed. Champaign, IL: Human Kinetics. 1983. pp. 56-98.

21. Kaplan, N.M. Dietary aspects of the treatment of hypertension. *Annu. Rev. Public Health* 7:503-519. 1986.

22. McCance, R.A. Experimental sodium chloride deficiency in man. *Proc. R. Soc. Lond.* 119:245-268. 1936.

23. McMillan, J., M.H. Stone, J. Sartain, D. Marple, R. Keith, D. Lewis, and C. Brown. The 20-hr hormonal response to a single session of weight-training. *J. Strength and Cond. Res.* 7(1):9-21. 1993.

24. Miller, D.S. Food intake and energy utilization. In: *International Series on Sports Sciences: vol. 7. Nutrition, Physical Fitness and Health*, J.V.A. Parizkova, ed. Baltimore: University Park Press. 1978.

25. Morris, J.N. Exercise and the incidence of coronary heart disease. In: *Exercise-Heart-Health*. London: The Coronary Prevention Group. 1987.

26. Nieman, D.C., D.E. Butterworth, and C.E. Nieman. *Nutrition*. Dubuque, IA: Brown. 1992.

27. Nieman, D.C. *Fitness and Your Health*. Palo Alto, CA: Bull. 1993.

28. Roy, S.R., and W. Irwin. *Sports Medicine*. Englewood Cliffs, NJ: Prentice Hall. 1983.

29. Saltin, B., and J. Stenberg. Circulatory response to prolonged severe exercise. *J. Appl. Physiol.* 19:833-838. 1964.

30. Scala, D., J. McMillan, D. Blessing, R. Ruzenek, and M.H. Stone. Metabolic cost of a preparatory phase of training in weightlifting: A practical observation. *J. Appl. Sports Sci. Res.* 1(3):48-52. 1987.

31. Smith, N.J. Gaining and losing weight in athletics. *JAMA* 236:149-151. 1976.

32. Sohar, E., and R. Adar. Sodium requirements in Israel under conditions of work in hot climate. In: *UNESCO/India Symposium on Environmental Physiology and Psychology*. Lucknow, India: UNESCO. 1962.

33. Stone, M.H., S.J. Fleck, W.J. Kraemer, and N.T. Triplett. Health- and performance-related potential of resistance training. *Sports Med.* 11(4):210-231. 1991.

34. Stone, M.H., R. Keith, J.T. Kearney, G.D. Wilson, and S.J. Fleck. Overtraining: A review of the signs and symptoms of overtraining. *J. Appl. Sports Sci. Res.* 5(1):35-50. 1991.

35. Stone, M.H., R.E. Keith, D. Marple, S.J. Fleck, and J.T. Kearney. Physiological adaptations during a one-week junior elite weightlifting training camp. *Conference Abstracts*, Southeast Chapter of the American College of Sports Medicine meeting. January 1989.

36. Stone, M.H., and H.S. O'Bryant. *Weight Training: A Scientific Approach*. Minneapolis: Burgess International. 1987.

37. Strauss, R.H., R.R. Lanese, and W.B. Malarkey. Weight loss in amateur wrestlers and its effect on serum testosterone levels. *JAMA* 254:3337-3338. 1985.

38. Tsai, A.C., and T-W. Gong. Modulation of the exercise and retirement effects by dietary fat intake in hamsters. *J. Nutr.* 117:1149-1153. 1987.

39. Vorobeyev, A. *Weightlifting*. (W.J. Brice, trans.). Budapest: International Weightlifting Federation (Medical Committee). 1978.

40. Walberg, J.L., M.K. Leidy, D.J. Sturgill, D.E. Hinkle, S.J. Ritchey, and D.R. Sebott. Macronutrient needs in weight lifters during caloric restriction. *Med. Sci. Sports Exerc.* 19(2[suppl.]):S70. 1987.

41. Wright, J.E., and M.H. Stone. NSCA statement on anabolic drug use. *NSCA Journal* 15(2):9-29. 1993.

CHAPTER 14

EATING DISORDERS

Michael H. Stone

Eating disorders are not uncommon and may result from a wide variety of sociocultural, familial, and physiological factors (4,9,10). Eating disorders affect a person's health and diminish his or her physical capabilities. The strength and conditioning professional should be able to recognize the symptoms of these disorders and provide assistance for the athlete in overcoming them, referring the athlete to health professionals when necessary.

Three types of eating disorders—obesity, bulimia nervosa, and anorexia nervosa—will be briefly discussed in this chapter. Although not technically classified as an eating disorder, obesity is a problem related to overeating and binge eating and is included in here. The number of cases of all three of these in the United States appears to be increasing (1). Bulimia and anorexia are common among women, including athletes, but also occur in males. Both bulimia and anorexia are more common among Caucasians than other races in the United States. The onset of these two eating disorders usually occurs between the ages of 14 and 30, with anorexia developing somewhat earlier than bulimia.

mass and the **body mass index**, the number of kilograms of body weight per unit of surface area (Table 14.1).

Obesity is a common problem, but one that is very difficult to treat because obesity and the ability to deposit fat are related not only to eating habits but also, possibly, to a low daily energy expenditure; there also appears to be a strong genetic component (7-9,11). Obesity is associated with a number of degenerative diseases, including cardiovascular disease, diabetes, and certain types of cancer (7-9,11). People with more fat in the upper body and abdominal area appear to be at greater risk for cardiovascular disease and diabetes than those with greater fat deposition in the lower body (6). Obesity can also be associated with reduced performance. Obese individuals usually fatigue faster than lean individuals, often have more difficulty with thermoregulation, and may be at greater risk for heat exhaustion and heat stroke (8,10,11).

In the United States great emphasis is placed on the idea that "thin is beautiful," and the general public often expresses negative stereotypes toward people deviating from this norm (10). At least partially because

OBESITY

Obesity is defined as a condition in which there is excess body fat (9), although "excess" can be difficult to pinpoint. Some physiologists and nutritionists categorize obesity based on specific percentages of body fat. Nieman (8), for example, suggests that males should be considered obese at a percentage of body fat of 25 or higher and women at 32% or higher. A three-level classification of obesity may also be made using body

Table 14.1 Classification of Obesity

Category	% over ideal weight	Body mass index (kg/m^2)	Prevalence (% of total obese population in U.S.)
Mild	20-40	25-30	90.5
Moderate	41-100	30-35	9.0
Severe	> 100	> 35	0.5

of the stereotype, obese people often develop guilt feelings and show signs of depression.

Treatment

Treatment for obesity usually involves four elements (7-9):

- Admission of the problem
- Diet, including reduced caloric and fat intake
- Increasing caloric expenditure through regular exercise and other physical activity
- Behavior modification, including self-monitoring of food intake so as to be aware of how much food is being eaten; learning to recognize and control events that lead to overeating; and developing a support group and a system of noncaloric rewards for helping to achieve weight reduction goals

Treatment can be assigned using the classification in Table 14.1. The treatment for mild obesity is usually behavior modification, including caloric restriction, and a change in food choices, so that less fat is eaten. Moderate obesity may respond best to very low calorie diets, moderate exercise, and behavior therapy. Severe obesity may require such surgical interventions as gastric stapling, in which the volume of the stomach is reduced (7). The strength and conditioning professional may encounter people with mild obesity and be of assistance in their reduction plans (see chapter 13). People with moderate or severe obesity should be referred to a physician.

Of great importance to the coach and athlete is the fact that many athletes would be classified as mildly to moderately obese by the body mass index. More appropriate criteria for determining obesity in an athletic setting, especially for the heavy athlete, are the percentage of body fat, the amount of lean body mass, and the ability to perform successfully. If an athlete's body fat interferes with performance, steps should be taken to correct this problem (i.e., reduce the body fat). In general, among most athletes a combination of appropriate training and sound nutrition produces optimal body composition values.

As noted in the previous chapter, athletes, especially heavier athletes such as football linemen and throwers, may continue to eat very high caloric diets after their athletic career is finished. Often, these retired athletes continue with their old eating patterns but with a reduced energy expenditure as a result of reducing the volume and intensity of their physical training program; this pattern will likely result in some level of obesity. Strength and conditioning professionals should be prepared to assist retired athletes to lose weight before obesity becomes a major health problem.

BULIMIA NERVOSA

Bulimia nervosa and anorexia nervosa are listed as mental disorders in *Diagnostic and Statistical Manual of Mental Disorders*, 3rd edition, revised (*DSM-IIIR*), published by the American Psychiatric Association (2). Neither condition was defined in previous editions of the manual (which were published before 1980), and bulimia in particular was considered a rare disorder before 1980. **Bulimia nervosa** may be defined as an abnormal and constant craving for food. Approximately 1% to 2% of American women and 0.1% to 0.2% of American men are bulimic (7-9). Bulimia usually begins in adolescence. In extreme cases, the bulimic patient may steal in order to maintain the expensive habit of food bingeing.

The *DSM-IIIR* diagnostic criteria for bulimia are listed as follows (2):

1. Recurrent episodes of binge eating (rapid consumption of a large amount of food in short periods of time, often less than 2 hr)
2. Three or more of the following:
   (a) Consumption of high-calorie food
   (b) Inconspicuous bingeing (often at night)
   (c) Termination of binges by abdominal pain, sleep, social interruption, or self-induced vomiting
   (d) Repeated attempts at losing weight by severely restrictive diets, self-induced vomiting, or use of cathartics or diuretics
   (e) Frequent weight fluctuations due to alternate binges and semistarvation
3. Awareness of abnormal eating patterns but a fear of not being able to stop the binges voluntarily
4. Depression and self-deprecating thoughts after binges

A primary characteristic of bulimia is the binge-purge eating pattern, which usually occurs more than once a week and often daily (1).

Bulimia may be a body image or self-concept disorder (3,10). The psychological manifestations of bulimia nervosa include

- preoccupation with food,
- pursuit of thinness,
- difficulty in expressing emotions,
- low tolerance for frustrations, and
- high need for approval.

Binge eating can create a number of medical problems, including

- stomach dilation and rupture,
- infection of the lungs from aspirating vomitus,

- infection and rupture of the esophagus,
- enlargement of the salivary glands,
- gum problems,
- tooth erosion and decay, and
- loss of electrolytes.

Among athletes, symptoms of bulimia in addition to those listed previously include unnecessary dieting and excessive exercise (beyond that needed for normal training); athletes may often "disappear" after eating (to vomit) (10). As a result of purging and loss of electrolytes, disturbance of the body's acid-base balance, poor thermoregulation (see chapter 13), and cardiac arrythmias can occur, which can markedly alter physical performance. Bulimic behavior can be especially prevalent in sports in which leanness is valued, such as gymnastics, diving, figure skating, and distance running (10). Bulimic behavior can also occur in sports in which the athlete must "make weight" on a regular basis, such as wrestling. It is not uncommon for athletes involved in these sports to purge, deprive themselves of food, abuse laxatives, and employ such thermal methods as saunas and rubber suits to make weight for competition. Even though most athletes use these methods only during the sport season, the practices should be discouraged by the strength and conditioning professional, because even performed intermittently or on an irregular basis they can affect the health of the athlete.

Treatment

Treatment of bulimia must begin with a discussion of the eating disorder with the affected person. Treatment usually includes psychological counseling aimed at behavior modification and nutritional and dietary guidance, the latter in conjunction with a registered dietician. Occasionally, a psychiatrist may prescribe drug therapy to assist in behavior modification (10).

The physical training programs of athletes with bulimia nervosa or bulimic behaviors may have to be modified, depending upon the health of the athlete. The strength and conditioning professional can work out appropriate modifications with the athletic trainer and team physician.

ANOREXIA NERVOSA

Anorexia nervosa is essentially self-starvation. Anorexia usually begins in adolescence, but may begin in childhood or adulthood (1). The *DSM-IIIR* diagnostic criteria for anorexia nervosa are listed as follows (2):

1. An intense fear of becoming obese, even as weight is lost and underweight is achieved

2. Disturbance of body image; claims of being or feeling fat even when emaciated
3. Loss of 25% or more of original body mass; in children, expected growth reduced by 15%
4. Amenorrhea (absence of three consecutive menstrual cycles) in women

Anorexia may consist of a single short-term episode or persist and become life threatening (1,10). In addition to weight loss, anorexia is often characterized by a deficit in the amount of body fat necessary to maintain good health (1).

The psychological characteristics of anorexia include

- preoccupation with food,
- irrational fear of being or becoming fat,
- a distorted body image,
- marked dissatisfaction with one's body,
- low self-esteem,
- depression, and
- irritability and anxiety (10).

Among athletes, additional symptoms often include claims of feeling fat, excessive exercise, resistance to weight gain, and unusual weighing behavior (excessive weighing or refusal to weigh oneself). Anorexia is associated with a variety of medical problems. The starvation and wasting affect every organ system and can result in death. Among athletes anorexia is associated with amenorrhea and connective tissue injuries.

Anorexia is not common among males. Between 1956 and 1958 the incidence of anorexic episodes in females was less than 4%; between 1973 and 1975 the incidence was about 17%, a fourfold increase. The current incidence of anorexia is believed to be somewhat higher (1,10). Part of the increase may be due to society's emphasis on thinness being beautiful. Among certain populations, such as female athletes—especially those involved in sports and other activities that demand low body mass, low body fat, or in which image is important (e.g., distance running, figure skating, and ballet)—the incidence is likely higher than in the nonathletic population (10). It should be noted that the exact influence that these sports have on the underlying psychological aspects of anorexia and bulimia is unclear. Information that these "thin" sports directly or indirectly cause eating disorders is lacking (5). It is possible that in many cases anorexics and bulimics are attracted to these sports because the sport allows their eating disorder to continue rather than causes it (4).

Treatment

Because anorexia nervosa stems from deep-seated emotional problems, long-term professional counseling, both psychological and nutritional, is necessary. Drug therapy may also be necessary to treat the psychological problems (4,10), and nutritional support is needed to reverse the effects of starvation.

More so than with other eating disorders in athletes, physical training programs must be greatly modified or stopped with anorexics; most anorexics should not be allowed to compete. However, modification of training and curtailing competition may worsen psychological symptoms (4,10). An athlete with anorexia (or bulimia) who is allowed to train or compete, even on a modified basis, should do so in conjunction with psychological and nutritional counseling and nutritional support if necessary (10).

APPROACHING AN ATHLETE WHO HAS AN EATING DISORDER

Identification of eating disorders can be difficult. Strength and conditioning professionals should familiarize themselves with the symptoms of eating disorders in order to better identify potential problems. Sometimes an athlete's eating disorder is brought to the coach's attention by a teammate. While the teammate should be reassured that the matter is not being taken lightly, discussing the problem with teammates is not appropriate, because gossip creates additional problems and may reinforce denial. It may be helpful to use a screening device such as the Eating Disorder Inventory with the entire team when eating disorders are suspected even in a single athlete (see reference 4). This would allow the athlete in question to take the first step in identifying a problem on his or her own.

When the strength and conditioning professional suspects an athlete of having an eating disorder, discussing the problem with the athlete can be difficult because the athlete often denies the problem, out of embarrassment or fear of disapproval by teammates or coaches, of not being allowed to compete, or of being dismissed from the team (10). Difficult as broaching the subject may be, someone should approach an athlete suspected of having an eating disorder as soon as possible. Care should be taken in selecting the person who approaches the athlete. It should be someone in a position of authority, but someone who has good rapport with the athlete, such as a coach, athletic trainer, or physician. A teammate is usually inappropriate, because he or she does not bear the authority of the athletic staff and may be more easily dismissed by the athlete. Furthermore, this could place a burden of responsibility on the teammate that he or she is not ready for emotionally or is simply not willing to accept (10). It is important that the person approaching the athlete realize the importance and implications of assisting the athlete in finding help. Too often, even a coach may join the athlete in denial because he or she does not want to lose the athlete from competition. Thus, if a strength and conditioning professional suspects an athlete of an eating disorder, it is important that he or she follow up with the person contacting the athlete to ensure that referral to a clinician (counselor or physician) was made and what treatment, if any, ensued.

The strength and conditioning professional should work with the clinician to make appropriate modifications in the athlete's training program, if necessary. Modifications in the training program may include reductions in volume and intensity or changing the type of exercises used. It should always be understood that the athlete's health takes precedence over his or her athletic career. However, it should be made clear to the athlete that every effort will be made to preserve his or her position and status on the team (4).

CONCLUSION

A strength and conditioning professional may encounter three types of eating disorders: obesity, bulimia nervosa, and anorexia nervosa. The most common of these is obesity. The strength and conditioning professional can assist the obese person in losing body mass and body fat by recommending a combination of diet and exercise (see chapter 13). Moderately or severely obese persons should be referred to a physician. The strength and conditioning professional must be able to recognize the difference between heavy athletes and obese nonathletes. The professional should be aware of the need for heavy athletes to permanently reduce body mass when they retire and be willing to assist them in carrying out a reduction program.

Individuals recognized as bulimics or anorexics should be encouraged to seek professional counseling and appropriate medical supervision.

Key Terms

anorexia nervosa	240	bulimia nervosa	239	obesity	238
body mass index	238				

Study Questions

1. Generally, obesity is defined as

   a. a body mass index above 35
   b. a body mass index below 25
   c. excess body fat
   d. a proportion of body fat above 32%

2. Among athletes, obesity is most accurately described as

   a. men with a proportion of body fat greater than 25
   b. women with a proportion of body fat greater than 32
   c. an amount of body fat that interferes with performance
   d. excess body fat

3. The primary characteristic of bulimia nervosa is

   a. a very low proportion (<5%) of body fat
   b. vomiting
   c. binge-purge eating
   d. loss of electrolytes

4. Purging can upset the body's acid-base balance and affect thermoregulation as a result of

   a. loss of body mass
   b. vasoconstriction
   c. loss of electrolytes
   d. cardiac arrythmias

5. Sports in which anorexics are most likely to be found competing include

   a. golf, figure skating, and archery
   b. diving, figure skating, and powerlifting
   c. diving, distance running, and gymnastics
   d. distance running, powerlifting, and gymnastics

Applying Knowledge of Eating Disorders

Problem 1

The body composition of a starting football lineman includes 23% fat. Although it appears, based on the training table, that he eats well, making reasonable food choices and taking appropriate amounts, he is gaining weight and fat. He trains hard, but his performance is getting poorer. The coaches are concerned that his performance will decrease further. What should be done?

Problem 2

A distance runner has been losing weight for almost the entire cross-country season—to the point of looking emaciated. She has become amenorrheic. However, her time for the 10,000-m race is improving. Should anything be done? If so, what?

References

1. Agras, W.S. *Eating Disorders: Management of Obesity, Bulimia and Anorexia Nervosa.* New York: Pergamon Press. 1987.

2. American Psychiatric Association. *Diagnostic and Statistical Manual of Mental Disorders*. Washington: American Psychiatric Association. 1987.

3. Fairborn, C.G., and D.M. Garner. The diagnosis of bulimia nervosa. *Int. J. Eating Disord.* 5:403-420. 1986.

4. Garner, D.M., and L.W. Rosen. Eating disorders among athletes: Research and recommendations. *J. Appl. Sports Sci. Res.* 5(2):100-107. 1990.

5. Gleaves, D.H., D.A. Williamson, and R.D. Fuller. Bulimia nervosa symptomatology and body image disturbance associated with distance running and weight loss. *Br. J. Sports Med.* 26(3):157-160. 1992.

6. Jequier, E. Energy, obesity and body weight standards. *Am. J. Clin. Nutr.* 45:1035-1047. 1987.

7. Nieman, D.C. *Fitness and Sports Medicine*. Palo Alto, CA: Bull. 1987.

8. Nieman, D.C. *Fitness and Your Health*. Palo Alto, CA: Bull. 1993.

9. Nieman, D.C., D.E. Butterworth, and C.E. Nieman. *Nutrition*. Dubuque, IA: Brown. 1992.

10. Thompson, R.A., and R.T. Sherman. *Helping Athletes with Eating Disorders*. Champaign, IL: Human Kinetics. 1993.

11. Schull, W.J. Heredity, fitness and health. In: *Exercise, Fitness and Health*, C. Bouchard, R.J. Shepard, T. Stephens, J.R. Sutton, and B.D. McPherson, eds. Champaign, IL: Human Kinetics. 1990. pp. 137-145.

PART II

TESTING
AND EVALUATION

OVERVIEW OF PART II

Strength and conditioning professionals base many of their decisions on the results of tests that they administer to athletes before, during, and after a training period. A **test** is a specific means of assessing someone's ability in a particular endeavor, in this case, a physical activity (1). Test results provide the strength and conditioning professional with a means of assessing athletic talent, screening for possible health risks that may preclude strenuous exercise, and identifying specific weaknesses; they may also serve as a basis for developing individual exercise prescriptions (2, 12). **Field tests** are tests that assess specific athletic talents in an applied setting (8). The term **measurement** refers to the collection of data upon which a decision is based (3), and **evaluation** is the process of analyzing test and measurement results for the purpose of making decisions; evaluation gives meaning to tests and measurements. (The terms *test*, *measurement*, and *evaluation* are often used interchangeably, but as the definitions here indicate, they have distinct meanings.)

The professional with a broad understanding of exercise science can effectively use the results of tests and measurements to make appropriate decisions concerning training methods for achieving program goals and helping athletes achieve their potential. Tests and measurements form the objective core of the evaluation process.

A systematic model for evaluating strength and conditioning programs should include these components:

1. **Program objectives** give direction to the training program. It is important at the outset to have a clear understanding of what is to be accomplished.
2. **Preassessment** tests allow the training and conditioning professional to determine the training level of the athletes and serve as a guide for program design and implementation.
3. The **training prescription** is thoughtfully designed to achieve overall program objectives and forms the heart of the conditioning regimen.
4. **Postassessment** tests involve the selection or development of specific measures of an athlete's achievement of the program objectives.
5. *Evaluation* of the training prescription uses the results of tests to make decisions as to whether or not the program objectives were achieved.

Evaluation that runs concurrent with the learning process is known as **formative evaluation** (5). Formative evaluations are tests that occur at regular intervals in the training program. They help the strength and conditioning professional and the athlete to determine the degree of mastery achieved so far and to pinpoint areas of the exercise prescription requiring emphasis relative to the individual needs of the athlete. Periodic testing also allows the strength and conditioning professional to evaluate different training methods, to collect normative data, and to evaluate his or her own effectiveness. Testing and evaluation also help athletes to assess their strengths and weaknesses while making the training prescription more interesting and intrinsically motivational.

This section will focus on basic abilities of the motor performance domain. However, in the design of training programs for athletes, testing in a broader sense will include a number of *parameters of physical fitness*, defined as follows:

• **Muscular strength** is the force that a muscle or muscle group can exert against a resistance in one maximal effort (2, 4, 6, 9). A practical test for muscular strength is a 1RM (repetition maximum) bench press.

• **Local muscular endurance** is the ability of a muscle or muscle group to perform repeated contractions against a light (submaximal) load for an extended period of time (2, 6, 9). A practical test for local muscular endurance is the maximum number of bent-knee sit-ups a person can do.

• **Aerobic power** is the amount of work a person can perform, normally determined by the rate at which oxygen is utilized during exercise (3). A practical test of aerobic power is Cooper's Timed 1.5-Mile Run (8).

• **Anaerobic power** is the amount of work performed using primarily anaerobic energy systems. Anaerobic power is strongly related to explosive movements (3, 5, 10, 11). A practical test of anaerobic power is the vertical (Sargent) jump.

• **Agility** is the ability to change the direction of the body or body parts rapidly under control (3). A practical test of agility is the T-test (13).

• **Speed** is the rapidity of movement (3). Most practical tests of speed involve running—for example, 60-m sprint (3).

• **Flexibility** is the range of motion about a joint (3). A practical test for flexibility is the sit-and-reach test. Other tests use a **goniometer**, which is a mechanical device that measures the range of motion about a joint.

• **Body composition** refers to the relative proportions by weight of body fat and lean mass. Skinfold measurements, for example, are used to determine percentage of body fat (3).

• **Anthropometry** is the measurement of the size (including height), weight, and proportions (including overall girth and limb girths) of the human body (7).

Chapters 15 to 18 offer guidelines for appropriate test selection, organization of test procedures, testing protocols, and evaluation of test data. A comprehensive testing and evaluation program allows the strength and conditioning professional to bridge the gap between exercise science knowledge and practical application (2).

Key Terms

References

1. Allerheiligen, B., J. Arce, M. Arthur, D. Chu, A. Vermeil, L. Lilja, D. Semenick, B. Ward, and M. Woicik. Testing for football. *NSCA Journal* 5(5):12-68. 1983.
2. Altug, Z., T. Altug, and A. Altug. A test selection guide for assessing and evaluating athletes. *NSCA Journal* 9(3):67-69. 1987.
3. Anderson, B. Flexibility testing. *NSCA Journal* 3(2):20-23. 1981.
4. Astrand, P., and K. Rodahl. *Textbook of Work Physiology: Physiological Basis of Exercise.* New York: McGraw-Hill. 1986.
5. Baumgartner, T., and A. Jackson. *Measurement for Evaluation in Physical Education and Exercise Science.* Dubuque, IA: Brown. 1987.
6. Behnke, A., and J. Wilmore. *Evaluation and Regulation of Body Build and Composition.* Englewood Cliffs, NJ: Prentice Hall. 1974.
7. Burke, E. *Toward an Understanding of Human Performance.* Ithaca, NY: Mouvement. 1980.
8. Chu, D., and A. Vermeil. The rationale for field testing. *NSCA Journal* 5(2):35-36. 1983.
9. Cooper, K. *The New Aerobics.* New York: Bantam Books. 1972.

10. Harmon, E., M. Rosenstein, P. Frykman, R. Rosenstein, and W. Kraemer. Estimation of human power output from maximal vertical jump and body mass. *J. Appl. Sport Sci. Res.* In press.

11. Kalamen, J. Measurement of maximum muscular power in man. Doctoral dissertation, The Ohio State University, 1968.

12. Kontor, K. Testing and evaluation. *NSCA Journal* 3(2):7. 1981.

13. Semenick, D. Tests and measurements: The T-test. *NSCA Journal* 12(1):36-37. 1990.

CHAPTER 15

SELECTING APPROPRIATE TESTS

Douglas M. Semenick

The three most important characteristics of a test are validity, reliability, and objectivity. If a test does not fulfill these requirements, it will not produce acceptable measurements for evaluation.

VALIDITY

Validity refers to the degree to which a test measures what it is supposed to measure and is the most important characteristic of testing (3, 12-14, 17). There are four types of validity: content validity, concurrent validity, predictive validity, and construct validity.

Content validity—a technique based on the subjectively established fact that the test measures the wanted content (also called face validity)

Concurrent validity—the degree to which scores on a test correlate with scores on an accepted standard

Predictive validity—the degree to which one measure can predict performance on a second measure

Construct validity—the degree to which a test measures some part of a whole skill or an abstract trait (3)

The primary interest of the strength and conditioning specialist in the selection of field tests is construct validity. The objective measurement tool for establishing construct validity is the **criterion variable**, which is the score used to represent a participant's ability at some part of a whole skill or an abstract trait. Examples of constructs encountered by the strength and conditioning professional include jumping ability, running ability,

and muscular strength of the arms (14). Construct validity assumes that the athletes who score high on a performance test (e.g., the vertical jump) will score higher on the criterion variable (e.g., demonstration of power by a baseball player) than athletes who score low on the performance test (1).

RELIABILITY

Reliability refers to the degree of consistency with which a test measures what it measures; it is essentially repeatability of the test (3, 14, 17). When an athlete whose ability has not changed is measured two times with a perfectly reliable test, the two scores will be identical. Any variance in the two scores represents **measurement error**, which can arise from any of the following factors (3):

- Lack of agreement among scorers
- Lack of consistent performance by the person tested
- Failure of an instrument to measure consistently
- Failure of the tester to follow standardized testing procedures
- Failure of the tester to calibrate the testing instrument

For a measure to be valid it must be reliable, but a reliable test may not be valid, because the test may not measure what it is supposed to measure. For example, both the 60-m dash and the 1.5-mile run are reliable field tests, but only the 1.5-mile run is considered a valid field test for cardiovascular fitness. It is also possible for a test to be highly reliable for one group (e.g., college tennis players) and to be only moderately reliable for another group (e.g., high school tennis players), due to physical maturity factors.

OBJECTIVITY

Objectivity is the degree to which multiple scorers agree on the magnitude of scores. This is also known as *interrater reliability* or *interrater agreement* (3, 14, 17). To enhance test objectivity, it is essential to have a clearly defined scoring system and a competent scorer. The scorer should be trained and have experience with the testing instruments being used. For example, if a scorer is measuring time in the 40-yd dash with a stopwatch, he or she should be familiar enough with a stopwatch to know precisely when and how to start and stop it; otherwise, an inaccurate score may be recorded for the test.

A high degree of objectivity is essential when two scorers are administering a test to two subgroups of athletes. If one scorer is more lenient than the other, his or her subgroup are at an unfair advantage. The same scorer should test a group at the beginning and the end of the training period. If there are two scorers and the scorer at the beginning is more or less lenient than the scorer at the end, the resultant measurements may be worthless for comparative purposes. Consider a situation in which an athlete is tested in the back squat. If the pretest scorer is more lenient (requiring less depth on the squat) than the posttest scorer, the athlete may achieve a lower test score on the posttest, even though he or she may have made significant strength improvement.

Perhaps the most common scenario in which objectivity is lacking involves the coach with a strong personal commitment to the athlete. The commitment may influence the coach to see what he or she wants to see, resulting in inflated test results (6, 13, 15). Accurate and consistent athletic testing should be the goal of all strength and conditioning professionals.

SELECTING VALID, RELIABLE, AND OBJECTIVE TESTS

When selecting tests for high levels of validity, reliability, and objectivity, the strength and conditioning professional must rely on his or her academic and practical experience in the sport. A thorough understanding of the three basic energy systems (ATP-CP, glycolytic, oxidative), their interrelationships, and the principle of

specificity of training will allow the professional to choose or design valid and reliable tests for measurement of athletic ability in a specific sport (7, 8, 11, 16, 18-20). A superficial understanding of these systems and principles (e.g., knowing the difference between aerobic and anaerobic power) is insufficient; an in-depth understanding of the scientific principles and the sport itself is required. For example, in choosing an appropriate test for running ability in basketball, the strength and conditioning professional must not only understand that basketball is predominantly an anaerobic running sport (9, 10), but should also understand the specific physical demands of a basketball game well enough to choose an appropriate anaerobic power test that simulates the energy demands of a real game.

By understanding the various levels of anaerobic field testing (see Table 17.2 on p. 260), a professional will be able to make defensible decisions with regard to which test to use (20). (Each of the categories in Table 17.2 refers to a discrete set of movements that define a subset of anaerobic performance.) The professional should give the same careful consideration when selecting field tests for measuring a parameter of athletic fitness relative to aerobic fitness, strength, and other major areas.

In choosing the most valid and reliable tests for a specific athletic activity, several additional considerations are warranted:

1. *Age-related factors.* The 1.5-mile run may be a valid and reliable field test of aerobic power for college-age males and females (5), but may not be appropriate for preadolescents, owing to lack of experience and motivation (2).

2. *Sex-related factors.* Chin-ups may be a valid and reliable test for upper body strength and endurance for male wrestlers, but they are not a valid and reliable test for females in any sport, because most females lack sufficient upper body strength to complete several chin-up movements.

3. *Experience-related factors.* The 25-m one-leg hop may represent a valid and reliable test of elastic strength for an experienced long jumper (4). However, for a novice long jumper it may not be appropriate.

4. *Environmental factors.* Be aware of environmental extremes, such as altitude, heat, and humidity, when choosing many athletic fitness tests.

5. *Positions within the sport.* A valid and reliable upper body strength test for basketball centers may be indicative of basketball playing ability. However, it may not be a valid and reliable test for measuring the playing ability of guards or forwards.

6. *Unbiased test.* An unbiased test is one that takes into account the activity for which the athlete

has been training and the energy requirements of that activity. It would not be fair, for example, to ask a baseball player to perform a 3-mile run test 1 week before the beginning of fall practice, because he has probably been doing interval training and relatively short runs (7). A strength test using free-weight equipment may not be fair to the athlete who has been training exclusively with isokinetic equipment. A lower body strength test using the parallel squat would not be a fair test for the athlete who has trained exclusively using the leg press.

The most important criterion in athletic testing is the ability to play the game. A valid and reliable test for assessing athletic ability in any sport should meet the following 10 criteria (1):

1. It should measure important abilities (be relevant).
2. It should involve gamelike situations.
3. It should encourage good form.
4. It should involve one performer only.
5. It should be interesting and meaningful.
6. It should be of suitable difficulty.
7. It should differentiate between levels of ability.
8. It should provide accurate scoring.
9. It should provide a sufficient number of trials.
10. It should be judged by statistical evidence.

Given the choice between two valid and reliable tests, the strength and conditioning professional should give consideration to simplicity and economy of test administration.

CONCLUSION

Only through valid, reliable, and objective tests can one accurately measure an individual's abilities. In order to select valid, reliable, and objective tests, the strength and conditioning professional must have thorough knowledge of the sport in which the athlete participates and the three basic energy systems.

Key Terms

concurrent validity	250	criterion variable	250	predictive validity	250
construct validity	250	measurement error	250	reliability	250
content validity	250	objectivity	251	validity	250

Study Questions

1. Which of the following would be the greatest source of measurement error?

   a. testing conducted by an inexperienced tester
   b. recording the average of three trials and not the best as the criterion score
   c. not allowing the participant any practice trials before testing
   d. failure of the tester to follow standardized testing procedures

2. The best test for assessing the running ability of high school basketball players 1 week before the beginning of preseason basketball practice in the fall would be

   a. a 1.5-mile run
   b. the line drill test
   c. a 12-min run
   d. a 40-yd dash

3. A high school soccer player has been training for 1 year by performing distance runs, short-interval sprints, and strength training with a multistation exercise machine. Which of the following batteries of tests would be the most valid and reliable for assessing strength, local muscular endurance, and aerobic capacity?

   a. 5RM leg press, 1.5-mile run, maximum number of chin-ups
   b. 5RM squat, 12-min run, maximum number of chin-ups
   c. 1RM leg press, 1.5-mile run, maximum push-ups in 2 min
   d. 2RM squat, 12-min run, maximum push-ups in 2 min

4. A swimming test whose mean score is consistently higher for an advanced swimmer compared with a novice swimmer would indicate

a. construct validity
b. predictive validity
c. content validity
d. concurrent validity

Applying Knowledge of Test Selection

Problem 1
You have been given the assignment to develop a testing battery for use in assessing the physical conditioning program of a high school soccer team. In deciding what tests to use, what preparatory information is necessary to choose the most appropriate test for the target group?

Problem 2
Why is it of prime importance that physical conditioning and sport-specific tests have a high degree of validity and reliability and that they be administered in an objective manner? What criteria would you consider when selecting the most valid and reliable tests for your target population?

References

1. Allerheiligen, B., J. Arce, M. Arthur, D. Chu, A. Vermeil, L. Lilja, D. Semenick, B. Ward, and M. Woicik. Testing for football. *NSCA Journal* 5(5):12-68. 1983.
2. American Alliance for Health, Physical Education, Recreation and Dance. *AAHPERD Health Related Fitness Test.* Reston, VA: Author. 1980.
3. Baumgartner, T., and A. Jackson. *Measurement for Evaluation in Physical Education and Exercise Science.* Dubuque, IA: Brown. 1987.
4. Chu, D., and A. Vermeil. The rationale for field testing. *NSCA Journal* 5(2):35-36. 1983.
5. Cooper, K. *The New Aerobics.* New York: Bantam Books. 1972.
6. Epley, B. The Nebraska timer: A simple, accurate way to measure the 40-yard dash. *NSCA Journal* 4(5):14-15. 1982.
7. Fleck, S., and M. Marks. Interval training. *NSCA Journal* 5(5):40-62. 1983.
8. Fox, E., and D. Mathews. *The Physiological Basis of Physical Education and Athletics.* Philadelphia: Saunders. 1981.
9. Garl, T., L. Rink, and B. Bomba. Evaluating basketball conditioning. *NSCA Journal* 10(4):46-47. 1988.
10. Gilliam, G. Basketball bioenergetics: Physiological basis. *NSCA Journal* 6(6):44-73. 1985.
11. Gilliam, G., and M. Marks. 300-yard shuttle run. *NSCA Journal* 5(5):46. 1983.
12. Hastad, D.N., and A.C. Lacy. *Measurement and Evaluation in Contemporary Physical Education.* Scottsdale, AZ: Gorsuch. 1989.
13. Hopkins, C. *Understanding Educational Research.* Columbus, OH: Merrill. 1980.
14. Johnson, B., and J. Nelson. *Practical Measurements for Evaluation in Physical Education*, 2nd ed. Minneapolis: Burgess. 1974.
15. Kontor, K. Truth in testing. *NSCA Journal* 3(6):11. 1982.
16. Kraemer, W., and S. Fleck. Anaerobic metabolism and its evaluation. *NSCA Journal* 4(2):20-21. 1982.
17. Safrit, M. *Evaluation in Physical Education.* Englewood Cliffs, NJ: Prentice Hall. 1980.
18. Stone, M., H. Newton, and H. O'Bryant. Anaerobic capacity. *NSCA Journal* 5(6):40-41. 1984.
19. Stone, M., and H. O'Bryant. *Weight Training: A Scientific Approach.* Minneapolis: Burgess. 1987.
20. Tesch, P. Anaerobic testing: Practical applications. *NSCA Journal* 6(5):44-73. 1984.

CHAPTER 16

ORGANIZING TESTING PROCEDURES

Douglas M. Semenick

Once the strength and conditioning professional has chosen appropriate tests, as explained in the previous chapter, he or she needs to organize and administer the battery of tests in a manner that will yield valid, objective, and reliable results. This chapter will serve as a practical guide for the organizing process that takes place prior to actual testing.

TEST AND EVALUATION FORMAT

The person planning the tests needs to decide how the test will be conducted. For example, will the athletes be tested all at once or in groups? Will one person do all the testing or will athletes test each other in pairs? If time and personal schedules permit, one competent test administrator (also called a test supervisor) should do all the testing. If this is not feasible, the test administrator can allow simple, well-defined tests (such as measuring sit-and-reach flexibility or counting correct chin-ups) to be tested by additional test supervisors or athletes in pairs and have more sophisticated tests (such as judging depth in the squat) be scored by the supervising test administrator. The strength and conditioning professional must be able to judge whether the athletes are capable of testing one another.

As a rule, the tester should judge only one test at a time, especially when complex judgments have to be made. It is permissible, however, to position one tester between certain testing stations to judge two tests. The

tester's undivided attention should be focused on only the test being performed.

ORGANIZING TIME

When time is limited and there is a large group of athletes, duplicate test set-ups may be employed to make efficient use of testing time. For example, when conducting the 300-yd shuttle run, two test courses can be made available (3). A tester may administer up to two nonfatiguing tests if test reliability can be maintained. For example, when administering a test battery that includes a two-test flexibility station with only 1 tester at the station, the athlete being measured could be instructed to perform the sit-and-reach test first, then assume a prone position to perform the shoulder elevation test before moving to the next testing station.

SEQUENCE OF TESTS

The strength and conditioning professional needs to draw on his or her knowledge of exercise science to determine the proper order of tests and the duration of rest periods between tests to ensure test reliability. For example, a test that maximally taxes the phosphagen energy system requires 3 to 5 min of rest for complete recovery (5, 6), whereas a maximal test of the lactic acid energy system requires at least 1 hr for complete recovery (2). Therefore, tests requiring high-skill movements, such as reaction and coordination tests, should be administered before tests that are likely to produce fatigue and confound the results of subsequent tests. Several trials of a nonfatiguing test are necessary to discern best performance. These tests should be followed by brief strength and power tests assuming these tests are in the testing battery. Very fatiguing anaerobic capacity tests, such as 400- or 800-m runs, should be performed last.

DEVELOPING SCORING FORMS

Individual scoring forms should be developed prior to the testing session. Each athlete should receive a form with his or her name and all the tests printed on it before the testing period begins. This allows resting time to be used more efficiently and reduces the incidence of recording errors. Individual scoring forms allow athletes to rotate among testing stations and to quickly record scores (1). An example of an individual scoring form is shown below.

TRAINING TEST ADMINISTRATORS

Test administrators should be trained sufficiently and have a thorough understanding of all testing procedures

Individual Scoring Form

Name: Joe Smith   Date: 3/7/94

Sport: Basketball

Test	Score
1.5-mile run (min:s)	_____
Line drill (min:s)	_____
Bench press (lb)	_____
Parallel squat (lb)	_____
Bent knee sit-ups (no. in 2 min)	_____
Vertical jump (in.)	_____
Edgren Side Step (points)	_____
Shoulder elevation (in.)	_____
Sit and reach (in.)	_____
Body composition (% body fat)	_____

and protocols. The strength and conditioning professional should give special attention to novice test administrators, particularly to their scoring objectivity. For example, a test administrator who is unfamiliar with using a stopwatch for timing speed tests or with judging depth in the back squat needs practice under the direction of a qualified person before testing begins.

The test administrator should read the test instructions and determine how he or she will present them and how the student will perceive them. The test administrator and support personnel should review test procedures and protocols at least once before testing begins. It is advisable to conduct a mock testing session prior to administering a complex testing battery to ensure smooth and efficient test administration when measurements are to be recorded. The test administrator should have a checklist of materials needed for testing and written test protocols to refer to before and during the testing process.

PREPARING ATHLETES

The date and time and the purpose of a test battery should be announced in advance of the test date to allow athletes to prepare physically and psychologically to perform at their best. To maximize test reliability, athletes should be familiar with test content and procedures. A short, supervised pretest practice session on the day before the test is often beneficial.

GIVING TEST INSTRUCTIONS

The clarity and simplicity of instructions have a direct bearing on the reliability and objectivity of a test (4). Instructions should specify policy concerning warm-up and practice attempts, how the test is to be performed, how many trials will be allowed, how the test will be scored, the policy regarding a subject's incorrectly performing any part of the test, and recommendations for maximizing performance.

The test administrator should demonstrate proper test performance when possible; this is much more effective than merely reading the instructions aloud. The administrator should anticipate questions and have answers prepared and motivate athletes equally and not give special encouragement to some.

CONCLUSION

Validity and reliability are highest when the test administrators are organized and competent, the athletes are informed in advance of testing, they are prepared physically and psychologically for testing, they are motivated to do well, and the testing environment is suitable for good performance.

Study Questions

1. Arrange the following tests in the proper sequence so that test reliability is not adversely affected:

   I.   1RM bench press
   II. 1RM power clean
   III. 400-m run
   IV. chin-ups
   V.   agility run

   a. V, II, I, IV, III
   b. II, I, V, III, IV
   c. I, II, V, IV, III
   d. V, I, II, III, IV

2. When scoring several tests with numerous athletes, the most efficient procedure would be to

   a. have one coach score all athletes with a master scoring form
   b. have one coach score all athletes with individual scoring forms
   c. have the athletes carry individual scoring forms and rotate among stations
   d. have the athletes sign up on a master scoring form and rotate among stations

3. Which of the following procedures would yield the most reliable test results with the most efficient use of time?

   a. vertical jump, rest 10 min, chin-ups, rest 10 min, push-ups, rest 10 min, 400-m run
   b. vertical jump, move directly to chin-ups, rest 2 min, push-ups, rest 2 min, 400-m run
   c. vertical jump, rest 10 min, push-ups, rest 10 min, chin-ups, rest 10 min, 400-m run
   d. vertical jump, move directly to chin-ups, rest 10 min, push-ups, rest 10 min, 400-m run

4. Which of the following groups of tests could best be conducted by pairs of athletes testing each other?

   a. 1RM squat, 1RM bench press, 1RM power clean
   b. push-ups, chin-ups, sit and reach
   c. 40-yd dash, push-ups, chin-ups
   d. push-ups, sit-ups, agility run

Applying Knowledge of Organizing Testing Procedures

Problem 1

You and an assistant are in charge of physical testing for the lacrosse team. After a general warm-up, the tests to be conducted are Edgren Side Step (agility), 40-yd dash (running speed), line drill (anaerobic capacity), and 1RM squat (lower body strength). There are 20 athletes to be tested and the testing is to be completed in one 2-hr practice session. Describe how you would organize the testing session (i.e., the testing order and rest periods necessary between trials and testing events).

Problem 2

You are preparing two assistants to administer the testing battery in problem 1. One administrator has two years of experience conducting athletic fitness tests, the other test administrator is a novice. Describe what steps you would follow to prepare these test administrators (i.e., pretest procedures, which tests would be assigned to each administrator, how the instructions and demonstrations should be presented, etc.). What preparations should the athletes make to ensure collection of valid and reliable data?

References

1. Baumgartner, T., and A. Jackson. *Measurement for Evaluation in Physical Education and Exercise Science*. Dubuque, IA: Brown. 1987.

2. Fox, E., and D. Mathews. *The Physiological Basis of Physical Education and Athletics*. Philadelphia: Saunders. 1981.

3. Gilliam, G., and M. Marks. 300-yd shuttle run. *NSCA Journal* 5(5):46. 1983.

4. Johnson, B., and J. Nelson. *Practical Measurements for Evaluation in Physical Education*, 2nd ed. Minneapolis: Burgess. 1974.

5. Kraemer, W., and S. Fleck. Anaerobic metabolism and its evaluation. *NSCA Journal* 4(2):20-21. 1982.

6. Margaria, R., P. Carretelli, P. diPrampero, C. Massori, and G. Torelli. Kinetics and mechanism of oxygen debt contraction in man. *J. Appl. Physiol.* 18:371-377. 1963.

CHAPTER 17

TESTING PROTOCOLS AND PROCEDURES

Douglas M. Semenick

The cornerstone of meaningful testing and evaluation is the selection and administration of valid and reliable tests, as well as the ability of the test administrators to perform with a high degree of objectivity.

ADMINISTERING TESTS

To administer valid tests that have a high degree of reliability and objectivity, the strength and conditioning professional needs to give consideration to the following seven areas, some of which were touched upon in the previous chapter.

Test Supervision

Test reliability is directly proportional to the quality of the test administrator. Always conduct athletic testing with a qualified, competent test supervisor present.

Warm-Up

Reliability improves with pretest warm-up (4). An appropriate organized warm-up consists of a general warm-up followed by a specific warm-up. Both types of warm-ups include movements similar to the particular skill to be tested. An instructor-led organized (general) warm-up ensures that all athletes have the same amount of practice. It is acceptable to allow the first two or three trials of a test to serve as the activity-specific warm-up and to record the best or average of subsequent

trials as the **criterion score** (the score actually recorded and used to represent the person's ability) (4).

Preparation

The athletes undergoing testing should have a thorough understanding of the purpose and procedures of all tests prior to actually performing them. If possible, the test administrator or a competent nonparticipant should demonstrate each test. The athletes should be given opportunities to ask questions before and after the demonstration. It is acceptable to allow the athletes to run through a practice trial before testing begins.

Motivation

Offer encouragement to all participants equally. Whenever possible, let athletes know test scores immediately after a test trial; this tends to motivate them to perform better on subsequent trials (4).

Safety

Anticipate and watch closely for safety problems. Be sure that the testing area is large enough and free of clutter. Running, throwing, and agility drills should be conducted on large nonslip surfaces. Proper footwear is essential; for example, an agility drill requiring intensive lateral change of direction performed in shoes designed for distance running is likely to result in an ankle injury. It is advisable to use soft, unbreakable marking devices; chairs, soda bottles, volleyball standards, and the like are not appropriate. When conducting lateral jumping tests, use cones, not a ball or rigid standard, which may cause the athlete to trip and fall.

Organize and supervise the testing session to prevent mishaps that could occur from a lack of alertness by the participants. Always have spotters appropriately stationed during testing. Do not allow an athlete to perform muscular-strength testing that puts weight on the vertebral column (e.g., the back squat) with near-maximum or maximum loads without having him or her wear a prescribed lifting belt (13).

Multiple Test Trials and Testing Batteries

When multiple trials of a test or a battery of tests are to be performed, allow the participant complete recovery between test trials and between the different tests. For example, when conducting multiple trials of a test of **1RM strength** (one repetition maximum: the maximum amount of weight a person can lift once) (31), allow at least 2 to 3 min of rest between attempts. When administering a testing battery (e.g., one in which wrestlers will perform maximal-repetition pull-up and push-up tests to assess strength and local muscular endurance), separate tests by at least 5 min to prevent the effects of fatigue from confounding test results. (See also "Sequence of Tests," p. 254.)

Cool-Down

Administer a supervised cool-down period to athletes after certain fatiguing tests and at the completion of the test battery. For example, after completion of the 300-yd shuttle run, the athlete should not lie down; low-intensity movement and light stretching will enhance the recovery process.

HEALTH AND FITNESS FIELD TESTS

Chapter 15 discussed the criteria to be used in selecting an appropriate test. Here we look at the purpose and protocols of several health and fitness field tests. Detailed protocols for most of the tests mentioned are on pages 262 to 271 at the end of this chapter. Table 17.1 summarizes appropriate tests for various fitness parameters.

Muscular Strength

Muscular strength is the force that a muscle or muscle group can exert against a resistance in one maximal effort (4). Typically, 1RM strength tests, including 1RM back squats and bench presses, are used to measure this parameter of fitness. In general, the athlete begins his

Table 17.1 Practical Analysis of Athletic Fitness Parameters

Athletic fitness parameter	Practical tests	Typical equipment	Suggested readings
Muscular strength	1RM tests	Free weights, dynamometer, isokinetic equipment (e.g., Cybex)	1, 4, 6, 9, 14, 15, 20, 21, 22, 27, 29
Local muscular endurance	Chin-ups, push-ups, dips	Chin-up/dip bars, free weights, isokinetic equipment	1, 15, 21, 22
Aerobic power	2-mile run, 12-min run, 3-min step test	Stopwatch, running track, treadmill, cycle ergometer, step, metronome	1, 5, 11, 14, 15, 16, 21, 22, 27, 30
Anaerobic power	Vertical jump, line drill, medicine ball put, Wingate Test, 300-yd shuttle run	Vertical jump scale, medicine ball, cycle ergometer, stopwatch, running track	1, 5, 9, 11, 13, 14, 15, 19, 22, 25, 27, 29
Agility	T-test, Edgren Side Step	Stopwatch, course, shoes, electronic timer	1, 7, 9, 15, 22, 24
Speed	10- to 60-yd dash	Stopwatch, track, shoes, electronic timer, gymnasium floor	1, 8, 9, 11, 14, 15, 22, 27
Flexibility	Sit and reach	Goniometer, sit-and-reach box, meter stick	1, 2, 3, 5, 14, 15, 21, 29
Body composition	Sum of skinfolds	Skinfold calipers	1, 5, 12, 14, 15, 21, 27
Anthropometry	Height, weight, girth measurements	Tape measure, Gulich tape, balance scale, right angle	1, 9, 15, 21, 27

or her single repetition attempts at 50% of subjective predicted maximum, then 75%, 90%, and finally 100% and above if successful. The test supervisor must be present during strength testing. Station one or more spotters where needed and enforce correct form at all times. Discourage improper procedures, such as bouncing the bar on the chest, lifting the hips off the bench during the bench press, and not achieving proper depth in the squat; warn athletes that such violations will result in automatic disqualification of the attempt (13).

Local Muscular Endurance

Local muscular endurance is the ability to persist in physical activity or to resist fatigue (4). Tests of local muscular endurance should require the athlete to perform the test in a continuous manner without advantageous rest periods or extraneous body movements. Examples of local muscular endurance tests are maximal repetitions of chin-ups, push-ups, and parallel bar dips. Procedures for local muscular endurance tests are found on pages 262 and 263.

Aerobic Power

Aerobic power is the amount of work a person can perform, normally determined by the rate at which oxygen is utilized during exercise (4). The test administrator should be fully aware of testing protocols, procedures, and equipment for aerobic field tests. Many aerobic tests may require the supervisor to be competent in the use of a **metronome** (a device that emits a regularly repeated tick) and in taking the athlete's pulse. To ensure test reliability, the tester should palpate the pulse with his or her fingertips, not the thumb. The pulse is easily located above the carotid artery in the neck, proximal

to the thumb on the dorsal side of the supinated wrist, and adjacent to the ear on the temple. Count the pulse for at least 10 s and convert to heartbeats per minute. Procedures for the 3-minute step test and the 2-mile run are found on pages 264 to 265.

Anaerobic Power

Anaerobic power is the ability to perform brief (< 2 min) maximal muscular activity. A variety of tests measure anaerobic power in the upper and lower body (30). The strength and conditioning professional should be familiar with the vertical jump test using a wall scale or a vertical jump scale (26). A disadvantage encountered with using a wall scale is the tendency of the athlete to hit the wall with his or her body while performing the jump.

Table 17.2 lists several other tests for anaerobic power. The Category III and V tests listed in the table require the tester to coordinate trial times with a second timer, who measures the predetermined rest interval between trials. Procedures for the vertical jump test, a basketball time-drill test, and a 300-yard shuttle run are on pages 265 to 267.

Agility and Speed

Agility and speed tests require proper footwear and a nonslip running surface. Agility is the ability to stop, start, and change direction of body movements of less than 10 s in duration. Examples of agility tests are the T-test and the Edgren Side Step, which are explained on pages 268 to 269. Speed tests measure the body's displacement per unit of time (1). Examples of speed tests are sprints with distances of multiples of 10 m, up to 100 m.

Table 17.2   Categories of Anaerobic Field Testing

Category	Characteristics	Field test examples
I	A single explosive movement of less than 1 s in duration	Vertical jump Medicine ball put
II	A continuous-sequence movement (i.e., running) of less than 15 s in duration	50-yd sprint with running start
III	Multiple continuous sequence movements of less than 15 s in duration, separated by timed relief intervals	30- to 50-yd sprints
IV	A continuous-sequence movement of 15 s–2 min in duration	220-, 440-, and 880-yd sprints and runs Swimming 50, 100, 200 m Bicycling 880 yd–1 mile
V	Multiple continuous-sequence movements of 15 s–2 min in duration, each separated by timed relief intervals	Multiple 220-yd sprints 300-yd shuttle run

Adapted from Semenick (1981).

Agility and speed tests usually require a stopwatch, a significant source of measurement error if the tester is not sufficiently trained. Experienced testers should give novice testers explicit instructions as to when to start, how to start, and when to stop the watch. The most reliable and objective hand-held–stopwatch times are achieved by starting and stopping the stopwatch with the index finger, not the thumb. Stopwatch-measured sprint times can result in errors of up to 0.24 s, compared with electronic timing, even under ideal conditions (9, 10). Procedures for speed tests are found on page 269.

Body Composition

Body composition refers to the relative proportions by weight of body fat and lean mass. Skinfold measurements are the most valid and reliable measures ordinarily available to the strength and conditioning professional for the assessment of body fatness; they have greater validity for athletes than body circumference measures. Trained testers have been shown to produce highly reliable skinfold measurements ($r = 0.99$) (19). The **Sloan formula** is used for assessing the body composition of high school and college athletes. The Sloan formula was developed specifically for the male and female population of this age group. The Sloan formula for prediction of body density and percentage fat is as follows (28):

Body density = 1.0764 − [.00081 (suprailiac)]
  − [.00088 (triceps)] for females

  1.1043 − [.00133 (thigh)]
  − [.00131 (subscapular)] for males

Percentage fat = 100[4.570/(body density)] − 4.1421

Procedures for reliable and objective skinfold measurements require the tester to be competent in the use of **skinfold calipers**, an instrument designed to measure subcutaneous fat thickness by exerting a constant pressure regardless of the amount of fat being measured. Procedures for measuring skinfolds and exact sites for selected skinfold measurements are listed on page 270.

Anthropometry

Anthropometric measurements involve assessment of height, weight, and selected body girths. Measurement of height requires a flat surface against which the subject stands, a measuring tape or marked surface, and an object to place on the subject's head that forms a right angle to the wall. Height is usually measured without shoes to the nearest quarter inch (18).

Accurate body weight measurement is performed with a certified balance scale. Balance scales are more reliable than spring scales and should be calibrated on a regular basis (18). Weigh the subject in a minimum amount of clothing (e.g., gym shorts), in the same outfit, and at the same time of day for any subsequent measurements. The most reliable body weight measurements are taken early in the morning upon rising, after elimination, before breakfast.

Reliable girth measures are usually performed with the aid of a Gulich tape, which is equipped with a spring-loaded attachment that permits a slight amount of constant tension on the tape and therefore yields a more consistent measurement (29). Take girth measurements at the beginning of a training period to serve as a baseline for comparison with subsequent measures. The sites and protocols for measuring various body girths are on page 271.

Flexibility

Flexibility is the range of motion about a joint (4). Typical devices for measuring flexibility include the goniometer, which measures the angle of a joint, and the **sit-and-reach box**, which evaluates the flexibility of the lower back and hamstrings. Flexibility measurements are more reliable when a period of warm-up and static stretching precedes the actual assessment of flexibility. When performing a test of flexibility, the athlete should move slowly into the fully stretched position and hold this position for a minimum of 3 s (3). Ballistic stretching—bouncing in an attempt to attain a greater range of motion—should be strictly prohibited and any measurement not counted. See page 271 for a description of a flexibility test.

CONCLUSION

A well-organized testing session, in which the athletes are aware of testing purpose and procedures, tends to promote reliability of test measures. Reliable measures obtained from valid tests are a great asset in assessing fitness levels and evaluating changes over a period of time.

LOCAL MUSCULAR ENDURANCE

Timed Sit-Ups

Equipment

Stopwatch or clock with a sweep second hand

Gymnastics mat

Procedure

1. Have the athlete assume the starting position by lying on his or her back with knees bent at 90°. Feet may be together or up to 12 in. apart. Another person holds the athlete's ankles with the hands only. The heel is the only portion of the foot that must remain in contact with the ground. The athlete's fingers are interlocked behind the neck, and the backs of the hands touch the mat.
2. On the "Go" command, the athlete begins raising the upper body to the up position shown in Figure 17.1b.
3. The athlete lowers the body until the upper portion of the back touches the mat. The head, hands, arms, and elbows do not have to touch the ground.
4. With each repetition, the scorer calls out the number of correct repetitions achieved so far.
5. Record the number of correct repetitions achieved in 1 min.
6. The up position is the only authorized rest position.

Reasons for Disqualification

If the athlete fails to reach the up position, fails to keep the fingers interlocked behind the neck, arches or bows the back and raises the buttocks off the ground to raise the upper body, or lets the knees exceed a 90° angle, that repetition will not count (the scorer repeats the number of the last correct repetition).

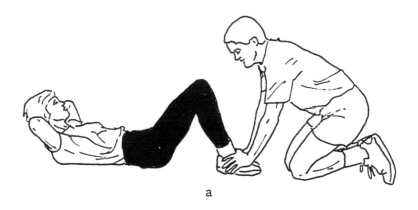

a

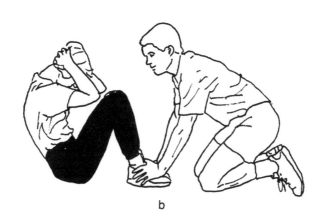

b

Figure 17.1   Sit-up: (a) starting position (down) and (b) up position.

LOCAL MUSCULAR ENDURANCE

Timed Push-Ups

Equipment
Stopwatch

Procedure
1. On the "Get set" command, the athlete assumes the front-leaning rest position by placing the hands where they are comfortable. The feet may be together or up to 12 in. apart. When viewed from the side, the body should form an essentially straight line from the shoulders to the ankles.
2. On the "Go" command, the athlete begins the push-up by bending the elbows and lowering the entire body as a unit until the upper arms are parallel to the ground.
3. The athlete returns to the starting position by raising the entire body until the arms are fully extended. The body must remain in a generally straight line and move as a unit for the entire repetition.
4. Record the number of repetitions correctly completed in 1 min.

Reasons for Disqualification
Failure to keep the body straight or to lower the entire body until upper arms are parallel to the ground results in disqualification. Incorrect movements will not be scored.

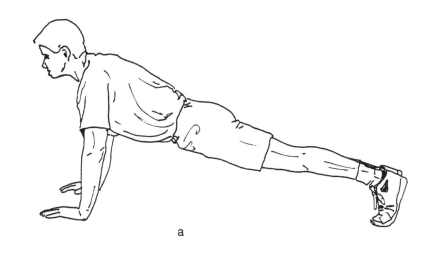

a

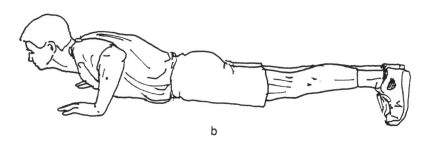

b

Figure 17.2 Push-up: (a) starting position (up) and (b) down position.

AEROBIC POWER

3-Minute Step Test

Equipment

Sturdy 12-in.-high bench

Metronome

Timer

Stethoscope

Procedure

1. Set the metronome at 96 beats/min.
2. Demonstrate the test: Face the bench and, in time with the metronome, step one foot up on the bench (first beat), step up with the other foot (second beat), step down with the first foot (third beat), and step down with the other foot (fourth beat). The sequence is alternating feet; at 96 beats/min, there will be 24 cycles/min. It does not matter which foot leads or if the lead foot changes during the test.
3. Explain to the athlete the importance of sitting down quickly at the end of 3 min and remaining still for 1 min so that the tester can count the heart rate.
4. Do not allow the athlete to practice; this would affect the heart rate.
5. Position the athlete facing the bench and allow him or her to pick up the beat of the metronome by marking time in place.
6. When the athlete starts stepping, start the timer. Check the rhythm and correct if necessary.
7. Inform the athlete of the time as it passes by saying, "One minute . . . two minutes."
8. As soon as the athlete sits down (after 3 min of the stepping) place the stethoscope on the chest, listen for the heart rhythm, and start counting for 1 min (use the same timer or a separate one to measure this minute). Begin the count on a beat, counting that beat as "zero." The recovery rate count must be started within 5 s, or the heart rate will be significantly different. The 1-min count reflects the heart's rate at the end of stepping as well as the rate of recovery.
9. Record this count.

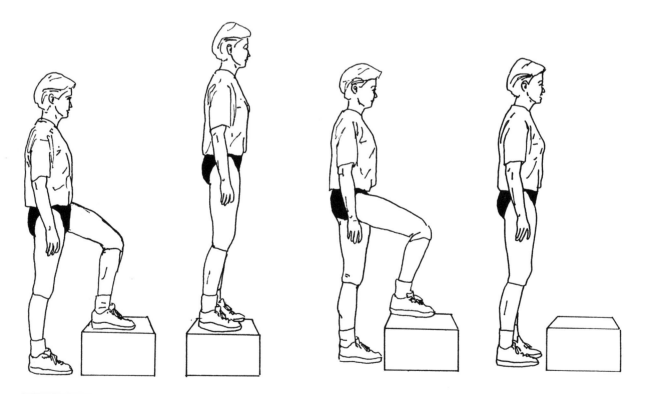

Figure 17.3   Three-minute step test.

AEROBIC POWER

2-Mile Run

Equipment

Stopwatch

Recording form

Quarter-mile running track or marked and measured 2-mile course

Procedure

1. At the start, all runners should line up behind the starting line.

2. Athletes are instructed to complete the 2-mile run and listen for their finish time. They should verify this time with the event recorder.
3. On the command of "Go," start the clock; runners will begin running at their own pace.
4. The event supervisor serves as timer for the event. As the runners near the finish line, the event supervisor calls off the time in minutes and seconds as follows: "Fifteen-thirty, fifteen-thirty-one, fifteen-thirty-two," and so on.
5. Event recorder notes each runner's time on the recording form.

ANAEROBIC POWER

Vertical Jump

Equipment

Yardstick

Ladder

Wall with a high ceiling and good landing area

Chalk

Person to measure reach and jump

(You may also use a vertical-jump measurement scale.)

Procedure

1. The athlete puts chalk on the fingertips of the right hand.
2. Athlete stands with his or her right side to the wall, making sure the feet and hips are next to the wall.
3. Athlete reaches as high as possible with feet flat and makes a chalk mark on the wall.
4. Athlete positions himself or herself comfortably, hand still as high as possible. Without moving the feet, the athlete flexes the knees, jumps, and places a second chalk mark as high on the wall as possible.
5. Measure the distance between the two chalk marks.
6. Record the best of three trials to the nearest 0.5 in.

Reasons for Disqualification

Any irregularity in placing the first mark on the wall, such as not having feet and hips next to the wall or not

having feet flat when reaching, results in disqualification, as does taking a step or shuffle-step before jumping.

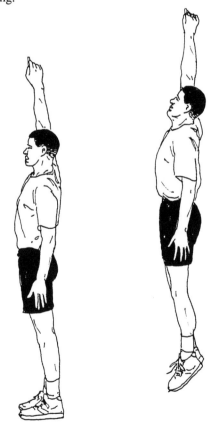

Figure 17.4 Vertical jump.

Adapted from Semenick (1990).

ANAEROBIC POWER

Line Drill for Basketball

Equipment

Lined basketball floor (94-ft long for college, 84-ft long for high school) or five cones to mark off the distances seen in the figure

Stopwatch

2 timers

Procedure

1. Ensure that athletes perform adequate stretching and warm-up.
2. Athletes are allowed one run through the course at submaximal speed.
3. Supervisor explains the testing procedure and emphasizes the requirement to touch each line with the foot and to be at the starting line 2 minutes after completion of each trial.
4. The athlete starts at point A (baseline on basketball floor).
5. On the "Go" command, start the stopwatch. The athlete sprints from point A and makes these four round trips without stopping:

    (a) From point A to point B (the near free-throw line) and back (38 ft)

    (b) From point A to point C (the midcourt line) and back (94 ft for college, 84 ft for high school)

    (c) From point A to point D (the far free-throw line) and back (150 ft for college, 130 ft for high school)

    (d) From point A to point E (the far baseline) and back (188 ft for college, 168 ft for high school)

    The total distance is 470 ft for college and 420 ft for high school.

6. Stop the watch when the athlete passes point A.
7. Upon completion of the course, the second timer starts his watch and gives the athlete a 2-min rest.
8. The athlete repeats the course three more times, with a 2-min rest between repetitions.
9. Sum all four times for the athlete to the nearest second and divide by 4.

Reasons for Disqualification

Disqualify the athlete if he or she does not touch any of the points with his or her foot during the run or does not begin repeated shuttle runs after exactly 2 min rest.

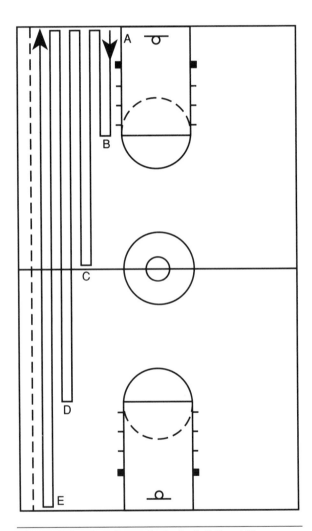

Figure 17.5 Floor layout for basketball line drill.
Adapted from Semenick (1990).

Adapted from Semenick (1990).

ANAEROBIC POWER

300-Yard Shuttle Run

Equipment

Five stopwatches (0.1 s)

Four clipboards

Two measured courses (see Figure 17.6)

Seven or eight coaches or managers

Recording charts and roster

Chart to keep track of 5-min rest interval

Whistle

Procedure

1. Ensure that athletes perform adequate stretching and warm-up.
2. Event supervisor explains the procedure, emphasizing that each line must be touched with the foot and the athletes must report to the starting line 5 min after the first trial to avoid disqualification.
3. The coaches are arranged to time the trials and rest periods, and to monitor compliance with line touches.
4. Pair off athletes of similar capability.
5. Position 2 athletes at the X's in the first course. (All athletes begin the first two trials at the first course.)
6. On the coach's signal, the athletes sprint to the 25-yd line and return to the starting line for a total of six round-trips (i.e., 12 × 25 yd = 300 yd).
7. Foot contact must be made on the starting line and 25-yd line when changing directions.
8. Upon completion of first trial, record both athletes' times to the nearest 0.1 s and start a 5-min clock to allow for a rest interval until the next trial. As each pair of runners completes the first trial, the runners may walk and stretch, and must stay alert for the starting time on the second course.
9. After 5 minutes of rest, the pair begins the second course. Record the times to the nearest 0.1 s.
10. Take the average of the two times and record it.
11. After all testing is completed, rank each athlete on the team by position and time, for future reference.

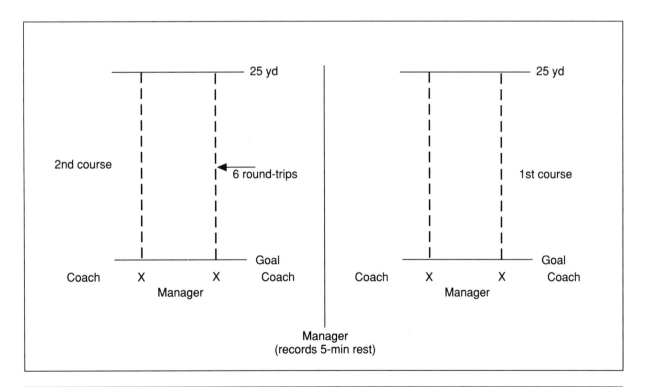

Figure 17.6   Ground layout for 300-yd shuttle run.
Adapted from Gilliam (1983).

Adapted from Gilliam (1983).

AGILITY AND BODY CONTROL

T-Test

Equipment

Four cones

Stopwatch (0.1 s)

Gymnasium basketball floor

1 timer, 1 spotter, 1 person to record times

Procedure

1. Arrange the four cones as seen in Figure 17.7 (points A, B, C, and D).
2. Ensure that athletes perform adequate stretching and warm-ups.
3. The athlete starts at point A.
4. On the ''Go'' command, the athlete sprints to point B and touches the *base* of the cone with the right hand.
5. Athlete shuffles to the left 5 yd and touches the base of the cone at point C with the left hand. When shuffling, athletes should always face front and not cross the feet.
6. Athlete shuffles to the right 10 yd and touches the base of the cone at point D with the right hand.
7. Athlete shuffles to the left 5 yd and touches the base of the cone at point B with the left hand.
8. Athlete runs backward past point A.
9. The timer stops the watch when the athlete passes the cone at point A.
10. For safety, have a spotter and gym mat several feet behind point A to catch the athlete if he or she should fall.

11. Each athlete should complete two trials for the T-test. Record the better trial to the nearest 0.1 s.

Reasons for Disqualification

Athletes are disqualified if they (a) do not touch the base of any cone, (b) cross the feet when shuffling, or (c) fail to face the front at all times.

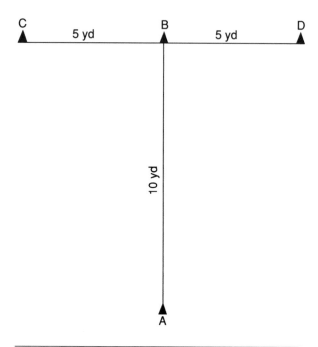

Figure 17.7   Floor layout for the T-test.
Adapted from Semenick (1990).

Adapted from Semenick (1990).

AGILITY AND BODY CONTROL

Edgren Side Step

Equipment

Gymnasium floor 12 ft wide, marked in 3-ft increments (see Figure 17.8)

Stopwatch (0.1 s)

1 timer, 1 counter, and 1 recorder

Procedure

1. Ensure that athletes perform adequate stretching and warm-up.
2. Allow each athlete to perform a submaximal trial run.
3. The athlete stands astride the center line. On the signal ''Go,'' the athlete sidesteps to the right until his or her right foot has touched or crossed the outside line.
4. Athlete then sidesteps to the left until his or her left foot has touched or crossed the left outside line.
5. The athlete sidesteps back and forth to the outside lines, as rapidly as possible, for 10 s.

Scoring

Each completion of a 3-ft increment (from center line to first increment, from first increment to outside line,

from outside line back to first increment, etc.) counts as 1 point.

Reasons for Disqualification

Impose a 1-point penalty for each time one foot crosses the other and for each failure to get the proper foot on or across the outside marker.

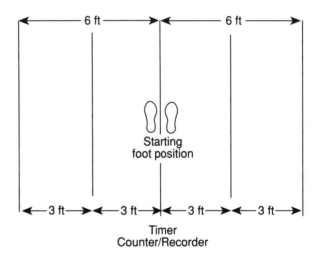

Figure 17.8 The Edgren Side Step.

RUNNING SPEED

40-Yard Sprint

Equipment

At least 60 yd of uncluttered, flat, safe running space

Stopwatch (0.1 s)

Procedure

1. Ensure that the athletes perform adequate stretching and warm-up.
2. Allow two practice runs at submaximal speed for specific warm-up.
3. Have the athlete position himself or herself behind the starting line with one or two hands on the line.
4. On the ''Go'' command, the athlete sprints the 40-yd distance and decelerates over the remaining 20 yd.
5. Timer should start the watch on the first movement of the athlete's hand and stop the watch as the athlete crosses the 40-yd line.

Scoring

Record two trials, average to the nearest 0.1 s and record as the criterion score.

BODY COMPOSITION

Measurement of Skinfolds

Equipment
Skinfold calipers

Felt-tip pen

Site Selection and Marking
Various skinfold sites and equations can be used to determine body composition. Take care to use the correct sites for the selected equation. Also realize that certain equations, such as the Sloan formula (28), are better suited for athletic populations than others.

Once a decision is made concerning what sites to include, take care to mark the skin at the specific locations described here for each site. It is easiest to mark all the sites before beginning skinfold measurements.

Measurement Procedures
1. For each site listed here, grasp the skinfold firmly by the thumb and index finger and place the caliper prongs perpendicular to the fold approximately 1 cm from the thumb and index finger.
2. Release the caliper grip so that full tension is exerted on the skinfold.
3. Read the dial on the caliper to the nearest 0.5 mm, 1 to 2 s after the grip has been released.
4. Take at least two measurements; if the measurements don't differ by more than 1 mm, use the lowest figure. Otherwise, take a third measurement

and use it. For increased validity and reliability, take skinfold measurements prior to exercise on dry skin (4). Obtain one measurement from each test site, and then repeat all test sites for a second trial.

Anatomical Sites for Measurement of Skinfolds (23)
Chest—A diagonal fold taken one half of the distance between the anterior axillary line and the nipple for men and one third of the distance from the anterior axillary line and the nipple for women.

Axilla—A vertical fold on the midaxillary line at the level of the xiphoid process of the sternum.

Triceps—A vertical fold on the posterior midline of the upper arm (over triceps muscle), halfway between the acromion and the olecranon processes. The elbow should be extended and relaxed.

Subscapular—A fold taken on a diagonal line that extends from the vertebral border to a point 1 to 2 cm from the inferior angle of the scapula.

Abdominal—A vertical fold taken about 2 cm to the left or right of the umbilicus.

Suprailium—A diagonal fold above the crest of the ilium at the spot where an imaginary line would come down from the anterior axillary line. It should be noted that many recommend the measure be taken more laterally, at the midaxillary line (5).

Thigh—A vertical fold on the anterior aspect of the thigh, midway between hip and knee joints.

ANTHROPOMETRY

Girth Measurements

Equipment

Gulich tape

Procedures

1. Use the Gulich tape to measure each site listed below.

Girth Measurements for Weight Training Applications (17, 29)

Neck girth—The circumference immediately below the larynx.

Chest girth—Measured at nipple level in males and at the level of maximum circumference in females. Two measurements should be taken: one at the end of a normal expiration, and another at the end of a maximal inspiration. Both measurements are noted and recorded.

Biceps girth—Two measures should be taken: one at the location of greatest circumference when flexed, and another when the arm is fully extended and muscles are relaxed.

Forearm girth—Measured at the point of greatest circumference between the elbow and wrist in an extended, relaxed position.

Waist girth—Located at the level of the umbilicus and just above the iliac crests; measured after a normal expiration.

Hip girth—Measured at a level of maximal protrusion of the buttocks.

Thigh girth—Located at the point of maximal circumference midway between the hip and knee.

Calf girth—Located at the level of maximal calf circumference between the knee and ankle.

FLEXIBILITY

Sit and Reach

Equipment

Yardstick or tape measure

Tape

(Inexpensive, easily stored equipment can be built to facilitate convenient administration of this test. In addition, a commercially available trunk flexion instrument may be used.)

Procedure

1. Ensure that athletes warm up.
2. Tell athletes to refrain from fast, jerky movements that may increase the possibility of an injury.
3. Place a yardstick on the floor and put one piece of tape about 12 in. long across it at a right angle to the 15-in. mark.
4. Have the shoeless athlete sit with the yardstick between the legs with the 0 mark toward the body and the legs extended and spread apart about 12 in. to the taped line on the floor. The heels of the feet should nearly touch the edge of the taped line and be about 10 to 12 in. apart.
5. Have the athlete slowly reach forward with both hands as far as possible on the yardstick, holding this position approximately 3 s. To get the best stretch, the athlete should exhale and drop the head between the arms when reaching. Be sure that the athlete keeps the hands parallel and does not stretch or lead with one hand. Fingertips should be in contact with the yardstick. Hold the athlete's knees down to keep them straight.
6. Have the athlete do three trials. For each, measure the most distant point (to the nearest 0.25 in.) reached on the yardstick with the fingertips. Record the best of the three.

Key Terms

criterion score	258	sit-and-reach box	261	Sloan formula	261
metronome	260	skinfold calipers	261	1RM strength	259

Study Questions

1. In the timing of sprint events, hand-held stopwatches can result in errors of up to ___ s compared with new electronic timing systems, even under ideal conditions.

   a. 0.20
   b. 0.24
   c. 0.34
   d. 0.40

2. Which of the following is *not* a proper testing procedure?

   a. muscular strength testing conducted by an experienced student
   b. instructor-led warm-up before testing
   c. having athletes run through a practice trial on the day of testing, before actual testing begins
   d. testing conducted by a novice test administrator

3. When conducting the 1RM back squat test,

   a. a lifting belt is mandatory
   b. a lifting belt is encouraged but optional
   c. lifting boots are mandatory
   d. knee wraps are mandatory

4. Which of the following represents an unsafe procedure for conducting a test involving intensive lateral change of direction?

   a. wearing shoes designed for basketball
   b. performing the test on a nonskid surface
   c. use of soft, unbreakable marking devices
   d. wearing shoes designed for distance running

5. When scoring running speed tests, the most reliable and objective hand-held–stopwatch times are achieved

   a. by starting and stopping the stopwatch with the thumb of the dominant hand
   b. by starting and stopping the stopwatch with the index finger
   c. by starting the stopwatch on the "Go" command of the starter
   d. by using a stopwatch accurate to 0.01 s

6. Taking a pulse is most reliable when the test administrator

   a. palpates the pulse at the jugular vein in the neck and counts the beats for at least 6 s
   b. palpates the pulse with his or her thumb and counts the beats for at least 10 s
   c. palpates the pulse with his or her fingertips and counts the beats for at least 10 s
   d. palpates the pulse at the carotid artery in the neck and counts the beats for at least 6 s

Applying Knowledge
of Testing Protocols and Procedures

Problem 1

What athletic fitness field tests would be considered appropriate for inclusion in a testing battery designed for high school–aged female soccer athletes to assess the following areas of general fitness:

- Aerobic power
- Agility
- Anaerobic power
- Lower body strength
- Speed
- Flexibility

Problem 2

There are several categories of anaerobic power field testing that span the spectrum of maximum anaerobic energy production. Category III includes multiple continuous sequence movements of less than 15 s in duration separated by timed relief intervals (i.e., repeated 30- to 50-yd sprints). Name three sporting activities for which this category of anaerobic field testing would be appropriate.

References

1. Altug, Z., T. Altug, and A. Altug. A test selection guide for assessing and evaluating athletes. *NSCA Journal* 9(3):67-69. 1987.
2. American Alliance for Health, Physical Education, Recreation and Dance. *AAHPERD Health Related Fitness Test.* Reston, VA: Author. 1980.
3. Anderson, B. Flexibility testing. *NSCA Journal* 3(2):20-23. 1981.
4. Baumgartner, T., and A. Jackson. *Measurement for Evaluation in Physical Education and Exercise Science.* Dubuque, IA: Brown. 1987.
5. Behnke, A., and J. Wilmore. *Evaluation and Regulation of Body Build and Composition.* Englewood Cliffs, NJ: Prentice Hall. 1974.
6. Cooper, K. *The New Aerobics.* New York: Bantam Books. 1972.
7. Costill, D., S. Miller, W. Myers, F. Kehoe, and W. Hoffman. Relationships among selected tests of explosive leg strength and power. *Res. Q.* 39(3):785-787. 1968.
8. Edgren, H. An experiment in the testing of ability and progress in basketball. *Res. Q.* 3(1):159-171. 1932.
9. Epley, B. The Nebraska Timer: A simple, accurate way to measure the 40 yard dash. *NSCA Journal* 4(5):14-15. 1982.
10. Epley, B. *Husker Power.* Lincoln: University of Nebraska Press. 1983.
11. Fleck, S. Percent of body fat of various groups of athletes. *NSCA Journal* 5(2):46-48. 1983.
12. Fleck, S., and M. Marks. Interval training. *NSCA Journal* 5(5):40-62. 1983.
13. Gotshalk, L. Discipline and strictness in testing and training. *NSCA Journal* 7(5):72-73. 1985.
14. Gould, D. Goal setting for peak performance. In: *Applied Sport Psychology*, 2nd ed., J.E. Williams, ed. Mountain View, CA: Mayfield. 1993. pp. 158-169.
15. Henschen, K.P. Athletic staleness and burnout: Diagnosis, prevention, and treatment. In: *Applied Sport Psychology*, 2nd ed., J.E. Williams, ed. Mountain View, CA: Mayfield. 1993. pp. 328-337.
16. Hopkins, C. *Understanding Educational Research.* Columbus, OH: Charles E. Merrill. 1980.
17. Jackson, A., M. Pollock, and L. Gettman. Intertester reliability of selected skinfold and circumference measurements and percent fat estimates. *Res. Q.* 49:546-551. 1978.
18. Johnson, B., and J. Nelson. *Practical Measurements for Evaluation in Physical Education*, 2nd ed. Minneapolis: Burgess. 1974.
19. Katch, F., and W. McArdle. *Nutrition, Weight Control and Exercise.* Boston: Houghton Mifflin. 1977.
20. Kontor, K. Editorial: Testing and evaluation. *NSCA Journal* 3(2):7. 1981.
21. Kraemer, W., and S. Fleck. Anaerobic metabolism and its evaluation. *NSCA Journal* 4(2):20-21. 1982.
22. Mayhew, J., B. Levy, T. McCormick, and G. Evans. Strength norms for NCAA Division II college football players. *NSCA Journal* 9(3):67-69. 1987.
23. Pollock, M., J. Wilmore, and S. Fox. *Exercise in Health and Disease.* Philadelphia: W.B. Saunders. 1984.
24. Safdrit, M. *Evaluation in Physical Education.* Englewood Cliffs, NJ: Prentice Hall. 1980.
25. Semenick, D. Anaerobic testing: Practical applications. *NSCA Journal* 6(5):44-73. 1984.
26. Semenick, D. Tests and measurements: The line drill test. *NSCA Journal* 12(2):47-49. 1990.
27. Semenick, D. Tests and measurements: The vertical jump test. *NSCA Journal.* In press.
28. Sloan, A., and J. Weir. Nomograms for prediction of body density and total body fat from skinfold measurements. *J. Appl. Physiol.* 28(2):221-222. 1970.
29. Stone, M., and H. O'Bryant. *Weight Training: A Scientific Approach.* Minneapolis: Burgess. 1987.
30. Tesch, P. Anaerobic testing: Practical applications. *NSCA Journal* 6(5):44-73. 1984.
31. Wade, G. Tests and measurements: Meeting the standards of professional football. *NSCA Journal* 4(3):23. 1982.

CHAPTER 18

EVALUATING TEST DATA

Douglas M. Semenick

Once the proper test or tests are chosen and administered and the scores collected, the next step is to analyze the data and answer questions about the athletes. For example, What was the overall performance of the group? Has the group improved from the beginning of the training period (this could be measured in months or years)? How has the group improved over the past one, two, or three training periods? How has this group scored as compared to similar groups tested in the past? How do the scores from each athlete compare to the group? How do the individual scores compare with local, state, and national norms? This chapter will attempt to answer these questions by illustrating individual and group descriptions and comparisons based on test scores.

Typically, the evaluation of athletes centers on difference scores, also known as "change scores," or "improvement scores." A **difference score** is the difference between an athlete's scores at the beginning and end of a training period, or between any two separate testing times. Difference scores can be part of the systematic measurement process, which provides information on the effectiveness of the conditioning program (4). Evaluation based purely on difference scores, however, has two major limitations that preclude their exclusive use. First, athletes who begin the training period at a higher fitness level and who therefore pretest well will not improve as much as untrained athletes who perform poorly at the beginning of the training period. For example, a wrestler who can bench press 150 lb (68 kg) at the beginning of training has a substantially greater opportunity for improvement than does a wrestler who initially can bench press 300 lb (136 kg). Second, athletes may deliberately perform poorly on a pretraining

test with the intent of achieving an inflated improvement score on the posttraining test, a practice commonly called sandbagging.

Evaluating athletic fitness using difference scores can be very deceptive if the initial test is not **normalized** (corrected at the beginning to equalize scores). For example, it is not unusual for a female basketball player to double her level of upper body strength in the course of her first year of strength training because of a low initial level of upper body strength. However, even with an excellent strength training program, during the rest of her training career she will probably not continue to achieve such dramatic improvement in upper body strength. Therefore, when evaluating athletic fitness, take into consideration not only the chronological age of the athlete but also his or her training age. Another practical example of deception common in the evaluation of athletic fitness involves an athlete's training status. For example, if an athlete is initially tested after a period of detraining, the difference scores, as measured after the training period, will be substantially higher than they would have been if the athlete had been in a trained state for the initial test. Therefore, coaches should interpret improvement scores cautiously.

STATISTICS

A working knowledge of statistics is helpful in making sound evaluations of test results. **Statistics** is the science of collecting, classifying, analyzing, and interpreting numerical data (9, 20). There are two main branches of statistics. **Descriptive statistics** summarizes or describes a large group of data. It is used when all the information about a population is known. For example, if all the members of a team are tested, statements can be made about the team using descriptive statistics. **Inferential statistics** makes general statements about a population from information collected in a sample of the population. For example, if the boys' ninth-grade gym class that meets at 10:00 a.m. is put through a battery of tests, and it is assumed that this class (sample) is representative of all the ninth grade boys in the school (the population), then the results of these tests can be used to infer generalizations about the population as a whole. Inferential statistics assume that the sample is truly representative of the population (19).

Descriptive statistics are commonly used by the strength and conditioning professional to evaluate a team's performance. There are four categories of numerical measurement in descriptive statistics: central tendency, variability, percentile rank, and standard scores. In the sections that follow we will define these terms and present examples of how to calculate the respective values and scores. Note, however, that many commercially developed computer programs are available that calculate values in these four categories, so that it is not necessary to perform all the calculations manually.

Central Tendency

Measures of **central tendency** attempt to find a numerical value about which the data tend to cluster. There are three measures of central tendency (1, 10, 20):

- The **mode** is the score that occurs with the greatest frequency. If each numerical score appears only once, there is no mode; if two or more scores are "tied" for greatest frequency, they are all modes. In general, the mode is the least useful measure of central tendency.
- The **median** is the middle score when a set of scores is arranged in numerical order. (If there happens to be an even number of scores, the median is the average of the two middle scores.) From this definition, it follows that half a group of scores falls above the median and half falls below the median.
- The **mean** ($\bar{x}$), the most commonly used measure of central tendency, is simply the average of the scores (i.e., the sum of the scores divided by the number of scores).

The "Descriptive Statistics Example" (p. 282) illustrates the measures of central tendency, as well as measures of variability.

Variability

Variability indicates the magnitude of the spread of scores in a group. Two common measures of variability are the range and the standard deviation. The **range** is simply the difference between the highest score and the lowest score. The advantage of the range is that it is easy to understand; its disadvantage is that it uses only the two extreme scores and so may not be an accurate measure of variability (1, 20).

The **standard deviation** (s) is a measure of the variability of a set of scores about their mean. The formula for the standard deviation of a sample is

$$s = \sqrt{\frac{\Sigma(x - \bar{x})^2}{n - 1}}, \qquad (18.1)$$

where Σ (Greek sigma) refers to a summation, x is a score, $\bar{x}$ is the mean of the scores, and n is the sample size (number of scores). A relatively small standard deviation would indicate that a set of scores is clustered about the mean; a large standard deviation would indicate a larger spread of scores about the mean. The standard deviation is most useful when the group of scores is "normally distributed," forming the bell-shaped curve seen in Figure 18.1 (1, 10, 18, 20).

The z-score will come in handy in our subsequent discussion of standard scores. The z-score for any particular score from a sample expresses, in units of standard deviations, how far that score is from the mean:

$$z = (x - \bar{x})/s. \qquad (18.2)$$

For example, if an athlete runs the 40-yd dash in 4.6 s, and the mean and standard deviation for the scores of all the athletes in the sample are 5.0 s and 0.33 s, Equation 18.2 gives a z-score for that athlete of −1.2. His or her score is 1.2 standard deviation units less than the mean.

Percentile Rank

Percentile ranks are **ordinal scores** (scores classified by rank, e.g., best to worst, smallest to largest) that indicate the relative position of an individual in a group; specifically, they indicate the percentage of scores below a given score. For example, if an athlete's test score has a percentile rank of 75, this means that 75% of the group scored below that athlete's score, and the athlete is said to be in the 75th percentile. Norms, performance standards based on the scores of a group of people, are often expressed in **percentiles**, that is, a score that has a specified percentage of scores below it. Percentiles are generally expressed in multiples of 5 (i.e., 5th, 10th, 15th, etc., percentiles) (1).

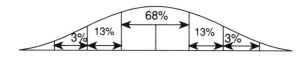

Figure 18.1 Normal bell curve.

The calculation of percentile ranks is a three-step process (4):

1. Order the scores in a simple frequency distribution, listing the best score first (see Table 18.1).
2. Make a cumulative frequency (cf) column by adding the frequencies, starting with the worst score and working upward to the best.
3. Calculate the percentile rank of a given score using the following formula:

$$PR_x = \left(cfb + \frac{fw}{2}\right)\left(\frac{100}{n}\right)$$

where PR_x is the percentile rank of score X, cfb is the number of scores below X (the entry in the cf column one level below X), fw is the frequency of X, and n is the number of scores (the sum of the frequency column).

An application of percentile ranking for football is seen in Table 18.2. After testing the whole team and developing percentile ranks, the mean score for each

Table 18.1   Simple Frequency Distribution of Standing Broad Jump Scores of 50 Junior High School Boys

x	f	x	f	x	f
90	2	72	1	60	1
84	1	71	2	59	1
83	2	70	1	58	2
82	1	68	6	56	3
79	1	67	1	55	1
78	2	66	2	54	1
77	1	65	3	49	1
76	3	64	1	48	1
75	3	63	1	47	1
73	1	62	2	46	1

Reprinted from Baumgartner and Jackson (1987).

Table 18.2   Percentile-Rank Norms for University Football Players

Percentile	0-5 yd	20-40 yd	0-40 yd	Percentage fat	Bench press	Leg press	
99	0.985	1.933	4.412	4.1	422	778	
95	1.029	1.995	4.626	6.5	389	726	
90	1.052	2.028	4.737	7.7	376	707	
85	1.067	2.049	4.812	8.7	360	681	
80	1.080	2.067	4.903	9.2	350	666	Linemen
75	1.091	2.083	4.926	9.8	342	653	
70	1.101	2.096	4.973	10.3	335	642	
65	1.109	2.108	5.013	10.7	329	632	
60	1.118	2.121	5.057	11.3	322	622	
55	1.126	2.131	5.094	11.6	316	613	Linebacker-Tight end
50	1.134	2.143	5.134	12.0	310	603	
45	1.142	2.155	5.174	12.3	304	593	
40	1.150	2.166	5.212	12.7	298	584	
35	1.159	2.178	5.255	13.2	291	574	Backs
30	1.167	2.190	5.295	13.6	285	564	
25	1.177	2.203	5.342	14.1	278	553	
20	1.188	2.219	5.394	14.6	270	540	
15	1.201	2.237	5.456	15.1	260	525	
10	1.216	2.258	5.531	15.9	244	500	
5	1.239	2.291	5.642	16.9	231	480	
1	12.83	2.353	5.856	18.8	198	428	
$\overline{x}$	1.134	2.143	5.134	12.0	310	603	
s	0.064	0.090	0.310	3.1			

Note. Data used with the permission of William F. Yeoman, Head Football Coach, University of Houston, Texas.

test for players at each position was plotted to yield a visual profile of the average athlete at that position. This kind of profile—for either a sport as a whole or a position within a sport—provides important information for exercise prescriptions. An understanding of where the athlete ranks relative to his or her peers (and past best performers) also provides a motivational tool for training. For example, consider a linebacker who scores 5.2 s in the 40-yd dash (slower than average), has 13% body fat (higher than average), bench presses 350 lb (159 kg) (better than average), and leg presses 680 lb (309 kg) (better than average). His conditioning program might be adjusted to emphasize speed work and lowering body fat through dietary adjustment and appropriate exercise, while maintaining upper and lower body strength.

Standard Score

A **standard score** is a calculated test score using the test mean and standard deviation; its purpose is to allow for comparing and combining scores having different units of measure. For practical purposes, standard scores are usually expressed as **T-scores**, which are standard scores usually used in sport and exercise with a mean of 50 and a standard deviation of 10. For example, a testing battery may include a long jump, a 50-yd dash, and pull-ups, which are measured in inches, seconds, and repetitions, respectively. Because the tests are in different units they must be converted to standard scores before they can be combined. Each athlete's T-scores for the three tests are totaled, giving an "athletic index" that can be compared among the athletes in the sample. For example, in Table 18.3, Athlete 13, with a total

Table 18.3   T-Scores[a] for Three Athletic Fitness Tests*

Athlete	Squat Score (lb)	Squat T-score	40-yd dash Score (s)	40-yd dash T-score	Vertical jump Score (in.)	Vertical jump T-score	Total T-score
1	315	36	4.70	65	29.0	60	161
2	465	66	5.15	43	27.0	55	164
3	450	63	4.65	68	30.0	62	193
4	300	33	4.85	58	25.5	51	142
5	435	60	4.70	65	30.0	62	187
6	550	83	5.00	50	28.0	58	191
7	480	69	5.10	45	26.0	52	166
8	350	43	4.60	70	32.0	67	180
9	400	53	4.85	58	29.0	60	171
10	405	54	5.05	48	24.0	48	150
11	415	56	4.90	55	27.5	56	167
12	285	30	4.75	63	29.0	60	153
13	475	68	4.65	68	33.0	70	206
14	385	50	4.50	75	32.0	67	192
15	425	58	5.35	33	24.0	48	139
16	290	31	4.65	68	35.0	75	174
17	405	54	4.95	53	26.5	53	160
18	450	63	5.05	48	26.0	52	163
19	395	52	5.15	43	25.0	50	145
20	290	31	4.70	65	28.0	58	154
$\bar{x}$	—	—	5.00	—	25.0	—	—
s	—	—	0.30	—	4.0	—	—

*The values in this table represent an example only; universal norms have not been established.

[a]T-score = $(10 \times z) + 50$

Note. Data presented in "Testing and Evaluation: Rational, Protocol, Data and Profile Analysis" by Douglas M. Semenick at the NSCA National Convention, Pittsburgh, 1984.

T-score of 206, would be objectively judged the best performer. (See ''Procedure for Computing T-Scores'' on p. 281.)

Another tool for evaluating athletic fitness is the T-score table, an example of which is illustrated in Table 18.4. From this table a numerical ''athletic index'' can be derived by adding T-scores across columns. This athletic index represents sport-specific athletic fitness as a single number.

If the testing battery has a high level of validity and reliability and athletes are at equal pretest training levels, the best athletes for the sport or position in question should tend to achieve the highest athletic indexes. Table 18.5 is an example of player position characteristics for basketball. Strength and conditioning professionals can develop such tables for any sport over several seasons and then use them to evaluate individual players.

The T-score totals for each athlete are appropriately placed on a T-score scale (Figure 18.2), which serves as a visual aid that allows the athlete to judge where he or she ranks relative to all players on the team and at the position in question. This has proven to be a strong motivational tool that encourages athletes to work on their weakest areas (lowest T-scores) and improve their relative standing on the team and at their position (15).

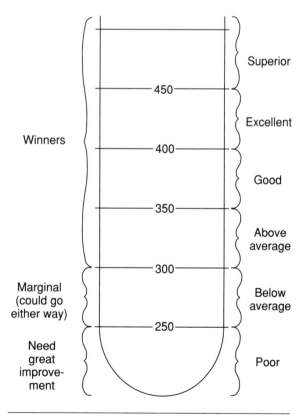

Figure 18.2   T-score scale for six athletic fitness tests.

DEVELOPING AN ATHLETIC PROFILE

To determine the sport-specific fitness of an athlete, the strength and conditioning professional can combine the results of selected tests to generate an athletic profile. When evaluating athletes, the professional should follow the following six steps:

1. Select tests that will measure the specific fitness parameters most characteristic of the sport or sports in question. For example, a testing battery for wrestlers should include tests for pulling and pushing strength and local muscular endurance.
2. Choose valid and reliable tests to measure these fitness parameters and arrange the testing battery in an appropriate order with sufficient rest between tests to promote test reliability. For example, appropriate tests for wrestling might include a maximum number of push-ups and sit-ups. These two tests should be separated by at least 5 min of rest to allow recovery from fatigue and thus promote reliable scores.
3. Administer the test battery to as many athletes as possible.
4. Calculate percentile ranks to present a visual profile.
5. Evaluate the athlete against these ranks and against his or her best performances from cumulative test results over past years, if possible.
6. Develop a T-score table to generate a numerical athletic index for each athlete (see Table 18.4).

Several percentile rank tables and T-score tables have been developed for male and females of different age groups for various sports, including football (4, 6, 11, 12, 15, 16, 21), basketball (8, 16, 17), volleyball (4, 16), and health-related fitness (2, 5, 13, 21).

GOAL SETTING

The importance of setting appropriate training goals cannot be overemphasized. Setting goals gives purpose and direction to the training program and helps promote athletes' intrinsic motivation, self-confidence, and sense of responsibility (14).

The strength and conditioning professional should consider the following guidelines when helping an athlete set goals:

- Help athletes organize their goals into realistic short-range performance goals (1-2 months), mid-range goals (for this season), and long-range goals (1-4 years or one's career).

Table 18.4   T-Score Table for University Football Players*

T-score points	Strength		Power	Speed	Muscular end.	Agility
	Bench press	Parallel squat	Vertical jump	40-yd dash	Sit-ups in 2 min	Edgren Side Step
20	120	235	13	5.6	48	29
21	125	240	13.5		49	
22	130	245	14		50	
23	135	250	14.5	5.55	51	
24	140	255	15			30
25	145	260	15.5	5.50	52	
26	150	265			53	
27	155	270	16		54	31
28	160	275	16.5	5.45	55	
29	165	280				
30	170	285	17	5.40	56	
31	175	290	17.5		57	32
32	180	295			58	
33	185	300	18	5.35	59	
34	190	305	18.5			
35	195	310	19	5.3	60	33
36	200	315	19.5		61	
37	205	320			62	
38	210	325	20	5.25	63	34
39	215	330	20.5			
40	220	335	21	5.20	64	
41	225	340	21.5		65	
42	230	345	22		66	
43	235	350	22.5	5.15	67	35
44	240	355				
45	245	360	23	5.10	68	
46	250	365	23.5		69	36
47	255	370			70	
48	260	375	24	5.05	71	
49	265	380	24.5			
50	270	385	25	5.00	72	37
51	275	390	25.5		73	
52	280	395	26		74	
53	285	400	26.5	4.95	75	
54	290	405				38
55	295	410	27	4.90	76	
56	300	415	27.5		77	
57	305	420			78	39
58	310	425	28	4.85	79	
59	315	430	28.5			

(co ed)

Table 18.4   *(continued)*

T-score points	Strength		Power	Speed	Muscular end.	Agility
	Bench press	Parallel squat	Vertical jump	40-yd dash	Sit-ups in 2 min	Edgren Side Step
60	320	435	29	4.80	80	
61	325	440	29.5		81	
62	330	445	30		82	40
63	335	450	30.5	4.75	83	
64	340	455				
65	345	460	31	4.70	84	41
66	350	465	31.5		85	
67	355	470	32		86	
68	360	475	32.5	4.65	87	
69	365	480				42
70	370	485	33	4.60	88	
71	375	490	33.5		89	
72	380	495			90	
73	385	500	34	4.55	91	43
74	390	505	34.5			
75	395	510	35	4.50	92	
76	400	515	35.5		93	44
77	405	520			94	
78	410	525	36	4.45	95	
79	415	530	36.5			
80	420	535	37	4.40	96	45
81	425	540	37.5		97	
82	430	545			98	
83	435	550	38	4.35	99	
84	440	555	38.5			
85	445	560		4.30	100	46
86	450	565	39		101	
87	455	570	39.5		102	
88	460	575		4.25	103	
89	465	580	40			47
90	470	585	40.5	4.20	104	

*Please note this is an example only, universal norms have not been established.

Note. Data presented in "Testing and Evaluation: Rational, Protocol, Data and Profile Analysis" by Douglas M. Semenick at the NSCA National Convention, Pittsburgh, 1984.

- When setting the goals, the athlete should ask four questions:
  a. Is it really my goal?
  b. Are my short-range goals consistent with my long-range goals?
  c. Can I commit myself physically, mentally, and emotionally to reaching these goals?
  d. Can I visualize myself reaching these goals?
- Have athletes put a copy of the goals where they will be seen daily—for example on the bedroom wall or in their locker—and carry a copy. Athletes should spend a few minutes reviewing and updating their goals daily, to keep focused on them.

Table 18.5 Physical Characteristics of Well-Conditioned Basketball Players Based on Performance Averages of Starting Varsity Athletes at Each Position

Parameter	Test	Male athletes			Female athletes		
		Center	Forward	Guard	Center	Forward	Guard
Aerobic power	1.5-mile run (min:s)	11:00	10:00	9:15	11:30	11:00	10:30
Anaerobic power	Vertical jump (in.)	28.0	31.0	32.0	19.0	19.0	20.5
	400-m run (s)	65	62	59	69	66	66
	Line drill (s)	29	28	26	34	32	30
Strength							
Upper body	Bench press (lb)	225	235	215	115	115	108
Lower body	Parallel squat (lb)	275	315	315	186	185	175
Local muscular endurance	Bent-knee sit-ups	75	75	80	68	72	77
Running speed	20-yd dash (s)	3.00	2.82	2.73	3.35	3.28	3.20
Agility	Edgren Side Step	38	42	44	35	27	39
	T-test (s)	9.8	9.3	9.1	11.4	10.8	10.6
Flexibility							
Upper body	Shoulder elevation (in.)	16	18	18	18	18	20
Lower body	Sit and reach (in.) (1)	14	14	14	16	16	16
Body composition	Body fat (%; skinfolds, Sloan formula)	12.0	10.7	8.2	19.5	18.0	17.0

- Have athletes share their goals with someone. Telling another person what the goals are helps solidify personal commitment. The athlete should consider writing, signing, and having a second party sign the list of goals in the form of a contract (see, for example, the form on p. 285).
- The coach should review the goals with each athlete at the end of the competitive season.

It is valuable to keep a folder with a longitudinal testing and evaluation record for each athlete (see the sample record on p. 286). This record can help the strength and conditioning professional evaluate the athlete's total program and can serve as a motivational tool when counseling the athlete. Girth measurements and pictures of the athlete in the anatomical position can be taken at the beginning and end of each training year to serve as an additional visual motivator for the athlete and should be kept with the longitudinal file. The individual longitudinal testing and evaluation record is also useful in identifying athletic staleness, burnout, and overtraining (7). The sooner the source of the problem is identified and effectively addressed, the more effective the total program will be for developing athletic potential.

CONCLUSION

Evaluation of an individual athlete's test scores is a valuable tool in aiding the strength and conditioning

professional in making exercise prescription adjustments and assessing the effectiveness of the conditioning regimen.

Procedure for Computing T-Scores

Step 1. Rank raw scores from lowest to highest.

Step 2. Compute the mean ($\bar{x}$) by summing the raw scores and dividing by the number of scores.

Step 3. Compute the standard deviation (s) using the formula

$$s = \sqrt{\frac{\Sigma(x - \bar{x})^2}{n - 1}}.$$

a. Subtract the mean from each raw score: $x - \bar{x}$.
b. Square each resulting value: $(x - \bar{x})^2$.
c. Sum the squares: $\Sigma(x - \bar{x})^2$.
d. Divide this number by the number of scores (n) minus 1.
e. Take the square root of this result.

Step 4. Compute z-scores using the formula

$$z = \frac{x - \bar{x}}{s}.$$

Step 5. Convert z-scores to T-scores using the formula

T-score = ($z \times 10$) + 50.

**Descriptive Statistics Example:
40-yd Dash Scores (in Seconds)
in 9th- and 12th-Grade Students**

	9th-graders' scores (x)	12-graders' scores (x)
	5.8	6.1
	5.7	6.0
	5.5	5.9
	5.3	5.9
	5.1	5.8
	5.1	5.7
	5.1	5.6
	5.0	5.3
	5.0	5.2
	5.0	5.2
	4.9	5.0
	4.9	4.9
	4.9	4.8
	4.8	4.8
	4.8	4.7
	4.8	4.7
	4.8	4.6
	4.7	4.6
	4.7	4.5
	4.6	4.5
	4.6	
n (sample size, or number of scores)	21	20
$\bar{x}$ (mean)	5.0	5.2
Median	4.9	5.1
Mode(s)	4.8	5.9, 5.2, 4.8, 4.7, 4.6, 4.5
Range	1.2	1.6
s (standard deviation)	0.33	0.56

Sample calculations:

Mean

$\bar{x} = \Sigma x/n$

$\quad = 105.1/21 \quad | \quad = 103.8/20$

$\quad = 5.0 \qquad\quad | \quad = 5.2$

Median

For the 9th-graders, the median is simply the middle score. For the 12th-graders, there is no single middle score, so the two scores closest to the middle, 5.2 and 5.0, are averaged to get the median.

Mode

The score that appears most frequently among the 9th-graders is 4.8 (four times). Six scores appear twice among the 12th-graders (and none more than twice) so there are six modes; this demonstrates that the mode is often rather useless.

Range

The range is simply the difference between the highest score and lowest score.

Standard deviation

$$s = \sqrt{\frac{\Sigma(x - \bar{x})^2}{n - 1}}$$

$\quad = 0.33 \quad | \quad = 0.56$

The larger standard deviation for the 12th-graders reflects the larger spread of their scores about the mean.

Key Terms

central tendency	275	mode	275	standard deviation	275
descriptive statistics	274	normalize	274	standard score	277
difference score	274	ordinal score	275	statistics	274
inferential statistics	275	percentile rank	275	T-score	277
mean	275	percentile	275	variability	275
median	275	range	275		

Study Questions

1. The personal physical goal for a female college volleyball player is to score in the 75th percentile for female college volleyball players. Her raw test scores and percentile rank are as follows:

Test	Raw score	Percentile rank
Vertical jump	18.5 in.	80
20-yd dash	3.60 s	20
Basketball throw	51.0 ft	30
Proportion of body fat	14.0%	75

Her conditioning program should be adjusted to emphasize which of the following to achieve her goals?

a. upper body strength and sprint work
b. plyometric jumping drills and aerobic conditioning
c. upper and lower body strength
d. sprint work and aerobic conditioning

2. A well-conditioned college-level defensive halfback in football has achieved the test scores listed here:

- Bench press, 285 lb
- Squat, 375 lb
- Vertical jump, 29 in.
- 300-yd shuttle run, 62 s
- Sit-ups (in 2 min), 65
- Proportion of body fat, 10%

Which of the following exercise recommendations is most appropriate?

a. Emphasis should be placed on interval sprint training and abdominal strength exercises.
b. Emphasis should be placed on interval sprint training and plyometric depth jumps.
c. Emphasis should be placed on aerobic fitness and plyometric depth jumps.
d. Emphasis should be placed on abdominal strength and plyometric depth jumps.

3. A mature college freshman female basketball guard recorded the following test results at the beginning of her first year of training in September (T1) and at the end of the training period in May (T2):

	T1	T2
Line drill test (s)	36	34
Vertical jump (in.)	17	20
Bench press (lb)	60	110
20-yd dash (s)	3.35	3.25

It is now June and you are helping her set appropriate goals for the beginning of practice in September of her sophomore year. In which of the following would she be most likely to make the greatest improvement and should she make a high priority area for her training?

a. line drill
b. vertical jump
c. bench press
d. 20-yd dash

Applying Knowledge of Evaluating Test Data

Problem 1

Data collection from testing batteries is useless unless the evaluative message is communicated properly to the coach and athletes. Difference scores are often reported from pretest and posttest measurements for evaluation purposes. This information can grossly misrepresent program efficacy and individual progress. Present the case for why difference scores should not be used alone for evaluation purposes. What would represent a more sound method of presenting the data?

Problem 2

When constructing a longitudinal athletic profile, raw data is generally recorded and treated in a manner that allows comparison of physical test data of differing fitness parameters (i.e., speed, muscular endurance, strength, etc.) with differing measuring units (i.e., seconds, repetitions, kilograms, etc.). Identify and describe this statistical method and discuss how it interrelates with measures of central tendency and standard deviation.

References

1. Altug, Z., T. Altug, and A. Altug. A test selection guide for assessing and evaluating athletes. *NSCA Journal* 9(3):67-69. 1987.
2. American Alliance for Health, Physical Education, Recreation and Dance. *AAHPERD Health Related Fitness Test.* Reston, VA: Author. 1980.
3. Baechle, T. Offseason strength and conditioning for basketball. *NSCA Journal* 5(1):19-55. 1983.
4. Baumgartner, T., and A. Jackson. *Measurement for Evaluation in Physical Education and Exercise Science.* Dubuque, IA: Brown. 1987.
5. Cooper, K. *The New Aerobics.* New York: Bantam Books. 1972.
6. Epley, B. *Husker Power.* Lincoln: University of Nebraska Press. 1983.
7. Henschen, K.P. Athletic staleness and burnout: Diagnosis, prevention, and treatment. In: *Applied Sport Psychology*, 2nd ed., J.E. Williams, ed. Mountain View, CA: Mayfield. 1993. pp. 328-337.
8. Hitchcock, H., and B. Pauletto. Tennessee's championship preseason conditioning program. *Coaching Women's Basketball* 5:10-14. 1987.
9. Hopkins, C. *Understanding Educational Research.* Columbus, OH: Merrill. 1980.
10. Johnson, B., and J. Nelson. *Practical Measurements for Evaluation in Physical Education*, 2nd ed. Minneapolis: Burgess. 1974.
11. Kurland, H. Isokinetic testing and training. *NSCA Journal* 2(2):34-35. 1982.
12. Mayhew, J., B. Levy, T. McCormick, and G. Evans. Strength norms for NCAA Division II college football players. *NSCA Journal* 9(3):67-69. 1987.
13. Pollock, M., J. Wilmore, and S. Fox. *Exercise in Health and Disease.* Philadelphia: Saunders. 1984.
14. Rees, R., and J. Blakey. Motivational strategies in offseason conditioning programs—making athletes work and making athletes want to work. *NSCA Journal* 5(5):20-21. 1983.
15. Semenick, D. Testing and evaluation. *NSCA Journal* 2(2):8-9. 1981.
16. Semenick, D. Anaerobic testing: Practical applications. *NSCA Journal* 6(5):44-73. 1984.
17. Semenick, D. Basketball bioenergetics: Practical applications. *NSCA Journal* 6(6):44-73. 1985.
18. Sifft, J. Using descriptive statistics in sport performance. *NSCA Journal* 5(5):26-28. 1983.
19. Sifft, J. Statistics for sport performance: Basic inferential analysis. *NSCA Journal* 8(6):46-47. 1986.
20. Thomas, J., and K. Nelson. *Introduction to Research in Health, Physical Education, Recreation and Dance.* Champaign, IL: Human Kinetics. 1985.
21. Wilkerson, G. Time expectations for a well-conditioned athlete in the 1-1/2 mile. *NSCA Journal* 5(5):44-45. 1983.

Personal Strength and Conditioning Goal Commitment

I, _____ , agree with the following physical strength and conditioning goals that
I and Coach _____ have established for me. I promise to achieve my goals by
committing myself to intensive consistent training. My goals will be achieved by _____ (date).

1.	Body weight	lose/gain _____ lb
2.	1.5-mile run	_____ min
3.	Edgren Side Step	_____ repetitions in 10 s
4.	Sit-and-reach stretch	_____ in.
5.	Vertical jump	_____ in.
6.	Bench press	_____ lb, one repetition
7.	Parallel squat	_____ lb, one repetition
8.	Medicine ball put	_____ ft and in.
9.	Chin-ups	_____ repetitions (maximum)
10.	Dips	_____ repetitions (maximum)
11.	Unanchored sit-ups	_____ repetitions (maximum in 2 min)

_____
Player's signature

_____
Coach's signature

_____
Date

University of Louisville Football Longitudinal Record (Sample)

(Name)

	1980 Aug.	1980 Dec.	1981 Apr.	1981 Aug.	1981 Dec.	1982 Apr.	1982 Aug.	1982 Dec.	1983 Apr.	1983 Aug.	Total change (% change)
Height (in.)	75	75	75.5	75.5	75.5	75.5	75.5	75.5	75.5	75.5	
Weight (lb)	231	239	245	248	246	252	255	255	258	255	+24 (+10.4%)
Body fat (%)	16.8	17.0	16.5	16.0	16.5	16.5	16.0	16.0	15.5	15.0	−1.8 (−10.7%)
Strength											
Power clean (lb)	—	215	240	—	240	265	—	255	270	—	+55 (+25.6%)
Bench press (lb)	—	290	325	—	315	345	—	330	365	—	+75 (+25.9%)
Squat (lb)	—	335	405	—	375	445	—	430	475	—	+140 (+41.8%)
Anaerobic power											
Vertical jump (in.)	25.0"	25.0"	25.5"	26.0"	26.0"	26.0"	26.5"	26.5"	27.0"	27.5"	+2.5 (+10%)
Medicine ball put (ft; in.)	18'10"	18'11"	19'8"	20'2"	20'0"	21'1"	21'0"	21'0"	21'5"	21'8"	+2'10" (+14.9%)
Speed											
40-yd dash (s)	5.05	5.05	5.05	5.00	5.00	5.00	4.95	5.00	4.90	4.90	−0.15 (−3.0%)
Agility											
Edgren Side Step (points)	38	37	40	42	40	40	42	41	42	42	+4 (+10.5%)
Aerobic power											
1.5-mile run (min:sec)	11:50	11:40	11:15	11:00	11:15	11:15	11:00	11:00	10:42	10:30	+1:20 (+12.0%)
Muscular endurance											
Dips (reps)	17	19	26	28	25	32	33	30	35	36	+19 (+112%)
Sit-ups (reps)	64	66	69	75	70	75	79	75	30	82	+18 (+28.1%)
Total points	—	463	532	—	529	581	—	576	635	—	
T-score improvements	—	—	69	—	—	52	—	—	59	—	+172
Team rank	58/119	51/122	40/122	40/120	38/119	18/119	16/116	12/118	9/118	6/116	6/116

PART III

EXERCISE TECHNIQUES

CHAPTER 19

STRETCHING AND WARM-UP

William B. Allerheiligen

This chapter briefly introduces the preexercise warming-up process, with a particular focus on stretching. A proper warm-up is specific to the sport or activity, and stretching should be an integral part of any warm-up. A total warm-up program includes the following components:

- It begins with a **general warm-up** period (9,12,41), which may consist of 5 to 10 min of slow jogging or riding a stationary bicycle. A general warm-up increases heart rate, blood flow, deep muscle temperature (16), respiration rate, viscosity of joint fluids (6), and perspiration. A warm muscle exhibits a greater amount of flexibility (42).
- It incorporates 8 to 12 min of sport or activity stretches, such as shoulder stretches for volleyball players.

Additionally, a warm-up is sometimes based on the dynamic movements of a specific sport or activity, i.e., low-intensity bounding for a long jumper. **Specific warm-up** uses movements that are similar to the movements of the athlete's sport. The more power necessary for the sport or activity, the more important the warm-up (17).

Flexibility is the range of possible movement in a joint (13,16) and its surrounding muscles (21); it may also be referred to as *static flexibility* (20). **Dynamic flexibility** refers to the resistance of a joint during movement (20). The ability to go through the full range of possible movement about a joint is called **range of motion (ROM)**.

Stretching is commonly credited with the prevention of injuries. Although not strongly supported by research (3,9), there is some evidence that stretching may aid in the prevention of injuries (7,45). (For a more detailed discussion, refer to chapter 35.) A loss or lack of flexibility can result from excessive periods of sitting or standing, limited ROM weight training exercises, and simple lack of stretching. Stretching twice a week for 5 weeks will significantly improve flexibility (20).

FACTORS AFFECTING FLEXIBILITY

The first three factors here deal with mechanics, structure, and age and gender and thus cannot be altered by training. It is therefore necessary to work on the remaining factors to enhance flexibility.

Joint Structure

The structure of a joint determines its ROM (27,31,48). Ball-and-socket joints, such as the hip and shoulder joints, yield the greatest ROM of all joints (5). The wrist, one of the least flexible joints, is an ellipsoidal joint (an oval-shaped condyle that fits into an elliptical cavity) (5) with a ROM of 80°; the knee's ROM, in contrast, is 130° (Figure 19.1).

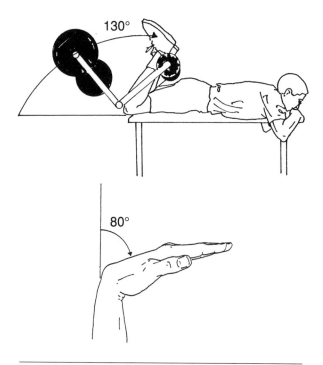

Figure 19.1   Range of motion of the knee and wrist joints.

Muscle Bulk

A large increase in muscle bulk may adversely affect ROM. A person with large biceps and deltoids, for example, may experience difficulty in stretching the triceps (16), racking a power clean, or holding a bar while performing the front squat. Weight training, if performed properly (with full ROM of both the agonist and antagonist muscles), does not adversely affect ROM (46). Although the amount of muscle bulk can be decreased by altering the training program, this may not be advisable for large power athletes such as shot-putters or offensive linemen.

Age and Gender

Young people tend to be more flexible than older people (47), and females more flexible than males (21,25,39). Differences in flexibility between young males and females may be due in part to anatomical differences and the type and extent of activities performed (22). Older persons also undergo a process called *fibrosis*, in which muscle fibers degenerate and are replaced by fibrous connective tissue (5).

Connective Tissue

Tendons, ligaments, fascial sheaths, and joint capsules may have a limiting influence on ROM, as does the skin (16,48). *Elasticity* (the ability to return to original form) and *plasticity* (the inability to return to original form) of connective tissue are other factors that determine ROM (42,47).

Weight Training With Limited Range of Motion

Although normal resistance training may increase flexibility (27-29,32,43), heavy resistance training with limited ROM in the exercises may result in restricted ROM (16). High-volume resistance training programs (i.e., bodybuilding) with limited ROM may also impair ROM improvement. To prevent loss of ROM, perform exercises that develop both agonist and antagonist muscles (19) and use full ROM specific to the joint.

Frequency and Duration of Stretching

Stretching for 2 min once a week is not adequate for increasing flexibility. Although the number of stretching sessions per week varies according to the sport and the time of year, on average each practice session should be preceded by 5 to 6 min of general warm-up and 8 to 12 min of stretching and concluded with 4 to 5 min of stretching.

Activity Level

An active person tends to be more flexible than an inactive one (21,34). Both men and women can increase their flexibility during a resistance training program (46).

WHEN SHOULD YOU STRETCH?

Ideally, stretching should be performed at the following times for optimum benefits (1):

• *Before practice and competition.* Stretching will aid in injury prevention and assist in warm-up. The duration of this stretching session should normally be 8 to 12 min, with some sports—gymnastics for example—requiring more time.

• *Following practice and competition.* Postpractice stretching facilitates ROM because of increased muscle temperature (42); it should be performed within 5 to 10 min after practice. If the sport or activity has required a high-volume or high-intensity workout involving the legs and low back, this is an excellent time to stretch the hamstrings and low back. Postpractice stretching may also decrease muscular soreness (41).

Additionally, for those who lack sufficient flexibility for their sport or activity, extra stretching sessions during free time may be both relaxing and beneficial.

INDIVIDUALITY OF STRETCHING

Stretching should not be viewed as a contest with another person, but as an individual activity. Athletes should work on increasing flexibility, only stretching to the point of discomfort, then backing off a little. One person may have superior ROM in the shoulder area, and another person poor ROM there. The less flexible person should not try to compete with the more flexible one; stretching does not increase flexibility if it causes pain. The only result may be damaged muscle or connective tissue.

STRETCH REFLEXES

This reflex is comprised of the **stretch reflex** and the **inverse stretch reflex**. Two *proprioceptors* that act to elicit the two reflexes are *muscle spindles* and *Golgi tendon organs (GTOs)*. Muscle spindles are sensory mechanisms located within intrafusal muscles that run parallel with extrafusal muscle fibers; they monitor the changes in length of a muscle (20). In a simple reflex, when a muscle spindle is stimulated by a rapid stretching movement, a sensory neuron from the muscle spindle innervates a motor neuron in the spinal column that is activated. The motor neuron then causes a contraction of the muscle (extrafusal fibers) that was previously stretched—this is the stretch reflex. If the muscle spindles are not stimulated, then the muscle will be relaxed. An example of the stretch reflex is the knee-jerk. When the patellar tendon is tapped, the tendon is quickly stretched, which causes the quadriceps muscle to contract. (The stretch reflex only responds to stretching, while the inverse stretch reflex responds to both stretching and contraction [9].) Because of the very slow movement during static stretching, the stretch reflex is not invoked. Rapid stretching movements (ballistic) may invoke the stretch reflex. GTOs respond to changes in the length of a muscle and muscle tension. They are very sensitive to tension that results from active contraction. A force as little as 0.1 g results in impulse propagation of the GTO (16). The inverse stretch mechanism is stimulated when the GTO prevents overstressing a muscle as a result of either overstretching or active contraction. A contraction of the agonist will result in a reflex relaxation of the antagonist; this is called **reciprocal inhibition**, or inverse stretch reflex inhibition. The GTO is a protective device that inhibits muscle contraction (2) and may cause contraction of the antagonists (10). A maximal isometric contraction of the agonist produces increased tension, which stimulates the GTO to effect a reflex relaxation of the agonist (41).

The relaxation of the agonist during a maximal isometric muscle contraction is called **autogenic inhibition** (42).

TYPES OF STRETCHING

Active stretches may be static, dynamic, or ballistic. Passive stretches are normally performed as static or dynamic (PNF).

Active Stretch

An **active stretch** occurs when the person stretching supplies the force of the stretch. During the sitting toe touch, for example, the athlete supplies the force for the forward lean that stretches the hamstrings and low back.

Passive Stretch

A **passive stretch** occurs when a partner or device provides the force for the stretch. **Proprioceptive neuromuscular facilitation (PNF)** stretching uses a partner to passively stretch a muscle, although a "device" may be used to passively stretch a muscle. For example, while stretching the hamstrings from a supine position and with one leg elevated, a towel (the device) may be placed behind the heel. By pulling the towel toward the upper body, the hamstrings will be stretched.

Static Stretch

A **static stretch** is a constant one in which the end position is held for 10 to 30 s. A static stretch includes the passive relaxation and concurrent elongation of the muscle (19). Static stretching is easy to learn and effective. It does not elicit the stretch reflex of the stretched muscle (10); the likelihood of injury is less than if ballistic stretching (discussed next) is used (5,42,44); and it helps relieve soreness (10,15,41) and is relaxing. Although injury to muscles or connective tissue may result if the intensity of the static stretch is carried too far, there are no real disadvantages to static stretching as long as correct methods are used. Athletes in a variety of sports use static stretching exercises.

The sitting toe touch is an example of a static stretch. Starting from a sitting position on the ground, with both legs straight and together, the upper body perpendicular to the legs and the feet in a vertical position (Figure 19.2), lean forward from the waist (18). Slowly reach toward the ankles with the hands (Figure 19.3). Gradually increase the intensity of the stretch, by leaning forward more, until discomfort in the hamstrings or lower back is felt (Figure 19.4). Hold this position for 10 to 15 s. Slowly return to a vertical sitting position. (A more general and complete set of instructions for static stretching begins on p. 298.)

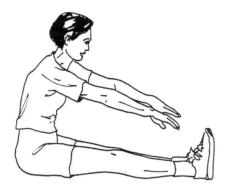

Figure 19.2   Start of the sitting toe touch.

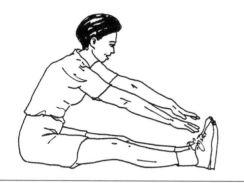

Figure 19.3   Easy stretch of the sitting toe touch.

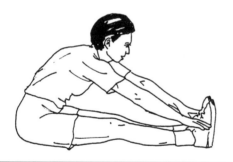

Figure 19.4   Developmental stretch of the sitting toe touch.

Stages of Static Stretching (18)

1. **Easy stretch**. During this stage the muscle stretches slightly (see Figure 19.3).
2. **Developmental stretch**. Intensity of the stretch is increased during this stage (see Figure 19.4). This may also be called "stretch by feel" (4).
3. **Drastic stretch**. This stage may result in pain. **WARNING**: If so, avoid this stage.

Steps in Static Stretching (2)

1. Get into the starting position of the stretching exercise. Remember to stay relaxed during the whole stretch and breathe normally.

2. Move the body or body segment into the stretching movement (easy stretch) until a stretching of the muscle is felt.
3. From the easy stretch, slowly increase intensity of the stretch for 10 to 15 s (developmental stretch). Do not bounce while stretching.
4. Do not stretch so far that pain is felt (drastic stretch) in the muscle or joint. If this happens, slowly decrease the intensity of the stretch.

Ballistic Stretch

A **ballistic stretch** involves a bouncing movement in which the end position is not held. Ballistic stretching involves active muscular effort (33,35,36). A dynamic movement is used to create ballistic movement in order to stretch the agonist. Ballistic and static stretches may encompass identical or nearly identical stretches (in terms of body movement and form); both types of stretches will yield nearly identical results in development of ROM (15,30). Ballistic stretching, however, may produce injuries to muscles or connective tissue, especially when there has been a previous injury (10). Injury may result if a person forcefully tries to go beyond his or her ROM for a particular area of the body. Ballistic stretching is normally performed only for the lower body (quadriceps, hamstrings, and hips) and lower torso (low back and external obliques); it may occasionally be used for the upper body.

As an example, let us look at the sitting toe touch performed as a ballistic stretch rather than as a static stretch. Start by sitting on the ground with legs straight and together, upper body perpendicular to the legs, feet in a vertical position, and arms extended in front of the upper body. Contracting the abdominal muscles, quickly reach toward the ankles (if the hands can reach the ankles then reach past the feet) and immediately return to a near vertical upper body position. Repeat this movement 10 times for one to three sets. Bounce at the end position, with each bounce extending further than the preceding one. The ballistic stretch is normally not the preferred technique and should not be used by those with low-back injuries or certain other injuries.

Dynamic Stretch

A **dynamic stretch** involves flexibility during sport-specific movements (16). Dynamic stretching is similar to ballistic stretching in that it utilizes movement, but dynamic stretching includes movements that may be specific to a sport or movement pattern; in a sense, dynamic stretching can be similar to a specific warm-up. Dynamic stretching is most common among track-and-field athletes, but is also used in other sports, such as basketball and volleyball. An example of dynamic stretching would be a track sprinter performing high knees with an emphasis on knee height and arm action and not on horizontal speed.

Proprioceptive Neuromuscular Facilitation Stretch

A proprioceptive neuromuscular facilitation (PNF) stretch combines alternating contraction and relaxation of both agonist and antagonist muscles; this causes neural responses that inhibit the contraction of the muscle being stretched. This interaction results in a decrease in resistance and increased ROM when stretching a muscle. Another benefit of PNF stretching is increased muscular strength owing to the isometric or concentric contraction of the agonist. PNF stretching usually requires a partner.

Static and PNF stretching techniques increase ROM, but PNF may be superior in producing improvements (13,24,40,42). Static stretching requires relaxation of the agonist while PNF utilizes relaxation and isometric or concentric action of the agonist (muscle being stretched) and relaxation and concentric contraction of the antagonist (muscle not being stretched). However, PNF techniques may often be impractical to use because many require a partner. It is imperative that the partner be experienced in PNF techniques; otherwise, injury may occur.

There are three basic types of PNF stretching techniques (26):

- **Hold-relax**
- **Contraction-relax**
- **Slow-reversal-hold-relax**

The following illustrate stretching the hamstrings with each PNF technique. First, here are the conditions for the starting position:

- Subject is on back with one leg raised 50° to 60°, knee locked, and the ankle flexed at 90° (Figure 19.5).

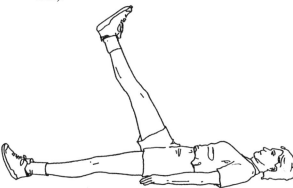

Figure 19.5   Starting position of PNF hamstring stretch.

- When stretching the right leg the partner places his or her right knee on the outside of the subject's left knee and the foot on the inside of the subject's left calf (Figure 19.6).
- Partner's left hand is on heel of the subject's right foot and the right hand on the subject's right knee (see Figure 19.6).

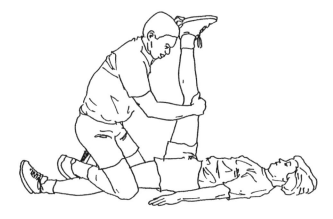

Figure 19.6   Partner and subject leg and hand positions for PNF stretching of the hamstrings.

Hold-Relax

1. Begin in the starting position. Partner performs a passive prestretch (or easy stretch) of the subject's right hamstring (Figure 19.7) (11,12,26).
2. When the partner says "push," subject performs a 3- to 4-s developmental isometric action (Figure 19.8) (the partner does not allow the subject's leg to move) of the hamstring followed by a 4- to 6-s near-maximal isometric action of the hamstring (11,12,26).
3. This is followed by a 10-s passive static stretch (partner says relax) of the hamstring as the part-

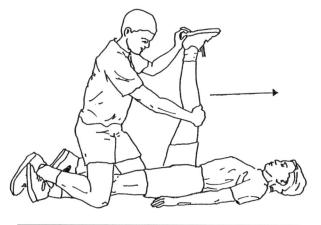

Figure 19.7   Passive stretch of hamstrings during hold-relax PNF stretching.

ner pushes backward on the subject's right leg (Figure 19.9) (11,12,26).

4. Without lowering the leg, repeat this process two to four times, then lower the leg to the starting position.

5. Repeat by starting at Step 1 for a total of three to five repetitions. Repeat with other leg.

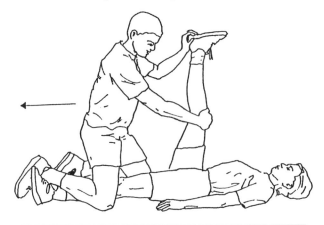

Figure 19.8 Isometric action of hamstrings during hold-relax PNF stretching.

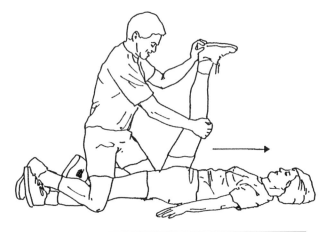

Figure 19.9 Increased ROM in the hamstrings during the passive stretch of hold-relax PNF stretching.

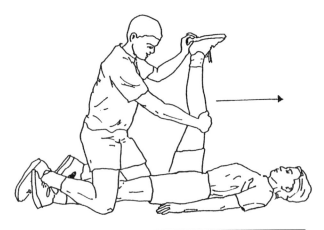

Figure 19.10 Passive stretch of the hamstrings during contract-relax PNF stretching.

Contraction-Relax

1. Begin in the starting position. Partner performs a passive prestretch of the subject's hamstring for 4 to 6 s (Figure 19.10) (11,12,26).

2. The partner says "back," and the subject performs a concentric contraction of the hip flexors for 4 to 6 s as the partner continues to push on the leg (Figure 19.11).

3. Partner then says "relax" and then performs a passive static stretch against the hamstring for 10 s (Figure 19.12) (11,12,26). Repeat this process two to four times.

4. The partner lowers the subject's leg to the starting position.

5. Repeat by starting at Step 1 for a total of three to five repetitions. Repeat with the other leg.

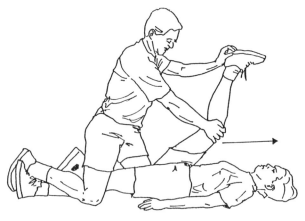

Figure 19.11 Concentric contraction of the hip flexors during contract-relax PNF stretching.

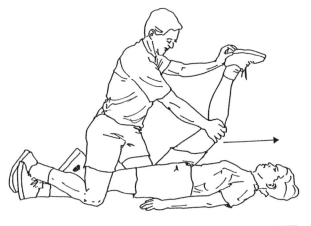

Figure 19.12 Increased ROM in the hamstrings during the passive stretch of contract-relax PNF stretching.

Slow-Reversal-Hold-Relax

1. Begin in the starting position. Partner performs a passive prestretch on the subject's straight leg (11,12,26) until there is slight discomfort in the hamstring (Figure 19.13).

2. Partner will feel some resistance in the leg being stretched. At this point, the partner tells the subject to "push" against the partner's hand for 6 to 10 s (isometric action of the hamstring) (Figure 19.14) (11,12,26).

3. The amount of tension generated by the subject should be enough to force the partner to use some resistive force. The subject will probably experience some discomfort while pushing downward.

4. While the subject continues to push against the hand, the partner says "back," at which time the subject immediately concentrically contracts (submaximally) the quadriceps and hip flexors to attempt to lift the heel off of the partner's hand (Figure 19.15) (11,12).

5. At the same time, the partner passively pushes back against the straight leg (Figure 19.16). It is during this time that the hamstring is relaxed and the ROM of the stretch is increased. The subject continues to contract the quadriceps and hip flexors until the partner says "relax."

6. The partner then finishes with a 10-s passive static stretch of the hamstring (11,12).

7. Steps 2 to 6 may be repeated two or three times before lowering the leg.

8. At the conclusion of the last passive static stretch, the partner slowly lowers the subject's leg to the starting position as subject slowly decreases tension in the hamstrings.

9. Repeat the process from Step 1 for a total of two to three repetitions. Repeat with the other leg.

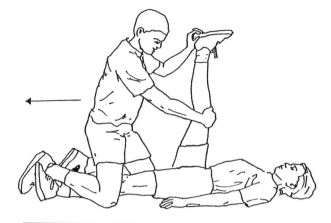

Figure 19.14 Isometric action of the hamstrings during slow-reversal-hold-relax PNF stretching.

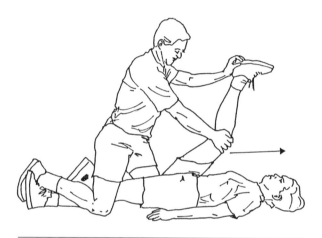

Figure 19.15 Concentric contraction of the quadriceps during slow-reversal-hold-relax PNF stretching.

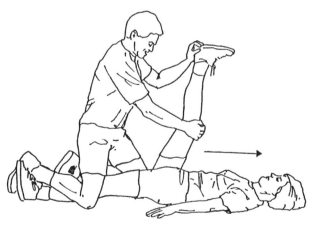

Figure 19.16 Increased ROM in the hamstrings during the passive stretch of slow-reversal-hold-relax PNF stretching.

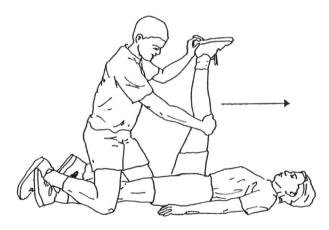

Figure 19.13 Passive stretch of the hamstrings during slow-reversal-hold-relax PNF stretching.

Common PNF Stretches With a Partner

- Calf and ankle (Figure 19.17)
- Chest (Figure 19.18)
- Groin (Figure 19.19)
- Hamstring and hip extensors (as described above)
- Quadriceps and hip flexors (Figure 19.20)
- Shoulder (Figure 19.21)

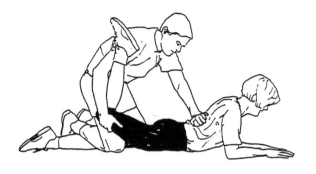

Figure 19.20 Passive stretch of the quadriceps and hip flexors during PNF stretching.

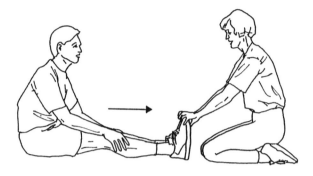

Figure 19.17 Isometric action of the calves during PNF stretching.

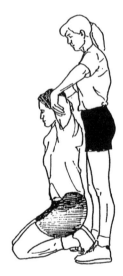

Figure 19.18 Passive stretch of the chest during PNF stretching.

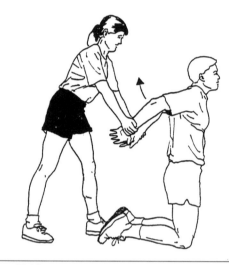

Figure 19.21 Passive stretch of the shoulder during PNF stretching.

Guidelines for Stretching

Do not perform ballistic stretches if the joint or an attached muscle is injured.

Do not perform ballistic toe touches with a sore back.

Do not perform static stretching with an intensity level that will cause reinjury.

Perform stretching exercises for the areas where increased ROM is desired (10).

Care should be taken during PNF stretching when a muscle is injured. Isometric actions and stretching of the agonist should be closely monitored for excessive intensity.

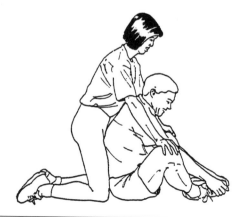

Figure 19.19 Concentric contraction of the groin muscles during PNF stretching.

BENEFITS OF STRETCHING

In general, PNF, static, and dynamic stretching stretch muscles, muscle sheaths, and tendons adequately in preparation for a workout. They also increase ROM in the joints. Although ballistic stretching will increase ROM, it is not the preferred method because of higher injury risks than other methods. Additional benefits of dynamic stretching are that it

- warms deep muscle fibers (16),
- warms joint fluids, lubricants, and synovial fluids (5),
- increases respiratory rate (depending on the type of warm-up), and
- elevates heart rate and therefore increases volume of blood flow (depending on the specific type of warm-up).

Stretching also

- decreases the chances and/or severity of injury (8,23,37,40),
- prepares the athlete mentally for the upcoming activity, and
- helps decrease joint inflexibility and pain after an athletic career.

STRETCHING TECHNIQUES

NECK

Look Right and Left

MUSCLE AFFECTED: *sternocleidomastoid*

1. Stand or sit with head and neck upright.
2. Turn head to the right using a submaximal concentric contraction. Hold for 10 s.
3. Turn head to the left using a submaximal concentric contraction. Hold for 10 s (14).

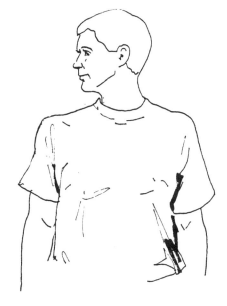

Rotational flexion of the neck.

Flexion and Extension

MUSCLES AFFECTED: *sternocleidomastoid, suboccipitals, and splenii*

1. Standing or sitting with head and neck upright, flex neck anteriorly (forward) by tucking chin in toward the chest; hold for 10 s.
2. If the chin touches the chest, try to touch lower on the chest with the chin.
3. Extend neck posteriorly (backward) by trying to touch the head to the trapezius; hold for 10 s.

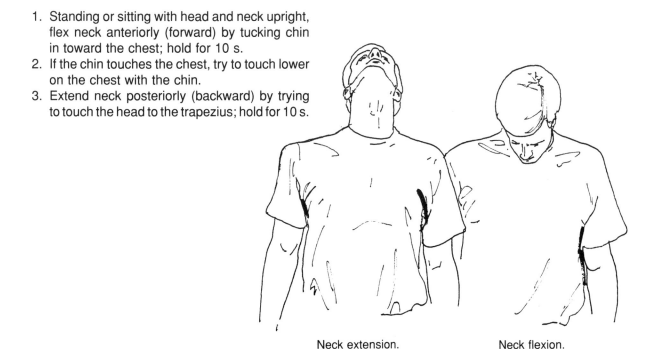

Neck extension.   Neck flexion.

SHOULDER

Straight Arms Behind Back

MUSCLES AFFECTED: *deltoids and pectoralis major*

1. Standing, place both arms behind back.
2. Interlock fingers with palms facing each other.
3. Straighten arms fully.
4. Slowly raise the straight arms.
5. Hold for 10 to 15 s.
6. Keep head upright and neck relaxed (2).

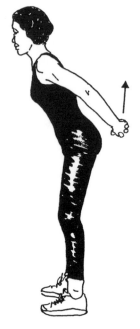

Stretching shoulder joints—standing.

Seated Lean-Back

MUSCLES AFFECTED: *deltoids and pectoralis major*

1. Sitting with legs straight and arms extended, place palms on floor about 1 ft (30 cm) behind hips.
2. Point fingers away (backward) from body.
3. Slide hands backward and lean backward.
4. Hold for 10 s (3).

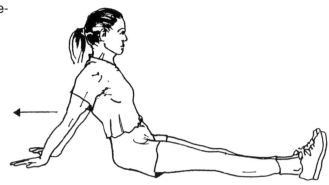

Stretching shoulder joints—sitting.

CHEST

Straight Arms Behind Back

MUSCLES AFFECTED: *deltoids and pectoralis major*

1. Standing, place both arms behind back.
2. Interlock fingers with palms facing each other.
3. Straighten arms fully.
4. Slowly raise the straight arms.
5. Hold for 10 to 15 s.
6. Keep head upright and neck relaxed (2).

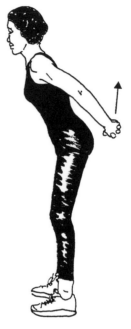

Stretching the chest.

POSTERIOR OF UPPER ARM

Behind-Neck Stretch (Chicken Wing)

MUSCLES AFFECTED: *triceps and latissimus dorsi*

1. Standing or sitting, flex right arm and raise elbow above head.
2. Reach the right hand down toward the left scapula.
3. Grasp right elbow with left hand.
4. Pull elbow behind head with left hand.
5. Hold for 10 s.
6. Repeat with left arm (1,3).

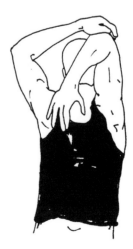

Stretching the triceps.

UPPER BACK

Cross Arm in Front of Chest

MUSCLES AFFECTED: *latissimus dorsi and teres major*

1. Stand or sit with the right arm slightly flexed (15°-30°) and adducted across the chest.
2. Grasp the upper arm just above the elbow, placing the left hand on the posterior side of the upper arm.
3. Pull the right arm across the chest (toward the left) with the left hand.
4. Hold for 10 s.
5. Repeat with the left arm.

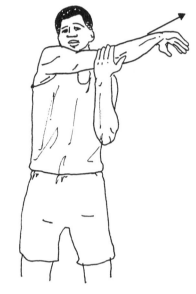

Stretching the upper back.

Arms Straight Up Above Head (Pillar)

MUSCLES AFFECTED: *latissimus dorsi and wrist flexors*

1. Stand with arms in front of torso, fingers interlocked with palms facing each other.
2. Slowly straighten the arms above the head with palms up.
3. Continue to reach upward with hands and arms.
4. While continuing to reach upward, slowly reach slightly backward.
5. Hold for 10 s (14).

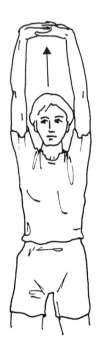

Stretching the shoulders, chest, and upper back.

LOWER BACK

Spinal Twist (Pretzel)

MUSCLES AFFECTED: *internal oblique, external oblique, and spinal erectors*

1. Sitting with legs straight and upper body nearly vertical, place right foot on left side of left knee.
2. Place back of left elbow on right side of right knee, which is now bent.
3. Place right palm on floor 30 to 40 cm behind hips.
4. Push right knee to the left with left elbow while turning shoulders and head to the right as far as possible. Try to look behind the back.
5. Hold for 10 s.
6. Repeat with the left leg (1).

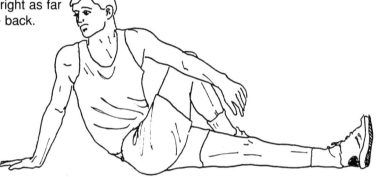

Stretching the low back and sides.

Semi–Leg Straddle

MUSCLES AFFECTED: *spinal erectors*

1. Sitting, knees flexed 30 to 50 degrees, let the legs totally relax.
2. Point the knees outward; the lateral side of the knees may or may not touch the floor.
3. Lean forward from waist and reach forward with extended arms. Hold position for 10 to 15 s.
4. Bending and relaxing legs decreases hamstring involvement and increases lower back stretch.

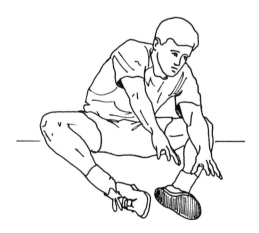

Stretching the low back from seated position.

HIPS

Forward Lunge (Fencer)

MUSCLES AFFECTED: *iliopsoas, rectus femoris*

1. Standing, take a long step forward (as with the lunge) with the right leg and flex the right knee until it is directly over the right foot.
2. Keep right foot flat on floor.
3. Keep back leg straight.
4. Keep back foot pointed in same direction as front foot; it is not necessary to have heel on floor.
5. Keep torso upright and rest hands on hips or front leg.
6. Slowly lower hips forward and downward.
7. Hold for 10 to 15 s.
8. Repeat with the left leg (1).

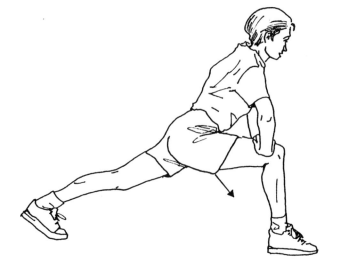

Stretching the hip flexors.

Supine Knee Flex

MUSCLES AFFECTED: *hip extensors (gluteus maximus and hamstrings)*

1. Lie on back with legs straight.
2. Flex right leg and lift knee toward chest.
3. Place both hands below knee and continue to pull knee toward chest.
4. Hold for 10 to 15 s.
5. Repeat with the left leg (1).

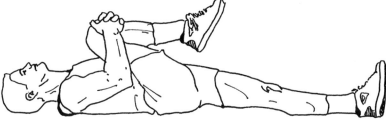

Stretching the gluteals and hamstrings.

SIDES

Side Bend With Straight Arms

MUSCLES AFFECTED: *external oblique, latissimus dorsi, and serratus anterior*

1. Stand with feet 35 to 40 cm apart.
2. Interlace the fingers with the palms facing each other.
3. Reach upward with straight arms.
4. Keeping arms straight, lean from waist to left side. Do not bend knees.
5. After moving as far as possible, hold for 10 s.
6. Repeat to the left side (1).

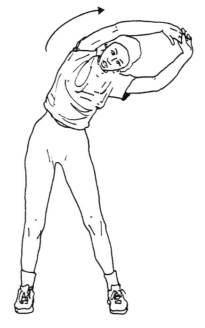

Stretching the sides, upper back, and shoulders.

Side Bend With Bent Arm

MUSCLES AFFECTED: *external oblique, latissimus dorsi, serratus anterior, and triceps*

1. Stand with feet 35 to 40 cm apart.
2. Flex right arm and raise elbow above head.
3. Reach the right hand down toward the left shoulder.
4. Grasp the right elbow (just above the elbow) with the left hand.
5. Pull elbow behind head.
6. Keeping arm bent, lean from waist to left side.
7. Do not bend knees.
8. After moving as far as possible, hold for 10 to 15 s.
9. Repeat with the left arm.

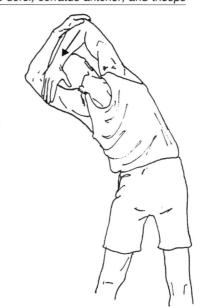

Stretching the sides, triceps, and upper back.

ANTERIOR OF THIGH AND HIP FLEXOR

Side Quadriceps Stretch

MUSCLES AFFECTED: *quadriceps and iliopsoas*

1. Lie on left side with both legs straight.
2. Place left forearm flat on floor and upper arm perpendicular to floor.
3. Place left forearm at 45° angle with torso.
4. Flex right leg with heel of right foot moving toward buttocks.
5. Grasp front of ankle with right hand and pull toward buttocks. **WARNING:** Do not pull on ankle so hard that pain or discomfort is felt in knee.
6. Move knee backward and slightly upward. The stretch occurs not so much from the excessive flexion of the knee but from moving the knee back and slightly up.
7. Hold for 10 to 15 s.
8. Repeat with the left leg (1).

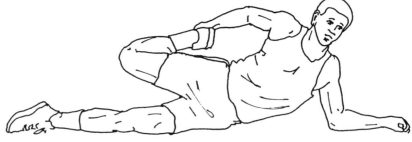

Stretching the quadriceps—on side.

Kneeling Quadriceps Stretch

MUSCLE AFFECTED: *quadriceps*

1. Kneel with the balls of the feet on the ground.
2. Keep hips straight (upper leg and torso should be in a straight line).
3. Place palms of hands on buttocks and push slightly forward.
4. With a straight body, lean slightly backward until developmental stretch is felt in quadriceps.
5. Hold for 10 to 15 s (1).

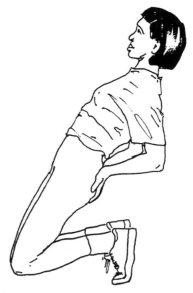

Stretching the quadriceps—kneeling.

POSTERIOR OF THIGH

Sitting Toe Touch

MUSCLES AFFECTED: *hamstrings, spinal erectors, and gastrocnemius*

1. Sit with the upper body nearly vertical and legs straight.
2. Lean forward from waist and grasp toes with each hand, slightly pull toes towards the upper body, and pull chest towards leg. (If you are very stiff, try to grasp the ankles.) Hold for 10 s.
3. Release toes and relax foot.
4. Grasp ankles and continue to pull chest toward legs. Hold for 10 s.
5. Still grasping the ankles, point toes away from body and continue to pull chest toward legs. Hold for 10 s (1).

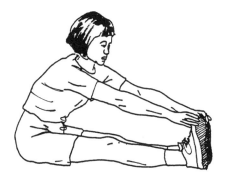

Stretching the hamstrings with emphasis on insertion of the hamstrings and calves.

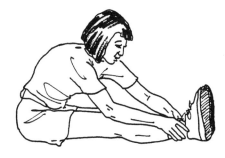

Stretching the hamstrings with emphasis on the middle portion.

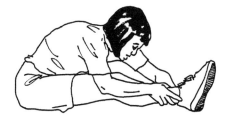

Stretching the hamstrings with emphasis on the upper portion.

Semistraddle (Figure Four)

MUSCLES AFFECTED: *gastrocnemius, hamstrings, and spinal erectors*

1. Sit with the upper body nearly vertical and legs straight.
2. Place sole of left foot on left side of right knee. The lateral side of left leg should be resting on the floor.
3. Lean forward from the waist and grasp toes with right hand and slightly pull toes toward the upper body as the chest is also pulled toward right leg. Hold for 10 s.
4. Release toes and relax foot.
5. Grasp ankle and continue to pull chest toward right leg. Hold for 10 s.
6. Point toes away from body and continue to pull chest toward right leg. Hold for 10 s.
7. Repeat with the left leg (1).

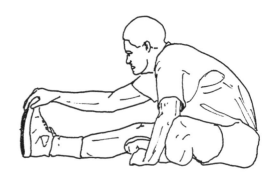

Stretching the hamstrings with emphasis on insertion of the hamstrings and calves.

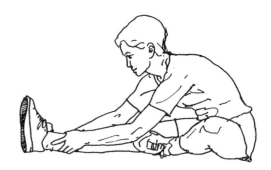

Stretching the hamstrings with emphasis on the middle portion.

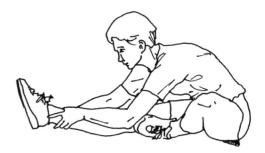

Stretching the hamstrings with emphasis on the upper portion.

GROIN

Straddle (Spread Eagle)

MUSCLES AFFECTED: *gastrocnemius, hamstrings, spinal erectors, adductors, and sartorius*

1. Sit with the upper body nearly vertical and legs straight, and spread legs as far as possible.
2. With right hand, grasp toes of right foot and pull on toes slightly, while pulling chest toward right leg. Hold for 10 s.
3. Release toes and relax foot.
4. Grasp ankle and continue to pull chest toward right leg. Hold for 10 s.
5. Point toes away from body and continue to pull chest toward right leg. Hold for 10 s.
6. Repeat process with the left leg.
7. Repeat process by grasping right toes with right hand and left toes with left hand. Move the torso forward and toward the ground (1).

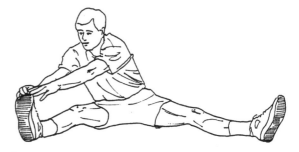

Stretching the hamstrings and groin with emphasis on insertion of the hamstrings and calves.

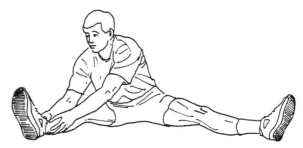

Stretching the hamstrings and groin with emphasis on the middle portion.

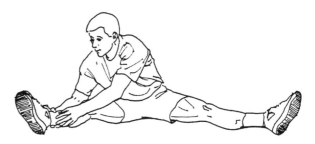

Stretching the hamstrings and groin with emphasis on the upper portion.

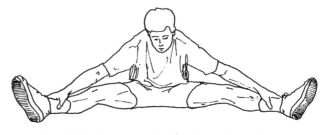

Stretching the groin, low back, and hamstrings.

Butterfly

MUSCLES AFFECTED: *adductors and sartorius*
---

1. Sitting with the upper body nearly vertical and legs straight, flex both knees as the soles of the feet come together.
2. Pull feet toward body.
3. Place hands on feet and elbows on legs.
4. Pull torso slightly forward as elbows push legs down.
5. Hold for 10 to 15 s (1,38).

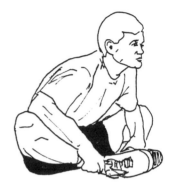

Stretching the groin.

POSTERIOR OF LOWER LEG

Bent-Over Toe Raise

MUSCLES AFFECTED: *gastrocnemius and soleus*
---

1. Stand with heel of right foot 15 to 20 cm in front of toes of left foot.
2. Flex right foot toward shin (dorsi-flexion) with heel in contact with floor.
3. Lean forward and try to touch right leg with chest while both legs are straight.
4. Continue to lean downward with upper body as the foot is dorsi-flexed near maximal toward the shin.
5. Hold for 10 to 15 s.
6. Repeat with the left leg (3).

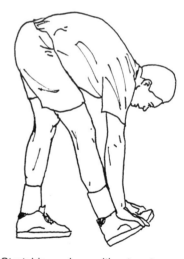

Stretching calves without a step.

Step Stretch

MUSCLES AFFECTED: *gastrocnemius and soleus; also, Achilles tendon*

1. Have ready a step or board 8 to 10 cm high.
2. Place balls of both feet on the step or board, 2.5 cm from its edge.
3. With straight legs, lower heels as far as possible.
4. Hold for 10 to 15 s.
5. To stretch Achilles tendon, raise heels slightly. Slightly flex the knees and then lower the heels. This stretch will be felt in the Achilles tendon.
6. Hold for 10 to 15 s.
7. For a more intense and individualized stretch, perform this stretch with one leg at a time.

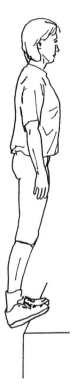

Stretching the calves standing on a step.

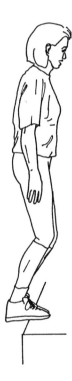

Preparing to stretch the Achilles tendon by slightly bending the knee.

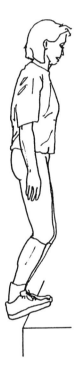

Stretching the Achilles tendon by lowering the heel.

Key Terms

Study Questions

1. When stimulated, the GTOs may be responsible for which of the following?

   a. relaxation of the agonist and contraction of the antagonist
   b. relaxation of the antagonist and contraction of the agonist
   c. contraction of the agonist only
   d. contraction of the antagonist only

2. Which of the following stretching methods will decrease the stimulation of muscle spindles?

   a. dynamic
   b. ballistic
   c. static
   d. drastic

3. Dynamic stretching is most similar to which of the following?

   a. specific warm-up
   b. general warm-up
   c. easy stretch
   d. static stretch

4. Stimulation of muscle spindles induces a

   a. relaxation of GTOs
   b. relaxation of the agonist
   c. contraction of the agonist
   d. contraction of the antagonist

Applying Knowledge of Stretching and Warm-Up

Problem 1
The postpractice cool-down should include a brief 4- to 5-min stretching program. Select three stretches that may be selected for cool-down to facilitate flexibility in the hamstring and lower back.

Problem 2
Explain the method and mechanism (physiological stretching principle) of increasing the intensity of the side quadriceps stretch.

References

1. Allerheiligen, W.B. *Weight Training and Conditioning*. Manhattan, KS: Ag Press. 1980.
2. Allerheiligen, W.B. *Poke Power Training Manual*. Ft. Collins, CO: Published by author. 1992.
3. Alter, M.J. *Sport Stretch*. Champaign, IL: Leisure Press. 1990.
4. Anderson, B. Flexibility: Roundtable. *NSCA Journal* 6(4):10-22, 71-73. 1984.
5. Anthony, C.P., and N.J. Kolthoff. *Textbook of Anatomy and Physiology*, 9th ed. St. Louis: Mosby. 1975.
6. Astrand, P.O., and K. Rodahl. *Textbook of Work Physiology*. New York: McGraw-Hill. 1970.
7. Beaulieu, J.E. *Stretching for All Sports*. Pasadena, CA: Athletic Press. 1980.
8. Beaulieu, J.E. Developing a stretching program. *Phys. Sportsmed.* 9(11):59-69. 1981.
9. Beaulieu, J.E. Flexibility: Roundtable. *NSCA Journal* 6(4):10-22, 71-73. 1984.
10. Corbin, C.B., L.J. Dowell, R. Lindsey, and H. Tolson. *Concepts in Physical Education*. Dubuque, IA: Brown. 1978.
11. Cornelius, W.J. Flexibility: Roundtable. *NSCA Journal* 6(4):10-22, 71-73. 1984.
12. Cornelius, W.J. The Effective Way. *NSCA Journal* 7(3):62-64. 1985.
13. Cornelius, W.J., and M.M. Hinson. The relationship between isometric contractions of hip extensors and subsequent flexibility in males. *Sports Med. Phys. Fitness* 20:75-80. 1980.
14. Croce, P. *Stretching For Athletics*. Champaign, IL: Leisure Press.
15. deVries, H.A. Evaluation of static stretching procedures for improvement of flexibility. *Res. Q.* 33:222-228. 1962.
16. deVries, H.A. *Physiology of Exercise for Physical Education and Athletics*. Dubuque, IA: Brown. 1974.
17. Dominguez, R.H. Flexibility: Roundtable. *NSCA Journal* 6(4):10-22, 71-73. 1984.
18. Epley, B. *The Strength of Nebraska*. Lincoln, NE: University of Nebraska Intercollegiate Athletics. 1974.
19. Fleck, S.J., and W.J. Kraemer. *Designing Resistance Training Programs*. Champaign, IL: Human Kinetics. 1987.
20. Fox, E.L. *Sports Physiology*. Philadelphia: Saunders. 1979.
21. Getchell, B. *Physical Fitness: A Way of Life*. New York: Wiley. 1979.
22. Haley, P.R. A comparative analysis of selected motor fitness test performance of elementary school boys. *Dissert. Abstr. Int.* 32:501A. 1972.
23. Holt, L.E. *Scientific Stretching for Sport*. Halifax, Nova Scotia: Sport Research. 1976.
24. Holt, L.E., T.M. Travis, and T. Okia. Comparative study of three stretching techniques. *Percept. Mot. Skills* 31:611-616. 1970.
25. Kirchner, G., and D. Glines. Comparative analysis of Eugene, Oregon, elementary school children using the Kraus-Weber test of minimum muscular fitness. *Res. Q.* 28:16-28. 1957.
26. Knortz, K., and C. Ringel. Flexibility Techniques. *NSCA Journal* 7(2):50-53. 1985.
27. Leighton, J.R. Instrument and technique for measurement of range of joint motion. *Arch. Phys. Med. Rehab.* 36:571-578. 1955.
28. Leighton, J.R. Flexibility characteristics of three specialized skill groups of champion athletes. *Arch. Phys. Med. Rehab.* 38:580-583. 1957.
29. Leighton, J.R. A study of the effect of progressive weight training on flexibility. *J. Assoc. Phys. Ment. Rehab.* 18:101. 1964.
30. Logan, G., and G.H. Egstrom. The effects of slow and fast stretching on sacrofemoral angle. *J. Assoc. Phys. Ment. Rehab.* 15:85-89. 1961.
31. Marshall, J.L., N. Johanson, T.L. Wickiewicz, H.M. Tishler, B.L. Koslin, S. Zeno, A. Myers. Joint looseness: A function of the person and the joint. *Med. Sci. Sports Exerc.* 12:189-194. 1980.
32. Massey, B.H., and N.L. Chaudet. Effects of heavy resistance exercise on range of joint movement in young male adults. *Res. Q.* 27:41-51. 1956.
33. McCue, B.F. Flexibility measurements of college women. *Res. Q.* 24:316-24. 1953.
34. McCue, B.F. Flexibility of college women. *Res. Q.* 30:297-316. 1953.
35. McFarland, B. Developing maximum running speed. *NSCA Journal* 6(5):24-28. 1984.
36. McFarland, B. (1984, June). *Developing maximum running speed*. Paper presented at NSCA National Conference.
37. Moore, M.A., and R.S. Hutton. Electromyographic investigation of muscle stretching techniques. *Med. Sci. Sports Exerc.* 12(5):322-329. 1980.
38. O'Neil, R. Prevention of hamstring and groin strain. *Athl. Training* 11:27-31. 1970.
39. Peterson, S.L. *The Woman's Stretching Book*. Champaign, IL: Leisure Press. 1983.
40. Phillips, M. Analysis of results from the Kraus-Weber test of minimum muscular fitness in children. *Res. Q.* 26:314-323. 1955.
41. Prentice, W.E. A comparison of static stretching and PNF stretching for improving hip joint flexibility. *Athl. Training* 18(1):56-59. 1983.
42. Prentice, W.E. Flexibility: Roundtable. *NSCA Journal* 6(4):10-22, 71-73. 1984.
43. Tanigawa, M.C. Comparison of the hold relax procedure and passive mobilization on increasing muscle length. *Phys. Ther.* 52:725-735. 1972.
44. Todd, T. Historical perspective: The myth of the muscle-bound lifter. *NSCA Journal* 6(4):37-41. 1985.
45. Walker, S.H. Delay of twitch relaxation induced by stress and stress relaxation. *J. Appl. Physiol.* 16:801-806. 1961.
46. Weiss, L.W., K.J. Cureton, and F.N. Thompson. Comparison of serum testosterone and androstenedione responses to weight lifting in men and women. *Eur. J. Appl. Physiol.* 50:413-419. 1983.
47. Wilmore, J.H., R.B. Parr, R.N. Girandola, P. Ward, P.A. Vodak, T.J. Barstow, T.V. Pipes, G.T. Romero, and P. Leslie. Physiological alterations consequent to circuit weight training. *Med. Sci. Sports* 10:79-84. 1978.
48. Wright, V., and R.J. Johns. Physical factors concerned with the stiffness of normal and diseased joints. *Johns Hopkins Hosp. Bull.* 106:215-231. 1960.

CHAPTER 20

SPEED DEVELOPMENT AND PLYOMETRIC TRAINING

William B. Allerheiligen

Speed and power are critical to many sports. Sports that require speed and power will benefit from training that is similar to the sport itself in movement, speed, power, and strength (11,44-46).

SPEED DEVELOPMENT

Some believe that a person is either born with speed or is not (29). This may be true to a certain extent because of inherited limb length, muscle attachments, and proportion of fast-twitch muscle fibers. However, although a person may inherently be unable to sprint well, most athletes can improve their running speed. Only a few athletes can run 100 m in under 11.0 s, but many athletes can improve from 13.0 s to 12.5 s. A slow athlete may not become ''fast'' but he or she may become ''faster'' (18). With the large number of average athletes in sports today, there is a tremendous potential for improving sprint speed among athletes in sports in which speed is required.

Components of Running Speed

The components of running speed are stride frequency, stride length (1), form, and speed-endurance (all discussed in detail in the following sections, as well as reaction time, acceleration, strength, power, and flexi-

bility (29). To improve all these components, a well-designed program should include strength training, assisted running, resistive running, plyometric activities (discussed in detail later), interval training, and running technique.

Stride Frequency. **Stride frequency** is the number of strides (steps) taken in a given amount of time. Improving stride frequency involves the ability to decrease the time between strides while maintaining or increasing stride length. Stride frequency may be developed by **sprint-assisted training**, which involves running at increased linear speed. Such training normally utilizes downhill running and towing. *Downhill running* should be performed on an even surface with a slope of 3° to 7° (1,29,36). For very short distances a downward slope of greater than 7° would result in a stride frequency that is too rapid, and the athlete could be injured because of losing control and falling. When stride frequency increases beyond what the athlete is capable of maintaining, he or she will begin landing on the heels rather than the balls of the feet. This is essentially a braking movement that eliminates the benefits of sprint-assisted training. A more gradual incline should be used if this occurs.

Prior to attempting downhill running the athlete should participate in a good sprint program for several weeks. Each session of downhill running should be preceded by a general warm-up, stretching, a specific warm-up, and several low- and medium-intensity acceleration sprints. Downhill running distances should range from 30 to 50 m (29).

Towing utilizes a mechanical device or a highly stretched surgical tube (5/8 in. by 50 ft, or 1.6 cm by 15 m) with a running harness securely attached at each end to pull the athlete so that he or she can run faster than usual. With a harness around the waist of 2 athletes, Athlete A walks away from Athlete B (the athlete to be ''towed'') until the distance between them is approximately 45 m (the distance is dependent upon the thickness, quality, and age of the surgical tube). With Athlete C holding the midpoint of the stretched tube, Athlete B runs for 10 m and then accelerates as rapidly as possible. Athlete C jogs in the same general direction, but slightly laterally, so that Athlete B does not trip on the tubing. The increase in running speed by this method may be 5% to 10% greater than that for nonassisted running.

Stride Length.

Stride length is simply the distance covered in one stride during running. It is developed by increasing the **speed-strength** (the ability to exert maximal force during high-speed movement) in the lower body (32,34,37). Strength training, pulling a weighted sled (resistive running), resistance applied by a running harness, running uphill, running up steps, plyometrics, and running chutes can be used to increase speed-strength. A speed development program should not, however, be based exclusively, or almost exclusively, on resistive running, because stride frequency might not improve. Some of the resistive drills may even decrease stride length or frequency if they are the only exercises performed. A well-designed program should use all the components of improving sprint speed.

Stride Analysis.

The running stride may be broken down into two phases (15): the support phase and the flight, or nonsupport, phase. The **support phase** starts at touchdown and ends with takeoff of the same foot. The support phase comprises the heel strike (or ground contact) (Figure 20.1a), midstance (Figure 20.1b), and takeoff (Figure 20.1c). The **flight phase** is the period when the feet are not in contact with the ground. The first subphase is when the foot of the driving leg leaves the ground and the center of gravity rises to its highest point (Figure 20.2). the second subphase is the descent of the center of gravity from the highest point to ground contact. Leg turnover is one complete cycle of a leg's movement (i.e., from contact of the right foot to contact of the right foot again) while running.

Form and Form Running.

Sprinting with good form is a motor learning process (36) that must be learned at slow speeds (60-75% of maximum) and transferred to high speeds. **Form running** (correct running form and drills that emphasize certain movements while running) is used to establish efficient and error-free movement.

Form Running Drills.

Form running drills are used to help ingrain neuromuscular movement patterns and increase *leg turnover* and therefore stride frequency. Leg turnover is the rate at which the recovery leg completes a cycle, that is, the period of time from when the foot leaves the ground and touches again.

''A''s and ''B''s are marching drills that emphasize high knee lift. All A drills use the same basic arm and leg movements. The major difference is the rate of arm and leg movement. To perform the As, lift the knee as high as possible while the other leg is fully extended. The elbows should be flexed at about 90° during the arm swing. During the arm swing the hands should

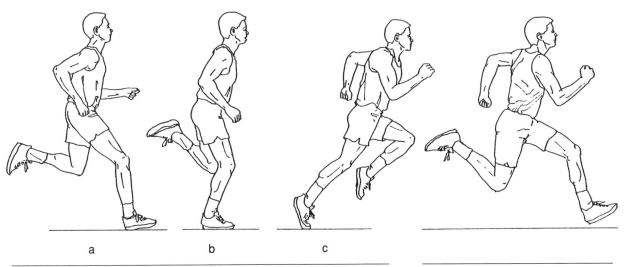

a   b   c

Figure 20.1 Stride analysis phases: (a) heel strike, (b) midstance, (c) takeoff.

Figure 20.2 Flight, or nonsupport, phase of stride analysis.

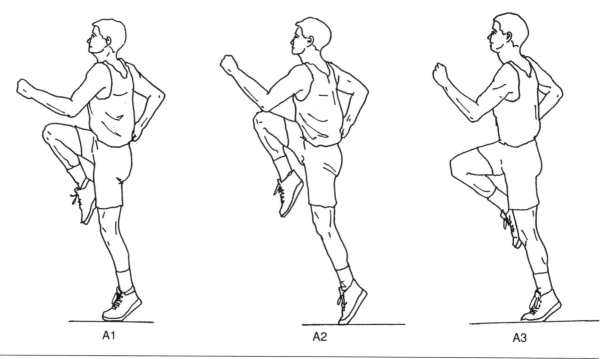

Figure 20.3　(A1) High knee marching drill. (A2) High knee marching drill with a skip. (A3) High knee marching drill with a rapid skip.

move from shoulder level to the hip. Use a snapping arm action. Think of the entire arm as a pendulum with the shoulder as the pivot point. As and Bs may also be performed without arm action by placing the hands on the hips.

A1 is a slow marching drill with emphasis on technique, knee lift, and arm action (A1, A2, and A3 are shown in Figure 20.3). All As should have approximately 3 foot-contacts per meter. The number of sets and the distances of the form running drills will depend on what other drills are being performed in each workout. Sets may range from two to four and distances from 10 m for high knees and rear heel kick to 30 m for As and Bs.

After the A1 is mastered, progress to the A2. The A2 is a marching drill at a moderate pace and uses a skipping action. While skipping keep the foot close to the ground. Progress to the A3 after the A2 is perfected. The A3 utilizes very rapid leg and arm movement with a rapid skipping action. While skipping keep the foot close to the ground. The A3 is similar in rate to sprinting but the emphasis is not on horizontal speed.

Bs are similar to As except that when the knee is slightly higher than waist level the leg is fully extended. After the leg is fully extended it is flexed as the foot moves toward the ground. The B1 is a slow marching drill and the B2 is performed at a moderate speed while skipping (Figure 20.4). Do not perform Bs rapidly.

Rear heel kicks (Figure 20.5) are used to help leg turnover rate. Increased leg turnover rate may increase running speed. To perform the rear heel kick, or butt kick, lean forward slightly from the waist. The arm action is the same as that of the As and Bs. While keeping the upper leg almost perpendicular with the ground (the knee is not lifted upward as in running), try to kick the right buttocks with the heel of the right foot, and as rapidly as possible perform a similar action with the left foot. Use a quick rhythm but horizontal movement should be slow.

High knees (Figure 20.6) are similar to the A3 but high knees do not use the rapid skipping action. The

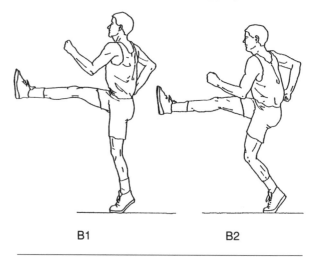

Figure 20.4　(B1) High knee marching drill with leg extension. (B2) High knee marching drill with leg extension and skip.

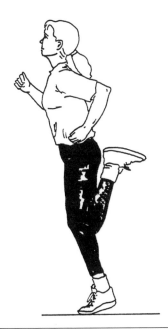

Figure 20.5 Rear heel kicks are the part of leg turnover that emphasizes leg flexion.

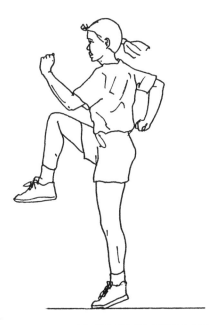

Figure 20.6 High knees are the part of leg turnover that emphasizes hip flexion.

knees should be lifted as high and as rapidly as possible. Emphasis is on knee height and rapid arm and leg movement, not on horizontal speed.

Some leg turnover drills (Figure 20.7) are similar to the rear heel kick, high knees, and running. Perform these drills by almost fully extending your arms and placing your hands on an object of approximately waist height, making sure there is room to lift the knees up and forward. Keep the torso nearly vertical. Perform the rear heel kick with one leg while maintaining the stationary position. Begin with a slow and fluid movement. Increase speed while maintaining good technique, but decrease speed if technique breaks down. Perform these drills for 5 to 10 s. Switch legs and repeat. Perform the high knees and leg turnover in the same manner. The leg turnover drill is a combination of the high knees and rear heel kicks in a running movement.

Errors in Form Running. The following list delineates form running errors and how to correct them:

Head sway—Do not let the head sway in any direction, but maintain a relaxed upright position.

Arm swing—Arm swing should be forward and backward with minimal lateral movement (or horizontal adduction) (9,43). Lateral movement causes a slight rotation at the shoulders, which decreases running speed, because the movement is lateral and not forward. The elbows should be flexed at about 90° and held in this position. Arm swing should come from the shoulder and not involve excessive flexion and extension of the arm itself. In general, the hands should not cross the midline of the body and go no higher than the armpits (Figure 20.8).

Rear heel kick action—The greater the speed, the higher the heel should kick up (50). This is a product of pushing off the ground and is known as heel recovery. Improper height of the rear heel kick action will hinder speed of proper leg turnover rate.

Upper body lean—The upper body should have a slight forward lean after the start (50).

Foot placement—The feet should point straight ahead and should not pronate excessively during the support phase (29). Foot contact should be ball-heel-ball, not on the balls of the foot only.

Relaxation—The runner must be able to relax the body during maximal or near-maximal sprint speed. Hands should not be clenched (43), and the jaw should be relaxed and loose.

Speed-Endurance. **Speed-endurance** is the ability to repeatedly perform maximal or near-maximal sprints with various sport-specific recovery intervals. The amount of speed-endurance required by an athlete is sport specific. The speed-endurance for the 100-m sprinter or shot-putter is different than that for the basketball player. Speed-endurance programs should be designed with reference to the sport's primary energy system (phosphogen, glycolytic, or oxidative), which involves the sport's duration.

Speed-endurance is normally enhanced by **interval training**, which involves high-intensity exercise bouts alternated with bouts of recovery (25). Interval running is the term used to describe a running program that utilizes interval training methods. Interval training in resistance training is called circuit training. As physical

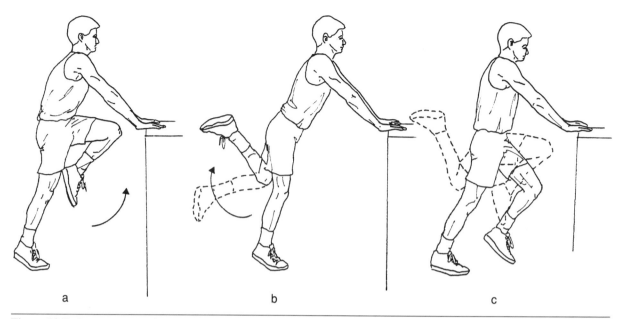

Figure 20.7 Leg turnover drills are specific speed drills performed from a stationary position and combine the rear heel kick and high knee (31). Shown here are (a) the high knee, (b) the rear heel kick, and (c) a leg turnover (or cycling) drill.

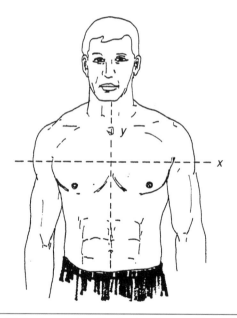

Figure 20.8 Arm swing: Hands should go no higher than *x* and not cross *y*.

conditioning improves, overall intensity is increased by increasing training distance, total training time, running intensity, and the number of repetitions, or decreasing the recovery period. Interval training, as compared to long slow distance running, normally involves more physical pain because of near-maximal efforts, which increase blood lactate (25).

Interval training may be used with various sports, including football, baseball, basketball, volleyball, running, swimming, cross-country skiing, and rowing. It may be designed to develop primarily the phosphogen, glycolytic, or oxidative energy systems or various combinations of these (22). This is accomplished by regulating the exercise time, training distance, and recovery times. In the context of running, interval training may improve speed and leg power and produces an aerobic base by anaerobic training. Ideal training distances of power athletes range from 40 to 400 m, depending on the sport-specific goals and the period in the overall training program. Training of this type develops the phosphogen and glycolytic energy systems, the ones primarily used in power sports (those lasting from 1-10 s).

Near-maximal intensities, and thus near-maximal heart rates—achieved with manipulation of exercise time, training distance, number of sets, recovery period, and number of repetitions—should be the goal of interval training, and a well-constructed speed-endurance program provides for both speed and cardiovascular development. The heart rate during work intervals is elevated over that of normal distance running (19). Recovery periods are inserted between work intervals; these allow the heart rate to return to baseline. An athlete should allow his or her heart rate to recover to about 65% of maximal heart rate before proceeding to the next work interval.

The recovery rate is calculated as follows:

$$220 - \text{age} = \text{theoretical maximal heart rate (beats/min)}$$

$$\text{theoretical maximal heart rate} \times 0.65 = \text{recovery heart rate (beats/min)}$$

The recovery heart rate for a 20-year-old athlete would be as follows:

$$220 - 20 = 200 \text{ beats/min}$$
(theoretical maximal heart rate)

$$200 \times \underline{0.65} \text{ (recovery factor} = 130 \text{ beats/min}$$

It is not unusual to see heart rates of 95% to 100% of maximal heart rate (190-200 beats/min for the 20-year-old athlete) near the end of some high-intensity workouts. When work intervals involve longer distances, for example, greater than 400 m, the heart rate may be near-maximal at the end of the second or third repetition.

The most efficient method of measuring the heart rate is to place the index and middle fingers on the carotid artery, which is located on the neck just under the joint of the jaw. Taking a 15-s heart rate and multiplying by four gives the 1-min heart rate.

Strength and conditioning professionals should have a working knowledge of the following interval training terminology:

Work interval—The part of the program consisting of the training time (i.e., 20 s) or the training distance (i.e., 100 m).

Training intensity—The integration of training time for specific training distance yields training intensity. For example, interval running with 100-m runs in 15 s may be high intensity while 100-m runs in 19 s may be low intensity. The training distance remains the same but the time is different. Training intensity may be expressed as a percent of maximal performance. For example, if maximal performance for the 100-m run is 12 s, then 80% = 14.4 s, 70% = 15.6 s, 60% = 16.8 s, etc.

Relief interval—Recovery period between work intervals. The relief interval may include walking or even slow jogging, with slow walking the norm.

Work-relief ratio—The ratio of the work interval to the relief interval. Work-relief ratios for distances of 40 m should be in the range of 1:5 to 1:6; for distances of 400 m they should be in the range of 1:3 to 1:4. Some recommend that the work-relief ratio be as low as 1:1 for distances of 400 m (31). While this ratio may be adequate for 3,000-m runners, it would be questionable for football players who require speed-endurance. As mentioned previously, the interval training program may be designed to develop primarily the phosphogen, glycolytic, or oxidative energy systems. Thus, if the goal is on speed-endurance (i.e., power), the recovery interval should be longer. If the goal of the program is endurance, the recovery interval may be shorter.

Set—A group of work and relief intervals—for example, five 100-m sprints and their relief intervals.

Repetition—One work interval and its subsequent relief interval. The five 100-m sprints just mentioned represent five repetitions.

Training time—The time of the work interval (i.e., 10 s). Training times vary with sport, body mass, and workouts within microcycles.

Training distance—The distance of the work interval. Training distance may be kept constant and training time varied. Training distance may also vary within a workout.

PLYOMETRICS

Plyometrics refers to exercises that enable a muscle to reach maximal strength in as short a time as possible. Such exercises usually involve some form of jumping, but other modes of exercise exist. The elements *ply* and *metric* come from Latin roots for "increase" and "measure," respectively; the combination thus means "measurable increase" (13; see 49 and 50 for Greek origins). Plyometric exercises utilize the force of gravity (e.g., you *step* off a box) to store energy in the muscles (potential energy). This energy is then utilized immediately in an opposite reaction (e.g., you immediately jump up upon landing), so the natural elastic properties of the muscle will produce kinetic energy (2,12). Elastic strength is the ability of muscles and connective tissues (muscle sheath and tendinous tissues) to rapidly exert a force in order to produce maximal power in linear, vertical, lateral, or combination movements (17).

Plyometric exercises are especially useful in sports that require speed-strength (33,35). Speed-strength is the ability to exert maximal force during high-speed movements. Sports that require speed-strength include track-and-field jumping, throwing, and sprinting; volleyball, basketball, football, baseball, and diving (which require maximal jumping ability); blocking and tackling in football; and racket sports, baseball, and softball (which require swinging movements). Plyometrics for the upper body include medicine ball throws, catches, and several types of push-ups. **In-depth jumps**, a form of plyometrics characterized by a shock-intensity level, have been shown to increase leg power and strength either on their own or in conjunction with resistance training (5,13,38-42). In-depth jumping may not improve vertical jumping ability (27), however. In-depth jumps are performed by stepping off a box and jumping immediately upon landing. Box heights range from 0.3 m to 0.9 m with 0.5 being the norm for many athletes. Athletes weighing over 100 kg should not perform in-depth jumps from over 0.5 m.

The ability to rapidly apply force (reactive force) is the major goal of plyometric training. Plyometrics are used to apply an overload to the muscles with speed-strength as a goal. Plyometrics should not be considered an end in themselves, but part of an overall program (stretching, running, strength training, nutrition, etc.). After the athlete has begun a proper strength and conditioning program, plyometrics are used to develop speed-strength.

Mechanics of Plyometric Exercise

To continue with the example mentioned earlier, if you were to stand on a box, step off, and, upon landing (with the knees flexing), immediately jump as high as possible, you would have performed a plyometric exercise (specifically, an in-depth jump). As soon as the balls of the feet touch the floor, the knees are quickly flexed, resulting in a rapid eccentric action of the quadriceps and hip extensors. A rapid deceleration (eccentric action) of a mass followed by a rapid acceleration (concentric contraction) of the mass in another direction (48) is the basis of plyometric training. The rapid eccentric movement evokes the stretch reflex, or stretch-shortening cycle, which results in greater concentric contraction of the same muscles. The main mechanism of the stretch reflex is the **muscle spindle**. Muscle spindles are sensory mechanisms located within intrafusal muscles that run parallel with extrafusal muscle fibers (21). Muscle spindles are sensitive to the rate and magnitude of a stretch. A sensory neuron from the muscle spindle innervates with a motor neuron in the spinal column. The motor neuron than causes a contraction in the muscle (extrafusal fibers) that was previously stretched. This process protects the muscle from excessive rapid stretching and injury.

The rate of the stretch is vital to plyometric training (3,38). A high stretch rate results in greater muscle tension and concentric contraction. Training movements that incorporate rapid eccentric movement (during sprinting, bounding, in-depth jumps, or lateral hops, for example), produce greater eccentric and concentric actions while one performs the exercise during a sport activity. The importance of the stretch rate may be illustrated by different vertical jump tests: a static squat jump, a countermovement with no steps, and an approach jump with several steps. A countermovement uses a rapid eccentric response followed immediately by a rapid concentric contraction. As the rate of stretch increases, one's absolute performance in these tests improves. The static squat jump will reveal the shortest jump and the approach jump the highest. The static squat jump does not utilize a countermovement (the countermovement involves the rapid eccentric response during the flexion of the ankles, knees, and hips) and the approach jump utilizes a more forceful countermovement than the countermovement only. Because plyometrics are active drills that produce high muscle

tension (eccentric), the stretch reflex will produce a greater force than a concentric contraction from a static position not preceded by a stretch (4,6,8,10,13,26,47).

During the stretch-shortening cycle (the result of the stimulation of the stretch reflex), the muscles and tendons elongate. It is during the elongation that the elastic tendencies of the muscle develops stored energy. If the eccentric response is followed immediately by a concentric contraction, the force produced by the concentric contraction will be increased (33). Speed-strength is thus increased.

The three main components of a plyometric drill are the eccentric phase, the amortization phase, and the concentric contraction. The amortization phase is the period of time from the initiation of the eccentric phase (touching the surface) to the initiation of the concentric contraction (start of the upward motion of the jump). As a result, the muscles in the leg become like a rapidly stretched rubber band. The "stretched rubber band" will result in a greater ability to develop power. In other words, the muscles are being trained to become more explosive. To take advantage of the stretch reflex, keep the amortization phase as brief as possible (11). Remember, the rate of stretch is more important than the magnitude. Greater power is produced when the depth of the countermovement is short and rapid rather than large and slow.

Besides in-depth jumps, there are other types of plyometric drills with various intensity levels and directional movements; these will be explained later. Jumping, hopping, skipping, and even running involve some degree of a stretch-shortening movement, in that all of them utilize a countermovement of varying degree. Examples of the countermovement in sports are a basketball player preparing to jump up for a rebound, a volleyball player preparing to jump up for a spike, a high jumper preparing to jump over the bar, and a wrestler preparing for the drop step.

Plyometric training is similar to progressive resistance training in that both incorporate overload principles. Drills should progress gradually from basic to difficult, and from low to high intensity. Form and technique should be emphasized at all stages of the program.

Pretraining Evaluation of the Athlete

To reduce the risk of injury and facilitate the performance of plyometric exercises, the athlete must first establish a strength and conditioning base. The following evaluation will help determine whether this condition has been met.

Physical maturity level—Don't judge physical maturity merely by chronological age. Athletes should have a sufficient sprint and resistance training base. The recommended strength level for the legs and hips is to be able to do the squat with 1.5 to 2.5 times the athlete's body weight, with 1.5 being the norm (13,23,30,45). These should be considered minimal standards for performing shock- and high-intensity level plyometrics. Regarding upper body strength, the athlete should be able to perform five clap push-ups in a row. Large athletes (weight >115 kg) should be able to bench press their body weight, smaller athletes (weight <75 kg) should be able to bench press 1.5 times their body weight, and athletes of intermediate body weight should use gradations of these guidelines (48).

Coachability—Does the athlete respond positively to the coach's instructions? If not, plyometric training should be postponed. Injury, overtraining, or undertraining may result if the athlete is inattentive to instructions.

Demands of the sport—Determine if the sport movements are mostly linear, vertical, lateral, or combinations of these. For example, volleyball players require an emphasis on vertical and lateral movement, while long jumpers must emphasize horizontal movement. The intensity and volume required for the sport should also be considered. During a training phase a shotputter may use low volume and high intensity while a 400-m hurdler may use moderate volume and intensity.

Fitness level—The strength (46) and conditioning level of the athlete must be considered prior to performing plyometrics. If the athlete does not possess sufficient muscular strength or a sufficient fitness level, plyometrics must be delayed until minimum standards are met.

Program Design

Equipment and Facilities. Use of the following guidelines to select appropriate equipment and facilities for plyometric training will enhance effectiveness and safety (24).

Proper footwear. Footwear with good ankle and arch support, good lateral stability, and a wide, nonslip sole is required. A crosstraining shoe is ideal because it helps prevent ankle rollover. Shoes with a narrow sole and poor upper support (such as running shoes) may create ankle problems (1), especially with lateral movements.

Resilient surface. To prevent injuries, the landing surface must possess good shock-absorbing properties. The best surface is a good grass field; the next-best surfaces are well-padded artificial turf and wrestling mats. Such surfaces as concrete, tile, and hardwood are not recommended, because they lack shock-absorbing properties (1). Excessively thick (≥15 cm) exercise mats may extend the amortization phase, thus not allowing efficient use of the stretch reflex. Minitrampolines are not effective for plyometric training because of the extended amortization phase while the athlete is in contact with the elastic surface.

Proper, sturdy equipment. Boxes used for box jumps and in-depth jumps must be sturdy and should have a nonslip top.

Sufficient training area. The amount of space needed depends on the drill. Long-response drills may require a straightaway of 100 m. For most of the bounding and running drills, at least 30 m of straightaway are required. For some of the vertical and in-depth jumps, only a minimum surface area is needed, but adequate height (3 to 4 m) is required.

Procedures. As with any training program, begin exercise sessions with a warm-up period that includes general warm-up, stretching, and specific warm-up.

It is easiest to think of a training program in 1-week units of time. The three basic features of a program, which determine the overall overload of the weekly training period, are frequency, volume, and intensity. (Overload refers to a greater than normal stress placed upon a muscle.) Alterations in any one of these may require adjustment to one or both of the others. Additional factors to consider are progression, recovery periods, and direction of motion.

Frequency. Frequency is simply the number of plyometric workouts per week. The usual range is one to three sessions, with two being the norm for most off-season sports, including football, and two to three for track and field. In season, one session/week is appropriate for football players and two or three for track-and-field athletes. The intensity of the daily workouts (practice, strength training, running, and plyometrics) may affect the number of workouts needed each week. Football players may not perform plyometrics in season because of the overall volume and intensity of practices. Three days of low-intensity drills may result in lower overall weekly training effect than 2 days of high-intensity drills. In any case, do not perform drills for the same body area 2 days in succession.

Volume. Volume is normally expressed as the number of foot contacts (each time a foot, or feet together, contact the surface) per workout. Volume should be 80 to 100 foot contacts/session for beginners, 100 to 120 contacts/session for intermediate-level athletes, and 120 to 140 contacts/session for advanced athletes. If intensity is high, volume should be low or medium. Volume may also be expressed as distance (i.e., 600 m).

Intensity. Intensity refers to the amount of stress placed upon muscles, connective tissue, and joints. Skipping places low stress on the muscles and joints whereas in-depth jumps place high stress on the muscles and joints. Generally speaking, as intensity increases, volume should decrease. In the early phases of training, both intensity and volume may increase, but once high-intensity drills form the base of the program, volume should decrease. The intensity of plyometric drills is related to a number of factors:

- Whether one or two feet make contact with the surface. Alternate leg bounds, which may emphasize a greater vertical than horizontal component, result in a large force when the athlete lands.
- The direction of the jump (vertical or horizontal).
- Horizontal speed.
- How high the center of gravity of the body is raised above the ground. The higher the center of gravity, the greater the force will be upon landing.
- Whether, and how much, external weight (in the form of weight vests, ankle weights, and wrist weights) is added to the body. Only experienced athletes should use such weights.

Because drills can vary so much in intensity, owing to these factors and other aspects of the drills themselves, careful consideration must be given to choosing optimal drills during a training cycle.

Progression. Assuming that the athlete has a proper strength and conditioning base, plyometric training should progress from low-intensity, in-place exercises to medium-intensity and then higher-intensity levels (1). Details of progression are discussed in a later section, after the various types of exercises have been defined.

Recovery. Because plyometric drills involve maximal efforts, adequate recovery between repetitions, sets, and workouts is required. Recovery for in-depth jumps may consist of 5 to 10 s of rest between repetitions and 2 to 3 min between sets. Drills should not be thought of as conditioning exercises but as speed-strength training. Recovery between workouts must be adequate (2 to 4 days depending on the sport and time of year); otherwise, overtraining or injury may occur.

Direction of Motion. Athletes require speed and power not only in the vertical plane but also in horizontal (straight ahead), lateral, and diagonal directions as well. Sports that are horizontal and/or lateral in execution include football, baseball, and sprinting. Sports that involve horizontal movement but also emphasize vertical movement include basketball and volleyball. The long and triple jumps are a combination of horizontal and vertical movement. Some sports utilize lateral movement or change of direction and include various degrees of horizontal and vertical components. Drills for different directional movements, as well as intensities, are given later in this chapter. Athletes involved in pushing, throwing, and swinging movements of the upper body benefit from plyometric drills for the upper body.

Safety. Because plyometric training emphasizes technique and form, it is advisable to have a strength and conditioning professional present to monitor and correct technique. Injuries occur when training procedures are violated and may be the result of an insufficient strength and conditioning base, inadequate warm-up, improper progression of lead-up drills, inappropriate volume or intensity for the phase of training, poor shoes or surface, or simple lack of skill. Injuries may occur in the joints of the back, knees, hips, and ankles (1). Although injuries may occur as a result of plyometric training, evidence exists that preseason plyometric training does not result in injury (7).

Individual and Sport Specificity. The strength and conditioning professional needs to monitor individual athletes carefully to help them avoid injury. For instance, large (>90-kg) athletes should avoid high-volume, high-intensity plyometric exercises. Take into account body structure—especially possible abnormalities of spinal alignment, the legs, and the feet—as well as previous injuries, when designing plyometric programs. Be aware that fatigue from high-volume training may lead to poor technique and injury.

A program should also take into consideration the athlete's sport. Large football players, for example, may be susceptible to injury because of the nature of their sport. During practice and competition they are constantly being placed in a variety of body positions that expose them to great stress and torque on the ankles, knees, and low back. This and the violent physical contact in general may require that these athletes refrain from performing high-intensity and shock drills.

In-Depth Jumping. There is a limit to the height at which an in-depth jump can be performed and be effective but not dangerous. A height of 1.2 m would provide a great overload on the muscles, but the resistance would be too great for many athletes to overcome while maintaining correct technique (45). Jumping from such a height increases the possibility of injury; furthermore, the amount of force to be overcome is so great that the amortization phase would be extended and thus the goal of the exercise lost. The recommended height for in-depth jumps ranges from 0.4 to 1.1 m, with 0.75 to 0.8 m being the norm (4,20,28,41,42,46). In-depth jumps for large (>100-kg) athletes should range from 0.5 to 0.75 m. Heights greater than this may not allow for the rapid switch from eccentric to concentric activity and may produce injuries.

Plyometric training has been criticized because of recommendations to perform in-depth jumps from great heights, such as 3.2 m (20). Such a height was part of one investigation to determine the most efficient jumping height. Stated simply, jumps from this height should not be performed.

Proper landing technique is particularly important for in-depth jumps. If the center of gravity is offset from the base of support, then performance will be hindered and injury may occur. The shoulders should be over the knees during the landing, by flexion of the ankles, knees, and hip.

Progressive Overload. Plyometrics is a form of progressive resistance training and thus must follow the principles of progressive overload. Progressive overload is the systematic increase in frequency, volume, and intensity by various combinations. There may be times when two of these variables may be increased or when one is increased and one or both of the others are decreased. As stated previously, as intensity increases, volume decreases, generally. The method of progressive overload is dependent upon the sport and training phase. Normally, except for some track athletes, frequency will stay the same during a training phase. An off-season plyometric program for football, for example, may be performed twice a week. The program may progress from (a) low to moderate volume of low-intensity plyometrics for two weeks, to (b) low to moderate volumes of moderate intensity, to (c) low to moderate volumes of moderate to high intensity. This is only a sample of the many possible combinations for different sports. In plyometric training the emphasis is on power development in which overloads are implemented.

Model Program. A "typical" plyometric program might take place over 8 to 10 weeks with two training sessions/week (Table 20.1). Proper progression means the following:

- The athlete has been evaluated
- Sport-specific goals have been established
- The length of the program has been established
- Proper technique is taught
- Proper warm-up is used
- Drills progress from low to high intensity
- Drills progress from low to high volume

The total number of sets, repetitions, and rest intervals is dependent on the intensity level of the drill, the sport, the time of year, and the physical condition of the athlete. The example in Table 20.1 is based upon an athlete who has all the prerequisites for plyometric training. Selection of specific drills must be based upon the required directional movements of the athlete. Table 20.2 provides an example of variation in volume based upon body weight and Table 20.3 is a model of variation in the number of foot contacts. These tables are only models and sport-specific programs will vary from these.

Table 20.2 Example of Variation in Volume Based on Body Weight

Exercise	Volume by body weight		
	150-200 lb	201-250 lb	>250 lb
Alternate leg bound	40	30	20
Double leg tuck jump	40	30	20
Split squat jump	30	20	10
Lateral cone hop	30	20	10
Total volume	140	100	60

Table 20.1 Example Off-Season Plyometric Program

	Drills	Set; repetitions per set	Rest period	Sessions/week
Weeks 1 and 2	Choose four low-intensity drills	2; 10	2 min between sets	2
Weeks 3 and 4	Choose two low- and two medium-intensity drills	2; 10	2-3 min between sets	2
Weeks 5 and 6	Choose four medium-intensity drills	2-3; 10	2-3 min between sets	2
Weeks 7 and 8	Choose two medium- and two high-intensity drills	Medium-intensity drills: 2-3; 10 High-intensity drills: 2; 10	2-3 min between sets Box jumps: 10-15 s between repetitions	2
Weeks 9 and 10	Choose four high-intensity drills	Nonbox jumps: 2-3; 10 Box jumps: 2; 10	3 min between sets	2

Table 20.3   Model of Variation in Number of Foot Contacts

Season	Beginning	Intermediate	Advanced	Intensity
Off-season	60-100	100-150	120-200	Low-moderate
Preseason	100-150	150-300	150-450*	Moderate-high
In-season	Sport-specific	Sport-specific	Sport-specific	Moderate
Championship season	Recovery only	Recovery only	Recovery only	

*An elite athlete performing low- to moderate-intensity level plyometrics.

Reprinted from Chu (1992).

Combining Plyometric and Strength Training.   A combination of plyometrics and strength training during a training cycle should be designed to allow for maximal efficiency and physical improvement. The following list and Table 20.4 provide guidelines for developing a combined program:

- Performing heavy strength training and plyometrics on the same day is not usually recommended (13,23). An exception is that some athletes, such as track-and-field participants, may benefit from "complex training" by performing high-intensity strength training followed by plyometrics. If this type of training is performed, ensure adequate recovery between the plyometrics and other high-intensity lower body training.
- Combine lower body strength training with upper body plyometrics, and upper body strength training with lower body plyometrics (1).
- Allow for adequate recovery between strength training and plyometric workouts. Recovery may range from 24 to 48 hr between high-intensity strength and plyometric workouts.

Table 20.4   Sample Schedule for Integrating of Strength Training and Plyometrics

Day	Strength training	Plyometrics
Monday	High-intensity upper body	High-intensity lower body
Tuesday	Low-intensity lower body	Low-intensity upper body
Thursday	Low-intensity upper body	Low-intensity lower body
Friday	High-intensity lower body	High-intensity upper body

Definition of Movements

The following are the basic types of plyometric drills. Table 20.5 gives specific examples classified by intensity.

Jump—A movement that concludes with a two-foot landing. A set may consist of 1 to 10 repetitions, but the jumps may be considered single repetitions.

Jump in place—Vertical jump performed in place. Examples: tuck, pike, split squat, squat, and power jumps.

Standing jump—A maximal jump that may be linear, vertical, or lateral and is a 1RM (repetition maximal) effort (19). Examples: standing long, triple, or lateral jumps.

Hop—A movement that starts and concludes with a one-foot or two-foot landing of the same foot or feet. Hops are repeated over a specific distance and/or a certain number of repetitions; they are not maximal jumps. Hops may be performed by number of repetitions (short response, 1-10) or distance (long response, 30 m or more).

Short-response hop—Plyometrics performed with 10 repetitions or less; a shock method may be added by adding external weights to the body. Examples: double and single leg—hop, speed hop, and lateral hop.

Long-response hop—Plyometrics performed for 30 m or more; a shock method may be added. Examples: double and single leg—hop and speed hop.

Bound—Series of movements in which the athlete lands successively on alternate feet. Bounds are normally measured in distance (long response, 30 m or more) but may also be performed as repetitions (short response, 10) for maximal distance.

Table 20.5 Plyometric Drills, Classified by Intensity Level

	Low intensity	Medium intensity	High intensity	Shock
In-place jumps	• Squat jump • Split squat jump • Cycled split squat jump (Also: ankle bounce, ice skater, lateral cone jump)	• Pike jump • Double leg tuck jump (Also: Jump-up, lateral hop)	• Double leg vertical power jump • Single leg vertical power jump • Single leg tuck jump	
Standing jumps		• Standing triple jump (Also: Standing long jump)		
Short-response hops		• Double and single leg zigzag hop and double leg hop	• Single leg hop and double and single leg speed hop	
Long-response hops		• Double leg hop	• Single leg hop and double and single leg speed hop	
Short-response bounds		• Alternate leg bound • Combination bound		
Long-response bounds		• Alternate leg bound • Combination bound		
Shocks				• In-depth jump • Box jump
Upper body plyometrics	• Medicine ball sit-up • Plyometric sit-up (Also: two-hand overhead forward throw, clap push-ups)	• Medicine ball push-up (Also: overhead backward throw, underhand forward throw, Russian twist)		• Drop-and-catch push-up

Note. Instructions are given in this chapter for the drills in the bulleted lists in this table. Additional drills are listed in parentheses for information.

Short-response bound—Plyometrics performed for 25 to 60 m; a shock method may be added. Examples: alternate leg, combination, or single leg.

Long-response bound—Plyometrics performed for more than 60 m; a shock method may be added. Examples: alternate leg, combination, or single leg.

Shock—In-depth jumps and box jumps. These are very highly intense nervous system activities that place great stress (shock) on muscle and connective tissues. The shock response is very high; few athletes (e.g., track and field, volleyball, and basketball) use this type of training. A set may consist of 1 to 10 repetitions.

Progression in a Plyometric Training Program

As noted earlier, a program should be initiated with low-intensity drills and low volume (up to 80 foot contacts).

Begin training neuromuscular reactivity with low- and medium-intensity jumps in place (see Table 20.5, and refer to the instructions beginning on p. 328). These emphasize the vertical component. The single leg tuck jump, a high-intensity jump, is also permitted at this stage. Jumps over cones may also be done.

Progress from jumps in place to standing jumps. These latter emphasize both linear and vertical components. Although standing jumps are 1RM efforts, they should be performed in sets of 5 to 10 repetitions. In addition to the standing triple jump, illustrated in this chapter, the standing long jump and jumps over cones and barriers may be performed.

Progress to multiple jumps and hops. These patterns involve repeated movements. Multiple jumps may be viewed as a combination of jumps in place and standing jumps. One possible multiple jump is repeat triple jumps (this will turn into combination bounding as soon as a long response is used).

Bounding involves movements with greater linear speed, compared to other drills, of preestablished distances or preestablished repetitions for maximal distance. Bounding drills are normally greater than 30 m and may include single and double leg bounds in addition to the ones illustrated in this chapter.

The next type of drills to be added, shocks, comprise in-depth jumps and box jumps. These make greater use of gravity than other plyometric drills because the body is elevated to a higher level, which increases the response of the stretch reflex. The height of the box depends on the size of the athlete, the landing surface, and the goals of the program during that phase of training. In-depth jumps may involve one or both legs; box drills may involve one, both, or alternating legs, as well as straddle jumps.

Upper body plyometric drills are the other part of a plyometric program. Upper body plyometrics are similar to lower body plyometrics because they both (a) use the stretch reflex, (b) should follow proper progression, and (c) will increase power in a specific area of the body.

Upper body plyometrics that incorporate a pushing movement from the chest (used in football and shotput) are considered 1RM efforts and are performed in sets of 5 to 10 repetitions. The overall design of the strength and conditioning program (strength training, running, plyometrics, and time of year) will determine on what day upper body plyometrics will be performed. Besides the pushing upper body plyometrics, some sports (baseball, discus, javelin, and tennis) may use upper body rotational plyometrics with medicine balls.

PLYOMETRIC DRILLS

JUMPS IN PLACE

Split Squat Jump

Intensity level: Low.

Starting position: Assume a stance with one leg extended forward and the other oriented behind the midline of the body as in a lunge position. The forward leg should be almost fully extended.

Direction of jump: Vertical.

Arm action: None, or double arm action.

Starting action: Start with a countermovement of approximately 6 to 10 in. (15-25 cm).

Ascent: Explosively jump off the front leg, using the calves (plantar flexion) of the back leg.

Descent: When landing, maintain the lunge position (same leg forward) and immediately repeat the jump.

Volume: 10 repetitions.

After completing a set, rest and switch front legs (1).

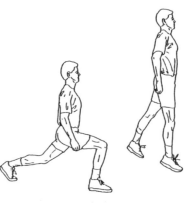
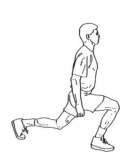
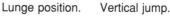

Lunge position.   Vertical jump.   Lunge position.

Cycled Split Squat Jump

Intensity level: Low.

Starting position: Assume a stance with one leg extended forward and the other oriented behind the midline of the body as in a lunge position. The forward leg should be almost fully extended.

Direction of jump: Vertical.

Arm action: None, or double arm action.

Starting action: Start with a countermovement of approximately 6 to 10 in. (15-25 cm).

Ascent: The jumping action is the same as that of the Split Squat Jump, except the legs are quickly switched from front to back while in midair before landing. Maximum height and power should be emphasized.

Descent: Land in the lunge position and immediately repeat the jump.

Volume: 10 repetitions (1).

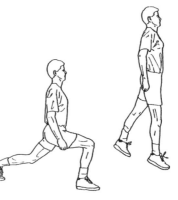
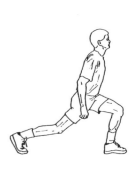

Lunge position.   Vertical jump.   Lunge position with legs switched.

Squat Jump

Intensity level: Low.

Starting position: Half-squat position (thigh parallel with the ground) with feet shoulder-width apart. Interlock fingers and place hands behind head.

Direction of jump: Vertical.

Arm action: None.

Starting action: Start movement by explosively jumping to maximum height.

Descent: Upon landing immediately go into half-squat position and, without pause, repeat exercise.

Volume: 10 repetitions.

The Squat Jump utilizes a deeper countermovement as compared to other jumps, so the amortization phase is the longest of all drills listed (1).

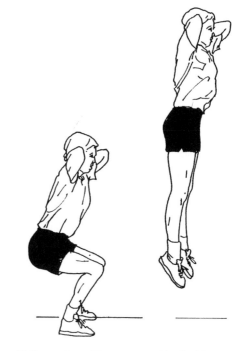

Half squat position.   Vertical jump.

Pike Jump

Intensity level: Medium.

Starting position: Assume a comfortable upright stance with feet shoulder-width apart.

Direction of jump: Vertical.

Arm action: Double arm action.

Starting action: Begin with a rapid countermovement as in performing a vertical jump.

Ascent: Immediately explode upward. Keeping the legs straight, try to lift them to a position parallel to the floor and touch the toes (pike position) with the hands.

Descent: Upon landing, immediately repeat this sequence, concentrating on lifting the straight legs upward.

Volume: 10 repetitions (1).

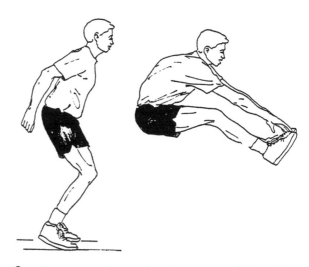

Counter movement.   Legs in near parallel position.

Perform the repetitions at the same semirapid rate, emphasizing minimum contact time on the ground.

Double Leg Tuck Jump

Intensity level: Medium.

Starting position: Assume a comfortable upright stance with feet shoulder-width apart.

Direction of jump: Vertical.

Arm action: Double arm action.

Starting action: Begin with a rapid countermovement.

Ascent: Immediately explode upward. Pull the knees high to the chest and quickly grasp the knees with the hands and release.

Descent: Upon landing, perform the next jump after minimal contact time on the ground.

Volume: 10 repetitions (1).

Concentrate on flexing and pulling the knees upward in this drill.

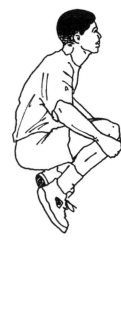
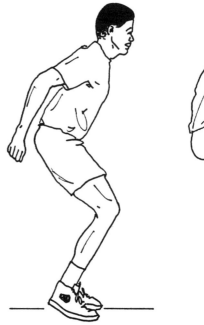
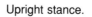

Upright stance.   Knees to chest.

Double Leg Vertical Power Jump

Intensity level: High.

Starting position: Stand with the feet shoulder-width apart.

Direction of jump: Vertical.

Arm action: Double arm action.

Starting action: Perform a rapid countermovement and jump as high as possible.

Ascent: Thrust arms upward vigorously and reach as high as possible with one or two hands.

Descent: When the feet hit the ground, jump again immediately without a stutter step.

Volume: 10 repetitions.

The jump is often performed against a wall or a free-standing device that measures jump height, with the athlete touching as high as possible (1).

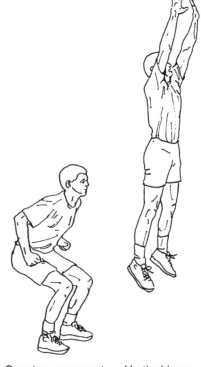

Counter movement.   Vertical jump.

Single Leg Vertical Power Jump

Intensity level: High.

Starting position: Stand with one foot on the ground.

Direction of jump: Vertical.

Arm action: Double arm action.

Starting action: Perform a rapid countermovement and jump as high as possible.

Ascent: The arms should be thrust vigorously upward with each jump and reach as high as possible with one or two hands.

Descent: When the feet hit the ground, immediately jump without a stutter step.

Volume: 10 repetitions.

Emphasis should be on maximum height and quick explosive takeoffs. Repeat this exercise with the opposite leg after a brief rest (15-30 s). This jump is often performed against a wall or free-standing device that measures jump height, with the athlete touching as high as possible (1).

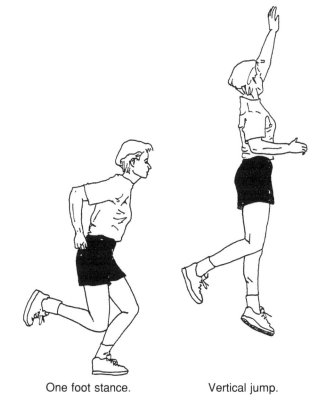

One foot stance.   Vertical jump.

Single Leg Tuck Jump

Intensity level: High.

Starting position: Assume a comfortable upright stance on one foot.

Direction of jump: Vertical.

Arm action: Double arm action.

Starting action: Begin with a rapid countermovement.

Ascent: Immediately explode upward. Pull the knee of the jumping leg high to the chest and quickly grasp the knee with the hands and release.

Descent: Upon landing, perform the next jump after minimal contact time on the ground.

Volume: 10 repetitions.

Concentrate on flexing and pulling the knee upward in this drill. Hold the nonjumping leg in a stationary position with the knee flexed during the exercise (1). Repeat this exercise with the opposite leg after a brief rest (15-30 s).

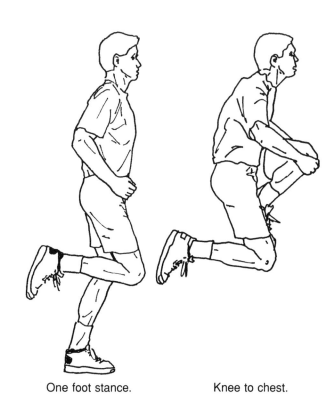

One foot stance.   Knee to chest.

STANDING JUMP

Standing Triple Jump

Intensity level: Medium.

Starting position: Stand with feet 15 to 20 cm apart—arms, ankles, knees, and hips slightly flexed and upper body with a slight forward lean.

Direction of jump: Horizontal, with a vertical component as well.

Arm action: Double arm action.

Starting action: Begin with a rapid countermovement and jump out and upward off of both feet. Try for maximum distance, as in a long jump.

Ascent: Prepare the right leg for initial contact with the surface.

Descent: Land on the right foot. Immediately jump off of the right foot and land on the left foot. Immediately jump off of the left foot and land on both feet. (This is the right-left method.) Strive for maximal distance on each jump.

Volume: 5 to 6 jumps.

After a short rest (30-60 s) perform another set as just described, and do another full set, this time landing on the left foot first (the left-right method).

One significant problem is that some athletes must learn how to jump off of both feet and land on one foot. It is more natural to jump off of two feet and land on two feet, or to jump off of one foot and land on one or two feet. (Some beginners will jump off of only one foot but believe that they have jumped off of two feet.)

The standing triple jump is an excellent test for horizontal power. After sufficient practice, take measurements of the total distance for the right-left or left-right methods. Although most athletes do about equally well with both methods, some have difficulty developing power from one leg and show a distance differential of up to 45 cm (1).

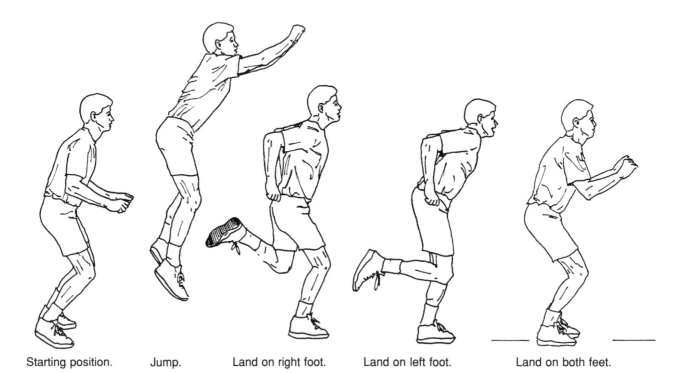

Starting position.   Jump.   Land on right foot.   Land on left foot.   Land on both feet.

HOPS

Double or Single Leg Zigzag Hop (short response)

Intensity level: Medium.

Starting position: Place about 10 cones (or bags) 45 to 60 cm apart in a zigzag pattern. Begin with the feet shoulder-width apart, arms flexed at a 90° angle and at the sides of the body.

Direction of jump: Diagonal.

Arm action: Double arm action.

Starting action: Jump diagonally over the first cone.

Ascent: Propel the body in a forward diagonal direction and keep the shoulders perpendicu-lar to an imaginary (or actual) straight line through the center of all cones.

Descent: Immediately upon landing, change direction and jump diagonally over the second cone. Continue, hopping over all the cones.

Volume: 10 repetitions.

Emphasize explosive hops and try to attain maximum height. Think about "hanging" in the air (1).

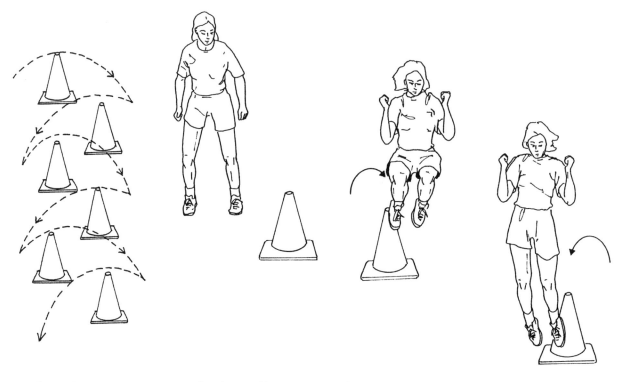

Cone placement.   Starting position.   Jump over first cone.   Jump over second cone—opposite direction.

Double Leg Hop

Intensity level: Medium.

Starting position: Stand with feet shoulder-width apart.

Direction of jump: Horizontal, with a vertical component as well.

Arm action: Double arm action.

Starting action: Jump off of both legs and strive for maximal distance.

Ascent: Think about "hanging in the air."

Descent: Land in the starting position and immediately repeat the movement.

Volume: 10 repetitions for short response, or 30 m or more for long response (1).

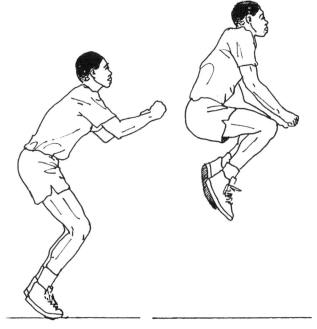

Starting position.   Jump for distance.

Single Leg Hop

Intensity level: High.

Starting position: Begin with one foot slightly ahead of the other as in initiating a step; arms are at the sides.

Direction of jump: Horizontal, with a vertical component as well.

Arm action: Double arm action.

Starting action: Use a rocker step to push off the front leg (or jog into the starting position) and drive the knee of the front leg up and out. The nonjumping leg is held in a stationary position with the knee flexed during the exercise.

Ascent: Think about "hanging in the air."

Descent: Land in the starting position (same leg) and immediately repeat the movement.

Volume: 10 repetitions for short response, or 30 m or more for long response (1).

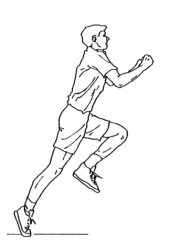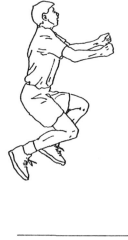

Starting position.   Drive knee up and out.

After a short rest, repeat with the other leg. The rest period for short response should be 1 to 1-1/2 min and 2 to 3 min for long response.

Double Leg Speed Hop

Intensity level: High.

Starting position: Stand with slight flexion in ankles, knees, and hips.

Direction of jump: Horizontal.

Arm action: Double arm action.

Starting action: Jump out and up, trying to reach maximal distance and some height.

Ascent: Jump as far as possible; flex the knees to bring the feet under the buttocks, but not as much as in the double leg hop.

Descent: Land in the starting position and immediately repeat the movement.

Volume: 10 repetitions for short response, or 30 m or more for long response.

Concentrate on keeping the feet together during the hops because the feet will want to spread to about shoulder width. When this occurs the feet will not touch the ground at the same time. In order of importance, the major goals of this drill are speed, distance, and height (1).

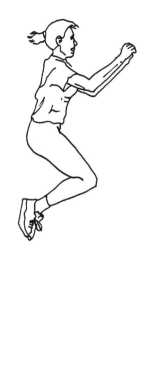

Starting position.   Jump for distance.

Single Leg Speed Hop

Intensity level: High

Starting position: Stand with one foot slightly in front of the other, with slight flexion in the ankles, knees, and hips. Arms should be flexed at 90° with upper arm close to upper body.

Direction of jump: Horizontal.

Arm action: Double arm action.

Starting action: Use a rocker step (or jog into the starting position) to push off the front leg and drive the knee of the front leg out and up. Jump out and up, trying to reach maximal distance and some height.

Ascent: Flex the legs to bring the feet under the buttocks, but not as much as in the leg bound.

Descent: Land in the starting position and immediately repeat the movement.

Volume: 10 repetitions for short response, or 30 m or more for long response. If this drill is used as a field test, the distance should be 25 m.

In order of importance, the major goals of this drill are speed, distance, and height (1). After a short rest repeat with the other leg. The rest period should be 1 to 1-1/2 min for short response and 2 to 3 min for long response.

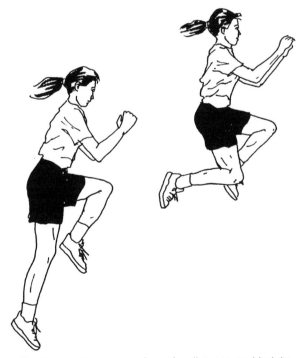

Starting position.   Jump for distance and height.

BOUNDS

Alternate Leg Bound

Intensity level: Medium.

Starting position: Begin with one foot slightly ahead of the other as in initiating a step; arms are at the sides.

Direction of jump: Horizontal, with a vertical component as well.

Arm action: An alternate arm action is preferred, but double arm action may be used.

Starting action: Use a rocker step (or jog into the starting position) to push off the front leg and drive the knee up and out.

Ascent: Think about "hanging" in the air to increase the distance covered.

Descent: Prepare the legs and arms for contact with the surface and execution of the next bound. Repeat with the opposite leg immediately upon landing.

Volume: 10 repetitions for short response, or 30 m or more for long response.

The goal is to cover maximal distance with each jump; this is not a race or sprint.

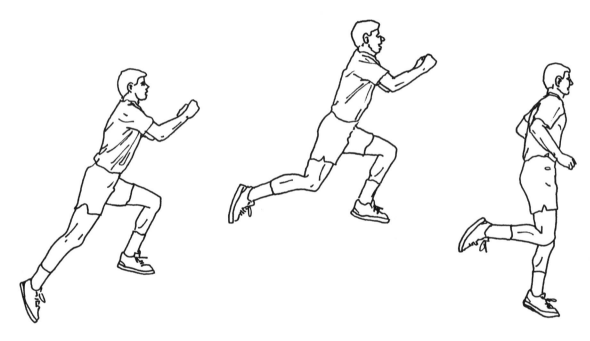

Drive knee up and out.   Hang time.   Land on opposite leg.

Combination Bound

Intensity level: Medium.

Starting position: Begin with one foot (e.g., the left) slightly ahead of the other as in initiating a step, arms to the sides.

Direction of jump: Horizontal, with a vertical component as well.

Arm action: Double arm action.

Starting action: Use a rocker step to push off the right leg and drive the right knee up and out.

Ascent: While "hanging" in the air, prepare the limbs for landing.

Descent: Upon landing on the right foot, immediately explode off the right foot and land on the right foot again. Immediately explode off the right foot again and then land on the left foot. After landing on the left foot, explode off the left foot and then land on the right foot. Repeat this process; foot contact is right-right-left.

Volume: 10 repetitions for short response, or 30 m or more for long response (1).

Repeat the drill in a left-left-right method. This drill may also be performed as right-right-left-left, left-left-right-right, left-right-right-right, or right-left-left-left.

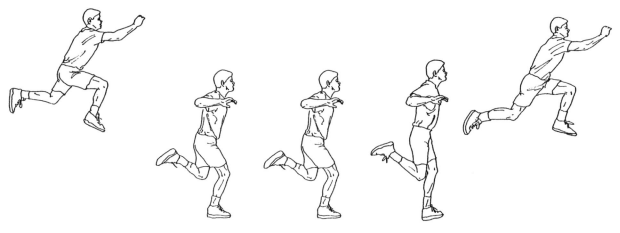

Drive knee up and out. Land on right foot. Land on right foot. Land on left foot. Jump from left foot.

SHOCKS

In-Depth Jump

Intensity level: Shock.

Starting position: Start with the balls of the feet on the edge of a box, knees slightly bent and arms relaxed at the sides.

Direction of jump: Either vertical or horizontal.

Arm action: Double arm action.

Starting action: Begin by *stepping* off the platform to land on the ground; do not jump off the platform.

Descent: While in the air, keep the knees very slightly bent. Land on the balls of the feet with the feet 20 to 30 cm apart. When landing, the body weight should cause the knees to flex more.

Ascent: As soon as possible upon landing on the ground, jump upward or forward, swing the arms in the desired direction, and propel the body as high or as far forward as possible. Concentrate on maximal effort.

Volume: 5 to 10 repetitions (1).

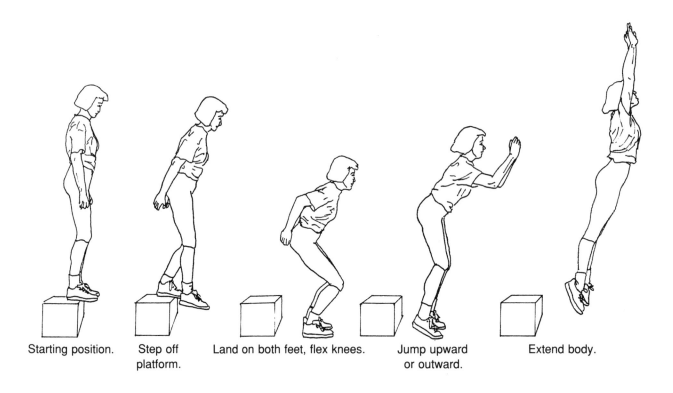

Starting position.   Step off platform.   Land on both feet, flex knees.   Jump upward or outward.   Extend body.

Box Jumps

Intensity level: Shock.

Starting position: Place four to eight wooden boxes evenly, 1 to 2 m apart; or one box may be used. Stand about 0.6 m in front of the first box. Feet should be shoulder-width apart; ankles, knees, and hips slightly flexed; head up; and arms at the sides.

Direction of jump: Vertical and horizontal.

Arm action: Double or single arm action.

Starting action: Jump upward and forward to land on the first box. Foot contact may be either one or two feet. (Only athletes of adequate strength and conditioning base, extensive background in plyometrics, and less than 100 kg should perform this drill with one leg.)

Ascent: Explode upward onto the first box.

Descent: As soon as you land on the box, explode again as high and/or far forward as possible. The distance between boxes depends on the amount of horizontal movement desired. Upon landing on the ground, immediately jump to the next box and continue. If only one box is used, when contacting the ground after jumping off the box immediately jump up or forward as far as possible.

Volume: Two to four sets of 5 to 10 repetitions (1).

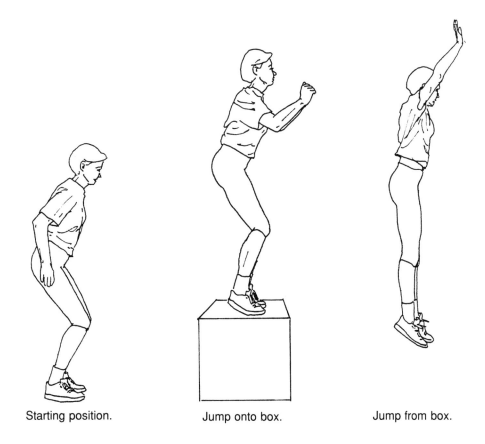

Starting position.   Jump onto box.   Jump from box.

UPPER BODY PLYOMETRIC DRILLS

Medicine Ball Sit-Up

Intensity level: Low.

Starting position: The subject sits on the floor with the knees flexed 90° and the upper body leaning slightly backward. A partner stands 1.5 to 2 m in front of the subject.

Direction of movement: Vertical.

Starting action: The partner passes the ball to the subject at the subject's chest level. The subject catches the medicine ball with arms slightly flexed.

Descent: The subject allows the force of the ball to push the upper body back and down. This movement causes an eccentric action of the abdominals.

Ascent: After the lower back touches the floor, the subject immediately sits up and performs a chest pass to the partner at the completion of the sit-up.

Volume: 10 repetitions (16).

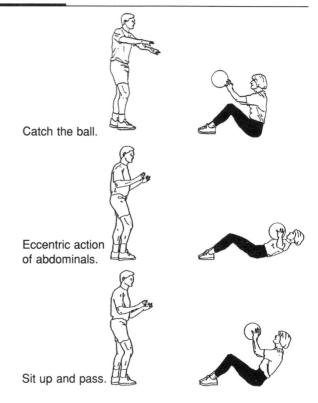

Catch the ball.

Eccentric action of abdominals.

Sit up and pass.

Plyometric Sit-Up

Intensity level: Low.

Starting position: Lie on the back with the legs slightly flexed and perpendicular to the floor. A partner stands with his or her feet on each side of the subject's head, facing the subject's feet. The partner grasps the subject's ankles and the subject grasps the partner's ankles.

Direction of the movement: Vertical.

Starting action: The partner thrusts the subject's legs toward the ground by rapidly extending the arms.

Descent: The subject provides slight resistance to the partner's push and allows the legs to slightly accelerate towards the floor.

Ascent: The subject quickly lifts the legs to the perpendicular position before they touch the floor.

Volume: 10 repetitions (16).

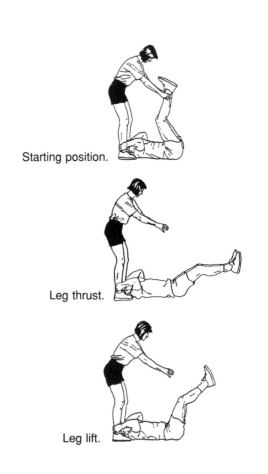

Starting position.

Leg thrust.

Leg lift.

Medicine Ball Push-Up

Intensity level: Medium.

Starting position: Lie in a push-up position, with the palms on the medicine ball and arms straight.

Direction of movement: Vertical.

Starting action: Quickly remove the hands from the medicine ball and drop down.

Descent: Move the hands slightly wider than shoulder-width. Contact the ground with the elbows slightly flexed. Allow gravity to further flex the elbows until the chest almost touches the medicine ball.

Ascent: Rapidly extend the arms to full extension so that the hands leave the ground. When the upper body is at maximal height the hands should be higher than the medicine ball (if not, flex the arms rapidly so palms are above the ball). Quickly place the palms on the medicine ball and repeat the exercise.

Volume: 10 repetitions.

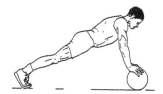

Starting position.

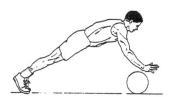

Drop down.

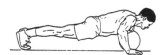

Flex elbows.

Drop-and-Catch Push-Up (or Drop Push-Up)

Note. Drop-and-Catch Push-Up is described, Drop Push-Up (without partner) is shown.

Intensity level: Shock.

Starting position: The subject kneels on the ground with a near vertical torso. The partner stands with feet on both sides of the subject's calves.

Direction of movement: Vertical.

Standing action: Partner grasps the subject under the armpits with hands on the anterior deltoid or chest. The partner lifts the subject to a 45° angle until the subject's knees come off the ground.

Descent: The partner then releases the subject, who, with extended but slightly flexed arms, contacts the ground, allowing the force to flex the elbows. The subject drops down until the chest almost touches the ground.

Ascent: The subject rapidly extends the arms to full length. The extension should be forceful enough to propel the upper body close to the starting position. The partner may either catch the subject in the air and repeat the exercise or, if the subject lacks power to obtain sufficient height, allow the subject to fall back to the ground and then repeat the exercise from the starting position.

Volume: 10 repetitions (14,16).

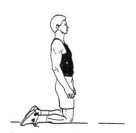

Starting position.

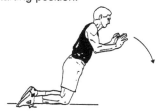

Drop down.

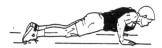

Bottom of push-up position.

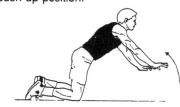

Extend arms.

Key Terms

Study Questions

1. After the start of a sprint the upper torso should be
   a. leaning slightly forward
   b. leaning forward at about 35° to 40°
   c. straight up
   d. leaning slightly backward

2. Which of the following is an assistive method for sprint training?
   a. downhill running
   b. maximal effort sprints
   c. pulling a weighted sled
   d. acceleration sprints

3. After catching the ball during the medicine ball sit-up, which type of muscle action is performed in the abdominals?
   a. isokinetic
   b. isometric
   c. eccentric
   d. concentric

4. Which of the following jumps will normally have the longest amortization phase?
   a. cycle split squat jumps
   b. split squat jumps
   c. squat jumps
   d. double-leg tuck jumps

5. Which of the following is most similar in execution to the standing triple jump?
   a. combination bound
   b. double-leg hop
   c. single-leg speed hop
   d. double-leg zigzag hop

6. Which of the following is *not* a technique error in performing an in-depth jump with a two-foot landing?
   a. using an alternate arm swing
   b. performing a full squat upon landing
   c. stepping out and dropping from the box
   d. landing with locked knees

Applying Knowledge of Speed Development and Plyometric Training

Problem 1
At what speed is correct running form best trained and corrected and why?

Problem 2
What techniques and drills may be used to increase stride frequency?

Problem 3
What are the most important program and athlete considerations prior to implementing a plyometric program?

References

1. Allerheiligen, B. *Poke Power Training Manual*. Ft. Collins, CO: Author. 1992.
2. Asmussen, E., and F. Bonde-Peterson. Storage of elastic energy in skeletal muscles in man. *Acta Physio. Scand.* 91:385-392. 1974.
3. Astrand, P., and K. Rodahl. *Textbook of Work Physiology*. New York: McGraw-Hill. 1970.
4. Aura, O., and J.T. Vitasalo. Biomechanical characteristics of jumping. *Int. J. Sport Biomech.* 5(1):89-97. 1989.
5. Blattner, S., and L. Noble. Relative effects of isokinetic and plyometric training on vertical jumping performance. *Res. Q.* 50(4):583-588. 1979.
6. Bobbert, M.F. Drop jumping as a training method for jumping ability. *Sports Med.* 9(1):7-22. 1990.
7. Borkowski, J. Prevention of pre-season muscle soreness: Plyometric exercise (abstract). *Athl. Training.* 25(2):122. 1990.
8. Bosco, C., J.T. Vitasalo, P.V. Komi, and P. Luhtanen. Combined effect of elastic energy and myoelectrical potentiation during stretch shortening cycle exercise. *Acta Physiol. Scand.* 114:557-565. 1982.
9. Brittenham, D.R. Speed development. *NSCA Journal* 5(6):12-20, 72-73. 1984.
10. Cavagna, G.A. Storage and utilization of elastic energy in skeletal muscle. In: *Exercise and Sport Science Reviews*, vol. 5. R.S. Hutton, ed. Santa Barbara, CA: Journal Affiliates. 1977. pp. 80-129.
11. Chu, D. Plyometrics: The link between strength and speed. *NSCA Journal* 5(2):20-21. 1983.
12. Chu, D. Plyometric exercise. *NSCA Journal* 5(6):56-59, 61-64. 1984.
13. Chu, D. *Jumping Into Plyometrics*. Champaign, IL: Human Kinetics. 1992.
14. Chu, D., and F. Costello. Jumping into plyometrics. *NSCA Journal* 7(3):65. 1985.
15. Chu, D., and R. Korchemny. Sprinting stride actions: Analysis and evaluation. *NSCA Journal* 11(6):6-8, 82-85. 1989.
16. Chu, D., and R. Panariello. Jumping into plyometrics. *NSCA Journal* 8(5):73. 1986.
17. Chu, D., and L. Plummer. Jumping into plyometrics: The language of plyometrics. *NSCA Journal* 6(5):30-31. 1984.
18. Costello, F. Training for speed using resisted and assisted methods. *NSCA Journal* 7(1):74-75. 1985.
19. deVries, H.A. *Physiology of Exercise for Physical Education and Athletics*. Dubuque, IA: Brown. 1974.
20. Dursenev, L., and L. Raeysky. Strength training for jumpers. *Soviet Sports Rev.* 14(2):53-55. 1979.
21. Fleck, S., and W. Kraemer. *Designing Resistance Training Programs*. Champaign, IL: Human Kinetics. 1987.
22. Fox, E.L. *Sports Physiology*. Philadelphia: Saunders. 1979.
23. Gambetta, V. Plyometric training. *Track and Field Q. Rev.* 80(4):56-57. 1978.
24. Gambetta, V. (1988). *Plyometric training: Understanding and coaching power development for sport* [Videotape]. Lincoln, NE: National Strength and Conditioning Association.
25. Getchell, B. *Physical Fitness: A Way of Life*. New York: Wiley. 1979.
26. Häkkinen, K., and P.V. Komi. The effect of explosive type strength training on electromyographic and force production characteristics of leg extensor muscles during concentric and various stretch shortening cycle exercises. *Scandinavian Journal of Sport Sciences*. 7:65-76. 1985.
27. Herman, D. (1976). *The effects of depth jumping on vertical jumping and sprinting speed*. Unpublished master's thesis, Ithaca College, Ithaca, NY.
28. Katschajov, S., K. Gomberaze, and A. Revson. Rebound jumps. *Modern Athlete and Coach* 14(4):23. 1976.
29. Klinzing, J. Improving sprint speed for all athletes. *NSCA Journal* 6(4):32-33. 1984.
30. Korchemny, R. Evaluation of sprinters. *NSCA Journal* 7(4):38-42. 1985.
31. Lamb, D.L. *Physiology of Exercise: Responses and Adaptations*. New York: Macmillan. 1978.
32. Luhtanen, P., and P. Komi. Mechanical factors influencing running speed. In: *Biomechanics VI-B*. E. Asmussen, ed. Baltimore: University Park Press. 1978. pp. 23-29.
33. Lundin, P. A review of plyometric training. *Track and Field Q. Rev.* 89(4):37-40. 1989.

34. Mann, R. Speed development. *NSCA Journal* 5(6):12-20, 72-73. 1984.
35. Matveyev, L. *Fundamentals of Sports Training*. Moscow: Progress Publishers. 1983.
36. McFarland, B. Speed: Developing maximum running speed. *NSCA Journal* 6(5):24-28. 1984.
37. McFarland, B. Special strength: Horizontal or vertical. *NSCA Journal* 7(1):64-66. 1985.
38. O'Connell, A., and E. Gardner. *Understanding the Scientific Bases of Human Movement*. Baltimore: Williams & Wilkins. 1972.
39. Parcells, R. (1977). *The effect of depth jumping and weight training on vertical jump*. Unpublished master's thesis. Ithaca College, Ithaca, NY.
40. Plattner, S., and L. Noble. Relative effects of isokinetic and plyometric training on vertical jumping performance. *Res. Q.* 50(4):583-588. 1979.
41. Polhemus, R., and E. Burkhardt. The effects of plyometric training drills on the physical strength gains of collegiate football players. *NSCA Journal* 2(1):13-15. 1980.
42. Polhemus, R., E. Burkhardt, M. Osina, and M. Patterson. The effects of plyometric training with ankle and vest weights on conventional weight training programs for men. *Track and Field Q. Rev.* 80(4):59-61. 1980.
43. Rosen, M. Speed development. *NSCA Journal* 5(6):12-20, 72-73. 1984.
44. Verkhoshanski, Y. Perspectives in the improvement of speed-strength preparation of jumpers. *Yessis Rev. Soviet Phys. Ed. Sports* 4(2):28-29. 1969.
45. Verkhoshanski, Y. Depth jumping in the training of jumpers. *Track Technique* 51:1618-1619. 1973.
46. Verkhoshanski, Y., and V. Tatyan. Speed-strength preparation of future champions. *Soviet Sports Rev.* 18(4):166-170. 1983.
47. Vitasalo, J.T., and O. Aura. Myoelectrical activity of the leg extensor musculature before ground contact in jumping. In: *Biomechanics X-B*, B. Johnsson, ed. Champaign, IL: Human Kinetics. 1987. pp. 695-700.
48. Wathen, D. NSCA position stand: Plyometric exercise. *NSCA Journal* 15(3): 1993.
49. Wilt, F. Plyometrics: What it is and how it works. *Athl. J.* 55(5):76, 89-90. 1975.
50. Wilt, F. Speed development. *NSCA Journal* 5(6):12-20, 72-73. 1984.

STRENGTH TRAINING AND SPOTTING TECHNIQUES

Thomas R. Baechle
Roger W. Earle
William B. Allerheiligen

This chapter provides guidelines for safe lifting and spotting conditions in the strength training facility. At the core of safe and effective strength training programs is proper exercise execution. Exercises that are performed correctly promote injury-free results, and do so in a more time-efficient manner than incorrectly performed exercises. The appropriate use of weight belts can also contribute to an injury-free environment. Their use primarily depends upon the type of exercise to be performed and the load to be used (see chapter 3). No belt is needed for exercises that do not stress the lower back (e.g., biceps curl, lat pulldown) or for exercises that do stress the lower back (e.g., back squat or dead lift) but involve the use of light loads. A belt should typically be worn when performing exercises that place stress on the lower back and involve the use of maximum or near-maximum loads. A weight belt may help avoid low back injuries, but only when proper exercise techniques are followed. Thus, the sole use of a weight belt is *not* a safeguard against injuries.

The first several sections of this chapter summarize the fundamental techniques involved in weight training exercises and spotting. The last section includes exercise and spotting checklists and illustrates many exercises. It is assumed that the reader is familiar with the exercises presented; therefore, the techniques presented are simply guidelines. If additional information is needed, refer to the selected readings presented at the end of the chapter.

EXERCISE TECHNIQUE FUNDAMENTALS

Follow the guidelines here when performing any exercise.

Establish the Proper Grip

There are two common grips used in strength training exercises; (a) the **pronated grip**, with knuckles up, also called the overhand grip, and (b) the **supinated grip**, with palms up, also known as the underhand grip (Figure 21.1). Two less common grips are the **alternated grip**, in which one hand is in a pronated grip and the other is in a supinated grip, and the **hook grip**, which is similar to the pronated grip except the thumb is positioned *under* the index and middle fingers. The hook grip is typically used when performing explosive/power exercises (e.g., snatch) where a stronger grip may be needed. Note that the thumb is wrapped around the bar in all of the grips shown. This positioning is called a closed grip. When the thumb does not wrap around the bar, it is called an open or false grip.

A proper grip also means that the **grip width**, that is, the spacing between the hands, is appropriate for the exercise. The three grip widths are common, wide, and narrow (Figure 21.2). Hand positioning should result in a balanced bar.

Some of the earlier work on the exercise checklists in this chapter was provided by Drs. Andrew Fry, Daye Halling, Chuck Stiggins, and Phil Allsen.

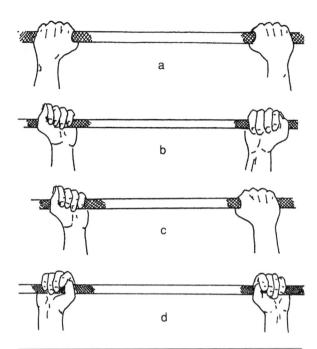

Figure 21.1   Bar grips: (a) pronated, (b) supinated, (c) alternated, (d) hook.

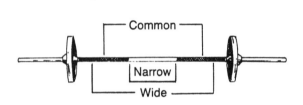

Figure 21.2   Grip widths.

Establish a Stable Position

Whether an exercise requires lifting a barbell or dumbbell from the floor or pushing while positioned in or on a machine, establishing a stable position is critical. A stable position enables the lifter to maintain proper body alignment during an exercise, which in turn places appropriate stress on muscles and joints.

Exercises performed while standing typically require that the feet be positioned slightly wider than hip-width, and that the balls of the feet and the heels be in contact with the floor (Figure 21.3). Establishing a stable position on machines sometimes calls for adjusting the seat or resistance arm and fastening belts snugly. Even though the directives to make these adjustments are not given in the checklists, the athlete should do so prior to beginning each exercise.

Move Through the Entire Range of Motion at the Proper Velocity

When the entire range of motion (ROM) is covered during an exercise, the value of the exercise is max-

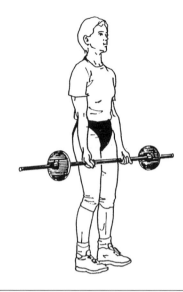

Figure 21.3   Hip-width during the biceps curl.

imized and the lifter maintains or improves flexibility. Repetitions performed in a slow, controlled manner increase the likelihood that the full ROM can be accomplished. When explosive or quick-lift exercises (e.g., the power clean, push jerk, and snatch) are involved, an effort should be made to maintain control of the bar throughout the entire ROM.

Inhale and Exhale at the Proper Times

The most strenuous time during an exercise is sometimes referred to as the sticking point. Teach lifters to exhale through the **sticking point** and to inhale during the less stressful phase of the repetition. The proper times for inhaling and exhaling are identified in the exercise checklist for each exercise.

For Exercises That Require Lifting a Barbell or Dumbbell From the Floor to the Shoulders or Overhead, Keep the Back Flat, the Bar Close, and Let the Leg Muscles do the Work

The position of the feet and back shown in Figure 21.4 enables the leg muscles to make a major contribution in lifting the bar off the floor. Keeping the bar close to the body and continuing to keep the back flat during the upward pull of the bar helps to avoid creating excessive strain on the lower back. (A more detailed explanation of this technique is presented in the exercise checklist section of this chapter.)

Handling Missed Lifts Appropriately

There may be occurrences when an athlete will ''miss'' or fail to complete an attempt with an exercise. In most

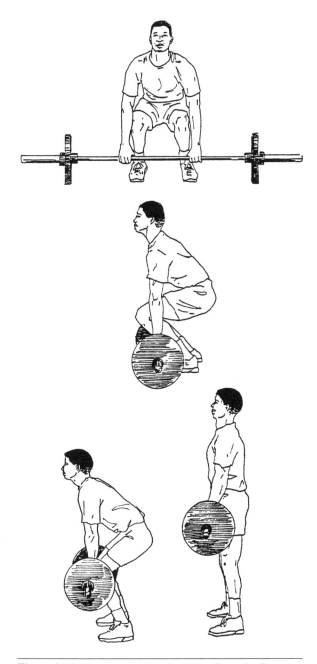

Figure 21.4 Correct position for lifting from the floor.

exercises assistance can be provided by a spotter who helps the lifter to manage a missed lift. Teaching the athlete how to get away from a bar that is unmanagable is important, especially during explosive (power) exercises that involve pushing or pulling the bar overhead. Spotting these types of exercises is typically *not* recommended. When the bar is missed in front, lifters should be instructed to push the bar away or simply drop it. If the bar is lost behind the head, lifters should be told to release the bar and jump forward. For these reasons the surrounding area or platform should be clear of other athletes and equipment prior to performing such exercises.

SPOTTING FREE-WEIGHT EXERCISES

A **spotter** is someone who assists the lifter in the execution of an exercise. Sometimes the spotter may help by recommending technique changes and assuming the role of a motivator. The spotter's primary role, however, is to protect the lifter from injury (and to avoid injury to himself or herself when doing so). The spotter must realize that poor execution of spotting responsibilities may result in very serious injury to the lifter.

Note that the term **spotting** as used in this chapter refers to the actions taken by the spotter to protect the lifter from injury. In contrast, actions of the spotter that enable the lifter to complete more repetitions or to encourage proper technique, such as a full ROM, are considered **partner-assisted actions**. Although partner-assisted actions are important in helping the lifter benefit from training, safety is of paramount importance. The checklists and illustrations on spotting techniques shown later in the chapter are for exercises that require a spotter or spotters for safety.

The remainder of this section should provide additional insight on spotting free-weight exercises. Although there are many relevant issues, we have limited our discussion to those indicated by the headings that follow.

Types of Exercises Performed and Equipment Involved

Free-weight exercises performed over the face (e.g., bench presses or lying triceps extensions), over the head (e.g., standing presses), or with the bar on the back (e.g., back squats) are more challenging for the lifter than those in which the bar or dumbbells are held at the sides or in front (e.g., standing dumbbell curls and shoulder shrugs, respectively). The over-the-face, over-head, and bar-on-the-back exercises also require more skill on the part of the spotter. With machine exercises, the primary responsibilities of the spotter shift from protecting the lifter to assisting in the completion of repetitions and perhaps motivation. Spotting dumbbell exercises typically requires more skill than spotting barbell exercises because there is an additional piece of equipment to observe and spot.

Spotting Overhead Exercises.
This type of exercise is potentially the most dangerous to spot. To insure the safety of the lifter, spotter, and other athletes, the following guidelines should be followed:

- All plates, bars, locks, and racks must be cleared from the area so they cannot be tripped over or run into.
- Other athletes must be instructed to stay clear of overhead lifting.

- Spotting overhead lifts is sometimes appropriate, such as when teaching the overhead press where the loads being used are very light. When spotting this exercise, only one spotter is involved and he or she should stand behind the lifter. The spotter should be at least as tall as the lifter, and at least as strong.
- Realize that performing overhead exercises with heavy weights is dangerous and that only well trained and experienced lifters should attempt them.

Spotting Dumbbell Exercises. It is important when spotting dumbbell exercises to spot as close to the dumbbell(s) as possible or, in a few exercises, to spot the dumbbell itself. Although some professionals may advocate spotting pressing movements by placing the hands on the upper arms or elbows (Figure 21.5a), this technique may lead to injury should the lifter's elbows collapse (i.e., flex); the spotter would then not be in a position to stop the dumbbells from striking the lifter's face or chest. Spotting above the elbow joint (Figure 21.5b) provides a safer technique.

For some exercises (pullovers, overhead dumbbell triceps extensions, and arm curls) it is necessary to spot with the hands on the dumbbell. Other exercises (bench presses, incline presses, shoulder presses, decline presses, chest flys, and shoulder raises) require the hands to be close to the dumbbell or on the wrist.

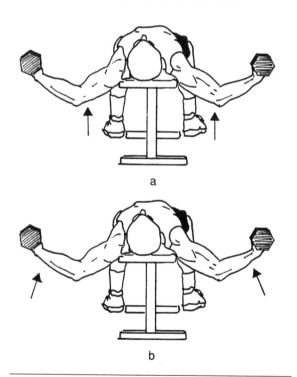

a

b

Figure 21.5 (a) Incorrect dumbbell fly spotting location. (b) Correct spotting for the dumbbell fly. (Arrows indicate the spotter's hand placement.)

How Many Spotters Are Needed?

The number of spotters needed is largely determined by the load being lifted, the experience and ability of the lifter and spotters, and the physical strength of the spotters. Obviously, with heavier loads the likelihood of injury increases as does the severity of the injury should an accident occur. Once the load exceeds the spotter's ability to effectively protect the lifter (or himself or herself), another spotter must become involved. On the other hand, one spotter is preferred if he or she can easily handle the load, because two or more spotters require coordination between themselves and with the lifter. As the number of spotters increases, so does the chance that an error in timing or technique may occur.

The exercise and spotting checklists that follow include suggestions for where and how spotters should be positioned. Where more than one spotter could be used in an exercise, only the most common approach to spotting is shown; the techniques involved in less-common approaches, however, are also listed.

Communication Between the Lifter and the Spotter

Communication is a responsibility for both the spotter and lifter. If the lifter does not tell the spotter how many repetitions will be performed, the spotter should ask prior to the beginning of the set. Spotters who do not have this information may take control of the bar too soon or too late and, consequently, disrupt or injure the lifter.

Use of the Liftoff. The term **liftoff** refers to moving the bar from a support to a position in which the lifter can begin the exercise. Usually the spotter helps to place the barbell or dumbbell(s) into the lifter's hands while the elbows are extended and helps to move the barbell or dumbbell(s) to the proper initial position(s). Some lifters want the spotter to provide a liftoff; others do not. If a liftoff is needed or requested, the lifter and spotter need to determine in advance a verbal signal; whether the command "Up" or some other phrase, such as, "I will give it to you on the count of three." Typically, the lifter signals that he or she is ready, the spotter says, "One, two, three," and on the "three" the bar is moved into position. Liftoffs are normally used in the bench press (off the rack) and the shoulder press (off the rack or off the shoulders) and in squatting exercises if the rack is nonadjustable and low. When two spotters are involved and the lifter wants a liftoff, as with a bench press, one spotter should assist with the liftoff and then quickly move to the end of the bar to spot (the other spotter is already at the other end). The spotter giving the liftoff must be sure that the lifter has complete control of the bar before moving to the end of the bar. Both spotters should help the lifter place the bar back onto the rack upon completion of the exercise.

How Much Help Is Needed? Knowing how much to help the lifter is an important aspect of spotting and requires experience. Most lifters typically need just enough help to successfully complete a repetition; other times they might need the spotter to assume the entire load. At the first indication that a lift will be missed, the lifter should quickly ask the spotter for help; the spotter needs to control the movement of the bar until it is racked. If the lifter cannot contribute anything to the completion of the repetition, the lifter should imme-diately tell the spotter to ''Take it'' or say some other phrase agreed upon before the lift. Regardless of when or why the spotter is needed to assist, he or she should take the bar from the lifter quickly and smoothly, trying to avoid abrupt changes in the amount of load being assumed by the lifter. The lifter should try to stay with the bar until it is racked or placed safely on the floor.

The checklists for spotting are appropriate to use with athletes using training loads. Spotting procedures may vary when excessively heavy loads are being used—such as 1RM (repetition maximum) attempts (as in pow-erlifting competitions)—because more spotters are needed.

STRENGTH TRAINING EXERCISES

ABDOMINALS

Bent-Knee Sit-Up

Beginning Position

☐ Lie face up on the mat.
☐ Flex knees to bring heels close to buttocks.
☐ Fold arms across chest or abdomen.

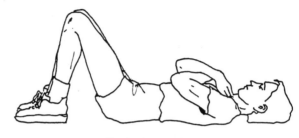

Beginning position.

Upward Movement Phase

☐ Tuck chin to chest.
☐ Curl upper body toward thighs until upper back is off mat.
☐ Keep feet flat on mat.
☐ Keep lower back flat on mat.

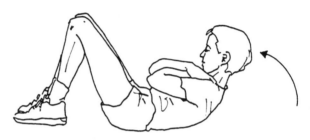

Upward movement.

Downward Movement Phase

☐ Lower shoulders slowly and with control.
☐ Keep feet flat on mat.
☐ Lower back to mat, then back of head to mat.
☐ Do not bounce or jerk body.

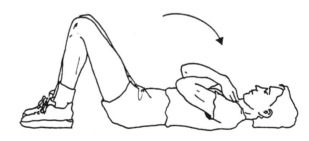

Downward movement.

Breathing

☐ Exhale through the sticking point of the upward movement phase.
☐ Inhale during the downward movement phase.

Crunch

Beginning Position

☐ Lie face up on the mat.
☐ Position calves and ankles on bench; hip and knees form a 90° angle.
☐ Fold arms across chest or abdomen.

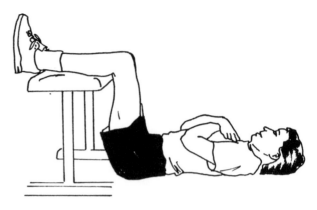

Beginning position.

Upward Movement Phase

☐ Tuck chin to chest.
☐ Curl upper body toward thighs until upper back is off mat.
☐ Keep calves and ankles on bench.

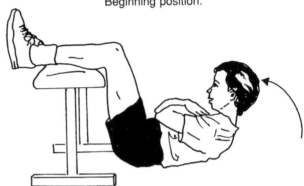

Upward movement.

Downward Movement Phase

☐ Lower shoulders slowly and under control.
☐ Keep calves and ankles on bench.
☐ Lower back to mat, then back of head to mat.
☐ Do not bounce or jerk body.

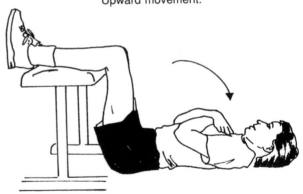

Downward movement.

Breathing

☐ Exhale through the sticking point of the upward movement phase.
☐ Inhale during the downward movement phase.

BACK

Bent-Over Row (Free Weight)

Before Beginning

☐ Grasp bar with a closed, pronated grip.
☐ Grip should be wider than shoulder-width.
☐ Using the floor-to-thigh lifting technique described in the Power Clean exercise (p. 392), pull the bar from the floor to the thighs.

Beginning Position

☐ Assume a shoulder-width stance with knees slightly flexed.
☐ Lean torso forward 10° to 30° above horizontal.
☐ Establish a flat-back position.
☐ Tilt head forward.
☐ Focus eyes ahead or slightly up.
☐ Lower bar until elbows are fully extended (but do not let the bar touch the floor).

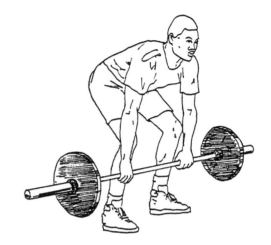

Beginning position.

Upward Movement Phase

☐ Pull bar up and touch the lower chest or upper abdomen.
☐ Point elbows up during movement.
☐ Maintain body position, flexed knees, and torso inclination.
☐ Keep the torso rigid and the back flat.

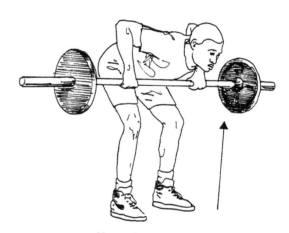

Upward movement.

Downward Movement Phase

☐ Keep the torso rigid and the back flat.
☐ Maintain body position, flexed knees, and torso inclination.
☐ Lower the bar slowly and under control until elbows are fully extended.

Breathing

☐ Exhale through the sticking point of the upward movement phase.
☐ Inhale during the downward movement phase.

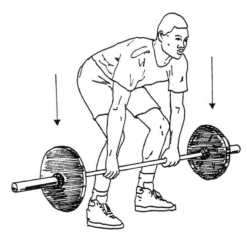

Downward movement.

Hyperextension

Beginning Position

☐ Lie face down on hyperextension bench.
☐ Position legs so that knees are level with hips.
☐ Position pads in contact with hips and back of ankles.
☐ Hang torso down to form a 90° angle at the hip.
☐ Place hands on each side of the head or crossed at the chest.

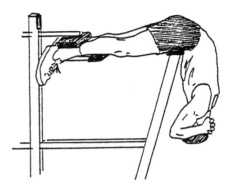

Beginning position.

Upward Movement Phase

☐ Raise trunk until upper torso is parallel to floor.
☐ Head faces forward.
☐ Once upper body is parallel to floor, the thighs and shoulders form a straight line.

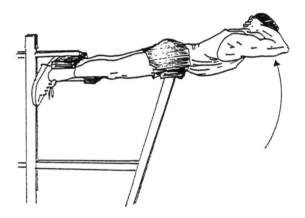

Upward movement.

Downward Movement Phase

☐ Lower upper body slowly to return to beginning position.

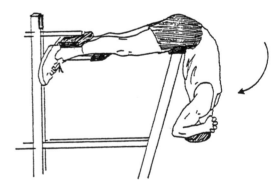

Downward movement.

Breathing

☐ Exhale through the sticking point of the upward movement phase.
☐ Inhale during the downward movement phase.

Lat Pulldown (Machine)

Beginning Position

☐ Grasp lat pulldown bar with a closed, pronated grip.
☐ Grip should be wider than shoulder-width.
☐ Pull bar down and position one knee on floor, with foot of other leg forward and on floor.
☐ Keep torso erect.
☐ Tilt head slightly down.
☐ Arms begin fully extended.

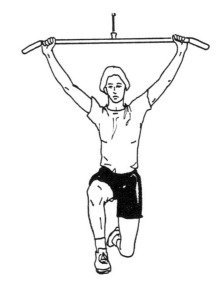

Beginning position.

Downward Movement Phase

☐ Pull bar down toward the neck.
☐ Maintain body position.
☐ Touch bar at base of the neck.
☐ Bar can also be pulled down in front to touch upper chest.

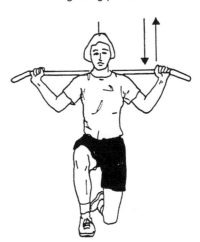

Pull bar down to base of neck.

Upward Movement Phase

☐ Allow arms to fully extend.

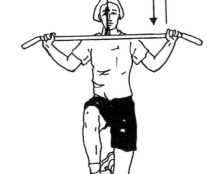

Breathing

☐ Exhale through the sticking point of the downward movement phase.
☐ Inhale during the upward movement phase.

Bar can also be pulled down to upper chest.

One-Arm Dumbbell Row (Free Weight)

Beginning Position

- ☐ Stand at one side of the bench.
- ☐ Kneel on the bench with the inside leg.
- ☐ Lean forward and place inside hand on the bench in front of the knee.
- ☐ Plant outside foot at side of bench and flex knee.
- ☐ Position torso parallel to floor.
- ☐ Grasp dumbbell with outside hand.
- ☐ Hang dumbbell at full elbow extension.

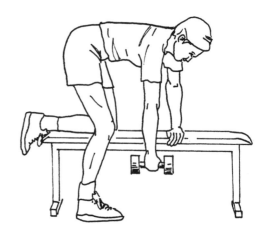

Beginning position.

Upward Movement Phase

- ☐ Pull dumbbell up toward the chest.
- ☐ Keep upper arm and elbow next to ribs.
- ☐ Keep back and shoulders even and parallel to floor.
- ☐ Touch dumbbell to outer chest and rib cage.

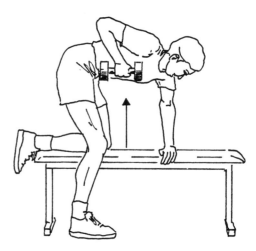

Bring dumbbell to chest.

Downward Movement Phase

- ☐ Lower dumbbell slowly and under control to a fully extended elbow position.
- ☐ Keep upper arm and elbow next to the ribs.
- ☐ Maintain body position.

Breathing

- ☐ Exhale through the sticking point of the upward movement phase.
- ☐ Inhale during the downward movement phase.

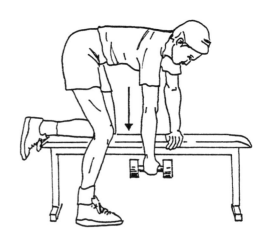

Downward movement.

Seated Row (Machine)

Beginning Position

☐ Assume a seated position facing the machine.
☐ Place feet on machine frame or foot supports.
☐ Position torso perpendicular to floor.
☐ Slightly flex knees.
☐ Grasp bar handle or bar with a closed grip.
☐ Fully extend elbows.

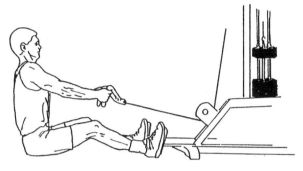

Beginning position.

Backward Movement Phase

☐ Keep body erect and stationary.
☐ Do not lean backward.
☐ Pull bar or handle toward chest/upper abdomen.
☐ Keep elbows next to ribs.

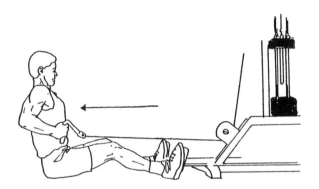

Backward movement.

Forward Movement Phase

☐ Allow bar or handle to move away from the body slowly and under control.
☐ Maintain body position.
☐ Keep elbows next to ribs.

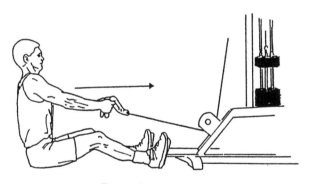

Forward movement.

Breathing

☐ Exhale through the sticking point of the backward movement phase.
☐ Inhale during the forward movement phase.

BICEPS

Biceps Curl (Free Weight)

Beginning Position

☐ Grasp bar using a closed, supinated grip.
☐ Grip should be slightly wider than shoulder-width.
☐ Little finger should be touching the outer thigh.
☐ Stand erect with feet shoulder-width apart, knees slightly flexed.
☐ Rest the bar on the anterior thigh, elbows fully extended.
☐ Position upper arms against the ribs and perpendicular to floor.

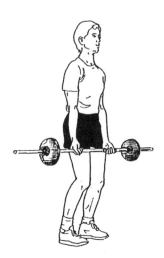

Beginning position.

Upward Movement Phase

☐ Raise bar in an arc by flexing arms at the elbows.
☐ Keep upper arms and elbows stationary.
☐ Maintain body position.
☐ Do not swing the bar upward.
☐ Raise bar to within 10 to 15 cm of the anterior deltoids.

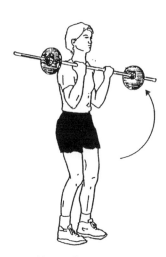

Upward movement.

Downward Movement Phase

☐ Lower the bar slowly and under control until elbows are fully extended.
☐ Maintain body position.
☐ Do not jerk or bounce the bar at the bottom of movement.

Breathing

☐ Exhale through the sticking point of the upward movement phase.
☐ Inhale during the downward movement phase.

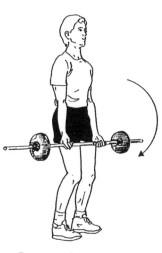

Downward movement.

Hammer Curl (Free Weight)

Beginning Position

☐ Grasp dumbbells using a closed, neutral grip.
☐ Palms should be facing outer thighs.
☐ Stand erect with feet shoulder-width apart, knees slightly flexed.
☐ Allow dumbbells to hang at the sides, elbows fully extended.
☐ Position upper arms against the ribs, perpendicular to floor.

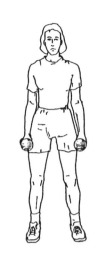

Beginning position.

Upward Movement Phase

☐ Raise one dumbbell in an arc by flexing the arm at the elbow.
☐ Keep upper arm and elbow stationary.
☐ Keep dumbbell in a neutral position.
☐ Maintain body position.
☐ Do not swing the dumbbell upward.
☐ Raise dumbbell to within 10 to 15 cm from the anterior deltoids.

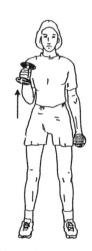

Upward movement.

Downward Movement Phase

☐ Lower dumbbell slowly and under control until elbow is fully extended.
☐ Keep dumbbell in a neutral position.
☐ Maintain body position.
☐ Do not jerk or bounce the dumbbell at the bottom of movement.
☐ Repeat upward and downward movement phase with other arm (alternate arms).

Breathing

☐ Exhale through the sticking point of the upward movement phase.
☐ Inhale during the downward movement phase.

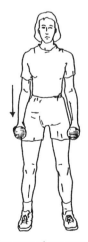

Downward movement.

CHEST

Dumbbell Incline Bench Press (Free Weight)

Note that this exercise can also be performed on a flat or decline bench.

Beginning Position

- ☐ Lie facing forward on incline bench.
- ☐ Position feet flat on floor.
- ☐ Position head, shoulders, and buttocks flat on bench.
- ☐ Grasp dumbbells with a closed grip, palms facing forward.
- ☐ Press both dumbbells to extended arm position above head.
- ☐ Point elbows out.

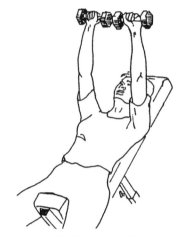

Beginning position.

Downward Movement Phase

- ☐ Lower dumbbells slowly and under control.
- ☐ Keep forearms parallel.
- ☐ Maintain body position on bench, feet on floor.
- ☐ Lower dumbbells to touch anterior deltoids or outer chest.

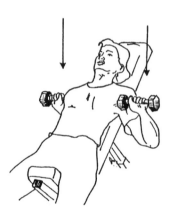

Downward movement.

Upward Movement Phase

- ☐ Push dumbbells to full elbow extension.
- ☐ Maintain body position on bench, feet on floor.
- ☐ Keep forearms parallel.

Breathing

- ☐ Inhale during the downward movement phase.
- ☐ Exhale through the sticking point of the upward movement phase.

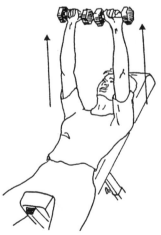

Upward movement.

Flat Bench Press (Free Weight)

Note that this exercise can also be performed using dumbbells and/or on a decline bench.

Beginning Position: Lifter

☐ Lie face up on a bench.
☐ Position feet flat on floor.
☐ Position head, shoulders, and buttocks flat on bench.
☐ Eyes should be below edge of the bar shelf.
☐ Grasp bar with a closed, pronated grip.
☐ Signal spotter.
☐ Move bar off bar shelf.
☐ Position bar over chest, elbows fully extended.

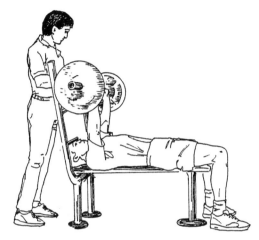

Beginning positions.

Beginning Position: Spotter

☐ Stand 15 to 20 cm from the head of the bench.
☐ Grasp bar with an alternated grip.
☐ Grip should be inside lifter's hands.
☐ Keep torso erect, knees slightly flexed.
☐ At lifter's signal, assist with moving bar from bar shelf.
☐ Guide bar to position over lifter's chest.
☐ Release bar smoothly.

Downward Movement Phase: Lifter

☐ Lower bar slowly and under control.
☐ Maintain body position on bench, feet on floor.
☐ Keep wrists straight.
☐ Lower bar to touch the chest near the nipples.

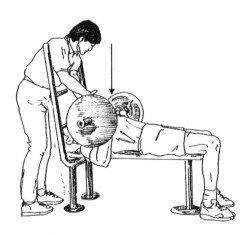

Downward movement positions.

Downward Movement Phase: Spotter

☐ Keep hands close to the bar as it descends.
☐ Maintain torso and knee position.

Upward Movement Phase: Lifter

☐ Push bar up to full elbow extension.
☐ Maintain body position on bench, feet on floor.
☐ Do not arch the lower back.
☐ At the completion of the set, signal spotter.
☐ Move bar to bar shelf.
☐ Keep grip on bar until racked.

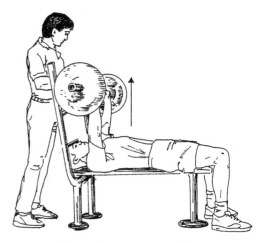

Upward movement positions.

Upward Movement Phase: Spotter

☐ Keep hands close to bar as it ascends.
☐ Maintain upright body position, knees flexed.
☐ At the lifter's signal at the completion of the set, grasp bar with alternated grip.
☐ Grip should be inside lifter's hands.
☐ Guide bar back into bar shelf.
☐ Keep grip on bar until racked.

Breathing

☐ Inhale during the downward movement phase.
☐ Exhale through the sticking point of the upward movement phase.

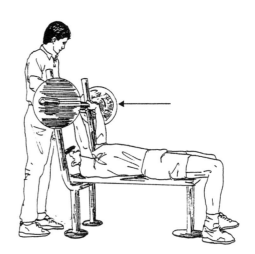

Racking the bar.

Flat Dumbbell Fly (Free Weight)

Note that this exercise can also be performed on an incline or decline bench.

Beginning Position

☐ Lie face up on a bench with feet flat on floor.
☐ Position head, shoulders, and buttocks flat on bench.
☐ Grasp dumbbells with a closed, pronated grip.
☐ Press dumbbells to extended arm position above chest.
☐ Rotate dumbbells so palms face each other.
☐ Point elbows out.

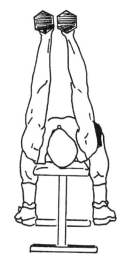

Beginning position.

Downward Movement Phase

☐ Slightly flex the elbows.
☐ Move dumbbells outward in wide arcs.
☐ Keep palms up and elbows pointed toward floor.
☐ Keep dumbbells in line with the shoulders as they are lowered.
☐ Lower dumbbells slowly and under control until they are level with the shoulders.

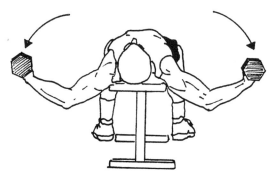

Downward movement.

Upward Movement Phase

☐ Pull dumbbells evenly toward each other in a wide arc to an extended arm position above chest.
☐ Keep the elbows slightly flexed until just prior to reaching the beginning position.

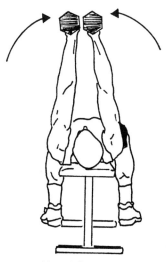

Upward movement.

Breathing

☐ Inhale during the downward movement phase.
☐ Exhale through the sticking point of the upward movement phase.

Incline Bench Press (Free Weight)

Beginning Position: Lifter

☐ Lie facing forward on incline bench.
☐ Position feet flat on floor.
☐ Position head, shoulders, and buttocks flat on bench.
☐ Grasp bar with a closed, pronated grip.
☐ Eyes should be ahead of bar shelf edge.
☐ Signal spotter.
☐ Move bar off bar shelf to fully extended elbow position.
☐ Position bar over clavicles/upper chest.

Beginning Position: Spotter

☐ Stand on spotter's platform.
☐ Grasp bar with an alternated grip.
☐ Grip should be inside lifter's hands.
☐ Keep torso erect, knees slightly flexed.
☐ At lifter's signal, assist with moving bar from bar shelf.
☐ Guide bar to position over lifter's clavicles/upper chest.
☐ Release bar smoothly.

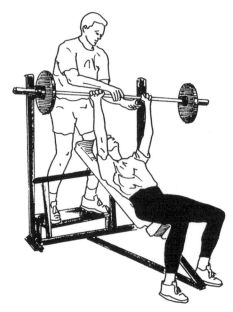

Beginning positions.

Downward Movement Phase: Lifter

☐ Lower bar slowly and under control.
☐ Maintain body position on bench, feet on floor.
☐ Keep wrists straight.
☐ Lower bar to touch upper chest below the clavicles.

Downward Movement Phase: Spotter

☐ Keep hands close to the bar as it descends.
☐ Maintain upright body position, knees flexed.

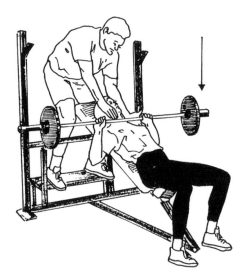

Downward movement positions.

Upward Movement Phase: Lifter

☐ Push bar up to full elbow extension.
☐ Maintain body position on bench, feet on floor.
☐ Do not arch lower back.
☐ At the completion of set, signal spotter.
☐ Move bar to bar shelf.
☐ Keep grip on bar until racked.

Upward Movement Phase: Spotter

☐ Keep hands close to bar as it ascends.
☐ Maintain upright body position, knees flexed.
☐ At lifter's signal at the completion of the set, grasp bar with alternated grip.
☐ Grip should be inside lifter's hands.
☐ Guide bar back onto bar shelf.
☐ Keep grip on bar until racked.

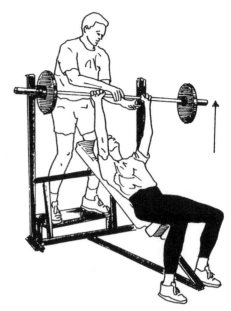

Upward movement positions.

Breathing

☐ Inhale during the downward movement phase.
☐ Exhale through the sticking point of the upward movement phase.

Chest Press (Machine)

Beginning Position

☐ Lie face up on the bench with the feet straddling the bench and flat on the floor.
☐ Position head, shoulders, and buttocks on bench.
☐ Allow a 5- to 10-cm space between head and weight stack.
☐ Grasp handles slightly wider than shoulders with a closed, overhand grip.
☐ Align handles with nipples on chest.

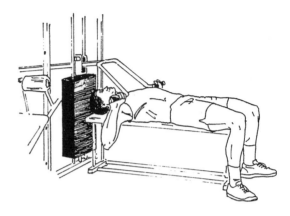

Beginning position.

Upward Movement Phase

☐ Push handles away from chest to a fully extended elbow position.
☐ Maintain body position on bench.
☐ Keep feet on floor and do not arch the lower back.

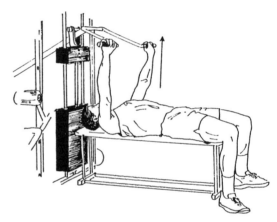

Upward movement.

Downward Movement Phase

☐ Lower weight slowly and under control.
☐ Maintain body position on bench.

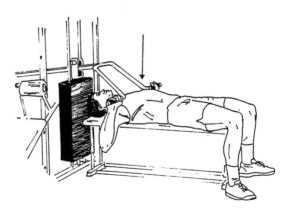

Downward movement.

Breathing

☐ Exhale through the sticking point of the upward movement phase.
☐ Inhale during the downward movement phase.

FOREARMS

Wrist Curl (Free Weight)

Beginning Position

- ☐ Sit on the end of a bench.
- ☐ Grasp bar with an open, supinated grip, hands 20 to 30 cm apart.
- ☐ Position feet flat on floor, thighs parallel to each other.
- ☐ Lean torso forward.
- ☐ Position elbows and forearms on the thighs.
- ☐ Extend wrists slightly beyond knees.

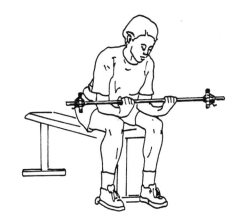

Beginning position.

Downward Movement Phase

- ☐ Open the hands and extend the wrists slowly and under control.
- ☐ Allow the bar to roll down to the ends of the fingers.
- ☐ Maintain body position.
- ☐ Keep elbows and forearms on the thighs.
- ☐ Keep the thighs parallel to each other.

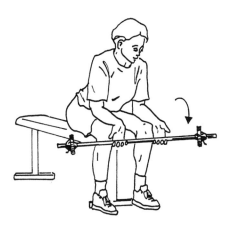

Downward movement.

Upward Movement Phase

- ☐ Raise the bar by flexing the fingers and wrists.
- ☐ Keep elbows on the thighs.
- ☐ Do not flex arm at the elbow during the movement.
- ☐ At the completion of the set, return bar to floor.

Breathing

- ☐ Inhale during the downward movement phase.
- ☐ Exhale through the sticking point of the upward movement phase.

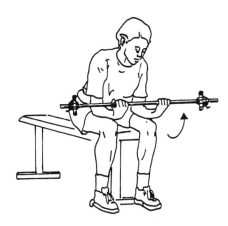

Upward movement.

Wrist Extension (Free Weight)

Beginning Position

- ☐ Sit on the end of a bench.
- ☐ Grasp bar with a closed, pronated grip, hands 20 to 30 cm apart.
- ☐ Position feet flat on floor, thighs parallel to each other.
- ☐ Lean torso forward.
- ☐ Position elbows and forearms on the thighs.
- ☐ Extend wrists slightly beyond knees.

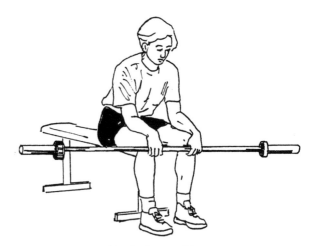

Beginning position.

Upward Movement Phase

- ☐ Raise the bar by extending the wrists.
- ☐ Keep elbows on the thighs.
- ☐ Do not flex arm at the elbow during the movement.

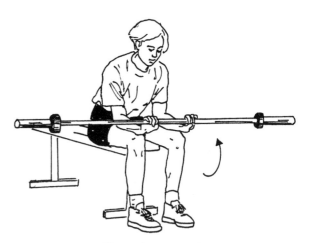

Upward movement.

Downward Movement Phase

- ☐ Flex wrists slowly and under control to allow bar to move toward floor.
- ☐ Maintain a closed grip.
- ☐ Maintain body position.
- ☐ Keep elbows and forearms on the thighs.
- ☐ Keep the thighs parallel to each other.
- ☐ At the completion of the set, return bar to floor.

Breathing

- ☐ Inhale during the downward movement phase.
- ☐ Exhale through the sticking point of the upward movement phase.

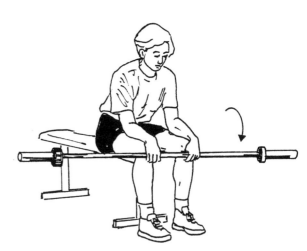

Downward movement.

LEGS

Back Squat (Free Weight)

Beginning Position: Lifter

☐ Grasp bar with a closed, pronated grip.
☐ Grip should be slightly wider than shoulder-width.
☐ Step under the bar and position feet parallel to each other.
☐ Move hips under bar.
☐ Position the bar in balanced position on the shoulders in one of two positions:

  1. *Low bar position*—across posterior deltoids at the middle of the trapezius
  2. *High bar position*—above posterior deltoids at the base of the neck

☐ Lift and hold chest up and out.
☐ Pull shoulder blades toward each other.
☐ Tilt head slightly up.
☐ Lift elbows up to create a "shelf" for the bar.
☐ Straighten both legs to lift bar out of racks.
☐ Take one or two steps backward.
☐ Position feet shoulder-width apart or wider, and even with each other.
☐ Point toes slightly outward.

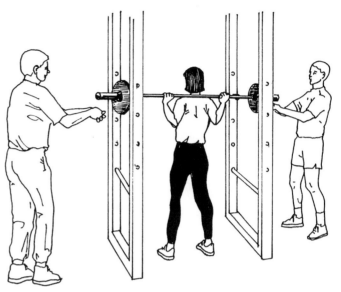

Beginning positions with bar in the high bar position.

Beginning Position: Spotters

☐ Two spotters stand at opposite ends of the bar, feet positioned slightly wider than hip-width.
☐ Cup hands with palms facing upward.
☐ Palms begin and are maintained in a position 5 to 8 cm below the ends of the bar.
☐ Spotters move sideways in unison with the lifter as lifter moves backward.
☐ Once in position, feet are slightly wider than hip-width, knees slightly flexed, back flat.

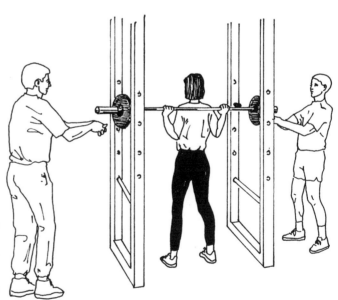

Beginning positions with the bar in the low bar position.

Downward Movement Phase: Lifter

☐ Focus eyes on wall 30 to 60 cm above eye level.
☐ Slowly and under control, lower bar by flexing at the hips and knees.
☐ Maintain erect body position.
☐ Keep weight over the middle of the foot and heels, not the toes.
☐ Keep heels on the floor.
☐ Keep knees aligned over the feet.
☐ Slowly lower hips until tops of thighs are parallel to floor.
☐ Do not bounce at the bottom of movement.

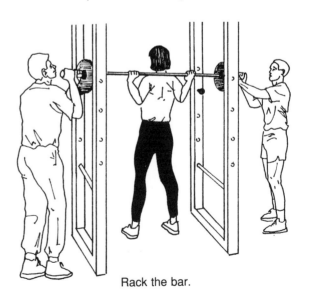

Downward movement positions.

Downward Movement Phase: Spotters

☐ Spotters squat down in unison with the lifter.
☐ Cup hands 5 to 8 cm below the bar and follow the bar downward.
☐ Maintain body position.

Upward Movement Phase: Lifter

☐ Keep eyes focused on wall 30 to 60 cm above eye level.
☐ Slowly raise bar by straightening the hips and knees.
☐ Maintain body position.
☐ Keep knees aligned over the feet.
☐ Do not let knees move in or out.
☐ Do not accelerate the bar at the top of movement.
☐ At the completion of the set, slowly step forward into the rack.
☐ Position hips beneath the bar.
☐ Squat down until the bar is resting in the rack.

Upward movement positions.

Upward Movement Phase: Spotters

☐ Stand up with the lifter.
☐ Keep hands 5 to 8 cm below and close to the bar.
☐ Assist only if necessary.
☐ Walk the lifter back into the rack.
☐ Spotters simultaneously grab onto the bar, keeping it level, and assist lifter with placing the bar in the rack.

Breathing

☐ Inhale during the downward movement phase.
☐ Exhale through the sticking point of the upward movement phase.

Rack the bar.

Front Squat (Free Weight)

Beginning Position

☐ Place hands evenly on the bar using one of two positions:

1. Forward elbow position
   ☐ Grasp bar with an open, pronated grip.
   ☐ Grip should be slightly wider than shoulder-width.
   ☐ Raise elbows, rotating the hands around bar.
   ☐ Place bar on front deltoids.
2. Crossed arm position
   ☐ Cross arms in front of chest.
   ☐ Support bar on front deltoids.
   ☐ Grasp bar with an open, pronated grip.

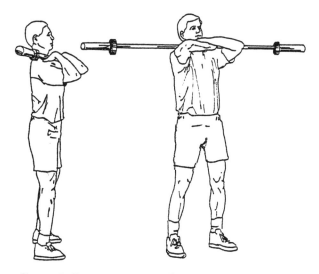

Forward elbow position.   Crossed arm position.

☐ Step forward and align hips under the bar.
☐ Keep elbows up and upper arms parallel to (or higher than) floor.
☐ Establish hip-width stance.
☐ Lift and hold chest up and out and pull shoulder blades toward each other.
☐ Tilt head slightly upward.
☐ Position feet approximately shoulder-width or wider apart and even with each other.
☐ Point toes slightly out.

Downward Movement Phase

☐ Focus eyes on wall about 30 to 60 cm above eye level.
☐ Slowly and under control, lower bar by flexing at the hips and knees.
☐ Maintain erect body position.
☐ Keep weight over the middle of the foot and heels, not the toes.
☐ Keep heels on the floor.
☐ Keep knees aligned over the feet.
☐ Slowly lower hips until tops of thighs are parallel to floor.
☐ Do not bounce at the bottom of the movement.

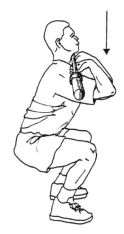

Downward movement.

Upward Movement Phase

☐ Keep eyes focused on wall about 30 to 60 cm above eye level.
☐ Slowly raise the bar by straightening the hips and knees.
☐ Maintain body position.
☐ Keep knees over the feet.
☐ Do not let knees move in or out.
☐ Do not accelerate the bar at the top of the movement.

Breathing

☐ Inhale during the downward movement phase.
☐ Exhale through the sticking point of the upward movement phase.

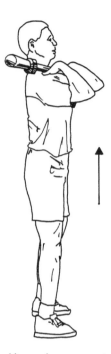

Upward movement.

Glute-Ham Raise

Beginning Position

☐ Lie face down on glute-ham raise bench.
☐ Position legs so knees are slightly below thighs.
☐ Position thighs and back of ankles in contact with pads.
☐ Hang torso down to form a 90° angle at the hip with the thighs over the thigh pad.
☐ Hips should be off thigh pad.
☐ Place a hand on each side of the head or cross at the chest.

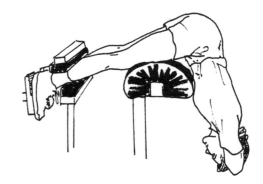

Beginning position.

Upward Movement Phase

☐ Raise trunk until upper torso is parallel to the floor.
☐ Face head forward.
☐ Once upper body is parallel to the floor, flex knees slightly by contracting the hamstrings until thighs and shoulders form a straight line.

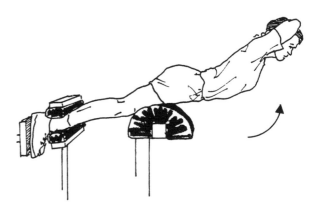

Upward movement to parallel position.

Downward Movement Phase

☐ Lower the upper body slowly to beginning position.

Breathing

☐ Exhale through the sticking point of the upward movement phase.
☐ Inhale during the downward movement phase.

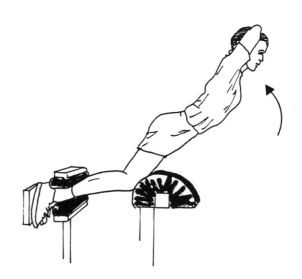

Upward movement flexing knees.

Leg Curl (Machine)

Beginning Position

- ☐ Lie face down on the bench.
- ☐ Position hips and chest flat on pads.
- ☐ Position knees below bottom edge of thigh pad.
- ☐ Position ankles under and in contact with heel roller pad.
- ☐ Align knees with axis of machine.
- ☐ Grasp handles or edge of torso pad.

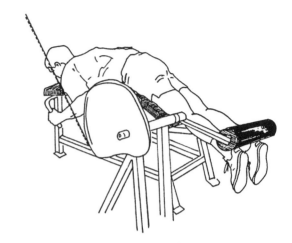

Beginning position.

Upward Movement Phase

- ☐ Maintain body position on the bench and roller pad.
- ☐ Keep hips in contact with bench.
- ☐ Flex the legs at the knees.
- ☐ Pull heels up and as close to the buttocks as possible.

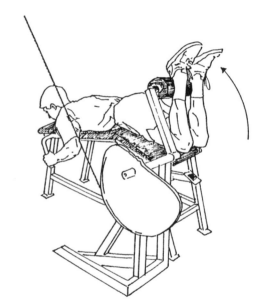

Upward movement.

Downward Movement Phase

- ☐ Maintain body position on the bench and roller pad.
- ☐ Lower roller pad slowly and under control to beginning position.

Breathing

- ☐ Exhale through the sticking point of the upward movement phase.
- ☐ Inhale during the downward movement phase.

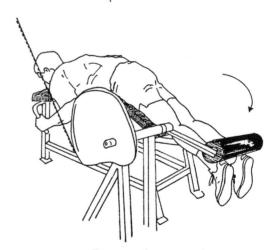

Downward movement.

Leg Extension (Machine)

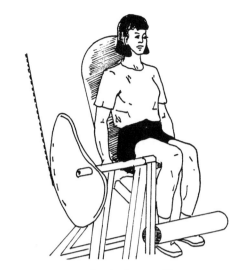

Beginning position.

Beginning Position

☐ Assume a seated position on the machine.
☐ Place ankles behind and in contact with roller pad.
☐ Position legs parallel to each other.
☐ Align knees with axis of machine.
☐ Grasp handles or sides of thigh pad.
☐ Keep torso erect.
☐ Keep back flat against back pad.

Upward Movement Phase

☐ Extend the legs at the knees.
☐ Move feet up to full knee extension.
☐ Maintain position on back and thigh pad.
☐ Keep buttocks in contact with the thigh pad.

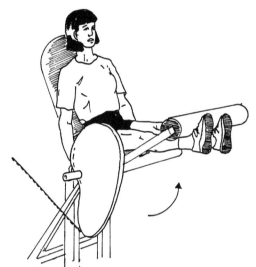

Upward movement.

Downward Movement Phase

☐ Lower pad slowly and under control.
☐ Maintain position on back and thigh pad.
☐ Lower roller pad to beginning position.

Breathing

☐ Exhale through the sticking point of the upward movement phase.
☐ Inhale during the downward movement phase.

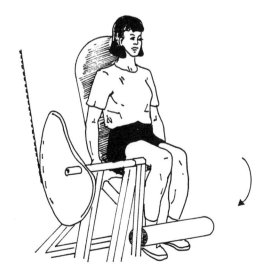

Downward movement.

Leg Press (Machine)

Beginning Position

- ☐ Assume a seated position on the machine.
- ☐ Place feet flat on pedals.
- ☐ Position thighs, lower legs, and feet parallel to each other.
- ☐ Grasp handles or sides of thigh pad.
- ☐ Keep torso erect.
- ☐ Keep buttocks on thigh pad and back flat against back pad.

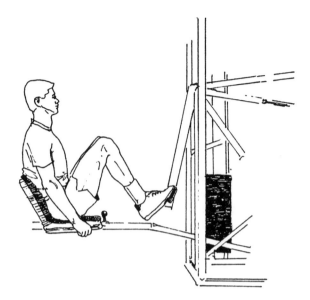

Beginning position.

Forward Movement Phase

- ☐ Push foot pedals forward.
- ☐ Maintain erect position on the seat and back pad.
- ☐ Keep buttocks in contact with the thigh pad.
- ☐ Keep thighs, lower legs, and feet parallel to each other.
- ☐ Avoid forcefully locking out the knees.

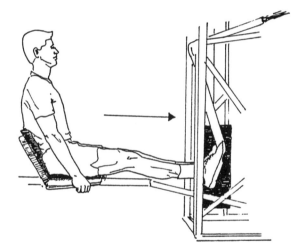

Forward movement.

Backward Movement Phase

- ☐ Maintain position on the pads.
- ☐ Move foot pedals backward slowly and under control to beginning position.

Breathing

- ☐ Exhale through the sticking point of the forward movement phase.
- ☐ Inhale during the backward movement phase.

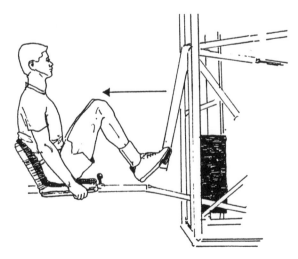

Backward movement.

Standing Heel (Calf) Raise (Free Weight)

Beginning Position

☐ Perform this exercise preferably inside of a squat rack and use two spotters, one on each side.
☐ Use a pronated grip with hands wider than shoulder-width.
☐ Position bar at base of neck.
☐ Use a hip-width stance and position balls of feet near edge of a raised surface.
☐ Position feet straight ahead.
☐ Establish position in which legs are parallel.
☐ Lock out knees.

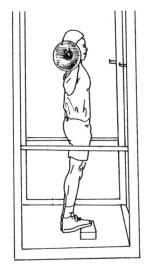

Beginning position.

Upward Movement Phase

☐ Push up on toes as high as possible (plantar flexion) in a slow, controlled manner, maintaining thigh and lower leg position.
☐ Hold "heels up" position momentarily before lowering.

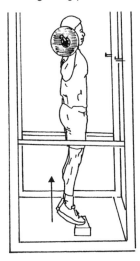

Upward movement.

Downward Movement Phase

☐ Lower heels until they are below toes.

Breathing

☐ Exhale through the sticking point of the upward movement phase.
☐ Inhale during the downward movement phase.

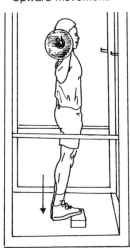

Downward movement.

Lunge (Free Weight)

Beginning Position: Lifter

☐ Grasp bar with a closed, pronated grip.
☐ Grip should be slightly wider than shoulder-width.
☐ Step under the bar and position feet parallel to each other.
☐ Move hips under bar.
☐ Position the bar in a balanced position on the shoulders (above the posterior deltoids at the base of the neck).
☐ Lift and hold chest up and out and pull shoulder blades toward each other.
☐ Tilt head slightly up.
☐ Lift elbows up to create a "shelf" for the bar.
☐ Extend both legs to lift bar out of racks.
☐ Take at least three steps backward.

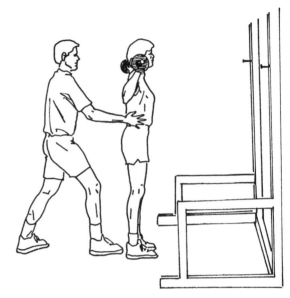

Beginning positions.

Beginning Position: Spotter

☐ Assist lifter with removing the bar from the rack.
☐ Step backward with lifter to beginning position location.
☐ Stand 15 cm behind lifter.
☐ Position feet hip-width apart.
☐ Position hands near the lifter's hips or sides or torso.

Forward Movement Phase: Lifter

☐ Take one exaggerated step directly forward with one leg (the "lead" leg).
☐ Keep lead knee and foot aligned, and toes pointing straight ahead or slightly inward.
☐ Plant lead foot squarely on floor.
☐ Flex the lead knee slowly and under control.
☐ Lower trailing knee toward floor.
☐ Bottom position for trailing knee is 2.5 to 5 cm above floor.
☐ Keep torso vertical to floor by "sitting back" on the trailing leg.
☐ Keep lead knee directly over lead foot.
☐ Keep lead foot flat on floor.
☐ Do not bounce in the bottom position.

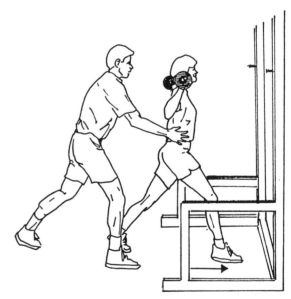

Beginning of forward movement positions.

Forward Movement Phase: Spotter

- ☐ Step forward with same foot as the lifter.
- ☐ Keep lead knee and foot aligned with lifter's lead foot.
- ☐ Plant foot 15 to 45 cm behind lifter's foot.
- ☐ Flex lead knee as lifter's lead knee flexes.
- ☐ Keep torso erect.
- ☐ Keep hands near lifter's hips or torso.
- ☐ Assist only when necessary to keep lifter balanced.

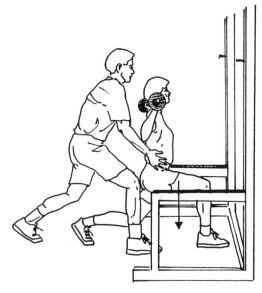

Completion of forward movement positions.

Backward Movement Phase: Lifter

- ☐ Forcefully push off with the lead leg.
- ☐ Maintain body position.
- ☐ Bring lead foot back to a position next to the trailing foot.
- ☐ Pause and stand erect.
- ☐ Alternate lead legs.
- ☐ At the completion of the set, slowly step forward into the rack.
- ☐ Position hips beneath the bar.
- ☐ Squat down until both ends of the bar are resting on the rack.

Backward Movement Phase: Spotter

- ☐ Push backward with lead leg simultaneously with the lifter.
- ☐ Bring lead foot back parallel to trailing foot.
- ☐ Keep hands near lifter's hips or torso.
- ☐ Assist only when necessary to keep lifter balanced.
- ☐ At the completion of the set, help lifter place the bar in the rack.

Backward movement positions.

Breathing

- ☐ Inhale during the forward movement phase.
- ☐ Exhale during the push-off of the backward movement phase.

Deadlift (Free Weight)

Beginning Position

- ☐ Assume a shoulder-width stance, knees inside arms.
- ☐ Position feet flat on the floor.
- ☐ Grasp bar with a closed, alternated grip.
- ☐ Grip should be slightly wider than shoulder-width.
- ☐ Squat down next to the bar, heels on the floor.
- ☐ Fully extend arms.
- ☐ Point elbows out to sides.
- ☐ Position bar over the balls of the feet; bar should be close to shins.
- ☐ Position the shoulders over or slightly ahead of the bar.
- ☐ Establish a flat back posture by

  - • pulling shoulder blades toward each other,
  - • holding chest up and out, and
  - • tilting head slightly up.

- ☐ Focus eyes ahead or slightly above horizontal.
- ☐ Keep torso tensed.

Upward Movement Phase

- ☐ Begin pull by extending the knees.
- ☐ Move the hips forward and raise shoulders at the same rate.
- ☐ Keep the angle of the back constant.
- ☐ Lift bar straight up.
- ☐ Keep bar close to the body, heels on the floor.

- ☐ Keep elbows fully extended.
- ☐ Keep shoulders back and above or slightly in front of bar.
- ☐ Keep head facing straight forward.
- ☐ Maintain torso position.
- ☐ Thrust hips forward and continue pulling until knees are under bar.
- ☐ Keep feet flat.
- ☐ Torso should be nearly vertical and erect.
- ☐ Keep shoulders positioned directly over the bar.
- ☐ Keep elbows fully extended.
- ☐ At full knee and hip extension, establish an erect body position.

Downward Movement Phase

- ☐ Flex hips and knees to lower bar slowly and under control.
- ☐ Squat down toward floor.
- ☐ Maintain erect torso position.
- ☐ Keep bar close to shins.
- ☐ Place bar on the floor.

Breathing

- ☐ Exhale through the sticking point of the upward movement phase.
- ☐ Inhale during the downward movement phase.

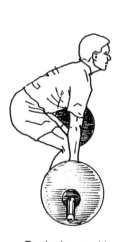 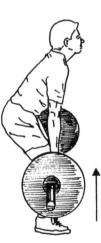 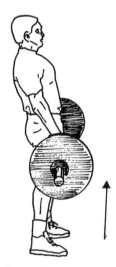

Beginning position.   Raise bar straight.   Thrust hips forward.

Step-Up (Free Weight)

Beginning Position

☐ Box should be 30 to 45 cm high (depending on which height creates a 90° angle at the knee joint when the foot is on the box).
☐ Position bar on shoulders.
☐ Stand about 30 to 45 cm from the box.
☐ Maintain an erect body position.

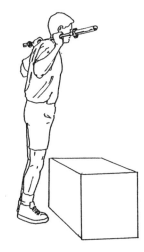

Beginning position.

Upward Movement Phase

☐ Step with one leg (the "lead" leg) onto top of box.
☐ Place entire foot on the center of the top of the box.
☐ Toes of lead foot should point straight ahead or slightly inward.
☐ Do not lean forward.
☐ Shift body weight to lead leg.
☐ Push with lead leg to move body to a standing position on top of the box.
☐ Do not push off with trailing leg/foot.
☐ Maintain erect body position.
☐ At the top position, the hips and knees should be fully extended with feet together and body weight distributed evenly.

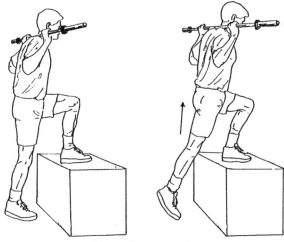

Upward movement.

Downward Movement Phase

☐ Shift body weight to same lead leg.
☐ With the same trailing leg, step off the box (30 to 45 cm away).
☐ Maintain erect body position.
☐ Place foot of trailing leg on floor.
☐ At full trailing foot contact with the floor, shift body weight to trailing leg.
☐ Step off the box with lead leg.
☐ Move lead foot next to trailing foot.
☐ Repeat, with other leg as lead leg.

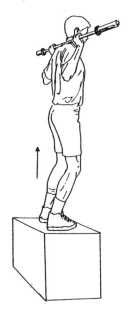

Highest position.

Breathing

☐ Exhale through the sticking point of the upward movement phase.
☐ Inhale during the downward movement phase.

SHOULDERS AND NECK

Shoulder Press (Free Weight)

Before Beginning

Execute the techniques described for the Power Clean exercise (p. 392) to move the bar from the floor to the shoulders. Then use the following techniques to press the bar overhead. At the completion of the set, use the Power Clean exercise techniques to return the bar to the floor. The movement can also begin from an initial bar position on shoulder-high racks as shown here.

An option is to perform this exercise in a seated position with the bar resting in the racks of a shoulder press bench. Realize that the seated shoulder press has the bar begin at full elbow extension so the first movement is to *lower* the bar.

Beginning Position: Lifter

☐ Grasp bar with a closed, pronated grip.
☐ Grip should be shoulder-width or slightly wider.
☐ Elbows should be under bar, wrists extended.
☐ Torso should be erect, back flat.
☐ Rest bar in hands on shoulders/clavicles.
☐ Signal spotter.
☐ Move bar off racks.
☐ Focus eyes straight ahead.

Beginning Position: Spotter

☐ Stand directly behind lifter.
☐ Keep torso erect, knees slightly flexed.
☐ Grasp bar and assist with moving bar from racks.

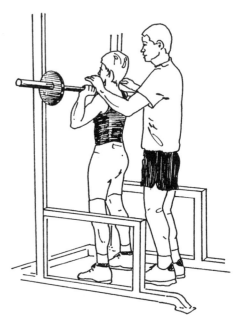

Beginning positions.

Upward Movement Phase: Lifter

☐ Push bar up to full elbow extension.
☐ Keep elbows pointed out to sides until arms are fully extended.
☐ Maintain body position.
☐ Do not forcefully lock out elbows.

Upward Movement Phase: Spotter

☐ Keep hands close and follow bar as it ascends.
☐ Maintain torso and knee position.
☐ Assist only if necessary.

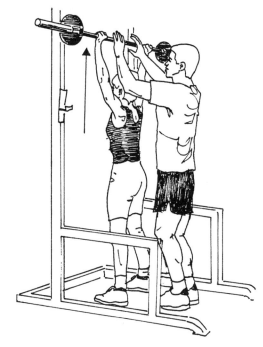

Upward movement positions.

Downward Movement Phase: Lifter

☐ Lower bar slowly and under control to shoulder level.
☐ Do not jerk or bounce at bottom of movement.
☐ At the completion of the set, signal spotter.
☐ Move bar to racks or to the floor.

Downward Movement Phase: Spotter

☐ Keep hands close and follow the bar as it descends.
☐ Maintain torso and knee position.
☐ At the lifter's signal, grasp bar and guide back to racks.

Breathing

☐ Exhale through the sticking point of the upward movement phase.
☐ Inhale during the downward movement phase.

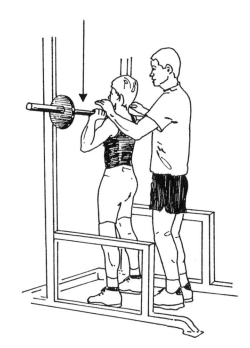

Downward movement positions.

Shoulder Press (Machine)

Beginning Position

☐ Grasp handles with a closed, pronated grip.
☐ Sit on seat and assume a flat back position.
☐ Position feet on floor or on the rungs of the seat.
☐ Focus eyes straight ahead.

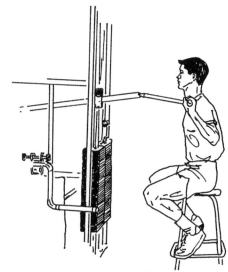

Beginning position.

Upward Movement Phase

☐ Push handles up.
☐ Keep elbows pointed out to sides until arms are fully extended.
☐ Maintain body position.
☐ Do not forcefully lock out elbows.

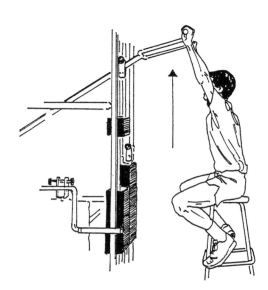

Upward movement.

Downward Movement Phase

☐ Lower handles slowly and under control to shoulder level.
☐ Do not jerk or bounce at bottom of movement.

Breathing

☐ Exhale through the sticking point of the upward movement phase.
☐ Inhale during the downward movement phase.

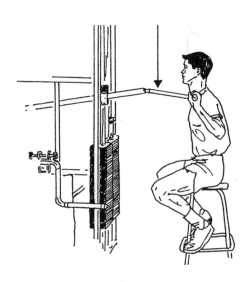

Downward movement.

Shoulder Shrug (Free Weight)

Beginning Position

☐ Grasp bar with a shoulder-width, closed, pronated grip.
☐ Establish upright standing position.
☐ Position feet shoulder-width apart.
☐ Flex knees slightly.
☐ Rest bar at arms' length on thighs.

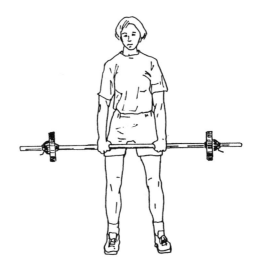

Beginning position.

Upward Movement Phase

☐ Lift bar by elevating shoulders toward ears.
☐ Maintain upright body position.
☐ Keep elbows fully extended.
☐ Shrug shoulders as high as possible.

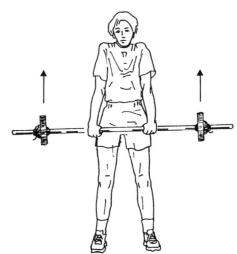

Upward movement.

Downward Movement Phase

☐ Lower bar slowly and under control.
☐ Maintain body position.
☐ Keep elbows fully extended.

Breathing

☐ Exhale through the sticking point of the upward movement phase.
☐ Inhale during the downward movement phase.

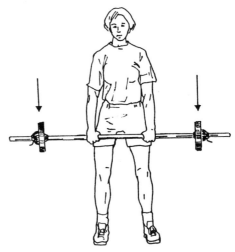

Downward movement.

Upright Row (Free Weight)

Beginning Position

- ☐ Grasp bar with a closed, pronated grip.
- ☐ Hands should be 20 to 30 cm apart.
- ☐ Rest bar at arm's length on front of thighs.
- ☐ Assume a shoulder-width stance.
- ☐ Flex knees slightly.
- ☐ Keep torso erect.
- ☐ Point elbows outward.

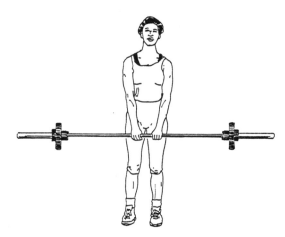

Beginning position.

Upward Movement Phase

- ☐ Pull bar upward along abdomen and chest toward chin.
- ☐ Keep bar very close to the torso.
- ☐ Maintain body position.
- ☐ At top position, elbows are higher than wrists and above shoulders.
- ☐ Do not jerk or swing bar upward.

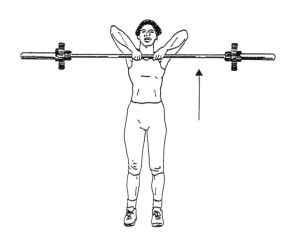

Upward movement.

Downward Movement Phase

- ☐ Lower bar slowly and under control.
- ☐ Keep bar very close to the torso.
- ☐ Lower bar to full elbow extension in front of thighs.

Breathing

- ☐ Exhale through the sticking point of the upward movement phase.
- ☐ Inhale during the downward movement phase.

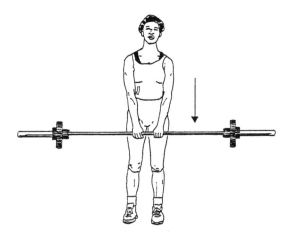

Downward movement.

Four-Way Neck (Machine)

Possible movements include left lateral flexion, hyperextension, right lateral flexion, and flexion. Note that the Upward Movement Phase refers to the execution portion of the exercise and the Downward Movement Phase is the action of returning to the beginning position.

Beginning Position: Left Lateral Flexion

☐ Sit in the neck machine with the left ear in the center of the pads.

Upward Movement Phase: Left Lateral Flexion

☐ Place the hands on the hand grips and flex the neck laterally to the left.

Downward Movement Phase: Left Lateral Flexion

☐ Relax the neck to allow the pad to move back until the plates slightly touch the weight stack.
☐ Do not allow the upper body to move or the shoulders to dip down.

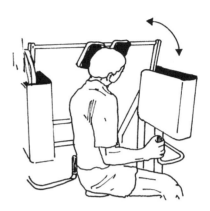

Left lateral flexion.

Beginning Position: Hyperextension

☐ Sit on the seat so that the back of the head is against the pad.

Upward Movement Phase: Hyperextension

☐ Place the hands on the hand grips and extend the head backward.

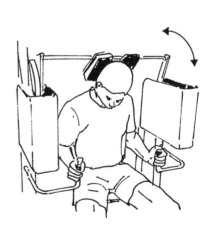

Hyperextension.

Downward Movement Phase: Hyperextension

☐ Relax the neck to allow the pad to move back until the plates slightly touch the weight stack.
☐ Do not allow the upper body to move or the shoulders to dip down.

Beginning Position: Right Lateral Flexion

☐ Sit on the seat so that the right ear is in the center of the pads.

Upward Movement Phase: Right Lateral Flexion

☐ Place the hands on the hand grips and flex the neck laterally to the right.

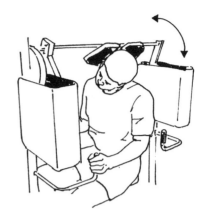

Right lateral flexion.

Downward Movement Phase: Right Lateral Flexion

☐ Relax the neck to allow the pad to move back until the plates slightly touch the weight stack.
☐ Do not allow the upper body to move or the shoulders to dip down.

Beginning Position: Flexion

☐ Place the hands on the hand grips and flex the neck laterally to the right.

Upward Movement Phase: Flexion

☐ Place the hands on the hand grips and flex the neck forward.

Flexion.

Downward Movement Phase: Flexion

☐ Relax the neck to allow the pad to move back until the plates slightly touch the weight stack.
☐ Do not allow the upper body to move or the shoulders to dip down.

Breathing (for all four exercises)

☐ Exhale through the sticking point of the upward movement phase.
☐ Inhale during the downward movement phase.

Behind-the-Neck Press (Free Weight)

Beginning Position: Lifter

☐ Sit on a bench with feet on floor.
☐ Grasp bar with a closed, pronated grip slightly wider than shoulder-width.
☐ Keep head facing forward.
☐ Signal the spotter to assist in lifting the bar from the racks to a position behind the head on the neck.
☐ Signal the spotter when full control of the bar is gained.

Beginning Position: Spotter

☐ Straddle the bench to a position behind lifter.
☐ Slightly flex knees.
☐ Grasp bar with alternated grip between lifter's hands.
☐ At the signal of the lifter, smoothly lift bar off racks to a position behind the lifter's head at the neck.
☐ Hold onto bar until lifter indicates that the bar is under control.

Upward Movement Phase: Lifter

☐ Press the bar overhead, keeping the elbows pointed outward.
☐ Tilt head up to neutral position during the ascent.
☐ Maintain body position.

Upward Movement Phase: Spotter

☐ Maintain body position.
☐ Follow bar path.
☐ Assist only when necessary.

Downward Movement Phase: Lifter

☐ Slightly tilt head forward during the descent.
☐ Slowly and under control, lower the bar to the bottom of the earlobes.
☐ Maintain body position.
☐ Forearms should be parallel to each other at the bottom position.
☐ At the completion of the set, signal the spotter and guide the bar back into the rack.

Downward Movement Phase: Spotter

☐ Maintain body position.
☐ Follow bar path.
☐ Assist only when necessary.
☐ At the signal of the lifter, guide the bar back into the rack.

Breathing

☐ Exhale through the sticking point of the upward movement phase.
☐ Inhale during the downward movement phase.

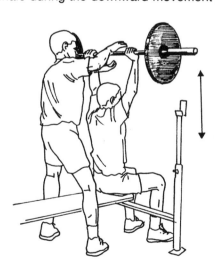

Beginning positions.

Upward and downward movement positions.

TRICEPS

Lying Triceps Extension (Free Weight)

Beginning Position: Lifter

☐ Sit on one end of the bench, then lay back so head rests on other end of bench.
☐ Position feet flat on floor.
☐ Position head, shoulders, and buttocks flat on bench.
☐ Grasp bar with a closed, overhand grip, hands 15 to 25 cm apart.
☐ Position arms parallel to each other, perpendicular to floor.

Beginning Position: Spotter

☐ Stand at the end of the bench near the lifter's head.
☐ Hand bar to lifter.

Downward Movement Phase: Lifter

☐ Maintain body position on bench.
☐ Lower bar slowly and under control, to the forehead.
☐ Upper arms remain perpendicular to floor and parallel to each other.

Downward Movement Phase: Spotter

☐ Keep hands under bar to protect lifter's head.

Upward Movement Phase: Lifter

☐ Push bar until elbows are fully extended.
☐ Upper arms remain perpendicular to floor and parallel to each other.
☐ Maintain body position on bench.

Upward Movement Phase: Spotter

☐ Assist lifter only if necessary.
☐ Take bar from lifter at the end of the set.

Breathing

☐ Inhale during the downward movement phase.
☐ Exhale through the sticking point of the upward movement phase.

Beginning positions.   Downward movement positions.   Upward movement positions.

Triceps Pushdown (Machine)

Beginning Position

☐ Grasp bar with a closed, pronated grip 10 to 15 cm apart.

☐ Position feet shoulder-width apart, knees slightly flexed.

☐ Establish upright body position.

☐ Move bar down to position elbows next to torso with forearms parallel to floor.

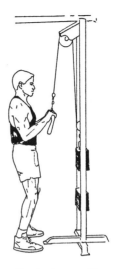

Beginning position.

Downward Movement Phase

☐ Keep elbows next to torso.
☐ Push bar down to full elbow extension.
☐ Maintain upright body position.
☐ Do not forcefully extend elbows.

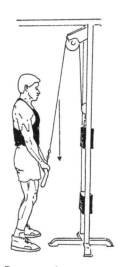

Downward movement.

Upward Movement Phase

☐ Keep elbows next to torso.
☐ Allow the bar to rise slowly under control.
☐ Maintain upright body position.
☐ Stop bar when forearms are parallel to floor.

Breathing

☐ Exhale through the sticking point of the downward movement phase.
☐ Inhale during the upward movement phase.

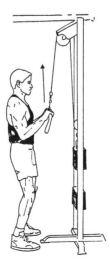

Upward movement.

EXPLOSIVE/POWER EXERCISES

Power Clean (Free Weight)

In other exercises that require the bar to begin at the thighs, perform the Beginning Position and the First Pull and Transition (Scoop) upward movements. To begin an exercise with the bar at the shoulders, perform the Power Clean checklist from the Beginning Position through the Catch.

Beginning Position

☐ Assume a shoulder-width stance, knees inside arms.
☐ Position feet flat on the floor.
☐ Grasp bar with a closed, pronated grip.
☐ Grip should be slightly wider than shoulder-width.
☐ Squat down next to the bar, heels on the floor.
☐ Fully extend arms.
☐ Point elbows out to sides.
☐ Position bar over the balls of the feet; bar should be close to shins.
☐ Position the shoulders over or slightly ahead of the bar.
☐ Establish a flat back posture by

 • pulling shoulder blades toward each other,
 • holding chest up and out, and
 • tilting head slightly up.

☐ Focus eyes ahead or slightly above horizontal.
☐ Keep torso tensed.

Upward Movement Phase: First Pull

☐ Begin pull by extending the knees.
☐ Move the hips forward and raise shoulders at the same rate.
☐ Keep the angle of the back constant.
☐ Lift bar straight up.
☐ Keep bar close to the body, heels on the floor.
☐ Keep elbows fully extended.
☐ Keep shoulders back and above or slightly in front of bar.
☐ Keep head facing straight forward.
☐ Maintain torso position.

Upward Movement Phase: Transition (Scoop)

☐ Thrust hips forward and continue pulling until knees are under bar.
☐ Keep feet flat.
☐ Torso should be nearly vertical and erect.
☐ Keep shoulders positioned directly over the bar.
☐ Keep elbows fully extended.

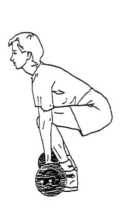

Beginning position.

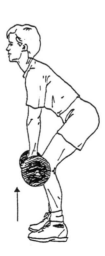

First pull.

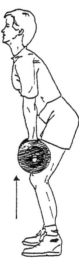

Scoop.

Upward Movement Phase: Second Pull

☐ Brush bar against the middle or top of the thighs.
☐ Keep torso erect and head facing straight or slightly up.
☐ Keep elbows straight.
☐ Move bar explosively by extending the hip, knee, and ankle joints in a "jumping action."
☐ Keep shoulders over the bar as long as possible and elbows out.
☐ Keep bar close to the body.
☐ At maximum plantar flexion, shrug the shoulders.
☐ At maximum shoulder elevation, flex and pull with the arms.
☐ Keep elbows high during pull; keep them over the wrists.
☐ Pull bar as high as possible.

Catch

☐ Rotate elbows around and under the bar.
☐ Hyperextend the wrists as the elbows move under bar.
☐ Point elbows forward or slightly up.
☐ Rack the bar across the front of shoulders.
☐ Keep torso erect.
☐ Flex hips and knees to absorb the weight of the bar.

Downward Movement Phase

☐ Lower bar slowly and under control to top of thighs.
☐ Flex hips and knees as bar lands on thighs.
☐ Squat down toward floor.
☐ Keep heels on floor.
☐ Maintain erect torso position.
☐ Keep bar close to shins.
☐ Place bar on the floor.

Breathing

☐ Inhale before the first pull of the first repetition.
☐ Hold breath until the second pull.
☐ Exhale through the sticking point (shrug) of the second pull.
☐ Inhale during the downward movement phase of succeeding repetitions.

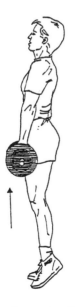

Second pull.

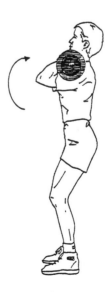

Catch.

Hang Clean (Free Weight)

This is a variation of the Power Clean. As noted, refer to the Power Clean checklist (p. 392) for parts of this exercise.

Beginning Position

☐ Using the floor-to-thigh lifting technique described in the Power Clean exercise (p. 392), move the bar from the floor-to-the thighs.

Upward Movement Phase

☐ Keep torso erect and head facing straight ahead or slightly up.
☐ Keep elbows straight.
☐ Move bar explosively from thighs by extending the hip, knee, and ankle joints in a "jumping action."
☐ Keep shoulders over the bar as long as possible and elbows out.
☐ Keep bar close to the body.
☐ At maximum plantar flexion, shrug the shoulders.
☐ At maximum shoulder elevation, flex and pull with the arms.
☐ Keep elbows high during pull; keep them over the wrists.
☐ Pull bar as high as possible.

Catch

☐ Follow the Catch phase of the Power Clean (p. 393).

Downward Movement Phase

☐ Lower bar slowly and under control to top of thighs.
☐ Flex hips and knees as bar contacts thighs.
☐ Keep torso erect.
☐ Begin succeeding repetitions with the bar on the thigh.

Breathing

☐ Inhale before the beginning of the upward movement phase of the first repetition.
☐ Hold breath until the sticking point (shrug) of the upward movement phase.
☐ Exhale through the sticking point (shrug) of the upward movement phase.
☐ Inhale during the downward movement phase of succeeding repetitions.

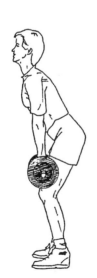
Beginning position.

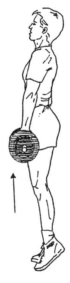
Upward movement.

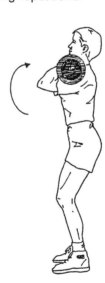
Catch.

Power Pull [High Pull] (Free Weight)

As noted, refer to the Power Clean checklist (p. 392) for parts of this exercise.

Beginning Position

☐ Using the floor-to-thigh lifting technique described in the Power Clean (p. 392), move the bar from the floor to the thighs.

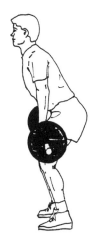

Beginning position.

Upward Movement Phase

☐ Keep torso erect and head facing straight ahead or slightly up.
☐ Keep elbows straight.
☐ Move bar explosively from thighs by extending the hip, knee, and ankle joints in a "jumping action."
☐ Keep shoulders over the bar as long as possible.
☐ Keep bar close to the body.
☐ At maximum plantar flexion, shrug the shoulders.
☐ At maximal shoulder elevation, flex and pull with the arms.
☐ Keep elbows out and as high and long as possible.
☐ Before bar slows, flex wrists and continue pulling the bar straight up.
☐ Pull bar as high as possible.
☐ The highest bar position should be at least neck-level with the wrists totally flexed.

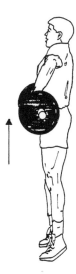

Jumping action.

Downward Movement Phase

☐ Follow the downward movement phase of the Hang Clean (p. 394).

Breathing

☐ Inhale before the beginning of the upward movement phase of the first repetition.
☐ Hold breath until the sticking point (shrug) of the upward movement phase.
☐ Exhale through the sticking point (shrug) of the upward movement phase.
☐ Inhale during the downward movement phase of succeeding repetitions.

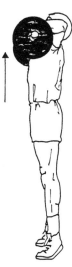

Highest position.

Push Press (Free Weight)

As noted, refer to the Power Clean checklist (p. 392) to move the bar from the floor to the shoulders. Then use the following techniques to move the bar from the shoulders to an overhead position. At the completion of the set, use the Power Clean exercise techniques to return the bar to the floor. The movement can also begin from an initial bar position on shoulder-high racks.

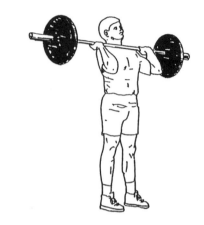

Beginning position.

Beginning Position

☐ Use the floor-to-shoulder lifting technique described in the Power Clean exercise (p. 392) to move the bar from the floor to the shoulders.

Upward Movement Phase

☐ Slightly flex the hips and knees, keeping torso erect.
☐ Immediately follow with an explosive push upward by extending the knees.
☐ Keep torso erect and tensed.
☐ At maximum hip and knee extension, shift body weight to balls of feet and extend ankle joints.
☐ At maximum hip and knee extension, shift body weight to balls of feet and extend ankle joints.
☐ At maximum plantar flexion, push bar from the shoulders.
☐ Push the bar with the arms to a fully extended elbow position overhead.

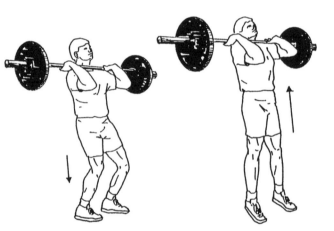

Flex hips and knees.   Extend knees.

Downward Movement Phase

☐ Lower bar to shoulders.
☐ Flex hips and knees slightly as bar touches shoulders.
☐ Straighten the hips and knees before the upward movement phase begins again.

Breathing

☐ Exhale through the sticking point of the upward movement phase.
☐ Inhale during the downward movement phase.

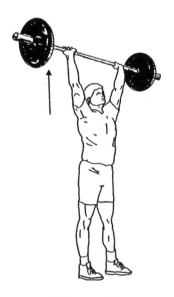

Highest position.

Snatch (Free Weight)

This exercise can also begin at the thighs (i.e., a power snatch). To perform a power snatch, use the floor-to-thigh lifting technique described in the Power Clean exercise (p. 392) to move the bar from the floor to the thighs. Begin successive repetitions from the thighs.

Beginning Position

☐ Assume a shoulder-width or slightly wider stance, knees inside arms.
☐ Position feet flat on the floor, toes pointed slightly outward.
☐ Grasp bar with a pronated closed or hook grip.
☐ The correct distance between hand placements should be determined by one of the following methods:

1. Elbow-to-elbow distance when arms are straight out at sides
2. Distance from edge of clenched fist of one hand to opposite shoulder when arm is straight out at side

☐ Squat down next to the bar, heels on the floor.
☐ Fully extend arms.
☐ Point elbows out to sides.
☐ Position bar over the balls of the feet; bar should be close to shins.
☐ Position the shoulders over or slightly ahead of the bar.
☐ Establish a flat back posture by

• pulling shoulder blades toward each other,
• holding chest up and out, and
• tilting head slightly up.

☐ Focus eyes ahead or slightly above horizontal.
☐ Keep torso tensed.

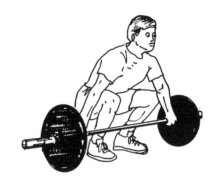

Beginning position.

Upward Movement Phase: First Pull

☐ Follow the First Pull upward movement phase of the Power Clean (p. 392).

Upward Movement Phase: Transition (Scoop)

☐ Follow the Transition (Scoop) phase of the Power Clean (p. 392).

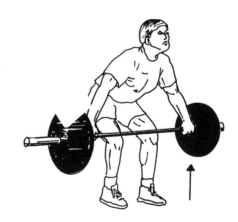

First pull.

Upward Movement Phase: Second Pull

☐ Follow the Second Pull upward movement phase of the Power Clean (p. 393).

Catch

☐ As the bar reaches maximum height, slightly flex the hips then the knees.
☐ Flex then rotate elbows around and under the bar.
☐ At maximum bar height, fully extend the elbows and hyperextend the wrists to lock bar overhead.
☐ Contact floor with feet before the bar is locked overhead.
☐ Catch bar by flexing at the knees and hips to absorb weight.
☐ Squat down slowly and under control.
☐ Keep torso erect.
☐ At lowest squat position, the bar should be over the shoulders, hips over the ankles, and the elbows locked.

Upward Movement Phase: Recovery

☐ Once under control in low squat position, slowly extend the hips and knees to move the body to a fully erect, standing position.
☐ Keep bar locked overhead.

Downward Movement Phase

☐ Follow the downward movement phase of the Power Clean (p. 393).

Breathing

☐ Inhale before the first pull of the first repetition.
☐ Hold breath until the second pull.
☐ Exhale through the sticking point (shrug) of the second pull.
☐ Inhale while lowering the body to the low squat position.
☐ Exhale through the sticking point of the recovery phase.
☐ Inhale during the downward movement phase of succeeding repetitions.

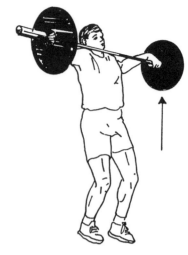

Second pull.

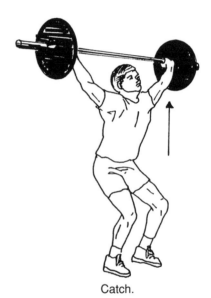

Catch.

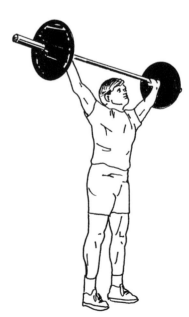

Recovery.

Key Terms

alternated grip	345	partner-assisted action	347	sticking point	346
grip width	345	pronated grip	345	supinated grip	345
hook grip	345	spotter	347		
liftoff	348	spotting	347		

Study Questions

1. All of the following exercises should employ the use of a spotter *except*

   a. dumbbell fly
   b. overhead triceps extension
   c. lunge
   d. triceps push-down

2. The spotter should place his/her hands on the lifter's wrists in which of the following exercises?

   a. bench press
   b. dumbbell incline bench press
   c. dumbbell pullover
   d. overhead triceps extension

3. Which of the following is a correct foot pattern in the step-up exercise?

   a. step up LEFT FOOT, step up RIGHT FOOT, step down LEFT FOOT, step down RIGHT FOOT
   b. step up RIGHT FOOT, step up LEFT FOOT, step down LEFT FOOT, step down RIGHT FOOT
   c. step up LEFT FOOT, step down LEFT FOOT, step up RIGHT FOOT, step down RIGHT FOOT
   d. step up RIGHT FOOT, step down LEFT FOOT, step up RIGHT FOOT, step down LEFT FOOT

4. What is the primary movement occurring in the "scoop" phase of the power clean?

   a. hip flexion
   b. hip extension
   c. knee flexion
   d. plantar flexion

Applying Knowledge of Strength Training and Spotting Techniques

Problem 1

A collegiate football player is attempting a 1RM in the squat exercise. Describe the number, positioning, and actions of the required spotters for each phase of the exercise.

Problem 2

Describe the similarities and differences between the following exercises: 1) power clean; 2) hang clean; 3) power pull; and 4) snatch. Discuss grip width and placement, initial bar position, feet/body position, the action phases of the exercises, and the final bar position.

Recommended Readings

1. Baechle, T.R., and R. Earle. *Weight Training: A Text Written for the College Student*. Omaha: Creighton University. 1989.
2. Baechle, T.R., and B.R. Groves. *Weight Training: Steps to Success*. Champaign, IL: Leisure Press. 1992.
3. Baechle, T.R., and B.R. Groves. *Weight Training Video: Steps to Success* [Video]. Champaign, IL: Human Kinetics. 1993.
4. Baechle, T.R., and B.R. Groves. *Weight Training Instruction: Steps to Success*. Champaign, IL: Human Kinetics. 1994.
5. Fleck, S., and W. Kraemer. *Designing Resistance Training Programs*. Champaign, IL: Human Kinetics. 1987.
6. Garhammer, J. *Sports Illustrated Strength Training*. New York: Harper & Row. 1986.
7. Getchell, B. *Physical Fitness: A Way of Life*, 3rd ed. New York: Wiley. 1983.
8. Hoeger, W.K. *Lifetime Fitness, Physical Fitness and Wellness*, 2nd ed. Englewood, CO: Morton. 1989.
9. Holloway, J., and T.R. Baechle. Strength training for female athletes. *Sports Med.* 9(4):216-228. 1990.
10. Kraemer, W., and T.R. Baechle. Development of a strength training program. In: *Sports Medicine*, 2nd ed. J. Ryan and F.L. Allman, Jr., eds. San Diego: Academic Press. 1989. pp. 113-127.
11. Lombardi, V.P. *Beginning Weight Training: The Safe and Effective Way*. Dubuque, IA: Brown. 1989.
12. O'Shea, J.P. *Scientific Principles and Methods of Strength Fitness*. Menlo Park, CA: Addison-Wesley. 1976.
13. Stone, M., and H. O'Bryant. *Weight Training: A Scientific Approach*. Minneapolis: Burgess International. 1987.

PART IV

PROGRAM DESIGN

CHAPTER 22

TRAINING METHODS AND MODES

Dan Wathen
Fred Roll

This chapter begins with a discussion of the various aspects included in a needs analysis. It then explains periodization in general, as a precursor to subsequent chapters. (Chapter 30 will culminate the periodization discussion by pulling all aspects together.) Finally, this chapter summarizes the methods and modes of training used to meet the needs of the individual in his or her sport and utilized within the context of periodization.

NEEDS ANALYSIS

You have just secured your first job as a strength and conditioning professional at a high school and now you must implement a total conditioning program for all men's and women's sports at the school. The school sponsors men's football, wrestling, baseball, and golf; women's volleyball, gymnastics, and field hockey; and men's and women's basketball, cross-country, tennis, and track and field. The first task is to develop a ''needs analysis'' for each sport. A **needs analysis** is when the professional analyzes the fitness needs of both the activity and the individual athlete involved in the sport.

To develop a needs analysis first analyze the physiological and biomechanical requirements of each sport. A physiological analysis will allow you to devise a program that addresses the aspects of strength, flexibility, power, endurance, and speed required for success in the sport. A biomechanical analysis will allow you

to choose training activities that develop the athlete in the manner most specific to the sport and also to determine the areas of critical stress in the sport. For example, a biomechanical analysis of sprinting and jumping would reveal a need for drills and exercises that develop the hamstring muscles. Tables 23.1 and 23.2 on pages 418 to 420 can be used to choose movement-specific resistance exercises and to discern which muscles are primarily used in particular sports, and many resources discuss physiological and biomechanical demands of sports (36,37,42). Obtain injury profiles for the sport from the medical personnel; you can then design training to address and prioritize areas of high injury rate.

You now need to assess each athlete's strengths and weaknesses. Different sports require various levels of fitness. Football players need more strength and muscle size than soccer players, for example, and wrestlers need more anaerobic endurance than gymnasts. All athletes should be tested for strength, flexibility, power, speed, and endurance. Discuss each athlete's injury profile with the medical personnel in order to determine specific needs with regard to injury prevention. When the data are in, a needs analysis for each athlete can be made and a specific program developed to address the needs of the sport and the athlete's strengths and weaknesses. For example, a soccer player with a low level of endurance will require more aerobic training than, say, a baseball player would, because soccer requires high levels of aerobic power and baseball does not.

Finally, available facilities (space) and equipment and monies budgeted for new equipment will affect the methods used in a conditioning program.

PERIODIZATION

Periodization is the gradual cycling (allocation of a specific period of time, whether days, weeks, or months) of specificity, intensity, and volume of training to achieve peak levels of fitness for the most important competitions. Periodization is discussed in detail in chapter 30. Training shifts from non–sport-specific activities of high volume and low intensity to sport-specific activities of low volume and high intensity over a period of many weeks. Training methods change to reflect the specific periods of training. A **macrocycle** (generally a year's training) is divided into two or more **mesocycles** (part of a year's training) that revolve

around dates of major competitions. Each mesocycle is subdivided into periods of preparation, competition, and transition (Table 22.1). Ideally, an athlete will complete a mesocycle of training prior to each major competition, with variations for lengthy competitive periods.

Preparatory Period

The first period of training is in preparation for competition. The period is divided into three phases: Hypertrophy/endurance and strength, which take place in the off-season, and power, which occurs during the preseason.

Phase I: Hypertrophy/Endurance. The hypertrophy/endurance phase occurs during the early stages of off-season preparation (14). This phase may last from 1 to 6 weeks. During this phase, training begins at a low intensity (power output) with high volume (amount

Table 22.1   Typical Training Mesocycle for a Sprinter

Season designation	Period/phase designation	Training schedule
Off-season	Preparatory period	
	• Hypertrophy/endurance phase	*Flexibility training*: ballistic, static, or proprioceptive neuromuscular facilitation (PNF) stretching
		Resistance training: specific or nonspecific exercises of high volume and low intensity
		Metabolic training: aerobic activities
		Speed training: high-volume, low-intensity technique training
	Transition (optional)	All training of low volume and low intensity
	• Strength phase	*Flexibility training*: ballistic, static, or PNF
		Resistance training: specific exercises of moderate volume and intensity
		Metabolic training: interval work
		Speed training: moderate-volume and moderate-intensity technique training, including towing and downhill activities
Preseason	• Power phase	*Flexibility training*: ballistic, static, or PNF stretching
		Resistance training: specific exercises of low volume and high intensity
		Metabolic training: short work intervals of maximal and near-maximal intensity with full recovery intervals
		Speed training: high-intensity, low-volume activities
	Transition period (optional)	All training of low volume and low intensity
In-season	Competition period	*Flexibility training:* ballistic, static, or PNF stretching
		All training of low volume and high intensity
		Resistance training: low-volume, high-intensity, sport-specific exercises
		Metabolic training: race-specific intervals with full or near-full recovery between intervals
Off-season	Transition period	*Optional*: recreational games; light, unsupervised training

of training time due to high repetitions of activity). The goal for this phase of training is to develop an endurance (muscular and metabolic) base for future, more intense training. Initially, the activities may be either specific or nonspecific relative to the athletic event. However, as the preparatory period continues over a number of weeks, the training activities become more specific in their relationship to the sport. For example, a sprinter may begin the preparatory period with long-distance runs at slow speeds, such low-level plyometrics as bounding and hopping, and weight training exercises not necessarily biomechanically similar to running (leg presses, leg curls, etc.) and done at high repetitions with low to moderate loads. After this phase, there may be a transitional phase of 1 week of low-intensity, low-volume training prior to commencing the next phase.

Phase II: Strength.   In the next phase, running programs progress to interval sprints of moderate distance, plyometrics activities become more complex, jumping activities may be introduced, and weight training becomes more specific to the event (squats and lunges with free weights). Intensity level is gradually increased to loads of over 80% of the athlete's 1RM (repetition maximum), or in the 5RM to 8RM range, and only a moderate volume of training is performed.

Phase III: Power.   As the cycle progresses, load increases to over 90% of 1RM (2RM-4RM), and speed work intensifies to near contest pace. Full recovery is allowed between bouts of exercise, and speed training drills, which may include sled towing, sprints against resistance, and uphill and downhill sprints, are incorporated.

Competition Period

The competition period is often preceded by a transition period, at which time the athlete usually performs all activities at a low level of intensity and volume, to allow for physical recuperation and mental preparation for competition. The competition period follows. The period generally lasts from 1 to 3 weeks. However, in the case of some team sports such as basketball, the competition (or in-season) period may last many months. The mesocycle should place the athlete in peak condition for a short competitive period. Longer periods will require some manipulation of the load intensity on a weekly basis, but in general the period is characterized by very high intensity and very low volume in training activities.

Transition

The last period in a mesocycle is a transition period, which refers to the early off-season period after the last contest of the season. During this time, activities are unstructured and nonspecific and are done at low intensity and low volume. A track sprinter might do some easy jogging, play various sports on a recreational basis, and do some low-intensity resistance exercise. During this period there should be no psychological stress from training or competition.

FLEXIBILITY TRAINING

Flexibility is a joint's range of motion (ROM). When assessing the needs of athletes in a particular sport, the ranges of motion involved in each sports movement must be determined (2,28,45). A variety of levels of flexibility are needed by participants in different sports and positions in the same sport (2,26,29,30). For example, gymnasts need more overall flexibility than other Olympic athletes to perform their activities successfully (26). Baseball pitchers need a greater range of motion in their throwing arm than players at other positions.

Once the flexibility needs of a sport and each participating athlete are determined, a flexibility program can be designed for each athlete. Athletes with normal levels of flexibility for their activity do not need additional flexibility to perform well or prevent injuries. In fact, excessive ROM in joints, called *laxity*, may predispose an athlete to joint injury (2,32). When an optimal level of flexibility is reached, athletes may spend training time more wisely on other factors needed for success. Athletes can maintain adequate levels of flexibility using proper warm-up procedures, flexibility training, and resistance training performed through the full, pain-free ROM (33,44).

Strength and conditioning professionals must assess functional ROM with properly taken measures. For example, external rotation of a thrower's arm should be measured in a position of abduction, with the athlete actively moving the joint through the ROM. When less-than-normal ROM is evident, the strength and conditioning professional should recommend a program to correct the deficit. There are three basic types of flexibility (stretching) programs currently in popular use: static, ballistic, and proprioceptive neuromuscular facilitation. These are covered in detail in chapter 19.

RESISTANCE TRAINING

A program of resistance training develops strength. The basis of all gains in any type of fitness endeavor is the **overload principle**, which means providing a greater stress or load on the body than it is normally accustomed to handling (8,11,14,19). For example, if an athlete can lift 50 kg in a movement for five consecutive repetitions, he would have to lift a greater mass for the same number of repetitions or increase the number of repetitions with the same mass to effect overload.

Specificity, stated as the **SAID principle** (for "specific adaptation to imposed demands"), must be integrated into a resistance training program. This means that the type of demand placed on the body controls the type of adaptation that will occur. For example, athletes engaged in high-speed events need to activate as many motor units as possible in the shortest amount of time. For specific adaptation to occur, the training program of these athletes should include resistance training exercise that recruits as many motor units as possible (13). Jumpers perform squats with near maximal weight; the forces and level of motor unit recruitment at the knee and hip are similar during training and the actual event. Training should become more specific as the competitive season approaches. Although only the activity itself provides 100% carryover to the event, the more related training activities are, the better the carryover effect. In the example of the jumper, we would introduce resistance training activities that are increasingly similar to jumping as competition nears.

For the greatest gains in muscular strength and power, the level of resistance should be at or near maximal (1RM) as the competitive season nears (3,5,11, 14,19,22,26,32). Prior to this, training should approach maximal resistances in a gradual, progressive, organized manner.

Muscle Actions

There are three major types of muscle actions in resistance training: isometric, concentric, and eccentric actions. *Isometric* muscle actions occur when force is produced by a muscle but no change in muscle length occurs. This happens when someone pushes or pulls on an immovable object. Isometric exercises were popularized for strength training in the 1960s by Hettinger (22) and Mueller. Studies found that the best results occurred with multiple sets of maximal or near-maximal muscle actions done for 3 to 10 s every day. Strength gains are generally plus or minus 20° on either side of the joint angle trained. An isometric leg press done at 90° of flexion would elicit similar strength gains between 70° and 110° of flexion. Strength gains are on the order of 0.5% to 1%/day in untrained nonathletes (14). Gains would be much smaller in well-trained athletes over many months of training. Isometric muscle actions are often used in rehabilitation when joint motion is contraindicated and in some PNF flexibility regimes. In athletes, isometric muscle actions naturally occur to stabilize joints. For example, the abdominal and low back muscles contract isometrically to keep the torso stable during running.

Isometric exercise is not extensively used in the training of athletes, mainly because the equipment—immovable objects—typically does not provide any feedback to the exerciser, thus dampening motivation. There are some expensive machines with isometric capabilities that provide the user with a visual display of force produced.

Concentric muscle actions occur when force is applied while a muscle shortens and a joint moves. All free-weight equipment and resistance machines have concentric–muscle action capabilities. Some machines that utilize hydraulics, air cylinders, or braking systems allow only concentric muscle action.

Eccentric muscle actions occur when force is produced while a muscle is lengthening, as when an athlete lowers a free-weight apparatus or the lever arm of a machine with weighted resistance. Higher increases in so-called dynamic, or isotonic, strength (constant external resistance) are seen when a combination of constant–external resistance concentric and eccentric muscle actions are utilized than when either is used alone. For this reason, when using constant external resistance, most athletes train with equipment that allows for both concentric and eccentric muscle actions.

Dynamic Resistance

Most athletic endeavors require the athlete to move his or her body or an object (e.g., ball, bat, or racquet) through a particular ROM. This is **dynamic resistance**, when the body or object provides resistance through a ROM. In training, we can use manual resistance, free-weight equipment, or resistance machines to provide dynamic resistance.

Manual Resistance. *Manual resistance* is supplied in a dynamic movement by a partner or an opposing limb of the exerciser. An example would be performing a knee extension movement against the resistance provided by the hands of a partner holding the ankle of the athlete, or by the athlete placing the opposite leg over the leg to be extended for resistance. This type of resistance is inexpensive, expedient, and sometimes more effective in developing strength than some other types of dynamic modes and methods, such as multiple sets with cam-type machines (25). Isometric muscle actions can also be utilized with manual resistance by not allowing movement in the joint exercised.

Free-Weight Equipment. *Free weights*—barbells and dumbbells—are generally inexpensive and allow multiple joint movements to be performed in more than one plane of motion. Using free-weight equipment requires greater proprioception, balance, and coordination than other modes. The athlete must balance the weight while exerting force to lift it in a pattern that will allow him or her to maintain balance.

A type of training that combines isometric muscle actions with dynamic free-weight exercise is termed **functional isometrics** (24). In this type of training, a power rack (Figure 22.1) is utilized so that a barbell can be loaded and placed at a position 15 to 30 cm below a pair of cross-pins set at or near the sticking point (angle of weakest joint leverage) in a dynamic movement. The barbell is loaded to approximately 80% of the athlete's 1RM effort in the movement. The athlete lifts the barbell 15 to 30 cm, until the cross-pins impede further movement; he or she then performs an isometric muscle action lasting 7 to 10 s, pulling or pushing the loaded bar against the pins. This type of training elicits strength gains superior to either isometric or dynamic training alone (24).

Resistance Machines. A virtual cornucopia of resistance training weight machines are found in today's market. They are generally more expensive than free weights and often limit the user to single-joint movements in fixed planes of motion. They do not require the proprioception, balance, and coordination required with free weights, but allow the user to isolate some areas of the body more easily. For example, it is nearly impossible to do knee curls with free weights, but there are a number of machines that allow this important

movement in a variety of positions (standing, prone, and seated). Many devices utilize a weight stack connected to a lever bar by chains or cables (Figure 22.2). Less expensive models require weight plates to be added to provide resistance (Figure 22.3). In the early 1970s the introduction of the offset cam (Figure 22.4) delivered "variable resistance": Changing the distance from the axis of rotation to the cable at the point where it leaves the cam changes the mechanical advantage and varies the resistance throughout the ROM. Shortly thereafter, a sliding-lever bar system (Figure 22.5) was introduced to achieve variable resistance. Rubber bands provide variable resistance either by themselves (Figure 22.6) or as part of resistance machines (Figure 22.7). As the bands are elongated, greater resistance results, which may be suitable to movements that have weaker joint force potential at the beginning of the movement and stronger joint force potential toward the end of the movement.

Although none of the machines examined by two researchers (16,21) matched the joint angle force production potential for any of the users in the studies, the machine age is upon us, and we have a wide variety of devices to choose from, depending on our likes and dislikes. Some machines are more biomechanically sound than others, in that they can be adjusted for different limb lengths and user sizes. The quality of machines can vary widely, so let the buyer beware.

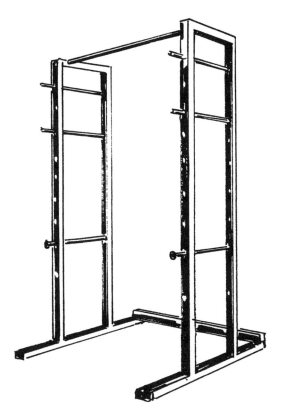

Figure 22.1 Power rack.

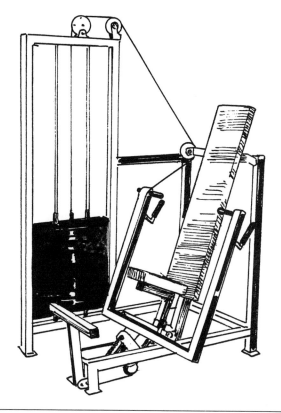

Figure 22.2 Selectorized weight stack machine.

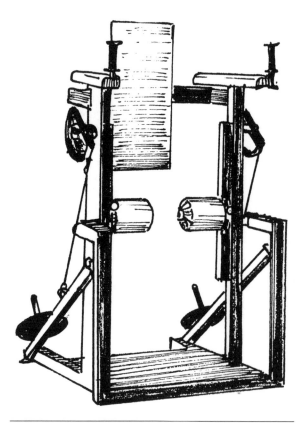

Figure 22.3 Weight plate loading machine.

Somewhat different from variable resistance devices are the accommodating-resistance devices. These machines utilize hydraulics (Figure 22.8), air cylinder shock absorbers (Figure 22.9), or braking systems (Figure 22.10) to provide resistance that increases as the user exerts force. This allows for maximal force to be erected through the available range of motion of the unit (34). As the force increases or decreases due to changing joint leverage potential in the exerciser, the resistance increases or decreases to match the effort (38). Some of the more sophisticated accommodating devices are called *isokinetic*. The term means "same speed or movement." In the more expensive models speed selection ranges from 300 to 500 degrees per second in most units and up to 1,000 degrees per second in one model. The speed selection only allows the user to go up to a certain angular velocity before much resistance is encountered. Many of these units have hardware that will record the magnitude of force at the various joint angles in a movement. Since the speed of movement can be varied, with the possible exception of the very slowest speed setting, there are no truly isokinetic units that allow for only one preset speed of movement. Most accommodating-resistance devices do not have the capability to allow for eccentric actions to alternate with concentric actions. While this may reduce muscle soreness in beginning trainees, it may also limit strength development (14).

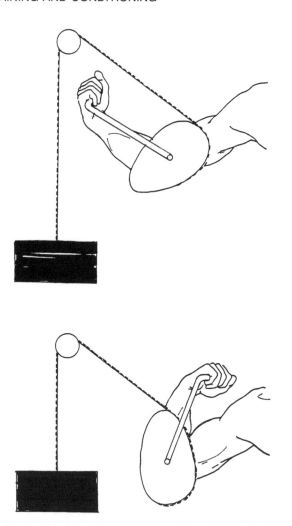

Figure 22.4 Offset cam.

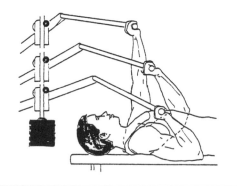

Figure 22.5 Sliding lever bar system.

Plyometric Training

Another type of resistance training is *plyometric* training. Chapter 20 explains plyometric principles and exercises. This type of training utilizes the stretch reflex and the accompanying stretch-shortening cycle to elicit more powerful concentric contractions. Research indicates that the faster a muscle is stretched with a rapid

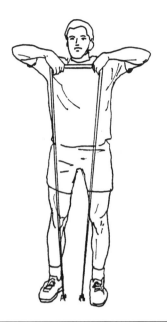

Figure 22.6 Rubber band resistance.

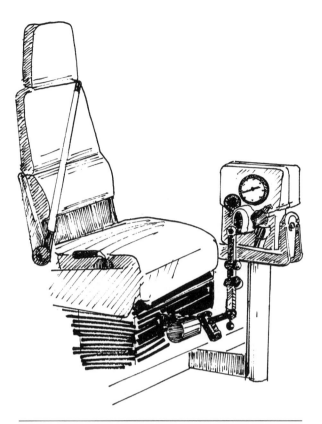

Figure 22.8 Hydraulic system.

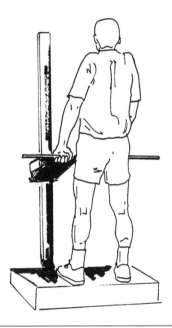

Figure 22.7 Rubber band in resistance machine.

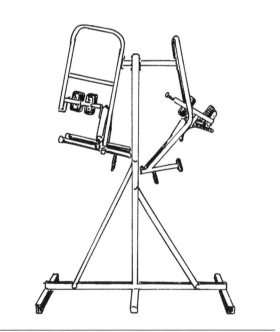

Figure 22.9 Air cylinder system.

eccentric loading, the more powerful its concentric contraction potential becomes (9,11,20). Armed with this information, cc ꞏhes can utilize a variety of bounding, hopping, and jum, ꞏ activities to train the lower body. Additional resistance ꞏeyond body weight is occasionally added by the use of weighted vests. Torso and upper extremity activities are accomplished by medicine ball throws and modified push-ups. Due to the high intensity of this type of training, it should be utilized judiciously 1 to 3 days/week for 15 to 20 min/session. Each set of activity should be followed by complete

recovery periods to avoid fatigue, which can cause degeneration of technique and possible injury. Activities should be conducted on yielding surfaces with proper footwear. Matching the athlete to the appropriate level of activity is critical to improving performance and

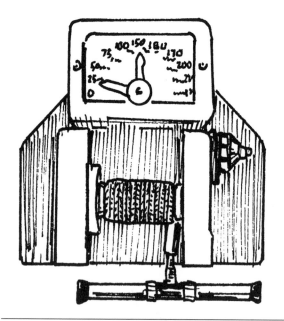

Figure 22.10   Braking system.

preventing injury. Progression from mastery at low-intensity activity to exercises of higher intensity and skill is vital. Many authorities feel that an adequate strength base is necessary prior to the introduction of plyometric exercises (6,44). Some activities, such as depth jumps, may not be appropriate for athletes who weigh over 100 kg. Various studies have purported the efficacy of one resistance training mode over another (4,16,25,27,39-41). Certainly strength gains can be produced from all types of training modes.

Individual preference, space availability, cost, level of training, and personal experience all play a role in the choice of training modes. The ideal program employs a variety of modes, depending on the sport and equipment availability. Lack of equipment should never deter an athlete from resistance training, because manual resistance techniques can always be used isometrically and dynamically, employing opposing limbs or a partner for resistance.

METABOLIC TRAINING

Metabolic training refers to activities that build up the energy stores needed for sports. Metabolic training is generally divided into two types: aerobic and anaerobic training.

Aerobic Training

Energy is derived aerobically when oxygen is utilized to metabolize substrates derived from food and liberate

energy. A sports event is termed *aerobic* when the majority of the energy needed is derived aerobically. Examples are such large–muscle group rhythmic activities as walking, jogging, rowing, nonsprint cycling, dancing, cross-country skiing, and swimming. Events are usually greater than 90 s in duration. In aerobic training, the activity should be performed continuously for a minimum of 15 to 20 min at a level of 70% to 90% of maximal heart rate for a minimum of three training sessions/week (1,12,26); athletes requiring high levels of aerobic fitness train aerobically 4 to 6 days/week (14). Some variation in these guidelines is permitted for age and fitness level. Specificity dictates that the training should closely resemble the event: Swimmers should swim and runners run, for example. Athletes involved in activities with a low aerobic component, such as football and power events in track, may see a decrease in power and strength with excessive aerobic training (10,23,35). These athletes should confine their aerobic training to the early preparation period of off-season training and then engage in a minimal amount of aerobic training to maintain good general fitness and body composition.

Athletes in running activities may find lower impact aerobic activities, such as cycling, swimming, and deep-water running in place, warranted as part of a weekly training regime to decrease common overuse and stress injuries. For example, a distance runner could run 3 days/week on the track and roads and either cycle or run in place in deep water on alternate days of training during the week. Deep-water running typically places a greater stress on the anaerobic energy systems than does land running (43). Just as with any other type of fitness, the intensity and duration of training must be increased gradually over time in a logical progression that allows the athlete to peak for the most important competitions.

Anaerobic Training

Anaerobic training and activities of less than 2 min in duration involve utilization of phosphagen and lactic acid energy sources. Events of under 6 s in duration rely almost exclusively on the phosphagen system; events lasting 30 to 90 s begin to rely heavily on lactic acid. These energy systems are effectively developed using an interval training system (15). It is important to remember that although one energy system may predominate for a given activity, all systems are in use at any time (Figure 22.11).

Interval Training

Interval training uses intervals that can consist of running, swimming, calisthenic exercises, or resistance training. Work intervals of less than 30 s are typically

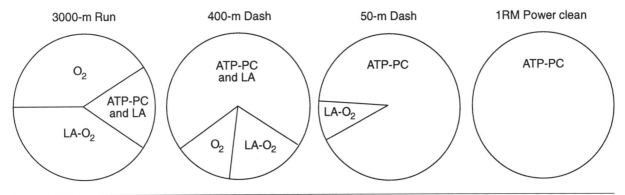

Figure 22.11 Energy source contributions to various activities.

done with rest intervals of approximately 3 times this duration. For example, a basketball player may sprint 20 yd in 2.9 s and then recover for 8 to 9 s before sprinting another 20-yd interval. This type of training does not allow for full recovery between bouts of work and is generally done during the middle to later part of the off-season preparatory period. As the competition period approaches, preseason interval training consists of longer rest intervals to accommodate near-maximal intensity or pace. The athlete should recover fully between exercise intervals; the exercise-to-rest ratio may approach 1:6 for short exercise intervals.

Exercise involving the lactic acid source generally has an exercise-to-rest ratio of 1:2. Thus, athletes running repeat 400-m sprints in 65 s would take approximately 130 s to recover before the next 400-m sprint. Full recovery is not achieved, but as athletes perform more of this type of training, they will be better able to tolerate and utilize increased concentrations of lactic acid. This type of training can be adapted to all types of running, cycling, swimming, rowing, and cross-country skiing.

Most athletes involved in strength-and-power activities, such as football, baseball, basketball, volleyball, running events of under 800 m, and swimming events of under 100 m, utilize both of the anaerobic energy sources to supply the majority of required energy. Interval training should comprise the bulk of their metabolic training. Some guidelines for interval training are presented in Table 22.2. Table 22.3 (15) provides an estimated percentage figure on the amount of time to be spent on the various types of metabolic training for a variety of sports. (These tables are guidelines based on the authors' experience and research.)

One type of interval training is called *circuit weight training*. This involves stations with either calisthenic movements (such as sit-ups, push-ups, pull-ups, squat thrusts, and jumping jacks) or resistance exercise equipment (machines and free weights). The stations are usually arranged so that different muscle groups are exercised in successive stations, thus allowing each muscle

Table 22.2   Guidelines for Interval Training

	Interval sprint training	Interval mid-distance training	Interval distance training
Energy system mainly involved	Phosphate	Lactic acid	Oxygen
Duration of load (s)	10-30	30-120	120-300
Duration of recovery (s)	30-90	60-240	120-310
Load:recovery	1:3	1:2	1:1
Repetitions	25-30	10-20	3-5

Reprinted from Kemper (1990).

group to recover. Successive stations are arranged near one another so athletes can move from station to station in an orderly manner and so large groups of athletes can work out simultaneously. An athlete may make one or more circuit through the stations, depending on time limits, goals of training, and the athlete's physical condition. Rest intervals are occasionally set up so that walking or slow running between stations may be employed to maintain a heart rate of 60% to 90% of maximum. This allows higher levels of aerobic endurance to be developed (17,18).

Circuit weight training is a compromise between endurance training and strength training. Intensity in strength training ranges from 40% to 70% of maximum capacity (17,18), levels that facilitate near-continuous activity but that do not elicit the strength gains seen in traditional strength training, which uses longer rest intervals and greater intensity. The heart rate fluctuations during and between stations can differ significantly, so that the endurance gains are not as great as those found in traditional aerobic exercise, in which a steady state heart rate is achieved and maintained for the duration of the workout. Circuit weight training

Table 22.3 Estimated Percentage of Time to Be Spent in Types of Metabolic Training

Sport	Phosphogen and lactic acid (Anaerobic)	Lactic acid and oxidative (Anaerobic and aerobic)	Oxidative (Aerobic)
	Emphasis according to energy systems (% of time)		
Baseball	80	20	—
Basketball	85	15	—
Fencing	90	10	—
Field hockey	60	20	20
Football	90	10	—
Golf	95	5	—
Gymnastics	90	10	—
Ice hockey			
Forwards, defense	80	20	—
Goalie	95	5	—
Lacrosse			
Goalie, defense, attack men	80	20	—
Midfielders, man-down	60	20	20
Rowing	20	30	50
Skiing			
Slalom, jumping, downhill	80	20	—
Cross-country	—	5	95
Pleasure skiing	34	33	33
Soccer			
Goalie, wings, strikers	80	20	—
Halfbacks or link men	60	20	20
Swimming and diving			
50 yd, diving	98	2	—
100 yd	80	15	5
200 yd	30	65	5
400 yd, 500 yd	20	40	40
1500 yd, 1650 yd	10	20	70
Tennis	70	20	10
Track and field			
100 yd, 220 yd	98	2	—
Field events	90	10	—
440 yd	80	15	5
880 yd	30	65	5
1 mile	20	55	25
2 miles	20	40	40
3 miles	10	20	70
6 miles (cross-country)	5	15	80
Marathon	—	5	95
Volleyball	90	10	—
Wrestling	90	10	—

Adapted from Fox and Mathews (1974).

typically has an exercise-to-rest ratio of 1:1 or greater and elicits greater aerobic gains if the relief interval contains traditional aerobic activity such as jogging (17,18). In a setting in which no aerobic activity occurs during the relief interval, the interval may be appreciably shorter. For example, an athlete performing an exercise at 60% of 1RM for maximal repetitions in a 30-s exercise interval can use a rest interval of 15 s or less. On the other hand, a very intense exercise interval may have a longer rest interval.

The intensity of the exercise interval and length of the rest intervals can be determined by monitoring the heart rate. Using the guidelines for aerobic exercise intensity (see p. 410), one may increase the level of exercise intensity or shorten the rest interval to increase heart rate or do the opposite to reduce heart rate. Circuit weight training is favored by athletes who have only very brief periods of time to train for both strength and endurance and do not need maximal levels of either.

SPEED TRAINING

Speed may be developed, but is in large part dependent upon a person's genetic ability. Chapter 20 explains the methods of speed development. Requirements for running speed are stride length, stride frequency, reaction time, acceleration, strength, power, endurance, flexibility, and running form. Improving swimming speed requires increases in stroke and kick frequency, strength, power, flexibility, endurance, and stroke technique. Of all these components, power is most important and may contribute most to speed (7,26).

Different variables may affect athletes at different levels. All the factors that determine speed may be trained for improvement. However, an elite athlete attempting to improve his or her speed may be able to improve only one or two areas, such as strength and stride frequency (13). Resistive training may be used to increase stride length. Resistive training methods vary from resistance-reliable techniques, such as uphill runs or sled towing, to techniques subject to inconsistent resistance variables, such as wind for parachute towing (7). Methods used to improve speed include

- weight training;
- running uphill or up stairs;
- towing someone or an object; and
- running in sand, water, or snow or against the wind.

Stride frequency may be improved with assisted training (7). Some exercises that help increase stride frequency are being towed at a pace faster than typical running, running downhill (a 4° downhill slope is the optimal and most practical method), and treadmill running (the most expensive method) at fast speeds (6,7).

Resistive training is utilized in swimming to improve stroke and kick power. Wearing panty hose or extra bathing suits and towing buoys or a cable attached to a resistance device are some of the methods used by swimmers to improve stroke and kick power. Assisted training includes using hand paddles and foot fins.

Reaction time, acceleration, strength, power, and endurance may be affected by weight training and plyometrics more than any other specific techniques because of the close relationship they both share with training of the neuromuscular system (31). Although many methods have been and are currently being practiced to improve speed, only increases in the strength of the muscles involved in running or swimming have been scientifically validated as effective.

CONCLUSION

The strength and conditioning professional must be well versed in all modes and methods of physical training. Once a needs analysis of a sport is performed, each athlete must be tested according to the criteria developed in the analysis and the proper application of training modes and methods developed. Each stage in an athlete's training requires modification of the various modes and methods of training according to the goals set by the athlete, skill coach, and conditioning specialist. The successful athlete has an optimal blend of training modes and methods.

Key Terms

dynamic resistance	406	mesocycle	404	periodization	404
functional isometrics	407	needs analysis	403	SAID principle	406
macrocycle	404	overload principle	405		

Study Questions

1. Each isometric muscle action should be held for _____ s.

    a. 10 to 20
    b. 3 to 10
    c. 1 to 3
    d. 20 to 30

2. Which of the following athletes requires the highest level of aerobic metabolism training?

    a. a basketball player
    b. a baseball player
    c. a gymnast
    d. a rower

3. Towing devices such as sleds and parachutes are used to develop

    a. speed
    b. endurance
    c. flexibility
    d. agility

Applying Knowledge of Training Methods and Modes

Problem 1

A collegiate freshman hammer thrower is presented to you. He is 196 cm tall, weighs 100 kg, and has 11% body fat. His 20-yd dash time is 2.85 s, his vertical jump is 66 cm, and his sit-and-reach test score is +8. He can bench press 111 kg, parallel squat with 141 kg, and power clean 86 kg. His 1.5-mile run time was 10 min flat. What modes and methods of training does this athlete need to emphasize?

Problem 2

Your first year on the job finds you with no equipment or budget. You have access to a gymnasium, and there are ample tumbling and wrestling mats along with an assortment of medicine balls. The Booster Club has donated $250.00 for equipment. Which modes and methods of training will not be available to you and how will you adjust training to compensate for this lack of equipment?

References

1. American College of Sports Medicine. *Guideline for Graded Exercise Testing and Exercise Prescription.* Philadelphia: Lea & Febiger. 1980.
2. Anderson, B., J.E. Beaulieu, W.L. Cornelius, R.H. Dominguez, W.E. Prentice, and L. Wallace. Flexibility. *NSCA Journal* 6(4):10-22. 1984.
3. Anderson, T., and J.T. Kearney. Muscular strength and absolute and relative endurance. *Res. Q. Exerc. Sport* 53:1-7. 1982.
4. Ariel, G. Barbell vs. dynamic variable resistance. *U.S. Sports Association News* 1:7. 1977.
5. Bompa, T.A. *Theory and Methodology of Training.* Kendall/Hunt: Dubuque, IA. 1983.
6. Chu, D. *Jumping Into Plyometrics.* Champaign, IL: Leisure Press. 1992.
7. Costello, F. Training for speed using resisted and assisted methods. *NSCA Journal* 7(1):74-75. 1985.
8. DeLorme, T.L., and A.L. Watkins. Techniques of progressive resistance exercise. *Arch. Phys. Med.* 29:263-273. 1948.
9. Desmedt, J.E., and E. Godaux. Ballistic contractions in man: Characteristic recruitment pattern of single motor units of the tibialis muscle. *J. Physiol.* 264:673-694. 1977.

10. Dudley, G.A., and R. Djamil. Incompatibility of endurance and strength training modes of exercise. *J. Appl. Physiol. Respir. Env. Exerc. Physiol.* 59:1336-1451. 1985.

11. Edgerton, V.R. Neuromuscular adaptation to power and endurance work. *Can. J. Appl. Sport Sci.* 1:49-58. 1976.

12. Fardy, P.S. Training for aerobic power. In: *Toward an Understanding of Human Performance*, E.J. Burke, ed. Ithaca, NY: Movement. 1978. pp. 10-14.

13. Fleck, S.J., and J.E. Falkel. Value of resistance training for the reduction of sports injuries. *Sports Med.* 3:61-68. 1986.

14. Fleck, S.J., and W.J. Kraemer. *Designing Resistance Training Programs*. Champaign, IL: Human Kinetics. 1987.

15. Fox, E.L., and D.K. Mathews. *Interval Training*. Philadelphia: Saunders. 1974.

16. Garhammer, J. Equipment for the development of athletic strength and power. *NSCA Journal* 3(6):24-26. 1981.

17. Gettman, L.R., J.J. Ayres, M.L. Pollock, and A. Jackson. The effect of circuit weight training on strength, cardiorespiratory function and body composition of adult men. *Med. Sci. Sports* 10:171-176. 1978.

18. Gettman, L.R., and M.L. Pollock. Circuit weight training: A critical review of its physiological benefits. *Phys. Sportsmed.* 9:44-60. 1981.

19. Gonyea, W.J., and D. Sale. Physiology of weight-lifting exercise. *Arch. Phys. Med. Rehabil.* 63:235-237. 1982.

20. Häkkinen, K., and P.V. Komi. Changes in neuromuscular performance in voluntary and reflex contraction during strength training in man. *Int. J. Sports Med.* 4:282-288. 1983.

21. Harman, E. Resistive torque analysis of 5 Nautilus exercise machines. *Med. Sci. Sports Exerc.* 15:113. 1983.

22. Hettinger, R. *Physiology of Strength*. Springfield, IL: Charles C Thomas. 1961.

23. Hickson, R.C. Interference of strength development by simultaneously training strength and endurance. *Eur. J. Appl. Physiol.* 45:255-263. 1980.

24. Jackson, A., T. Jackson, J. Hnatek, and J. West. Strength development: Using functional isometrics in an isotonic strength training program. *Res. Q. Exerc. Sport* 56:234-237. 1985.

25. Jacobson, B. A comparison of two progressive weight training techniques on knee extensor strength. *Athletic Training* 21(4):315-318. 1986.

26. Jensen, C., and G. Fisher. *Scientific Basis of Athletic Conditioning*. Philadelphia: Lea & Febiger. 1979.

27. Lander, J.E., B.T. Bates, J.A. Sawhill, and J.A. Hamill. Comparison between free-weight and isokinetic bench pressing. *Med. Sci. Sports Exerc.* 17:344-353. 1985.

28. Leighton, J. Instrument and technique for measurement of range of joint motion. *Arch. Phys. Mental Rehabil.* 36:571-578. 1955.

29. Leighton, J. Flexibility characteristics of four specialized skill groups of college athletes. *Arch. Phys. Med. Rehabil.* 38:24-28. 1957.

30. Leighton, J. Flexibility characteristics of three specialized skill groups of champion athletes. *Arch. Phys. Med. Rehabil.* 38:580-583. 1957.

31. Luhtanen, P., and P. Komi. Mechanical factors influencing running speed. In: *Biomechanics VI-B*, E. Asmussen, ed. Baltimore: University Park Press. 1982.

32. Marshall, J.L., N. Johanson, T.L. Wickiewicz, H.M. Tishler, B.L. Koslin, S. Zeno, and A. Myers. Joint looseness: A function of the person and the joint. *Med. Sci. Sports Exerc.* 12:189-194. 1980.

33. Massey, B.H., and N.L. Chaudet. Effects of heavy resistance exercises on range of joint movement in young male adults. *Res. Q.* 27:41-51. 1956.

34. Moffroid, M., R. Whipple, J. Hofkosh, E. Lowman, and H. Thistle. A study of isokinetic exercise. *Phys. Ther.* 49:735-747. 1969.

35. Nelson, A.G., R.K. Conlee, D.A. Arnall, S.F. Loy, and L.J. Silvester. Adaptations to simultaneous training for strength and endurance. *Med. Sci. Sports Exerc.* 16:184. 1984.

36. O'Shea, J.P. *Scientific Principles and Methods of Strength Fitness*. Reading, MA: Addison-Wesley. 1976.

37. Pearl, B. *Getting stronger: Weight training for men and women*. New York: Random House. 1988.

38. Perrine, J.A., and V.R. Edgerton. Isokinetic anaerobic ergometry. *Med. Sci. Sports* 7:78. 1975.

39. Silvester, L.J., C. Stiggins, C. McGown, and G. Bryce. The effect of variable resistance and free-weight training programs on strength and vertical jump. *NSCA Journal* 3(6):30-33. 1983.

40. Smith, M.J., and P. Melton. Isokinetic versus isotonic variable resistance training. *Am. J. Sports Med.* 9:275-279. 1981.

41. Stone, M.H., R.C. Johnson, and D.R. Carter. A short term comparison of two different methods of resistance training on leg strength and power. *Athletic Training* 14:158-160. 1979.

42. Stone, W.J., and W.A. Kroll. *Sports Conditioning and Weight Training*, 2nd ed. Carmel, IN: Brown & Benchmark. 1986.

43. Svedenhag, J., and J. Seger. Running on land and in water: Comparative exercise physiology. *Med. Sci. Sports Exerc.* 24(20):1155-1160. 1992.

44. Wathen, D. Flexibility: Its place in warm-up activities. *NSCA Journal* 9(5):26-27. 1987.

45. Williams, M., and L. Stutzman. Strength variation throughout the range of joint motion. *Phys. Ther. Rev.* 39:145-152. 1959.

CHAPTER 23

EXERCISE SELECTION

Dan Wathen

Exercise selection is a critical variable in an athlete's training program. Other variables in an exercise prescription may not be able to compensate for improperly chosen exercises (3-6). To make an informed decision on exercise selection, the strength and conditioning professional must first perform a sport-specific needs analysis, which includes the following (2):

- A general biomechanical analysis of the sport for which the athlete is training
- An analysis of the energy sources utilized in the sport, broken down by percent
- An analysis of the common injury sites for the sport

With this information, the strength and conditioning professional can answer the following questions on the specificity of training for a sport:

- What muscle groups need to be trained?
- What are the predominant types of muscle actions utilized (concentric, eccentric, isometric)?
- What are the motor patterns and speeds of motion?

At this point a general choice of exercises can be made.

Next, the strength and conditioning professional needs to perform an individual needs analysis. The individual analysis should use the sport-specific testing procedures covered in chapter 15 to identify an athlete's strengths and weaknesses. For example, tests of a baseball pitcher find that he has adequate flexibility in the internal and external rotators of the shoulder but his external rotators are weak both overall and in comparison to his internal rotators. His conditioning program

should reflect this; it would include a flexibility maintenance program and strength development of the external shoulder rotators.

MUSCLE BALANCE

Keep in mind muscle balance between joint agonists and antagonists when choosing exercises. For example, testing might reveal that the hamstrings are extremely weak compared with the quadriceps. The exercise choice may have more movements for the hamstrings to compensate for the imbalance. Remember, though, that an athlete needs to spend time on all major muscle groups to insure overall development (2-6,8). (Muscle balance is addressed in more detail in chapter 24.)

EQUIPMENT

The availability of training equipment must be taken into consideration when selecting exercises (2,3,8). A lack of certain equipment necessitates changes or deletions in desirable exercises. For example, lack of Olympic-type barbells with revolving sleeves would preclude the performance of power cleans and snatches. Lack of floor space would hamper many free-weight movements, such as overhead lifts, in which a dropped barbell would be very dangerous. Lack of sufficient barbell plates may force athletes to perform exercises that do not require a great amount of resistance, such as front squats instead of back squats, or power cleans instead of deadlifts. Rubber floor mats may have to be used if lack of funding precludes purchase of bumper plates.

Some machines may not allow for multidimensional training specific to the type of activity in which an athlete is engaged. Other machines may not be adjustable for shorter or taller athletes to train safely or effectively.

TRAINING BACKGROUND

Be certain to review an athlete's training background when prescribing exercises. Beginning trainees are often introduced to resistance training with machine or simple free-weight movements (2,3,8). Machines, although not necessarily safer, are easier to use because the athlete need not be overly concerned with balance and coordination (2,3,6,8). As the trainee progresses, introduce him or her to more complex free-weight activities.

One must weigh the value of certain exercises in terms of movement specificity versus the time it takes to learn the exercise (2,3,6,8). For example, it is more difficult to learn a squat snatch than a power snatch. The movement specificity of the power snatch is equal to, if not superior to, the squat snatch in terms of its effect on most athletic performance. Unless the athlete is interested in competitive weightlifting, the power snatch would be the more efficient activity to learn in terms of learning time and exercise specificity.

SPECIFICITY

Specificity refers to mechanical similarity between a training activity and a sport. The more similar the training activity is to the actual sport movement, the greater the likelihood of positive carryover to performance (2-7).

Use of Resistance Exercises

Specificity is a somewhat controversial area. Some trainers feel that because no resistance training exercise exactly duplicates an athletic movement, the only concern in exercise selection should be to isolate and develop the muscles used in the activity (8). This is true to a degree. However, the conditioning activities that have the greatest positive effect on the skill improvement are those that most closely duplicate the skill movement (2-7). For example, the prime movers in the standing vertical jump are the hip and knee extensors. These muscles could be exercised by performing either seated leg presses or barbell squats. Which exercise is preferable? Certainly both exercises would strengthen the hip and knee extensors. Because the standing vertical jump is done standing, with balance a factor, the barbell squat would be preferable. For general physical preparation, however, bodybuilding and general conditioning of nonathlete populations, this distinction may not be a major concern.

Use of Weighted Implements

An area of similar controversy is the use of weighted vests, ankle weights, and weighted implements (e.g., bats and racquets) in the performance of skills. Many trainers feel that heavier (or lighter) objects cause the athletes to alter their technique, which would bring about a decrement in performance. Certainly, if this practice altered correct technique significantly, it would be contraindicated. There is some evidence that using weighted bats causes impaired performance (1). However, the use of weighted implements remains a popular practice among athletes in many sports, primarily baseball and track and field.

Biomechanics of Equipment

One further controversy relative to specificity is the type of equipment used. Because most activities require an athlete to balance his or her body, and often another object or person, while exerting force in three dimensions, free-weight apparatus may be preferred to machines (2-7). However, as long as machines are available, their manufacturers will continue to extol their virtues. The consumer must be careful when purchasing equipment, because manufacturers have been known to cite pseudoscientific advertising rather than legitimate scientific studies.

It may be worthwhile having equipment that allows for acceleration and deceleration of the resistance similar to the motion of the actual sporting activity; such equipment may be of particular value in events in which the athlete or objects (e.g., a ball, racquet, or javelin) must be accelerated quickly in a controlled manner (2-4,6,7). The design of many machines, however, does not allow rapid acceleration (3,6,8). Free-weight equipment can be used in a number of activities that require controlled rapid acceleration (3-7). Most free-weight and some machine exercises require the athlete to accelerate the weight to allow the apparatus to pass through weak joint angles and then often require a deceleration phase when the apparatus reaches a position of favorable joint leverage near full joint extension. For example, an athlete has to accelerate a barbell during the initial ascent in the squat or bench press to allow the barbell to pass through the sticking point (area of weak joint leverage) and then decelerate the barbell near terminal extension. It is argued that greater force is created with weights that require near-isometric (very slow) movement and therefore develop greater strength (7). Certainly, heavy resistance that allows only slow movement should be a part of every athlete's training (2,3,8), because this may allow for more motor units to be recruited to complete the lift. However, most events requiring speed and power reward the athlete who can develop the most force in the shortest span of time. Therefore, such exercises as plyometrics, power cleans and snatches, and pulls that have a speed component also have a prominent place in many athletes' choice of exercises.

Each type of equipment has a role in the physical preparation of the athlete. Free weights can be utilized to more closely approximate sport movements, and machines can often more easily isolate certain muscle groups for physical development and injury prevention (2,3,5,6,8). Table 23.1 provides examples of resistance exercise specificity for various movement patterns.

There are many less specific activities that can be done with free weights and machines for general muscle development. Table 23.2 can act as a guide for exercise

selection by muscle group and sport. Both sport-specific and non–sport-specific exercises are listed.

PERIODIZATION CONCERNS

Specific and nonspecific exercises for muscle groups used in sports can be interchanged during various phases of the yearly periodization model, which is detailed in chapter 30. Generally, a mesocycle begins with a transitional phase of active rest, in which the athlete performs low-volume, low-intensity resistance training, or no exercises at all (1,2,5). As the preparatory period begins, the athlete uses nonspecific muscle exercises in ever-increasing intensities to induce general muscle hypertrophy and endurance (3,5,6). Athletes not interested in muscle hypertrophy keep this phase short and reduce volume by performing fewer repetitions and sets. As the competition period nears, the athlete incorporates

Table 23.1 Movement-Specific Resistance Exercises

Sport or movement pattern	Appropriate resistance exercises
Blocking	Power snatches and power cleans (FW)
Crew	Seated rowing (M)
Discus throwing	Supine flys (FW/M)
Gymnastics	Dips and chin-ups (FW/M)
Hand gripping sports (all)	Dynamic and isometric elbow and finger flexion (FW/M)
Jumping	Barbell squats, barbell/dumbbell lunges, step-ups, straight- and bent-knee calf raises, power snatches, power cleans, power/push jerks (FW)
Lateral running and shuffling	Standing, unilateral hip adduction/abduction (M)
Pole vault	Power/push jerks, chin-ups (FW)
Racquet serving and overhead throwing	Standing internal/external shoulder rotation with the humerus abducted (FW/M)
Racquet strokes	Standing shoulder horizontal abduction/adduction, and wrist curls (for all strokes) (FW/M)
Running	Straight- and bent-knee calf raises (M)
Shot put	Power/push jerks (FW)
Soccer kicks	Standing, unilateral hip adduction/abduction (M)
Sprinting	Barbell/dumbbell lunges, step-ups (FW)
Tackling	Power snatches and power cleans, torso rotation with free weights or machines, supine flys, wrist curls (FW/M)
Throwing	Standing internal/external shoulder rotation with the humerus abducted, simultaneous and alternating bent-arm pullovers, torso rotation with free weights or machines, wrist curls (FW/M)
Volleyball	Dynamic and isometric front shoulder raises and alternating lateral shoulder raises (for bumps and digs), supine flys (for digs), push press (for setting) (FW/M)
Wrestling	Torso rotation with free weights or machines, supine flys; power snatches and power cleans (for take-downs) (FW)

FW = free weight, M = machine

Table 23.2   Strength Training Exercises and Their Characteristics

Exercise	Prime mover	Synergist	Equipment	Sport
Knee extension	Quadriceps	—	Machine, iron boot	All sports
Knee curl	Hamstrings	Gastrocnemius	Machine, iron boot	All sports
Calf raise	Gastrocnemius, soleus	—	Machine, barbell	All sports
Leg press	Quadriceps, gluteals	Hamstring	Machine	All sports
Lunge	Quadriceps, gluteals	Hamstring	Barbell, dumbbells	All sports
Squat	Quadriceps, gluteals	Hamstring	Barbell	All sports
Step-up	Quadriceps, gluteals	Hamstring	Bench, barbell, dumbbell	All sports
Front squat	Quadriceps, gluteals	—	Barbell	All sports
Clean	All but pectorals and triceps	—	Barbell	All sports
Snatch	All but pectorals and triceps	—	Barbell	All sports
High pull	All but pectorals and triceps	—	Barbell	All sports
Deadlift	All but pectorals and triceps	—	Barbell	All sports
Push press	All but pectorals and triceps	—	Barbell	Volleyball, gymnastics, shot put
Push jerk	All but pectorals and triceps	—	Barbell	Volleyball, gymnastics, shot put
Split jerk	All but pectorals and triceps	—	Barbell	Volleyball, gymnastics, shot put
Gluteal-hamstring-gastrocnemius raise	Spinal erector, gluteals, hamstrings, gastrocnemius	—	Modified Roman chair	All sports
Sit-ups	Iliopsoas	Abdominals	Floor, machine	All sports
Leg raise	Iliopsoas	Abdominals	Floor, machine	All sports
Front/back torso rotation	Obliques	Abdominals	Roman chair machine	All sports
Bench press	Pectoralis major, anterior triceps, deltoid	Spinal erectors	Barbell, bench, machine, dumbbells	Football, basketball, wrestling, shot put, hockey, rowing, boxing, gymnastics
Dip	Pectoralis major, triceps	Anterior deltoid	Parallel bars	Football, basketball, wrestling, shot put, hockey, rowing, boxing, gymnastics
Incline press	Anterior pectoralis major, deltoid, triceps	—	Barbell, dumbbells, incline bench, machine	Football, basketball, wrestling, shot put, hockey, rowing, boxing, gymnastics
Fly (supine)	Pectoralis major	Deltoid	Dumbbells, machine	Football, tennis, discus throw, baseball, softball, wrestling, backstroke
Overhead press	Deltoid, triceps	Trapezius	Barbell, dumbbells, machine	Gymnastics, shot put
Behind-neck press	Deltoid, triceps	Trapezius	Barbell	Gymnastics, shot put

(continued)

Table 23.2   *(continued)*

Exercise	Prime mover	Synergist	Equipment	Sport
Bent-over rowing	Latissimus dorsi, rhomboids	Deltoid, elbow flexors	Barbell, dumbbells, pulley machine	Wrestling, rowing, baseball, basketball, bowling
Upright rowing	Trapezius	Deltoid, elbow flexors	Barbell, dumbbells, pulley machine	All sports
Lat pull-down	Latissimus dorsi	Elbow flexors	Pulley machine	Basketball, baseball, swimming, tennis, volleyball, wrestling
Pullover	Latissimus pectoralis major	Serratus anterior	Barbell, dumbbells, machine	All throwing, stroking, and racquet sports; soccer; volleyball; basketball
Internal/external shoulder rotation	Rotator cuff	—	Barbell, dumbbell, machine	All sports
Front shoulder raise	Anterior deltoid	—	Barbell, dumbbell	All sports
Bent-over lateral raise	Posterior deltoid	Rhomboids, Latissimus	Dumbbells, machine	All sports
Lateral shoulder raise	Deltoid	Trapezius	Dumbbells, machine	All sports
Shoulder shrug	Trapezius	—	Barbell, dumbbells, machine	All sports
Elbow curl	Elbow flexors	Forearm muscles	Barbell, dumbbells, pulley machine	All sports
Tricep extension	Triceps	—	Barbell, dumbbells, pulley machine	All sports
Wrist flexion	Wrist flexors	—	Barbell, dumbbells, machines	All sports
Wrist extension	Wrist extensors	—	Barbell, dumbbells, machines	All sports
Wrist roller	Forearm muscles	—	Roller and cord, machine	All sports
Grip squeeze	Finger flexors	—	Tennis ball, machines	All sports
Neck movements	Neck muscles	—	Head strap, machine	Football, wrestling, soccer

Adapted from Garhammer (1986).

more sport-specific exercises in the training schedule and phases out less specific exercises (3,6,7). This exercise variation may provide a psychological boost beyond the physical benefits (2,3,5,6).

A basketball player, for example, might take a 3-week transition period of active rest at the end of the competitive season. During this time she could play occasional games of racquetball and volleyball and, once or twice weekly, might perform one or two sets of 10 repetitions at 50% of 1RM of a circuit weight training regime consisting of knee extension and flexion exercises, bench presses, seated rows, hip and low back extension and hip flexion machine exercises, hanging leg raises, and chin-ups. After this period she would embark on a 6-week hypertrophy/endurance phase, part of the preparatory period, concentrating on distance running and high-volume weight training. Exercises would include incline presses, barbell curls, upright rows, abdominal curls, wrist curls, leg presses, calf raises, knee curls, and lat pull-downs. A shift can now be made to higher resistances, less training volume, and more sport-specific exercise movements. This strength phase may last up to 10 weeks, with a few (once a month) microcycle (weekly) fluctuations of unloading with the low-intensity, nonspecific exercises used in the transition period and hypertrophy/endurance phase. During the strength phase, more sport-specific core, or structural, exercises will be utilized. These are multiple-joint, multiple–muscle group movements such as squats, lunges, power cleans and snatches, pulls, bench and incline presses, push jerks/presses, and deadlifts, which are generally performed with free-weight equipment. Interval running is gradually introduced during this phase, along with plyometric sessions. Some single-joint movements are retained during this phase to give injury-prone areas continued attention. These would include calf raises and hamstring curls for running and jumping activities and rotator cuff exercises for throwing, swimming, and racquet sports.

In the final phase of the preparatory period, the shift is toward power with low volume and high loads. Exercise choice is similar to the previous phase, but some exercises can be changed as long as they are movement specific. During this phase, intervals of near full speed are incorporated along with weekly plyometric drills for power events.

When the competition, or in-season, period arrives, conditioning activities are reduced to their lowest total training time of the entire cycle. Skill and strategy sessions make up the majority of the athletes' training. Training intensity (load) is kept high during this phase and total volume is at its lowest point. Exercises are reduced to a few core multiple-joint movements that work all major muscle groups in the shortest amount of time: power cleans, snatches, and pulls; squats and lunges; bench, incline, and push presses; and supine torso rotations. The various multiple-joint exercises can be varied if the competition period is prolonged.

COMMUNICATING THE NEED FOR PARTICULAR EXERCISES

Effectively communicating to the athlete the need for particular exercises may be the most difficult skill to develop. Many athletes have misconceptions as to which exercises are important for their sport or the importance of conditioning in general. For example, males often engage only in exercises that develop the frontal plane muscles that can be seen in a mirror from the waist up (i.e., the chest, abdominals, and biceps). Their "program" is dominated by bench and incline presses, elbow curls, flys, lat pulldowns, and a variety of triceps press movements, and the ideas of lower body development and muscle balance are eschewed. This may be especially difficult to deal with if the athlete runs fast and jumps well. An injury prevention strategy, rather than a skills improvement approach, may have to be employed to rationalize an exercise program to this athlete. If the athlete is open-minded, he will see the value of a properly chosen exercise regime after being exposed to several training sessions.

Sometimes athletes' misconceptions are deeply ingrained and may require a team approach to convince an athlete of the value of certain exercises at certain times during the training cycle. The team may consist of coaching personnel, medical personnel, and other athletes in the same or a similar activity.

CONCLUSION

Exercise selection is similar to the selection of warm-up activities. General conditioning activities are initiated at the beginning of a training mesocycle, much as general warm-up activities are utilized at the beginning of a warm-up period. As competition approaches, more specific conditioning movements are incorporated; this is similar to the specific warm-up patterns that are undertaken after a general warm-up prior to an event.

Choosing proper exercises and deploying them at the proper time during an athlete's training cycle is an art. It requires a thorough knowledge of the fitness demands of various sporting activities, along with knowledge of which exercises are most appropriate for the athlete at a certain time during the training cycle.

Study Questions

1. Which of the following exercises most closely simulates the javelin-throwing motion at the shoulder joint?

   a. seated one-arm pullovers on a pullover machine
   b. lunges with a barbell
   c. one-arm bench presses with dumbbells
   d. power cleans with dumbbells

2. Which of the following exercises are most specific to volleyball?

   a. squats, front raises, lateral raises, push presses, calf raises, shoulder rotations
   b. lunges, bench presses, knee extensions, power cleans, chins, dips
   c. leg presses, incline presses, knee curls, calf raises, front shoulder raises, pullovers
   d. squats, bench presses, deadlifts, power snatches, knee extensions, arm curls

3. During the preparation period (hypertrophy phase), which of the following exercises would be most appropriate for a hockey player?

    a. leg presses, incline presses, flys, back extensions, upright rowing, sit-ups
    b. power cleans, squats, bench presses, knee curls, calf raises, torso rotations
    c. lunges, pulls, push jerks, knee extensions, arm curls, wrist curls
    d. power snatches, push presses, squats, calf raises, leg raises, lateral raises

4. During the competition phase of training, which of the following exercises could most effectively be substituted for lunges?

    a. step-ups
    b. push jerks
    c. power snatches
    d. safety bar squats

5. Which of the following exercises does not stress the hip, knee, and low back (trunk) extensors?
    a. leg presses
    b. squats
    c. lunges
    d. snatch pulls

Applying Knowledge of Exercise Selection

Problem 1

You have taken a position at a high school that has a multistation unit allowing for leg presses, chest presses, shoulder presses, dips, chins, lat pulldowns, low pulleys, back extensions, knee curls, knee extensions, neck harness, gripper/wrist roller; 5- to 25-kg dumbbells; three 180-cm exercise bars, and 160 kg of miscellaneous plates; and a pair of adjustable squat stands. You will have no budget for the next 9 months to buy additional equipment. The coach of the 20-member freshman football team is anxious to have the team begin working out to gain size and strength. The average weight-lifting values for the team are 135 kg for the leg press and 75 kg for the bench press (on the machine); their average body weight is 55 kg. It is August, and the freshmen have a four-game schedule from mid-September to late October. You will have 40 min 3 days/week to work with the team. You decide to utilize a circuit training format, with 10 groups (2 boys per station), giving each group 4 min at a station to perform two or three sets of 10 repetitions. Considering lifting safety, which exercises would you select?

Problem 2

A freshman female discus thrower is 183 cm tall, weighs 102 kg, and has 19% body fat. Her vertical jump score is 61 cm, and she runs 40 yd in 5.15 s. She bench presses 138 kg, but refuses to perform any squatting exercises or pulling because of a back injury suffered when squatting 2 years earlier. Because the athlete's family is poor, she did not consult a physician at the time of the injury. Flexibility exams reveal a normal low back and normal range of motion (ROM) in the hamstrings. The athlete is suffering no pain or disability. X-rays and the findings of the team orthopedist are normal. The athlete played basketball and threw the discus for 2 years after her injury with no problems. The track coach and medical personnel are consulted about the problem, and all agree that the athlete will never reach her potential without attention to strengthening her knee, hip, and low back extensor in a specific manner. What action should be taken?

References

1. DeRenne, C., K.W. Ho, R.K. Hetylev, and D.X. Chai. Effects of warm-up with various weighted implements on baseball bat swing velocity. *J. Appl. Sports Sci. Res.* 6(4):214-218. 1992.
2. Fleck, S.J., and W.J. Kraemer. *Designing Resistance Training Programs.* Champaign, IL: Human Kinetics. 1987.
3. Garhammer, J. *Sports Illustrated Strength Training.* New York: Harper & Row. 1986.
4. O'Shea, J. *Scientific Principles and Methods of Strength Fitness.* Reading, MA: Addison-Wesley. 1976.
5. Pauletto, B. Choice and order of exercise. *NSCA Journal* 8(2):71-73. 1986.
6. Stone, M., and H. O'Bryant. *Weight Training.* Minneapolis: Burgess International. 1987.
7. Verhoshansky, Y. *Fundamentals of Special Strength Training in Sport.* Livonia, MI: Sportivny Press. 1976.
8. Westcott, W. *Strength Fitness.* Boston: Allyn & Bacon. 1982.

CHAPTER 24

MUSCLE BALANCE

Dan Wathen

Muscle balance is the strength, power, or endurance of one muscle or muscle group relative to another muscle or muscle group. Balance is usually expressed in terms of relative strength. Joint agonists and antagonists (e.g., biceps curl vs. triceps press) are most often compared, although *contralateral* (e.g., right vs. left biceps) comparisons and comparisons of upper and lower body muscles (e.g., bench press vs. squat) are also made.

HISTORICAL BACKGROUND

Early strength and conditioning professionals felt that performance would be diminished if all the muscles of the athlete were not developed proportionally. Since the advent of isokinetic testing devices in the late 1960s, the concept of a certain ratio between contralateral limbs and between joint agonists and antagonists has been expounded in the medical and rehabilitation literature. One study (2) asserted that a difference of greater than 10% in contralateral limb strength of the knee joint would predispose an athlete to injury. This study has since been refuted (15), but still remains a standard criterion in many clinics. Other researchers have advanced the concept of having a hamstring-to-quadriceps strength ratio of 40:60 to prevent injuries (21), but many studies have noted ratios of 20% to 200% in healthy populations (1,5,6,7,9,10,13-19,22,24,27-31,33-35,37). It becomes confusing for the practitioner who would like to assign a specific value for strength ratios. Should such values be determined and used?

Many activities cause a strength increase in one muscle group without a concomitant increase in its antagonist. Examples are the quadriceps of sprinters and the internal rotators of the shoulder in throwers (5). As the prime mover for a movement becomes stronger, the antagonist is placed under increased stress as a joint stabilizer. Theoretically, the antagonist should then be trained to aid in both performance enhancement and injury prevention.

CONCERNS IN REHABILITATION

Muscle balance is especially important in the rehabilitation setting, where a certain percentage of pre-injury muscle strength must be met prior to advancing the athlete to the next level of rehabilitation or returning the athlete to activity. There are, however, no exact figures for muscle ratios that correlate accurately to injury prevention or performance enhancement for all athletes (11,14-18,22,23).

When recommending muscle balance ratios in rehabilitation, the athlete's gender, type of activity, body position, joint angle, and speed at which the values were derived must be considered (1,3-6,9,10,15,16,18,19,25, 28,30,33,35). It is fairly well established that as speed of movement increases, agonist-antagonist differences in concentric torque production diminish (5,9,25,33). Athletes engaged in power activities need more strength and power compared to their body weight than athletes involved in endurance activities. Men typically exhibit more strength with respect to body weight then women, although these differences diminish when expressed relative to lean mass (1,4). Isolated muscle testing is typically done on an isokinetic dynamometer in a position that is often very different from what is functional. For example, knee extension and flexion values are universally tested in a seated position, even though very few sports are performed from a seated position. The test speed is often far lower than the speed at which actual activities are performed. For example, hip extension in jumping movements may exceed 500°/s, but few devices are capable of testing above 300°/s (5,23).

To use specific ratios as anything but a general guideline may be erroneous. For example, some athletes with knee injuries can perform functionally—run, jump, turn, and change direction—with no problem at a slow-speed isokinetic torque of 80% of the uninjured knee. Other athletes with similar knee injuries may not be able to perform functionally with 95% of isokinetic torque in the injured versus the uninjured knee (23). This is especially true if the previous level of strength was insufficient with respect to body weight or athletic activity.

MUSCLE BALANCE RATIOS

Muscle balance ratios are difficult to measure accurately. However, once they have been measured, they can be key in designing training programs. Measuring strength at high speeds of limb movement seems to be a logical, sport-specific approach to injury prevention, rehabilitation, and performance enhancement. Certainly it will be difficult for strength and conditioning professionals to determine muscle balance ratios without adequate testing equipment, although it is possible to use selectorized or plate-loading weight machines to determine the strength of a muscle group. High-speed comparisons are virtually impossible without expensive isokinetic equipment. Much like body composition values, muscle balance ratios only give general guidelines that can vary greatly even among athletes of similar size and activity.

Table 24.1 lists commonly reported values for joint agonist-antagonist ratios at slow isokinetic (30°-60°/s) speeds. These ratios may vary from 5% to 33%, depending on the study cited. The torque ratio indicates which movement is stronger. For example, at the ankle, the plantar flexors are three times as strong as the dorsiflexors. In many cases it should be obvious that, because of muscle volume and muscle-bone leverage relationships, certain muscle groups will likely produce more torque than their joint antagonists. The prime movers in sprinting and jumping are the knee extensors, the hip extensors, and the ankle plantar flexors—muscles that develop extensively as a result of activity alone. Moreover, by their sheer mass the knee extensors should be stronger than the flexors, given equal conditioning. There is even more disparity between the posterior leg compartment muscles (plantar flexors) and the anterior compartment muscles (dorsiflexors).

Table 24.1   Agonist-Antagonist Ratios for Slow Concentric Isokinetic Movements

Joint	Strength training	Torque ratio
Ankle	Plantar flexion/dorsiflexion (gastrocnemius, soleus/ tibialis anterior)	3:1
Ankle	Inversion/eversion (tibialis anterior/peroneals)	1:1
Knee	Extension/flexion (quadriceps/hamstrings)	3:2
Hip	Extension/flexion (spinal erectors, gluteus maximus, hamstrings/iliopsoas, rectus abdominus, tensor fascia latae)	1:1
Shoulder	Flexion/extension (anterior deltoids/trapezius, posterior deltoids)	2:3
Shoulder	Internal rotation/external rotation (subscapularis/ supraspinatus, infraspinatus, teres minor)	3:2
Elbow	Flexion/extension (biceps/ triceps)	1:1
Lumbar spine	Flexion/extension (psoas, abdominals/spinal erectors)	1:1

Note. The values expressed are a summary of numerous studies (1, 2, 5-37) of slow-speed (30°-60°/s) concentric isokinetic movements.

One study (25) makes recommendations for strength levels according to body weight, sport, and position (Table 24.2).

The further the joint agonist-antagonist muscle balance ratio is from 1:1, the more concern there may be for joint imbalance. If the average quadriceps-to-hamstring ratio is 3:2, a ratio of 2:1 might alert the individual to concentrate on hamstring work. Do not use these ratios as absolute guidelines for anything. They are only a part of the athlete's profile when determining training protocol. Individual variations, sport played, and previous injury have a role in determining muscle balance and in allocating training time for various muscle groups. Take, for example, a football lineman with a body weight of 283 lb, a right quadriceps torque at slow speed of 372 ft-lb and a right hamstring torque of 149 ft-lb. The rate of his quadriceps torque to body weight, at 0.76, is excellent for his sport and position (see Table 24.2), but the hamstring torque (ratio to quadriceps torque = 0.40) is low. Thus, a program that deemphasizes the

Table 24.2 Strength Ratio Goals for Athletes in Several Sports

| Ratio | Speed | American-football players | | | Male and female basketball players | | | | |
		Offensive and defensive lines	Tight end and linebacker	Receiver and back	Center	Forward	Guard	Male sprinters, hurdlers, jumpers	Female sprinters, hurdlers, jumpers
Quadriceps strength to body weight	60°/s	1.20	1.20-1.30	1.30-1.40	1.20	1.20	1.30	1.30-1.50	1.20-1.40
	180°/s	0.75	0.80	0.85-0.90	0.75	0.80	0.85	0.90-1.20	0.80-0.95
	300°/s	0.60	0.65	0.70-0.75	0.55	0.65	0.70	0.70-0.80	0.60-0.70
Hamstrings-quadriceps	60°/s	0.70	0.70	0.70	0.70	0.70	0.70	0.65-0.70	0.65-0.70
	180°/s	0.83	0.83	0.83	0.83	0.83	0.83	0.77-0.82	0.77-0.82
	300°/s	1.00	1.00	1.00	1.00	1.00	1.00	0.95-1.00	0.95-1.00

Note. To get the quadriceps and hamstring strength goals for the 60°/s speed for a 180-lb male basketball guard (for example), perform the following calculations. (All measures are in lbs and ft-lbs.)

Quadriceps goal: body weight × ratio from table = 180 lb × 1.30 = 234 ft-lb

Hamstring goal: quadriceps goal × ratio from table = 234 lb × 0.70 = 164 ft-lb

Adapted from Moore and Wade (1989).

quadriceps and focuses on the hamstring would be advisable. Certain areas susceptible to injury may require priority in training, depending on the sport and athlete—for example, the hamstrings in sprinters, jumpers, and other power athletes and the external rotators of the shoulder in swimmers, players of racquet sports, and throwers.

CONCERNS IN RESISTANCE TRAINING PROGRAMS

It is helpful to know the strengths and weaknesses of joints and muscle groups—as general trends and for individual athletes—when assigning frequency and volume of exercises. The sequence of exercises, as well, is often dependent on which areas need priority in individual athletes. The ratios of left limbs to right limbs, agonists to antagonists, and upper body to lower body need to be considered, as does strength compared to the athlete's body weight. Weak areas need priority (done first in a workout) and more sets and exercises, whereas strong areas require maintenance.

Muscle balance can be considered in comparisons of multiple-joint exercises and upper and lower body muscle groups. For example, world records in powerlifting for the squat are 90 to 135 kg higher than bench press records for the same weight class; the higher the body weight, the more disparity between bench press and squat records. It is not unusual to find many large power athletes (such as American-football players, shot putters, and sprinters) who bench press within 45 kg of their squat. This could indicate that a greater percentage of their training time should be spent on lower body exercises.

INCORPORATING MUSCLE BALANCE IN PROGRAM DESIGN

A well-designed program includes exercises for all the major muscle groups. Testing can identify muscle imbalances and allow the strength and conditioning professional to focus on weak areas and deemphasize stronger ones. Because athletes tend to work with their strengths and avoid their weaknesses in training, the strength and conditioning professional needs to ensure that an athlete addresses his or her weaknesses and imbalances at the outset of a workout—and with greater frequency—with stronger areas receiving less attention and placed later or last in the training session. The following is a case study of a program incorporating muscle balance considerations.

CASE STUDY

Name: **Jason Marshall**

Sport: **Baseball**

Position: **Infielder/right-handed**

INITIAL TEST RESULTS

Body weight: 190 lb

Parallel squat: 295 lb

Bench press: 280 lb

Vertical jump: 23 in.

20-yd dash: 3.1 s

1.5-mile run: 10 min 5 s

Isokinetic knee extension:flexion at slow speed (60°/s): right, 144 ft-lb:132 ft-lb; left, 188 ft-lb:126 ft-lb

Shoulder flexion:extension at slow speed (60°/s): right, 72 ft-lb:99 ft-lb; left, 69 ft-lb:93 ft-lb

Shoulder internal:external rotation (position of abduction) at slow speed (60°/s): right, 52 ft-lb:46 ft-lb; left, 50 ft-lb:46 ft-lb

Body fat: 13.0%

Sit-and-reach: +12

Jason had suffered a Grade 2 medial collateral ligament knee sprain (5-10 mm abnormal valgus laxity) 6 months prior to testing; the sprain was treated nonsurgically. The doctor has cleared Jason for full participation in training and games. Testing indicates general weakness in the lower body relative to upper body strength, body weight, and sport position. The skill/position coach notes that Jason is a strong-armed athlete who hits well but is slow on the base paths. Low levels of speed and power are noted.

In view of these data, the design of Jason's program should emphasize lower body strengthening activities, right knee extension exercises, plyometrics, sprint form, and speed drills. Short-term goals for Jason are getting his squat lift 100 lb over his bench press, and increasing his right knee extension strength until it is equal to that of the left, increasing jump height, and lowering his 20-yd dash time. A maintenance program for upper body strength and flexibility can be placed at the end of the workout 1 or 2 days/week.

The type and order of exercises for a 3-day/week strength training program for Jason are as follows.

Day 1: Squats, knee extensions (right leg only), knee curls, calf raises, power cleans, lateral raises, dumbbell external shoulder rotations, chin-ups, wrist curls (palm-up and palm-down)

Day 2: Leg presses, knee extensions (right leg only), knee curls, calf raises, high pulls, prone flys, front raises, supine pullovers (bent-arm), barbell curls, incline presses, gripping

Day 3: (Same as Day 1)

Running activities would include interval sprints of 60 yd and under. Once the difference between left and right knee extension is corrected and leg strength and power increase, plyometric bounding, hopping, and jumping should be introduced and performed 2 days/week.

CONCLUSION

Muscle balance is the relationship of a muscle or muscle group to another muscle or muscle group; usually it is expressed in terms of ratios of strength. Muscle balance may have a bearing on performance and injury prevention. A needs analysis and athlete testing procedures can determine areas in which muscle balance needs improvement. Several factors influence the exercise prescription: sport and position, body size, gender, type of testing device used, speed of testing, and injury status. Areas of stress or obvious weakness must be given priority in the training program.

Key Terms

muscle balance   424

Study Questions

1. At higher speeds of isokinetic testing (above 200°/s), joint agonist:antagonist ratios begin to approach

   a. 1:1
   b. 2:1
   c. 3:1
   d. 1:2

2. A tennis player with a shoulder flexion:extension ratio of 1:3 in his racquet arm should concentrate on which of the following exercises?

   a. lateral raises, front raises, bent-over lateral raises, elbow curls
   b. cable flys, lat pulldowns, pullovers
   c. upright rows, straight-arm lat pulldowns, internal rotations with dumbbells
   d. external dumbbell shoulder rotations, triceps extensions, pullovers

3. What would be a good quadriceps torque goal for a 200-lb decathlete tested at 60°/s on an isokinetic knee extension unit?

   a. 1.3 times body weight
   b. body weight
   c. two times body weight
   d. one half of body weight

4. A collegiate discus thrower weighing 240 lb has 1RM values of 450 lb in the squat and 390 lb in the bench press. His training priority should be

   a. upper body strength
   b. gaining body weight
   c. lower body strength
   d. *a* and *c*

Applying Knowledge of Muscle Balance

Problem 1
A program for a swimmer that includes squats, knee extensions, calf raises, lat pulldowns, back extensions, internal shoulder rotations, pullovers, and upright rows should also contain what exercises to achieve or maintain muscle balance?

Problem 2
A right-handed guard in basketball injured her left knee and required reconstructive surgery of her anterior cruciate ligament. Her weight and fitness marks before the injury and at present—6 months after the surgery—are seen in the accompanying table. What should she do at this stage of her rehabilitation?

Fitness parameter	Value prior to injury	Value 6 months after surgery
Body weight (lb)	133	129
1RM squat (lb)	185	110
1 RM power clean (lb)	120	90
20-yd dash (s)	2.9	3.7
10-yd shuttle run (s)	4.5	6.1
300-yd shuttle run (s)	57	75
Right-knee extension, flexion (at 60°/s; ft-lb)	148, 102	145, 100
Left-knee extension, flexion (at 60°/s; ft-lb)	141, 99	139, 95

References

1. Beam, W.C., R.L. Bartels, and R.W. Ward. The relationship of isokinetic torque to body weight and to lean body weight in athletes. *Med. Sci. Sports Exerc.* 14:178. 1982.
2. Burkett, L.N. Causative factors in hamstring strains. *Med. Sci. Sports Exerc.* 2:39-42. 1970.
3. Cybex, Division of Lumex, Inc. *Isolated Joint Testing and Exercise: A Handbook for Using Cybex II and U.B.X.T.* Bay Shore, NY: Author. 1980.
4. Christensen, C.S. Relative strength in males and females. *Athletic Training* 10:189-192. 1975.
5. Davies, G.J. *A Compendium of Isokinetics in Clinical Usage*, 2nd ed. LaCrosse, WI: S&S Publishers. 1985.
6. Davies, G.J., D.T. Kirkendall, D.H. Leigh, M.L. Lui, T.R. Reinbold, and R.K. Wilson. Isokinetic characteristics of professional football players: Normative relationships between quadriceps and hamstring muscle groups and relative to body weight. *Med. Sci. Sports Exerc.* 13:76. 1981.
7. Dibrezzo, R., B.E. Gench, M.M. Hinson, and J. King. Peak torque values of the knee extensor and flexor muscles of females. *J. Orthop. Sports Phys. Ther.* 7:65-68. 1985.
8. Falkel, J. Plantar flexor strength testing using the Cybex Isokinetic Dynamometer. *Phys. Ther.* 58:847-850. 1978.
9. Figoni, S, C.B. Christ, and B.H. Mossey. Effects of speed, hip and knee angle and gravity on hamstring to quadriceps torque ratios. *J. Orthop. Sports Phys. Ther.* 9(8):287-291. 1988.
10. Fillyaw, M., T. Bevins, and L. Fernandez. Importance of correcting isokinetic peak torque for the effects of gravity when calculating knee flexor to extensor muscle ratios. *Phys. Ther.* 66:23-29. 1986.
11. Fugl-Meyer, A.R. Maximum isokinetic ankle plantar and dorsal flexion torques in trained subjects. *Eur. J. Appl. Physiol.* 47:393-404. 1981.
12. Fugl-Meyer, A.R., L. Gustafsson, and Y. Burstedt. Isokinetic and static plantar flexion characteristics. *Eur. J. Appl. Physiol.* 45:221-234. 1980.
13. Gilliam, T.B., S.P. Sady, P.S. Freedon, and J. Valamacci. Isokinetic torque levels for high school football players. *Arch. Phys. Med. Rehabil.* 60:110-114. 1979.
14. Goslin, B.R., and J. Charteris. Isokinetic dynamometry: Normative data for clinical use in lower extremity (knee) cases. *Scand. J. Rehabil. Med.* 11:105-109. 1979.
15. Grace, T., E.R. Sweetser, M.A. Nelson, L.R. Ydens, and B.J. Skipper. Isokinetic muscle imbalance and knee joint injuries. *J. Bone Joint Surg.* 66A:734. 1984.
16. Haymes, E.M., and A.L. Dickinson. Characteristics of elite male and female ski races. *Med. Sci. Sports Exerc.* 12:153-158. 1980.

17. Housh, T.J., W.G. Thorland, G.O. Tharp, G.O. Johnson, and C.J. Cisar. Isokinetic leg flexion and extension strength of elite adolescent female track and field athletes. *Res. Q.* 55:347-350. 1984.

18. Hunter, S., T.E. Cain, and C. Henry. Preseason isokinetic knee evaluation in professional football athletes. *Athletic Training* 14:205-206. 1979.

19. Imwold, C.H., R.A. Rider, E.M. Haymes, and K.D. Green. Isokinetic torque differences between college female varsity basketball and track athletes. *J. Sports Med.* 23:67-73. 1983.

20. Ivey, F.M., J.H. Calhoun, K. Rusche, and J. Bierschenk. Normal values for isokinetic testing of shoulder strength (abstract). *Arch. Phys. Med. Rehabil.* 66:384-386. 1984.

21. Klein, K., and F. Allman. *The Knee in Sports.* Baltimore: Williams & Wilkins. 1970.

22. Laird, D.E. Comparison of quadricep to hamstring strength ratios of an intercollegiate soccer team. *Athletic Training* 16:66-67. 1981.

23. Lehman, R., and A. Delitto. *Clinics in Sports Medicine: Rehabilitation*, vol. 8, no. 4. Philadelphia: Saunders. 1989.

24. Liemohn, W. Factors related to hamstring strains. *J. Sports Med.* 18:71-76. 1978.

25. Moore, J., and G. Wade. Prevention of anterior cruciate ligament injuries. *NSCA Journal* 11(3):35-40. 1989.

26. Murray, M.P., G.M. Gardner, L.A. Molinger, and S.B. Sepic. Strength of isometric and isokinetic contractions. *Phys. Ther.* 60:412-419. 1980.

27. Nosse, L.J. Assessment of selected reports on the strength relationship of the knee musculature. *J. Orthop. Sports Phys. Ther.* 4:78-84. 1982.

28. Osternig, L.R., J.A. Sawhill, B.T. Bates, and J. Hamill. Function of limb speed on torque ratios of antagonist muscles and peak torque joint position. *Med. Sci. Sports Exerc.* 13:107. 1981.

29. Parker, M.G., D. Holt, E. Bauman, M. Drayna, and R.O. Ruhling. Descriptive analysis of bilateral quadriceps and hamstring muscle torque in high school football players. *Med. Sci. Sports Exerc.* 14:152. 1982.

30. Rankin, J.M., and C.B. Thompson. Isokinetic evaluation of quadriceps and hamstring function: Normative data concerning body weight and sport. *Athletic Training* 18:110-113. 1983.

31. Schlinkman, B. Norms for high school football players derived from Cybex data reduction computer. *J. Orthop. Sports Phys. Ther.* 5:410-412. 1984.

32. Scudder, G.N. Torque curves produced at the knee during isometric and isokinetic exercises. *Arch. Phys. Med. Rehabil.* 61:68-73. 1980.

33. Sherman, W.S., M.J. Plyley, D. Vogelgesang, D.L. Costill, and A.J. Habansky. Isokinetic strength during rehabilitation following arthrotomy: Specificity of speed. *Athletic Training* 16:138-141. 1981.

34. Smith, D.J., H.A. Quinney, H.A. Wenger, R.D. Steadward, and J.R. Sexsmith. Isokinetic torque outputs of professional and elite amateur ice hockey players. *J. Orthop. Sports Phys. Ther.* 3:42-47. 1981.

35. Thomas, L. Isokinetic torque levels for adult females: Effects of age and body size. *J. Orthop. Sports Phys. Ther.* 6:21-24. 1984.

36. Wong, D.L.K., M. Glasheen-Wray, and L.F. Andrews. Isokinetic evaluation of the ankle inverters. *J. Orthop. Sports Phys. Ther.* 5:158-164. 1984.

37. Wyatt, M.P., and A.M. Edwards. Comparison of quadriceps and hamstring torque values during isokinetic exercise. *J. Orthop. Sports Phys. Ther.* 3:48-56. 1981.

CHAPTER 25

EXERCISE ORDER

Dan Wathen

The sequence in which exercises are performed within a workout interacts with all other program design variables. Should exercises be in less than an optimal sequence, the athlete's ability to perform the desired load (average weight/repetitions) and volume (total repetitions × average load) of each exercise may be compromised. This chapter presents guidelines for sequencing exercises within workouts, depending on the period of the training cycle. The current physical condition of the athlete may play a role in determining the order of exercise during all periods of the training cycle. Another consideration during all periods is the individual's strengths and weaknesses. The areas of weakness should demand priority in the workout sequence (2-6).

PREPARATORY PERIOD

Exercise sequence during the three main phases of the preparatory period are discussed in the following sections.

Phase I: Hypertrophy/Endurance Phase

The first phase of the preparatory period is largely devoted to developing a conditioning base, which most often consists of nonspecific exercises that train all major muscle groups. During this phase volume is high and intensity low, and traditional circuit weight training may be employed. The sequence of exercises in circuit weight training and other regimes normally alternate upper body and lower body exercises, to allow muscles to rest while other muscles are being exercised.

Because muscle endurance, hypertrophy, or both are the goals of this phase of training, general muscle-building techniques may be employed (1-4). Several techniques are possible:

- **Super setting** involves alternating agonists and antagonists of a joint with minimal rest between exercises. Examples are biceps curls and triceps presses, and knee extensions and leg curls.

- **Compound setting** involves performing two different exercises for the same muscle group in an alternating fashion with little to no rest between exercises; this, of course, is more intense than super setting. Examples are barbell curls followed by dumbbell alternating curls, and dumbbell side bends followed by torso rotations.

- **Preexhaustion** is a training technique that is often employed when the athlete feels that multiple-joint movement is not completely exhausting or developing the targeted muscle. In this technique, a muscle is fatigued in a single-joint, isolated movement prior to performing a multiple-joint exercise involving the same muscle. An example is preceding squats with leg curls to give hamstring fatigue.

Athletes in poor physical condition may find super setting, compound setting, and preexhaustion techniques too strenuous in the early stages of training. They would be better served with an alternation of muscle groups until their physical condition improves to the point where they can perform the activities without undue stress (2).

Other training activities, such as running, swimming, cycling, and rowing, may also be done at high volume and low intensity. In order to gain the most benefit from each activity, they should be performed on separate days or as far apart during the day as time permits (1). (This holds true for all phases of a mesocycle.)

Phase II: Strength Phase

During the strength phase of the preparatory period, more activity-specific movements are introduced. Many of these exercises involve multiple joints and therefore require more energy expenditure than single-joint movements; for free-weight exercises, greater balance and coordination are also required. Most authorities recommend that the multiple-joint exercises be placed first in the exercise order during this phase of training (2-6). Some further contend that multiple-joint lifts requiring the most skill, speed, and coordination be done first (3-5). For example, squats would be placed ahead of knee curls, and power cleans and snatches ahead of squats. The reasons for this sequence are as follows (2-6):

- The more difficult exercises should be performed when the athlete is fresh.
- Single-joint exercises may unduly fatigue some of the muscles critical for success in the multiple-joint movement.
- The gross motor activity can serve as a warm-up for the single-joint activities to follow in the workout.
- Maximal power may not be derived if the muscles involved in a movement are prefatigued by single-joint exercises (2-6).

These are all reasonable points to justify exercise order. For example, power cleans require a large energy expenditure, so it may not be possible to handle the prescribed loads if the exercise is done later in the workout. It is also reasonable to expect a decrement in performance if upright rows are done before power cleans, but power cleans serve as a good warm-up for upright rows, shrugs, calf raises, and back extensions.

There are occasions during the strength phase in which exercise order is varied so that a different training stimulus is provided to the muscles and the demands of competitions simulated (2, 4, 6). For example, many field events, as well as football games, often span a number of hours during which the athlete must give maximal effort after he or she has already become somewhat fatigued. A sequence such as hip flexion and extension, knee flexion and extension, hip adduction and abduction, and calf raises could serve as a warm-up, at an intensity high enough to cause some fatigue, for squats. The single-joint movements would be performed with moderately heavy loads (8RM-10RM range).

Many prefer to continue alternating muscle groups during the strength phase to further enhance recovery of each muscle group (3). An example of exercise order during this phase might be:

1. power snatches
2. incline presses
3. front squats
4. wrist curls
5. calf raises
6. torso rotations
7. glute-ham-gastroc raises

Phase III: Power Phase

During the final phase of the preparatory period, sport-specific gross motor activities should be placed first in the workout (2-5). This includes such multiple-joint and structural exercises as power cleans and snatches, push jerks, squats, plyometrics, and speed drills. Single-joint exercises follow, with weaker-joint exercises given sequential priority over stronger-joint exercises, for injury prevention. The power phase is characterized by higher loads and intensity and lower volume of work than the strength phase, with high rest-to-work ratios. High-speed running, swimming, and cycling intervals along with high-intensity plyometric drills are incorporated in this phase and should be conducted on separate days from resistance training.

COMPETITION PERIOD

The competition period follows the preparatory period; in it, little time is given to conditioning activities. Strength training is abbreviated in frequency, number of exercises, and volume, while loads are kept high (2-6). Multiple-joint exercises predominate during the workouts, owing to time constraints since it takes less time to do one multiple-joint exercise rather than several single-joint exercises. One to three sets of two to eight repetitions are generally utilized. The number of repetitions can be modified so that the greatest loads are used prior to the most important competitions to maximize strength-and-power levels. Also, the competition period should have the most important activities first in the workout. For example, a track sprinter with 4 weeks of dual meets prior to a regional competition would employ power cleans, power jerks, and lunges, in that order. Activities such as plyometrics and single-joint exercises are usually deleted from training during this period because they require additional training time or recovery time.

WARM-UPS AND COOL-DOWNS

Warm-up activities should precede each training session, which should end with a cool-down period of low-intensity activity. During the early part of the preparatory period the high number of repetitions requires only one or two warm-up sets; use warm-ups similar to the actual exercises, but with less resistance. As one enters more specific phases of the preparatory period, the significantly greater loads necessitate more warm-up activities to ensure optimal performance (2,4-6). This is true of relatively complex motor activities, such as power cleans and snatches. Multiple-joint activities may act as a warm-up for any subsequent single-joint movements involving the same muscles. Low-intensity single-joint movements may act as cool-down activities, because they require considerably less energy expenditure (2,3,6). More specific warm-up regimes are covered in chapter 19.

CONCLUSION

Exercises placed first in a workout are performed relatively well, owing to higher energy levels and less fatigue. Exercises placed later in a workout will not be performed with the same level of intensity that they would have been if they were placed first. Generally, multiple-joint, structural, large–muscle mass exercises precede single-joint, isolation, small–muscle mass exercises in most phases of training. An exception is the early part of the preparatory phase; additionally, the sequence may be altered in other phases for variation. Warm-ups with less weight than the actual training exercise should be performed, especially for multiple-joint movements. Cool-down can be achieved with single-joint activities of low intensity.

Key Terms

compound setting	431	preexhaustion	431	super setting	431

Study Questions

1. During the Phase I preparatory period of an athlete's training, she wishes to engage in traditional endurance circuit weight training. Which of the following sequences would be in the proper order?

    a. lat pulldowns, knee extensions, wrist curls, hip adductions, triceps presses, knee curls, chest flys, hip abductions
    b. chest presses, triceps presses, knee curls, leg presses, pullovers, chin-ups, arm curls, calf raises
    c. knee extensions, squats, chest flys, dips, arm curls, lat pulldowns, incline presses, triceps presses
    d. arm curls, triceps presses, chest presses, lat pulldowns, leg curls, leg extensions, leg raises, leg presses

2. Which of the following exercise sequences provides the best warm-up and cool-down progression?

    a. squats, bench presses, deadlifts, chin-ups, knee curls, lat raises, calf raises
    b. power cleans, incline presses, knee extensions, front raises, arm curls, leg presses
    c. hip adductions, leg curls, arm curls, triceps presses, wrist curls, bench presses, squats
    d. front squats, leg curls, deadlifts, dips, push presses, arm curls

3. To develop the most overall body power, which of the following sequences is most appropriate?

    a. power snatches, push presses, front squats, glute-ham-gastroc raises, wrist curls
    b. power squats, deadlifts, bench presses, calf raises, lat raises, chin-ups
    c. lunges, lat pulldowns, knee extensions, triceps presses, shrug pulls, push presses
    d. shrugs, arm curls, leg curls, power cleans, good mornings, leg presses

Applying Knowledge of Exercise Order

Problem 1

A tennis player has a test profile that identifies him as generally weak with low power in both upper and lower extremities. Flexibility is average in all joints, and endurance is good to excellent. The athlete has a history of ankle injuries. Place the following exercises in the order that would be most appropriate during the strength and power phases of the preparatory period of training: torso rotations, squats, pullovers, clean pulls, push presses, knee curls, lat raises, calf raises, supine flys.

Problem 2

A female gymnast with excellent flexibility and power but poor endurance and a history of low back injury is participating in the hypertrophy/endurance phase of the preparatory period of training. She will be engaged in traditional circuit training during this phase. Place the following exercises in the most appropriate order: calf raises, dips, back extensions, lat pulldowns, torso rotations, leg curls, abdominal curls, straight-arm pullovers, knee extensions.

References

1. Craig, B.W., J. Lucas, R. Pohlman, and H. Schilling. The effect of running, weightlifting and a combination of both on growth hormone release. *J. Appl. Sports Sci. Res* 5(4):198-203. 1991.
2. Fleck, S.J., and W.J. Kraemer. *Designing Resistance Training Programs*. Champaign, IL: Human Kinetics. 1987.
3. Pauletto, B. Choice and order of exercises. *NSCA Journal* 8(2):71-73. 1986.
4. Stone, M., and H. O'Bryant. *Weight Training*. Minneapolis: Burgess International. 1987.
5. Verhoshansky, Y. *Fundamentals of Special Strength Training in Sport*. Livonia, MI: Sportivny Press. 1976.
6. Westcott, W. *Strength Fitness*. Boston: Allyn & Bacon. 1982.

CHAPTER 26

LOAD ASSIGNMENT

Dan Wathen

Training *intensity* is recognized as the most critical aspect of a conditioning regime (5,6,12,17). Intensity of training is often synonymous with training **load** (amount of weight per repetition). Scientists describe **intensity** as the power output of an exercise (5,6,10,17); *power* is work per unit of time, or force times the velocity of movement. Power output, and thus intensity, is dependent upon the load and the speed of movement in the exercise.

For most athletes, intensity is most easily represented as a percentage of one's **repetition maximum (RM)** for an exercise. RM refers to the maximal number of repetitions that can be performed with a load. For example, if an athlete can do five (but not six) repetitions of a certain exercise with a load of 100 kg, he is said to have a 5RM of 100 kg. The accuracy of the RM is increased with proper warm-up, rest intervals, motivation, and familiarity with the exercise. In addition to being described in absolute terms of power output, intensity may be stated in relative terms, that is, as a percentage of an athlete's 1RM. For example, if an athlete's 1RM for the bench press is 100 kg, a *relative* intensity of 60% of 1RM for this exercise means doing repetitions with 60 kg.

Relative intensity varies with age, sex, physical condition, and health status. A heavy load for one athlete may not tax another, even when represented in relative, not absolute, terms. For example, an athlete who has a 1RM of 40 kg in an exercise and who has been training for a few weeks may not be highly taxed with a 70% load for 10 repetitions at slow speeds. An athlete with 8 years of training and a 1RM of 240 kg in the same exercise may be heavily taxed with a 70% load for 10 repetitions at any speed. This is in part due to a decrease in relative muscular endurance as absolute strength improves (1,11,13).

Load, speed, volume, and rest period length influence each other. Heavy-load and high-volume workouts with short rest periods are difficult. High speed of movement usually requires low to moderate loads. Exceptions would be such activities as power cleans, snatches, and pulls and plyometrics, in which speed is necessary to properly perform the activity. Training frequency also depends upon load. High-intensity workouts cannot be done as frequently as moderate- to low-intensity workouts without risking overtraining (5,10,12,17).

Using a percentage of the RM is one of the simplest methods of determining the load that an athlete should use. (Details of this determination are discussed in a later section.) Athletes with little background in resistance training often establish a new RM with whatever repetition scheme they are using, which changes from workout to workout, until their neural adaptations are developed. No matter what percentage of RM an athlete is using, he or she should attempt to perform as many repetitions in as good a form as possible with each heavy set. Experienced athletes usually find that there is very little variation in their RM capabilities over the short term, so that using percentages of their RM for a predetermined specific number of repetitions is usually accurate.

DETERMINING THE RM

Determining an athlete's RM is a relatively simple task when he or she is experienced and well rested. However, beginning trainees sometimes have not developed the skill, balance, and other neurological attributes that would allow for a safe and effective RM testing procedure. In the early stages of training, it may be appropriate to use a higher RM value (e.g., 10RM). Estimating a 1RM or higher is a relatively easy process when a table such as Table 26.1 is used.

Table 26.1 Estimating One–Repetition Maximum

% of 1RM:	100.0	93.5	91.0	88.5	86.0	83.5	81.0	78.5	76.0	73.5
Repetitions:	1	2	3	4	5	6	7	8	9	10
Weight lifted (lb): 0.0	0.0	0.0	0.0	0.0	0.0	0.0	0.0	0.0	0.0	0.0
5.0	4.7	4.5	4.4	4.3	4.2	4.1	3.9	3.8	3.7	
10.0	9.4	9.1	8.9	8.6	8.4	8.2	7.9	7.6	7.4	
15.0	14.0	13.7	13.3	12.9	12.5	12.2	11.8	11.4	11.0	
20.0	18.7	18.2	17.7	17.2	16.7	16.2	15.7	15.2	14.7	
25.0	23.4	22.8	22.1	21.5	20.9	20.2	19.6	19.0	18.4	
30.0	28.1	27.3	26.6	25.8	25.1	24.3	23.6	22.8	22.1	
35.0	32.7	31.9	31.0	30.1	29.2	28.4	27.5	26.6	25.7	
40.0	37.4	36.4	35.4	34.4	33.4	32.4	31.4	30.4	29.4	
45.0	42.1	41.0	39.8	38.7	37.6	36.5	35.3	34.2	33.1	
50.0	46.8	45.5	44.3	43.0	41.8	40.5	39.3	38.0	36.8	
55.0	51.4	50.1	48.7	47.3	45.9	44.6	43.2	41.8	40.4	
60.0	56.1	54.6	53.1	51.6	50.1	48.6	47.1	45.6	44.1	
65.0	60.8	59.2	57.5	55.9	54.3	52.7	51.0	49.4	47.8	
70.0	65.5	63.7	62.0	60.2	58.5	56.7	55.0	53.2	51.5	
75.0	70.1	68.3	66.4	64.5	62.6	60.8	58.9	57.0	55.1	
80.0	74.8	72.8	70.8	68.8	66.8	64.8	62.8	60.8	58.8	
85.0	79.5	77.4	75.2	73.1	71.0	68.9	66.7	64.6	62.5	
90.0	84.2	81.9	79.7	77.4	75.2	72.9	70.7	68.4	66.2	
95.0	88.8	86.5	84.1	81.7	79.3	77.0	74.6	72.2	69.8	
100.0	93.5	91.0	88.5	86.0	83.5	81.0	78.5	76.0	73.5	
105.0	98.2	95.6	92.9	90.3	87.7	85.1	82.4	79.8	77.2	
110.0	102.9	100.1	97.4	94.6	91.9	89.1	86.4	83.6	80.9	
115.0	107.5	104.7	101.8	98.9	96.0	93.2	90.3	87.4	84.5	
120.0	112.2	109.2	106.2	103.2	100.2	97.2	94.2	91.2	88.2	
125.0	116.9	113.8	110.6	107.5	104.4	101.3	98.1	95.0	91.9	
130.0	121.6	118.3	115.1	111.8	108.6	105.3	102.1	98.8	95.6	
135.0	126.2	122.9	119.5	116.1	112.7	109.4	106.0	102.6	99.2	
140.0	130.9	127.4	123.9	120.4	116.9	113.4	109.9	106.4	102.9	
145.0	135.6	132.0	128.3	124.7	121.1	117.5	113.8	110.2	106.6	
150.0	140.3	136.5	132.8	129.0	125.3	121.5	117.8	114.0	110.3	
155.0	144.9	141.1	137.2	133.3	129.4	125.6	121.7	117.8	113.9	
160.0	149.6	145.6	141.6	137.6	133.6	129.6	125.6	121.6	117.6	
165.0	154.3	150.2	146.0	141.9	137.8	133.7	129.5	125.4	121.3	
170.0	159.0	154.7	150.5	146.2	142.0	137.7	133.5	129.2	125.0	
175.0	163.6	159.3	154.9	150.5	146.1	141.8	137.4	133.0	128.6	
180.0	168.3	163.8	159.3	154.8	150.3	145.8	141.3	136.8	132.3	
185.0	173.0	168.4	163.7	159.1	154.5	149.9	145.2	140.6	136.0	
190.0	177.7	172.9	168.2	163.4	158.7	153.9	149.2	144.4	139.7	
195.0	182.3	177.5	172.6	167.7	162.8	158.0	153.1	148.2	143.3	

(continued)

Table 26.1 *(continued)*

% of 1RM:	100.0	93.5	91.0	88.5	86.0	83.5	81.0	78.5	76.0	73.5
Repetitions:	1	2	3	4	5	6	7	8	9	10
Weight lifted (lb): 200.0	187.0	182.0	177.0	172.0	167.0	162.0	157.0	152.0	147.0
205.0	191.7	186.6	181.4	176.3	171.2	166.1	160.9	155.8	150.7
210.0	196.4	191.1	185.9	180.6	175.4	170.1	164.9	159.6	154.4
215.0	201.0	195.7	190.3	184.9	179.5	174.2	168.8	163.4	158.0
220.0	205.7	200.2	194.7	189.2	183.7	178.2	182.7	167.2	161.7
225.0	210.4	204.8	199.1	193.5	187.9	182.3	176.6	171.0	165.4
230.0	215.1	209.3	203.6	197.8	192.1	186.3	180.6	174.8	169.1
235.0	219.7	213.9	208.0	202.1	196.2	190.4	184.5	178.6	172.7
240.0	224.4	218.4	212.4	206.4	200.4	194.4	188.4	182.4	176.4
245.0	229.1	223.0	216.8	210.7	204.6	198.5	192.3	186.2	180.1
250.0	233.8	227.5	221.3	215.0	208.8	202.5	196.3	190.0	183.8
255.0	238.4	232.1	225.7	219.3	212.9	206.6	200.2	193.8	187.4
260.0	243.1	236.6	230.1	223.6	217.1	210.6	204.1	197.6	191.2
265.0	247.8	241.2	234.5	227.9	221.3	214.7	208.1	201.4	194.8
270.0	252.5	245.7	239.0	232.2	225.5	218.7	212.0	205.2	198.5
275.0	257.1	250.3	243.4	236.5	229.6	222.8	215.9	209.0	202.1
280.0	261.8	254.8	247.8	240.8	233.8	226.8	219.8	212.8	205.8
285.0	266.5	259.4	252.2	245.1	238.0	230.9	223.7	216.6	209.5
290.0	271.2	263.9	256.7	249.4	242.5	234.9	227.7	220.4	213.2
295.0	275.9	268.5	261.1	253.7	246.3	239.0	231.6	224.2	216.8
300.0	280.5	273.0	265.5	258.0	250.5	243.0	235.5	228.0	220.5
305.0	285.2	277.6	269.9	262.3	254.7	247.1	239.4	231.8	224.2
310.0	289.9	282.1	274.4	266.6	258.9	251.1	243.4	235.6	227.9
315.0	294.5	286.7	278.8	270.9	263.0	255.2	247.3	239.4	231.5
320.0	299.2	291.2	283.2	275.2	267.2	259.2	251.2	243.2	235.2
325.0	303.9	295.8	287.6	279.5	271.4	263.3	255.1	247.0	238.9
330.0	308.6	300.3	292.1	283.8	275.9	267.3	259.1	250.8	242.6
335.0	313.2	304.9	296.5	288.1	279.7	271.4	263.0	254.6	246.2
340.0	317.9	309.4	300.9	292.4	283.9	275.4	266.9	258.4	249.9
345.0	322.6	314.0	305.3	296.7	288.1	279.5	270.8	262.2	253.6
350.0	327.3	318.5	309.8	301.0	292.3	283.6	274.8	266.0	257.3
355.0	331.9	323.1	314.2	305.3	296.4	287.6	278.7	269.8	260.9
360.0	336.6	327.6	318.6	309.6	300.6	291.6	282.6	273.6	264.6
365.0	341.3	332.2	323.0	313.9	304.8	295.7	286.5	277.4	268.3
370.0	346.0	336.7	327.5	318.2	309.0	299.7	290.5	281.2	272.0
375.0	350.6	341.3	331.9	322.5	313.1	303.8	294.4	285.0	275.6
380.0	355.3	345.8	336.3	326.8	317.3	307.8	298.3	288.8	279.3
385.0	360.0	350.4	340.7	331.1	321.5	311.9	302.2	292.6	283.0
390.0	364.7	354.9	345.2	335.4	325.7	315.9	306.2	296.4	286.7
395.0	369.3	359.5	349.6	339.7	329.8	320.0	310.1	300.2	290.3

(continued)

Table 26.1 *(continued)*

% of 1RM:	100.0	93.5	91.0	88.5	86.0	83.5	81.0	78.5	76.0	73.5
Repetitions:	1	2	3	4	5	6	7	8	9	10
Weight lifted (lb): 400.0	374.0	364.0	354.0	344.0	334.0	324.0	314.0	304.0	294.0
405.0	378.7	368.6	358.4	348.3	338.2	328.1	317.9	307.8	297.7
410.0	383.4	373.1	362.9	352.6	342.4	332.1	321.9	311.6	301.4
415.0	388.0	377.7	367.3	356.9	346.5	336.2	325.8	315.4	305.0
420.0	392.7	382.2	371.7	361.2	350.7	340.2	329.7	319.2	308.7
425.0	397.4	386.8	376.1	365.5	354.9	344.3	333.6	323.0	312.4
430.0	402.1	391.3	380.6	369.8	359.1	348.3	337.6	326.8	316.1
435.0	406.7	395.9	385.0	374.1	363.2	352.4	341.5	330.6	319.7
440.0	411.4	400.4	389.4	378.4	367.4	356.4	345.4	334.4	323.4
445.0	416.1	405.0	393.8	382.7	371.6	360.5	349.3	338.2	327.1
450.0	420.8	409.5	398.3	287.0	375.8	364.5	353.3	342.0	330.8
455.0	425.4	414.1	402.7	391.3	379.9	368.6	357.2	345.8	334.4

Example for Estimating the 1RM

To estimate 1RM from a 10RM test-measured value, have the athlete perform a set of 10 repetitions with a light weight. Depending on the ease with which this is completed, add additional weight and have the athlete perform another set of 10 repetitions. A rest of 2 to 4 min should be allowed between trials to insure adequate recuperation. Continue the process until a weight allowing *only* 10 repetitions is discovered. An experienced instructor can aid the athlete by supervising the process so that the 10RM value can be discovered in fewer than five trials. The athlete can then consult a table (such as Table 26.1) and find in the 10-repetition column the weight he or she achieved and then find the weight on the same line in the 1RM column to estimate his or her 1RM. For example, 10 repetitions with 305 lb yields in Table 26.1 a 1RM of 415 lb. Values may vary somewhat from table to table.

These tables are controversial as to their accuracy for different athletes and different lifts (7); they seem to be more accurate for free-weight and multiple-joint exercises than for machine exercises. They are intended to provide a general guide until the trainee has developed the neural and proprioceptive attributes that would make testing at low RMs (1RM-5RM) safe and effective (5,10,17). For example, after 2 weeks of introductory training (2 to 6 sessions), an RM could be established with a weight that allows for, say, 10 repetitions. Tables can be consulted to estimate the 1RM for further load assignment over the coming weeks. After 6 weeks (12-18 training sessions), a 1RM to 5RM test can be conducted. Strength-and-power athletes may benefit from

training with percentages of an established 1RM; other athletes may equally benefit from training with percentages of a 5RM or 10RM. The results obtained from lower RM testing are generally more accurate when an athlete has been training with low-RM resistances for a few training sessions prior to testing.

Excessive trials (sets) may fatigue the trainee to the point where an accurate estimate cannot be made. Some exercises, such as power cleans and snatches, do not lend themselves well to RM testing above five repetitions, owing to rapid deterioration of technique with fatigue. However, lower RM determinations can be made once the athlete has sufficient technique and experience. A very simple alternate method for estimating a low RM has been proposed (5); this method utilizes an RM continuum (Figure 26.1). Through trial and error, the athlete determines and utilizes weights at a variety of RMs to train with, depending on the phase or period of the training cycle. For example, early in a training cycle, weights at 10 RM to 12RM would be determined and utilized. As more repetitions are able to be performed with the 10RM to 12RM weight, the athlete adds weight. As the cycle progresses, the trainee adds intensity (resistance) as he or she moves through the RM continuum from high to low RMs.

Determining weights at various RMs is easier with machines than with free-weight equipment. This is due to the motor learning factor, which has more of an influence with free weight apparatus; balance and coordination are not critical with machines. Most athletes are able to accurately find their 5RM to 10RM weights after a week or so of machine training. Many weeks may be needed to accurately and safely determine the

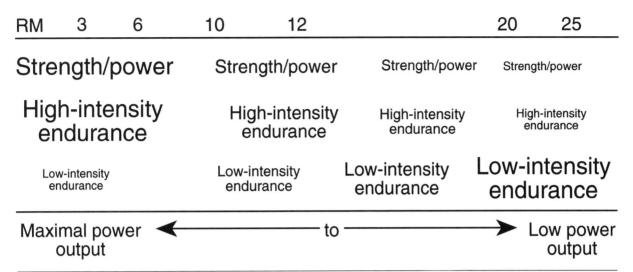

RM	3	6	10	12		20	25

Strength/power   Strength/power   Strength/power   Strength/power

High-intensity endurance   High-intensity endurance   High-intensity endurance   High-intensity endurance

Low-intensity endurance   Low-intensity endurance   Low-intensity endurance   **Low-intensity endurance**

Maximal power output ◄———————— to ————————► Low power output

Figure 26.1   Theoretical repetition maximum continuum.
Reprinted from Fleck and Kraemer (1987).

weights of lower RMs with free-weight apparatus, especially with multiple-joint movements, such as squats and power cleans.

It is more accurate to exercise with percentages of a test-established RM weight than it is to estimate one (5,8,9,11,14). A table such as Table 26.2 can be posted strategically in the weight room so that athletes can quickly determine how much weight corresponds to a given percentage of the weight at the RM at which they are training.

Precautions

Athletes desiring RM testing should be cleared by a physician for unlimited activities. A safety check of equipment should be made prior to testing. An adequate number of trained spotters or equipment with safety catches, such as power racks, must be employed with such free-weight exercises as squats and bench presses. Athletes to be tested should be properly dressed, rested, and very familiar with the exercises. Supervisors and other personnel should know emergency medical procedures in case an accident or injury occurs (10).

Warm Up

A safe and accurate RM test requires warm-up sets. Warm-up allows for optimal muscle contraction and elasticity (5,6,10,11,17,21). Stronger athletes usually need more warm-up sets prior to RM attempts. Although there is no scientifically supported best warm-up regime for RM attempts, enough warm-up sets should be employed to raise core temperature and allow for mental readiness and focus on the task (5,6,10,11,17). Generally, the first set of warm-up activities should be with

weights of 50% to 70% of the RM weight to be attempted. A second warm-up, at 75% to 80%, may be employed, with further warm-up sets in 5 to 10 percentage point increments. Lifts requiring a high level of skill, such as power cleans and snatches, usually require numerous warm-ups and more gradual increments than less complex activities such as bench presses. For example, Spassov recommends 10 to 18 warm-up attempts before a maximum effort in Olympic lifts (16). (Yet a former superheavy world-record holder in the squat used a three-set workout consisting of 450 lb for three repetitions for the first warm-up set, 700 lb for three repetitions for the second warm-up set, and 900 lb for the actual 3RM [22].) An example of progressive warm-up weights for various loads used at the University of Tennessee is seen in Table 26.3 (12). Trial and error will eventually produce the warm-up scheme that best suits an individual athlete.

LOAD ASSIGNMENT

Once the weight for a given RM has been established, assigning the load to be used in subsequent workouts is relatively simple: A percentage of the RM is utilized in each workout for a specific number of sets and repetitions or for sets of RM at the assigned load.

The amount of resistance required for strength gains is not known for all populations. Studies (5) indicate that inexperienced trainees can make strength gains with loads as low as 35% of isometric 1RM in isometric training and loads of 45% of 1RM in circuit training. Some trainers feel that elite athletes require a load of at least 80% of 1RM for strength gains (7,14,17). Pioneering studies (5,6,10,11,17) indicate that an athlete

Table 26.2 Weight Training Percentages (Rounded to 5 lb)

1RM weight (lb)	40%	45%	50%	55%	60%	65%	70%	75%	80%	85%	90%	95%	105%
50	20	25	25	30	30	35	35	40	40	45	45	45	55
60	25	30	30	35	35	40	40	45	50	55	55	55	65
70	30	35	35	40	40	50	50	55	55	60	60	65	75
80	30	40	45	50	50	55	60	65	70	70	75	75	85
90	35	40	45	50	55	60	65	65	75	80	80	85	95
100	40	45	50	55	60	65	70	75	80	85	90	95	105
110	45	50	55	60	65	70	75	85	90	95	100	105	115
120	50	55	60	65	70	80	85	90	95	100	110	115	125
130	55	60	65	70	80	85	90	100	105	110	115	125	135
140	55	65	70	75	85	90	100	105	110	120	125	135	150
150	60	70	75	85	90	100	105	115	120	130	135	145	160
160	65	75	80	90	95	105	110	120	130	135	145	150	170
170	70	80	85	95	100	110	120	125	135	145	155	160	180
180	70	80	90	100	110	115	125	135	145	155	160	170	190
190	75	85	90	105	115	125	135	145	150	160	170	180	200
200	80	90	100	110	120	130	140	150	160	170	180	190	210
210	85	100	105	115	125	135	145	155	170	180	190	190	220
220	90	100	110	120	130	145	155	165	175	185	200	210	230
230	95	105	115	125	140	150	160	175	185	195	205	220	240
240	95	110	120	130	145	155	170	180	190	205	215	230	255
250	100	115	125	140	150	165	175	190	200	215	225	240	265
260	105	120	130	145	155	170	180	195	210	220	235	245	275
270	110	125	135	150	160	175	190	200	215	230	245	255	285
280	110	125	140	155	170	180	195	210	225	240	250	265	295
290	115	130	145	160	175	190	205	220	230	245	260	275	305
300	120	135	150	165	180	195	210	225	240	255	270	285	315
310	125	140	155	170	185	200	215	230	250	265	280	295	325
320	130	145	160	175	190	210	225	240	255	270	290	305	335
330	135	150	165	180	200	215	230	250	265	280	300	315	345
340	135	155	170	185	205	220	240	255	270	290	305	325	360
350	145	160	175	195	210	230	245	265	280	300	315	335	370
360	140	160	190	200	220	230	250	270	290	310	320	340	380
390	160	180	200	210	230	250	270	290	310	330	350	370	410
420	170	190	210	230	250	270	290	320	340	360	380	400	440
450	180	200	230	250	270	290	320	340	360	380	410	430	475
480	190	220	240	260	290	310	340	360	380	410	430	460	505
510	200	230	260	280	310	330	360	380	410	430	460	490	535
540	220	240	270	300	320	350	380	410	430	460	490	510	570
570	230	260	290	310	340	370	400	430	460	480	510	540	600
600	240	270	300	330	360	390	420	450	480	510	540	570	630

(continued)

Table 26.2   *(continued)*

1RM weight (lb)	40%	45%	50%	55%	60%	65%	70%	75%	80%	85%	90%	95%	105%
630	250	280	320	350	380	410	440	470	500	540	570	600	660
660	260	300	330	360	400	430	460	500	530	560	590	630	695
690	280	310	350	380	410	450	480	520	550	590	620	660	725
720	290	320	360	400	430	470	500	540	580	610	650	680	755
750	300	340	380	410	450	490	530	560	600	640	680	710	790

Table 26.3   **Warm-Up and Load Progression Chart**

Warm-up (lb)			Workload				Warm-up (lb)				Workload		
75	85	95	105	115	125			135	225	275	325	355	375
75	90	105	115	125	135			135	225	275	335	365	385
85	95	110	125	135	145			135	225	315	345	375	395
85	105	115	135	145	155			135	225	315	355	385	405
95	110	125	140	155	165			135	225	315	365	395	415
95	115	130	145	160	175			135	225	315	375	405	425
95	125	140	155	170	185			135	225	315	385	415	435
95	135	150	165	180	195			135	225	315	385	415	445
135	145	160	175	190	205			135	225	315	385	425	455
135	155	170	185	200	215			135	225	315	405	435	465
135	155	180	195	210	225			135	225	315	405	445	475
135	155	185	195	215	235		135	225	315	365	425	455	485
135	155	185	205	225	245		135	225	315	365	435	465	495
135	155	185	215	235	255		135	225	315	365	445	475	505
135	155	185	225	245	265		135	225	315	405	455	485	515
135	155	195	235	255	275		135	225	315	405	465	495	525
135	185	225	245	265	285		135	225	315	405	465	505	535
135	185	225	255	275	295		135	225	315	405	475	515	545
135	185	225	265	285	305		135	225	315	405	485	525	555
135	185	225	275	295	315		135	225	315	405	485	525	565
135	185	245	285	305	325		135	225	315	405	495	535	575
135	225	255	295	315	335		135	225	315	405	495	545	585
135	225	255	305	325	345		135	225	315	405	495	555	595
135	225	275	315	335	355		135	225	315	405	495	565	605
135	225	275	325	345	365								

Adapted from Pauletto (1986).

must attempt a maximal effort set once a week and perform workouts of light to moderate intensity (50% - 90% of RM) on the other days during the week. The studies indicate that RM training during all workouts is not as effective as performing such training once weekly. One study (2) reports greater absolute strength gains when athletes perform each repetition of a 10-repetition set with maximal resistance compared with a 10RM set. This type of training is difficult to do without trained spotters or special equipment that allows for resistance reduction during each repetition of a set.

A schedule such as that seen in Table 26.4 (17) serves as a useful guide for spacing workouts of varying intensities, to provide optimal recovery from heavy workouts. This approach works well with an athlete's other training, in that heavy-lifting days can fall on light–metabolic training days, and light-lifting days on heavy–metabolic training days. The periodization training model found in chapter 30 employs this model.

When an athlete performs a workout at the assigned load, new RMs can be estimated on a workout-by-workout basis. For example, an athlete with a 1RM of 500 lb does a set at 85% of 1RM (i.e., 425 lb) and is able to manage eight repetitions. A check of Table 26.2 reveals that eight repetitions with 425 lb is at the 80% level for a 1RM of 530 lb. Subsequent workouts could

Table 26.4   Sample 4-Week Lifting Schedule

Week	Mon.	Tues.	Wed.	Thurs.	Fri.	Sat.	Sun.
1	MH	L	Rest	ML	Rest	L	Rest
2	H	ML	Rest	M	Rest	ML	Rest
3	VH	M	Rest	H	Rest	M	Rest
4	L	L	Rest	ML	Rest	L	Rest

Key:

Intensity designation	Percent of 1RM
VH (very heavy)	95-100+
H (heavy)	90-95
MH (moderately heavy)	85-90
M (moderate)	80-85
ML (moderately light)	75-80
L (light)	70-75
VL (very light)	65-70

Note. To ensure adequate recovery, the intensity of the session following a heavy or very heavy day is no higher than moderate intensity.

Adapted from Stone and O'Bryant (1987).

use the 530-lb figure for the athlete's 1RM to estimate future workout loads. The athlete must also occasionally attempt a 1RM measurement, to get a more accurate measure of absolute strength in an exercise. The level will be dependent on the goal of training for that day.

Outcomes of Different Training Levels

Fleck and Kraemer's RM continuum (Figure 26.1) graphically depicts the outcomes from RMs at various levels (5).

Most studies have found that RMs that allow for six or fewer repetitions (i.e., low RMs) provide the most strength and power benefits; that weights based on 6RM-12RM provide moderate strength, power, and endurance gains; and that weights based on RMs of 20 and above provide primarily muscular endurance gains with no strength gains (5). High-intensity is usually considered 90% of the given RM or higher, moderate intensity at 70% to 90% of the RM, and low intensity at below 70% of the RM (5,6,10-12,14,17,20). The range in intensities takes into account individual variables, as well as variable load schemes. For example, some athletes may be highly taxed with a load that is 90% of 1RM but only moderately taxed with a load that is 90% of a 10RM. A similar variation may occur with low-intensity loads. Gains in absolute strength (1RM) are inversely related to gains in relative endurance, but highly related to gains in absolute endurance (1,11,13). Relative endurance is the number of contractions that can be performed at a certain submaximal intensity level in relationship to the highest intensity level (1RM). Absolute endurance is the highest number of contractions that can be performed with a certain load regardless of the maximum load capability (1RM). This may account for the fact that athletes who improve their absolute strength show gains in endurance activities without concomitant gains in maximal oxygen uptake (6). The implications are that athletes who wish to improve their absolute endurance should engage in strength training sessions of high intensity. Athletes who engage primarily in high-load training display selective extreme (3 times normal) hypertrophy of Type II (fast twitch) muscle fibers, whereas athletes who engage primarily in higher volume (repetitions) training with moderate loads (8RM-12RM level) have more general (Type I and II) muscle hypertrophy (18,19). Athletes interested in attaining both types of hypertrophy outcomes should engage in a combination of the two types of training, detailed in chapter 30. The outcomes for various load assignments are that strength and power are best derived from loads over 80% of 1RM, whereas general muscle hypertrophy and muscular endurance are best gained from moderate to low loads (60%-80% of 1RM) with higher volumes (2,6,10,11,17,20).

Health Status and Load Assignment

The strength and conditioning professional needs to consider variables besides training outcomes when assigning loads. Initially, a physician must determine the health of the athlete. Certain organic conditions, such as hypertension, and musculoskeletal conditions, like joint weakness from previous injury, should be taken into consideration when assigning loads for resistance training programs. Fortunately, there are only a few conditions that permit the athlete to participate in a sport but prevent him or her from engaging in conditioning activities. There is no evidence that participation in a resistance training program causes or aggravates chronic hypertension (15).

Circuit weight training has been used with cardiac patients recently with favorable results (15). People training in a cardiac rehabilitation program can follow the prescribed standard circuit training protocols using intensities of 40% to 60% of 1RM (15). Cardiac patients can do 1RM testing without a Valsalva maneuver with less symptoms than in graded exercise testing. Patients who had good left ventricular function were able to perform sets of seven repetitions at 75% of 1RM, indicating that more stressful weight training may not be problematic for some cardiac patients (4). It is unlikely that cardiac factors will exclude many competitive athletes from any type of strength training regime.

Prior to working with an injured athlete, the strength and conditioning professional should seek guidance from the medical staff responsible for the athlete about whether the athlete is ready for strength training. Musculoskeletal injuries and inflammatory conditions may require a lowering of the percentage of RM at which an athlete is training, once the acute phase of the injury subsides enough to allow the athlete to return to training. It is prudent to begin an athlete who has not trained for an extended period of time with a light load (50%-60% of 1RM) and increase intensity gradually over time. Use pain and inflammation as guidelines for injured athletes; intensity can be gradually increased as long as no pain and inflammation occur from training. Detraining, a condition in which physiological capacity (e.g., strength, endurance, flexibility, speed, and power) diminishes due to prolonged loss of training stimulus (5), occurs in an athlete who has not been training for whatever reason for a period of time.

Training Level and Load Assignment

An athlete's current condition is a very important consideration when assigning loads. Individuals who are starting a weight training program or who have been in a detraining period should begin at a low intensity and gradually build up. A periodized program, as described in chapter 30, serves as an excellent model of gradually increasing load over time. The urge to add too much too soon should be discouraged, to allow for structures that adapt slowly, such as bone and connective tissue, to catch up to neuromuscular gains. There is no reason to believe that detrained subjects will not benefit from a periodized loading regime after a few weeks of low- to moderate-load training sessions (23).

Prepubescent children can gain significant muscular strength and endurance but do not generally display muscle hypertrophy (5,6,10,17). Children should engage in a program of low to moderate intensity, with a moderate to high number of repetitions, until they reach puberty (3). It has been hypothesized but not proven that heavy loads might damage the epiphyseal centers; a small percentage (<10%) of epiphyseal injuries results in growth impairment to long bones (3).

Sport-Specific Load Assignment

Training goals for athletes may vary considerably from sport to sport. Many sports—wrestling, tennis, running and jumping events in track, gymnastics, rowing, and weightlifting—see gains in strength or power without gains in body mass. Young athletes gain weight as they mature in most sports, but no athlete wants to sacrifice speed for gains in mass. To avoid excessive overall hypertrophy, keep volume low (one to six repetitions) and loads high to moderate ($\geq$80% of 1RM). American-football players and weight throwers may benefit from muscle mass gains if these do not cause a decrement in speed. Load assignments should also reflect the goals of the individual athlete and the strength levels required in the sport. The goals of the strength-and-power athlete are to improve performance through increased strength and, secondarily, to prevent injury.

Endurance athletes (distance runners and swimmers, and soccer players) also seek to improve performance, but injury prevention may be a greater motivation, because performance improvement may not be as acute from resistance training as it is for the power athlete. A limiting factor in training is the number of intense workouts that can be performed in a given period of time; endurance athletes train in their particular sport more often and at higher volumes than power athletes do in theirs, which makes endurance athletes susceptible to overuse injuries. Strengthening a distance athlete's joints will allow the athlete to bear greater stress during more frequent and intense running or swimming workouts.

Most athletes seek increases in strength, which necessitates weekly RM efforts coupled with days of moderate- to light-load training. Some athletes who require high-metabolic efforts, such as wrestlers, middle-distance and distance runners and swimmers, and rowers, often employ circuit training with short rest periods between bouts of resistance exercise. These high-metabolic workouts necessitate loads lower than normally used with priority training; typically, these athletes use loads 40% to 60% of 1RM for moderate to high (10-20) repetitions. This type of loading can be used occasionally, possibly as an unloading phase after a period of heavy loading. For example, in Table 26.4, Week 4 is an unloading week from the previous 3 weeks of heavy loading and could be used for high-metabolic training. The more the lactic acid energy source is utilized in a sport, the more often high-metabolic and/or circuit training should be employed in the off-season and preseason phases of training.

Periodization Concerns

The loads employed in various parts of athletes' yearly training cycle often depend upon when major contests are held. Most training is divided into off-season, preseason, and in-season periods (see Table 22.1, p. 404). The overall goal of each period is to bring the athlete to a physical peak for major competitions. During the off season, training may be higher in volume, in part because the athlete is spending less time on skill acquisition and strategy sessions. As the preseason approaches, volume tapers off and higher loads are employed to bring the athlete to a peak in strength and power. The highest loads are employed directly before competition, with an adequate number of days (1 to 10 days, depending on the athlete) of unloading to ensure recuperation prior to the contest.

Sports with long seasons (e.g., football, basketball) have in-season programs designed to maintain peak or near-peak condition for many months. Maintaining peak condition is difficult, because skill and strategy training takes up a large portion of an athlete's time, leaving little time for weight training. Weight training at heavy loads and low volume allows most athletes to maintain a large percentage of acquired strength. However, athletes who are not yet at an acceptable level of strength need to train for two or more sessions/week (2,5,6,10,11,17,21). Owing to time constraints, high-load, low-volume sessions of predominantly multiple-joint movements should be employed. All team members could engage in a session of heavy-load training on the lightest skill acquisition and strategy practice day of a week; athletes who need further strength gains would have a moderate-load session 2 or 3 days later. For weekly games played on Fridays, the heavy-load session could be on Sundays and the moderate-load session on Wednesdays. When two games are played each week, on Tuesdays and Fridays, the heavy-load session could be done on Saturdays and the moderate-load session on Wednesdays. Volume remains low during the in-season period of training.

Some experts (5) feel that athletes not engaged in strength-and-power events benefit from resistance exercise of lower load and higher volume in each phase of training. For example, these athletes would use 1.5 to 2 times the volume used by a strength-and-power athlete during the same phase of training. It should be noted that endurance athletes are usually engaged in a considerably higher volume of other types of training (running, swimming, etc.), so to increase the volume of resistance training significantly may lead to overtraining. Other experts (17) would point out that the main goal of resistance training is to add strength and power for all athletes despite the relative contributions that strength and power make to the event.

CONCLUSION

In order to determine proper load assignments, an athlete's RMs (10RM, 5RM, 3RM, 1RM, etc.) should be determined by testing. Testing should include proper warm-up and logical progression of intensity until the desired RM is determined. A trial-and-error method within the training program can also be used.

Different load assignments result in different outcomes. High intensities (above 80% of 1RM) produce more strength and power gains than do lower intensities (below 80% of 1RM), which tend to produce more hypertrophy and endurance (local muscular) gains.

The health status and training status of an athlete affect the load that should be assigned to him or her. Ill or injured athletes and athletes who are coming out of prolonged detraining or just starting training should have loads modified to meet their current health and training status.

The fitness requirements of various sports will necessitate a variety of load assignments to fit the needs of the activity and the athletes. At every phase of training, each athlete should strive to improve their RM levels over previous cycles.

Key Terms

| intensity | 435 | load | 435 | repetition maximum | 435 |

Study Questions

1. A 5RM load refers to a weight that

   a. can be lifted five but not six times with good technique
   b. is 85% of a 1RM
   c. is lifted a maximum number of times for five sets
   d. can be lifted at least five consecutive times

2. For novice trainees, the most accurate RM should be established

   a. after adequate skill acquisition has occurred
   b. with free weights before machines
   c. with very little warm-up, to insure little fatigue
   d. from a chart estimation based on 10RM

3. To improve lactic acid energy systems with traditional circuit weight training, employ loads of _____ of 1RM.

   a. 40% to 60%
   b. 20% to 40%
   c. 60% to 80%
   d. 80% to 100%

4. In estimating a 1RM from a 6RM test result of 260 lb using Table 26.1, you would have a 1RM estimate of

   a. 275 lb
   b. 215 lb
   c. 320 lb
   d. 312 lb

Applying Knowledge of Load Assignment

Problem 1
Assuming a 10RM of 310 lb in a free-weight exercise, what load assignments would be most appropriate for an untrained athlete during the first phase of the preparatory period of training?

Problem 2
What load assignments in the power snatch would be most appropriate for an injured but now medically cleared female volleyball player who had previously been lifting for 8 weeks with a 6RM power snatch of 75 lb?

References

1. Berger, R. Relationship between dynamic strength and dynamic endurance. *Res. Q.* 41:115-116. 1970.
2. Berger, R. (1972, August). Strength improvement. *Strength & Health*, pp. 44-45, 70-71.
3. Bilcheck, H. Epiphyseal injuries in young athletes. *NSCA Journal* 11(5):60-65. 1989.
4. Faigenbaum, A.D., G.S. Skrinar, W.F. Cesare, W.J. Kraemer, and H.E. Thomas. Physiologic and symptomatic responses of cardiac patients to resistance exercise. *Arch. Phys. Med. Rehabil.* 71:395-398. 1990.
5. Fleck, S.J., and W.J. Kraemer. *Designing Resistance Training Programs.* Champaign, IL: Human Kinetics. 1987.
6. Garhammer, J. *Sports Illustrated Strength Training.* New York: Harper & Row. 1986.
7. Hatfield, F. The wisdom behind Soviet training. *Powerlifting U.S.A.* 9(2):15. 1985.
8. Hickson, R., M.A. Rosenkoetter, and M.M. Brown. Strength training effects on aerobic power and short-term endurance. *Med. Sci. Sports Exerc.* 12:336-339. 1980.

9. Hoeger, W., S.L. Barette, D.F. Hale, and D.R. Hopkins. Relationship between repetitions and selected percentages of one repetition maximum. *J. Appl. Sport Sci. Res.* 1(1):11-13. 1987.
10. Lombardi, V. *Beginning Weight Training.* Dubuque, IA: Brown. 1989.
11. O'Shea, J. *Scientific Principles and Methods of Strength Fitness.* Reading, MA: Addison-Wesley. 1976.
12. Pauletto, B. Intensity. *NSCA Journal* 8(1):33-37. 1986.
13. Shaver, L. Maximum dynamic strength, relative dynamic endurance and their relationship. *Res. Q.* 42:460-465. 1971.
14. Simmons, L. Training by percents. *Powerlifting U.S.A.* 12(2):21. 1988.
15. Sparling, P., and J. Cantwell. Strength training guidelines for cardiac patients. *Phys. Sportsmed.* 17(3):190-196. 1989.
16. Spassov, A. Qualities of strength and their applications to sports, Part II. *NSCA Journal* 11(1):60-62. 1989.
17. Stone, M., and H. O'Bryant. *Weight Training.* Minneapolis: Burgess International. 1987.
18. Tesch, P., and L. Larson. Muscle hypertrophy in body builders. *Eur. J. Appl. Physiol.* 49:301-306. 1982.
19. Tesch, P., A. Thorsson, and P. Kaiser. Muscle capillary supply and fiber type characteristics in weight and power lifters. *J. Appl. Physiol. Respir. Env. Exerc. Physiol.* 56:35-38. 1984.
20. Verhoshansky, Y. *Fundamentals of Special Strength Training in Sport.* Livonia, MI: Sportivny Press. 1979.
21. Westcott, W. *Strength Fitness.* Boston: Allyn & Bacon. 1991.
22. White, J. My squatting routine. *Powerman* 3(1):17. 1973.
23. Willoughby, D. The effects of mesocycle-length weight training programs involving periodization and partially equated volumes on upper and lower body strength. *J. Strength and Cond. Res.* 7(1):2-8. 1993.

CHAPTER 27

TRAINING VOLUME

Dan Wathen

Volume describes the total amount of weight lifted in a workout session. (The total number of repetitions with various loads in a training session is also termed **volume**.) The weight per repetition determines the volume allowable in a set. For example, heavy weights cannot be lifted for a large number of repetitions in a single set. Therefore, high-volume training (i.e., a high number of repetitions per set) is usually done with low to moderate loads. In this sense, volume can be calculated by multiplying the number of sets by the number of repetitions times the weight lifted per repetition. Two sets of 10 repetitions with 50 lb would be expressed as $2 \times 10 \times 50$ lb = 1,000 lb of volume. Of course, if different sets are done with different amounts of weight, the volumes per set are calculated and then added up to obtain the total workout volume. (Recall from chapter 26 that the load is the number of repetitions times the weight lifted per repetition. Thus, volume can be calculated by multiplying the number of sets performed by the load.)

INDIVIDUAL VARIATIONS

Each athlete has a different capacity for training with various volumes. Records from each training cycle should indicate the relative success of various volumes on the final performance outcome of the cycle. Some athletes may make substantial progress with longer or more frequent periods of high-volume training sessions; others may not. The goals of the cycle (whether increased strength, power, endurance, speed, or some other attribute) can be compared to the results of past

cycles to better determine volume considerations for individual athletes. It is not advisable to adopt the results of one athlete's response to a training cycle for other athletes.

Some experts (2) feel that athletes who do not rely greatly on strength and power but have more need for endurance (e.g., distance runners and swimmers) should have higher volumes of training at all phases of a cycle. For example, if a strength-and-power athlete performs sets of 10 repetitions during a phase, then the endurance athlete would perform sets of 15 to 20 repetitions during the comparable phase. This relatively elevated volume would be consistent throughout a cycle and, for the endurance athlete, there may be very little if any power phase that utilizes 1RM to 3RM weights in training. In any event, however, endurance may be better developed from more sport-specific activities, such as running or swimming itself, than from resistance training.

VOLUME ADAPTATION

Like other training variables, volume of training in successive mesocycles may increase with the adaptation of the athlete and require greater levels to achieve further gains in performance.

Periodization Concerns

Volume may be gradually increased with each mesocycle as loads increase. Volume is high during the early phase of the preparatory period and is reduced with the addition of higher training loads during the later phases of the preparatory period. In most cases, the increase in training volume is achieved over time by increasing the number of sets in a workout. Higher volumes of training are also associated with higher levels of relative muscular endurance (2,3,5,6,12). Figure 27.1 illustrates how volume and load are manipulated in an 11-week training cycle (12). Each week's training follows a similar pattern of alternating high, medium, and light days of load and volume to allow for adequate recuperation and avoidance of overwork or overtraining. Generally, periods of high volume are done early in a training cycle to build up endurance for future enhancement of training recuperation in addition to increases in vascularization and lean body mass (13,14).

Some resistance training experts feel that high-volume training places more stress on connective tissue than low-volume, high-load training does (7,10,15). These experts advocate an early period of high-volume training to strengthen the ligaments and tendons for subsequent higher intensity phases, which, they feel, stresses mainly the muscles. This theory is somewhat supported by scientific data (11,12).

When the athlete has advanced past the initial stages of training and has developed a good level of strength, he or she can undertake higher volumes of training. The duration of high-volume training will be controlled somewhat by the amount of lean body mass and the muscle endurance the athlete desires. Athletes who desire more lean body mass should engage in longer and more frequent periods of high-volume training than those who are primarily training for strength and power increases (2,5,12-16).

The early phases of a preparatory period usually consist of higher volumes of training with gradually increasing loads to prepare the athlete for the greater levels of intensity to follow as the athlete moves closer to a competition period. As the ability to accept higher load levels increases, volume is reduced to allow for loads that facilitate greater gains in strength and power. For example, during the last week of high-volume training in the preparatory period, an athlete may perform three sets of 10 repetitions in an exercise with 75% of his 1RM of 300 lb. The total volume would be 3 × 10 × 255 lb = 6,750 lb, a heavy day's training for the week in that exercise. Subsequent training weeks may find the weight increased to 85% of 1RM for five sets of five repetitions. This would yield a total volume of 5 × 5 = 25 × 255 lb = 6,375 lb, lower than before. (The volume in terms of number of repetitions, 25 vs. 30, is also lower.)

Volumes remain low during phases that emphasize power or skill acquisition. As a competition approaches, the greatest amount of time is spent on skill acquisition, refinement, and competition strategy in many sports. This leaves little time for high volumes of physical training. A graphic illustration of the relationship between intensity, volume, and technique training is seen in the classic model of Matveyev's periodization as modified by Stone and O'Bryant (12) (Figure 27.2).

To maintain strength and attain higher levels of power, the volume is reduced with gradually increasing load intensity. In some team sports with prolonged seasons (e.g., football and basketball), volumes remain low but the load varies as outlined in chapters 26 and 30.

Effects of Age, Health Status, and Conditioning Level

Some conditioning professionals feel that the decrease in testosterone seen as men age is a reason for reduction

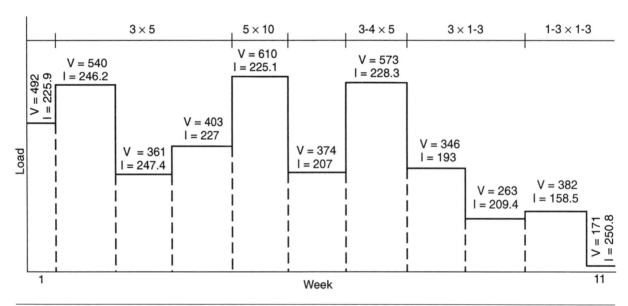

Figure 27.1 Example of load, volume, and intensity estimates. The basic training program is presented at the top of the figure. V = volume (repetitions) = workload, I = intensity (average weight lifted) = power output.
Adapted from Stone and O'Bryant (1987).

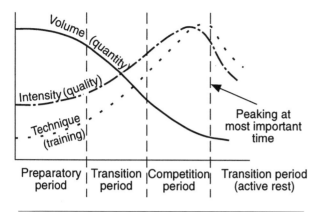

Figure 27.2 Matveyev's model of periodization (modified). Adapted from Stone and O'Bryant (1987).

in training volume as the age of the athlete increases. Spassov (9) believes that athletes should begin decreasing training volume in their mid-20s. Although Western research does not validate this concept, it would seem reasonable to reduce skill training volume as the skill of the athlete improves and then emphasize conditioning. As the athlete ages, arthritic conditions of the joints will be a factor in volume and in frequency of training. There are few elite athletes past the age of 40 who do not have to deal with the effects of arthritic joint wear

(4). The extent of volume decrease may be very gradual up to the age of 40 or 50 and then steeper declines may be warranted, depending on the physical condition of the athlete.

Beginners in a resistance training program should utilize moderate volumes of exercise in the early stages of training: workouts of one to three sets of 6 to 12 repetitions each. As mentioned in chapter 26, hypertensive trainees should utilize moderate loads (7RM-15RM), giving moderate volumes of work (8). A regime of this level is advised for athletes who resume training after musculoskeletal injuries and for prepubescent athletes (1,2,5,12,16).

CONCLUSION

Volume is kept at a moderate level in the beginning stages of training for novice trainees and athletes who are resuming training after illness or injury. Volume is increased during the first phase of the preparatory period. Gradual reductions in volume begin as the load of training increases in the strength and power phases of the preparatory period. The lowest volumes are seen in the late part of the power phase of the preparatory period and in the competition period of training.

Key Terms

volume   447

Study Questions

1. As an athlete's capability to train with high volumes improves, his or her _____ may improve.

   a. muscular hypertrophy
   b. local muscular endurance
   c. cardiovascular endurance
   d. *a*, *b*, and *c*

2. After a period of detraining of a joint or muscle group due to injury, training should be resumed at _____ volume.

   a. moderate (6-10 repetitions/set)
   b. low (1-6 repetitions/set)
   c. high (10-20 repetitions/set)
   d. very low (1-3 repetitions/set)

3. Volume can be calculated by multiplying sets times

   a. load times time
   b. total training time
   c. repetitions times weight
   d. average weight on the bar

4. Volume of training decreases

    a. during the hypertrophy/endurance phase of the preparatory period

    b. for athletes whose events require high levels of aerobic endurance with low levels of strength and power

    c. as the competition period approaches

    d. with younger athletes

Applying Knowledge of Training Volume

Problem 1

During the off-season, a 21-year-old softball pitcher's training sessions averaged between 275 and 350 repetitions/session, 4 days/week. She had been training consistently for 3 years and had good levels of strength in all exercises. As the competitive season approaches, how should she adjust the volume of training to allow for higher loads?

Problem 2

A 6-ft, 10-in basketball player has enrolled in your school. He weighs 190 lb and has a limited background in strength training. He is 19 years old and can perform a 30-in. standing vertical jump. Which phase of the preparatory period should he emphasize?

References

1. Bilcheck, H. Epiphyseal injuries in young athletes. *NSCA Journal* 11(5):60-65. 1989.
2. Fleck, S.J., and W.J. Kraemer. *Designing Resistance Training Programs*. Champaign, IL: Human Kinetics. 1987.
3. Garhammer, J. *Sports Illustrated Strength Training*. New York: Harper & Row. 1986.
4. Herrick, R., M. Stine, and S. Herrick. Injuries in strength-power activities. *Powerlifting U.S.A.* 7:7-9. 1983.
5. Lombardi, V. *Beginning Weight Training*. Dubuque, IA: Brown. 1989.
6. O'Shea, J. *Scientific Principles and Methods of Strength Fitness*. Reading, MA: Addison-Wesley. 1976.
7. Siff, M. (1987, June). *Physiologic and biomechanical aspects of safe exercise*. Paper presented at the annual meeting of the National Strength and Conditioning Association, Las Vegas, NV.
8. Sparling, P., and J. Cantwell. Strength training guidelines for cardiac patients. *Phys. Sportsmed.* 17(3):190-196. 1989.
9. Spassov, A. (1989, June). *Bulgarian training methods*. Paper presented at the symposium of the National Strength and Conditioning Association, Denver, CO.
10. Spassov, A. Qualities of strength and their application to sports, Part II. *NSCA Journal* 11(1):60-62. 1989.
11. Stone, M. Implications for connective tissue and bone alterations resulting from resistance exercise training. *Med. Sci. Sports Exerc.* 20(5 [Suppl.]):S262-S268. 1988.
12. Stone, M., and H. O'Bryant. *Weight Training*. Minneapolis: Burgess International. 1987.
13. Tesch, P., and L. Larson. Muscle hypertrophy in body builders. *Eur. J. Appl. Physiol.* 49:301-306. 1982.
14. Tesch, P., A. Thorsson, and P. Kaiser. Muscle capillary supply and fiber type characteristics in weight and power lifters. *J. Appl. Physiol. Respir. Env. Exer. Physiol.* 56:35-38. 1984.
15. Verhoshansky, Y. *Fundamentals of Special Strength Training in Sports*. Livonia, MI: Sportivny Press. 1979.
16. Westcott, W. *Strength Fitness*. Boston: Allyn & Bacon. 1982.

CHAPTER 28

REST PERIODS

Dan Wathen

Rest periods between sets of exercise are critical in the success of any training program. They are highly dependent upon possible volumes and loads and should reflect the goals of the athlete. Training for absolute strength (1RM [repetition maximum]) requires significantly longer rest periods between sets of exercise than training for muscle hypertrophy or local muscular endurance (2,3,6,7,9,12).

ENERGY UTILIZATION

In order to determine how long to rest between sets of exercise in a workout session, one must know the energy source being utilized. For bouts of high-intensity exercise of less than 30 s in duration, the primary energy sources are adenosine triphosphate (ATP) and creatine phosphate, which are stored in the muscles. Intense training can deplete these phosphagen stores in 15 s; it takes about 2.5 to 3 min to replenish the phosphagen stores needed for the next set of high-intensity effort (10).

TRAINING FOR ABSOLUTE STRENGTH

Training may enhance an athlete's ability to train with less rest (2,6,8-10,12), but athletes who seek to accomplish maximal or near-maximal repetitions with a heavy load usually need to take 3 to 5 min between heavy sets of exercise. This procedure works best for absolute strength (1RM) gains and is widely employed by weight-

lifters and powerlifters (2,3,6,9,11,12). This protocol is applicable to athletes interested in gaining strength and power but not necessarily interested in extensive muscle hypertrophy or relative endurance. It also appears that long rest periods and their higher accompanying loads of training are responsible for greater testosterone levels in experienced strength athletes performing large–muscle group exercises such as deadlifts (5).

TRAINING FOR HYPERTROPHY AND LOCAL ENDURANCE

Athletes who are interested in hypertrophy, local muscle endurance, or both need to perform higher volumes of exercise, use more exercises, train in the 8RM to 12RM range, and take brief rest periods—30-60 s—between sets of exercise. This represents a work-rest ratio of about 1:1 (2-5,7,9). Bodybuilders employ this ratio in order to achieve muscle "pump," which refers to the tight feeling in a muscle when it is being exercised, becomes engorged with blood, and fatigues to the point at which further activity is very difficult.

Activities such as wrestling, long-sprint running (400-1,000 m), and swimming (100-200 m), which require all-out bursts of activity for 1 to 3 min with very little or no rest require athletes who can withstand lactate accumulation. These athletes may benefit from periods of high-volume training with work-rest ratios of 1:1 or more, since such training creates very high lactate concentrations in the exercising muscles (2). Furthermore, human growth hormone concentration levels are

451

increased in individuals who train with high volumes and short rest periods when compared to those using longer rest periods (5).

CIRCUIT TRAINING

Circuit training is a good example of how rest periods between sets of exercise can be manipulated to give a variety of results. Traditional circuit training employs a work-rest ratio of 1:1 or more and has been shown to moderately increase both strength and aerobic endurance. The increases are 30% to 50% less than those achieved with traditional strength training and endurance training (resulting in a 4%-8% increase in both strength and aerobic endurance as opposed to a 15%-20% increase gained in traditional training) but are above average and significant (2,3,6,9). Athletes interested in moderate increases in both strength and aerobic endurance will find traditional circuit training to consume less time than training for both strength and endurance on separate occasions. Athletes interested in the highest levels of strength and endurance possible, however, have to train each separately. For example, sporting activities that demand high levels of both strength and anaerobic endurance, such as basketball, wrestling, and 400-m running, require athletes to train for strength on one day and endurance on an alternate day, or each at different times of the day (2,6,9). Because traditional circuit training alternates body parts in each set of exercise, the previously exercised muscle groups recuperate while other muscle groups are being exercised, allowing for shorter rest periods.

Rest periods between sets of exercise should be shortened gradually; this helps prevent nausea, which results from the disruption in the acid-base balance that accompanies dramatic increases in lactate accumulation. Athletes who become nauseated during a workout will tend to avoid that type of workout in the future if not gradually acclimated to it. Research suggests that a protocol of 15 s of high-intensity work followed by an equal time of rest allows for the most work to be performed in the shortest amount of time; this has proved to be superior to both longer and shorter rest and work periods (1).

OTHER FACTORS

After illness or any period of unavoidable detraining, the rest time between sets of exercises should be increased to allow for adequate recovery. As an athlete's condition improves, he or she will recover at a faster pace and need less rest between sets.

More highly conditioned athletes may be able to train with less recovery time between sets of exercise. Stone and O'Bryant (9) report that more highly trained lifters took less rest time between sets of exercise than lesser trained individuals (Table 28.1). Advanced bodybuilders take very little rest between sets of exercises and train daily, if not twice daily in many instances (2,3,6,9,10,12).

Some trainers utilize heart rate to determine when the athlete should perform the next set (8). When the heart rate returns to a certain level after a set, the next set is initiated. The heart rate to which the athlete must recover prior to the next set is often 100 to 110 beats/min. It usually takes heavier athletes longer to reach this heart rate level than lighter ones (8). Research indicates that the resting heart rate is achieved more quickly after exercise in more highly endurance trained athletes (2,9). Caution must be exercised when using heart rate levels to measure stress, because heart rates can soar with short rest protocols and not reflect true exercise intensity (4). People beginning a resistance training program require longer rest periods between sets until they adapt to training demands. This is especially true with older people, because it may be dangerous to elevate their heart rates significantly for prolonged periods of time, which occurs with traditional circuit weight training, for example. Individual athletes will adapt to training at different paces and be able to accept more intense training with adaptation.

CONCLUSION

Athletes who are in good health, have an adequate training background, and desire to gain muscle size and local

Table 28.1 Approximate Time of Training and Rest Periods for Various Exercises and Repetitions Per Set Using a Priority System*

Exercise	Repetitions per set	Exercise time (s)	Rest time between sets (min)	
			Untrained	Olympic weightlifters
Squats	10	45-60	4.0	3.5
	5	20-30	3.5	3.0
	3	10-15	3.0	3.1
Clean pulls	10	45-50	4.3	3.5
	5	25-30	3.2	3.0
	3	12-16	3.0	3.2
Bench presses	10	35-40	3.3	3.4
	5	15-20	3.0	3.1
	3	8-16	2.9	3.1

*In a priority system, all sets of an exercise must be completed before moving on to the next exercise.

Reprinted from Stone and O'Bryant (1987).

muscular endurance need to take less rest between bouts of exercise than athletes who have only a limited training background, are returning to training after illness or injury, or who desire to gain strength and power by utilizing heavy loads. Strength-and-power athletes require more time between sets of exercises to replenish energy stores.

Study Questions

1. To replenish phosphagen stores, rest between sets should last

   a. 3 min
   b. 1 min
   c. 30 s
   d. 6 min

2. A high jumper performing sets of three repetitions with 90% of his 1RM capacity in strength training exercises should rest _____ min between sets.
   a. 1-2
   b. 3-5
   c. 7-9
   d. 10-15

3. Traditional circuit weight training has a work-rest ratio of approximately

   a. 1:2
   b. 2:1
   c. 1:1
   d. 3:1

4. Athletes returning to training after prolonged periods of detraining should begin by resting _____ usual between sets of exercise.

   a. less than
   b. the same as
   c. more often than
   d. longer than

Applying Knowledge of Rest Periods

Problem 1

A baseball team is engaged in a nontraditional circuit weight training program during the strength and power phases of the preparatory period of training. The team has been divided into groups of 3 according to 1RM in various exercises. How much time should you allow at each station for each player to achieve a minimum of three sets with the last set being done at 90% of the 1RM with maximum repetitions?

References

1. Ballor, D.L., M.D. Becque, C.R. Marks, K.L. Nau, and V.L. Katch. Physiological responses to nine different exercises, rest protocols. *Med. Sci. Sports Exerc.* 21(1):90-95. 1989.
2. Fleck, S.J., and W.J. Kraemer. *Designing Resistance Training Programs.* Champaign, IL: Human Kinetics. 1987.
3. Garhammer, J. *Sports Illustrated Strength Training.* New York: Harper & Row. 1986.
4. Kraemer, W.J., B.J. Noble, M.J. Clark, and B.W. Culver. Physiologic responses to heavy resistance exercise with very short rest periods. *Int. J. Sports Med.* 8:247-252. 1987.

5. Kraemer, W.J. Endocrine responses and adaptations to strength training. In: *Strength and Power in Sports*, P. Komi, ed. Oxford: Blackwell Scientific. 1992. pp. 291-304.

6. Lombardi, V. *Beginning Weight Training*. Dubuque, IA: Brown. 1989.

7. Pauletto, B. Rest and recuperation. *NSCA Journal* 8(3):52-53. 1986.

8. Spassov, A. (1989, June). *Bulgarian training methods*. Paper presented at the symposium of the National Strength and Conditioning Association, Denver, CO.

9. Stone, M, and H. O'Bryant. *Weight Training*. Minneapolis: Burgess International. 1987.

10. Tesch, P., and L. Larson. Muscle hypertrophy in body builders. *Eur. J. Appl. Physiol.* 49:301-306. 1982.

11. Weiss, L. The obtuse nature of muscular strength: The contribution of rest to its development and expression. *J. Appl. Sports Sci. Res.* 5(4):219-227. 1991.

12. Westcott, W. *Strength Fitness*. Boston: Allyn & Bacon. 1982.

CHAPTER 29

TRAINING FREQUENCY

Dan Wathen

Training frequency refers to the number of training sessions completed in a given period of time. It is dependent upon the volume and load of exercises, the type of movement (multiple-joint vs. single-joint) that predominates in the workout, the training level of the athlete (probably the most critical factor in training frequency), the goals of training, and the health status of the athlete. Without proper training frequency, training may be unproductive and possibly dangerous.

PRINCIPLES OF FREQUENCY

Training frequency turns out to be a very individual matter. Some empirical findings on frequency may be summarized as follows:

- Traditionally, athletes engage in resistance training on alternating days in the early stages of training to allow for sufficient recovery from training bouts. As an athlete adapts to training and becomes more fit, more frequent sessions may be employed. Pioneering work (1) indicated that training on 3 alternating days/week was superior to other frequencies in previously untrained college-age subjects.

- When weightlifters and powerlifters use maximum and near-maximum resistance in multiple-joint movements done with few repetitions, more recuperation time (compared to all other protocols) is needed prior to another heavy loading session (2,3,6-9).

- The ability to train more frequently may be enhanced by lighter loading sessions spaced between heavy sessions (2,3,6,9).

- Trained athletes who have engaged in resistance training over a period of time may be able to benefit from more frequent sessions than athletes without long training backgrounds.

- There is also evidence that certain muscle groups recuperate faster than others in the same athlete (9). For example, upper body muscles seem to be able to handle more frequent heavy-loading sessions than lower body muscles (9).

- Athletes seem to recover more slowly from multiple-joint exercises than from single-joint exercises (9).

- During the first 2 weeks of training, eccentric loading causes muscle damage that requires more recuperation time than exercise incorporating only concentric loading (2,3,6,9,12). Programs that emphasize eccentric loading require less frequent sessions to avoid injury and overtraining (2,6,9,11).

Much of this information makes it clear why advanced bodybuilders train daily or during multiple daily sessions that emphasize predominately single-joint exercises, why they tend to exercise upper body muscles more often, and why they usually allow 1 or more days of recuperation for a muscle group prior to exercising that group again.

Although most trainers advocate 1 or more days of recuperation between bouts of heavy, multiple-joint exercise, one study (5) found that exercising 3 consecutive days and resting 3 consecutive days to be superior to a simple alternating-day frequency. Westcott (12) reports that there were no significant differences in strength gains between training 1, 2, 3, or 5 days/week when the total volume of work was kept constant. In practice, however, most trainees engage in more frequent training sessions to increase the weekly volume of exercise.

One study (4) found that when football players were allowed to select their own training frequency, players training 4 or 5 days/week made greater progress than those training 3 to 6 days/week. Some highly trained Olympic-style weightlifters train from two to five sessions/day before competition (8). Spassov (8) reported that the ability to do more work at higher intensity can be derived from multiple sessions of short duration in both bodybuilding and weightlifting. Such sessions would be about 45 min long and would be followed by sessions of rest, massage, sauna, cold plunges, nutritional supplements, and electrical stimulation to facilitate rapid recovery. These techniques need further substantiation. Early research by Berger (1) found that one workout/week with maximal resistance was sufficient to maintain a high percentage of strength in previously untrained college-age subjects. This may or may not hold true for highly trained strength athletes.

Ideally, an athlete will have the time and financial and family support to experiment with a variety of training frequencies to determine which works best for their training goals. In general, athletes training for strength and power should engage in less frequent workouts of high resistance and low volume, whereas those seeking gains in muscle size or muscular endurance need to engage in more frequent workouts of higher volume and lower resistance.

HEALTH STATUS

Individuals suffering from illness, lack of sleep, or undernourishment or malnutrition are not able to train as frequently as healthy, well-rested, nourished individuals. Until their health status is upgraded, these athletes need more recuperation between bouts of exercise than their healthy counterparts. Injuries may require an athlete to cease training during the acute injury phase and return gradually to a higher frequency during the rehabilitation phase. An athlete recovering from injury or illness should resume training at 50% to 60% of preillness frequency and increase the frequency 10 percentage points/week; for example, if the athlete had been training 6 days/week, she could begin with 3 or 4 days/week and each week add a day until she is up to previous levels. While there is no scientific data to support this modification of training frequency after periods of detraining, clinical experience and common sense support this approach. Athletes who train with a restricted caloric intake because of participation in a sport with weight

classes cannot put in as many training periods during caloric restriction.

NEURAL ADAPTATION

As strength gains begin to slow due to increased neurological efficiency, variation in frequency may be warranted (2,3,6,9,10,12). The first variation should usually take place from 6 weeks to 6 months after the onset of basic training. At this time a variety of training frequencies may be attempted to determine which ones are most advantageous to a particular athlete. Occasional periods of active rest should be incorporated after periods of intense training or competition (see chapter 30, on periodization). For example, if an athlete begins to make fewer additional gains during a 3 day/week program, he or she can try a 2 or 4 day/week program. When gains begin to slow or cease with the new regime, another frequency can be instituted. Often 1 to 3 weeks of active rest is helpful when gains begin to plateau from either physiological or psychological burnout. These periods can consist of low-intensity and low-volume weight training or other activity.

TRAINING GOALS

Training goals influence training frequency. Athletes training for power and strength generally train less frequently and with heavier resistance (1RM-6RM), lower volumes, and longer rest periods between sets of exercise. Athletes seeking muscular endurance or hypertrophy need to train more often, with higher volume, and with lower loads (8RM-12RM).

CONCLUSION

Training frequency varies according to training status, health status, goals, and types of exercises being performed by the athlete. Generally, healthy athletes with sufficient training background who are engaged in training for hypertrophy or muscular endurance need to train more frequently. Athletes who are in questionable health, have a limited training background, or are engaged in training for strength and power using predominately multiple-joint exercises should train less frequently. Two or more training sessions/week is necessary to make strength and power gains; training once weekly maintains them.

Key Terms

training frequency   455

Study Questions

1. In order to maintain muscle strength in an exercise, you need to engage in the exercise at least

   a. 2 days/week
   b. 1 day/week
   c. 3 days/week
   d. 4 days/week

2. When utilizing multiple-joint exercise training, frequency should be _____ single-joint exercises.

   a. lower than
   b. greater than
   c. the same as
   d. decreased one week and increased the next compared to

3. In general, strength gains are best facilitated by using RM training _____ per week.

   a. three alternating days
   b. three consecutive days
   c. once
   d. six times

4. If the volume of work performed is equal over a week's training, which of the following weekly training frequencies is superior for strength gains?

   a. five days per week
   b. twice per week
   c. three times per week
   d. *a, b,* and *c* are equally effective

Applying Knowledge of Training Frequency

Problem 1
A high school baseball outfielder has been training 4 days/week for the past 6 months without any breaks. He made good progress during the first 4 months, but over the past 2 months he has been stalled by training injuries and frequent colds. After his body fat was measured at 9% the athlete lost 4 kg. The baseball season begins in 1 month. Should any modifications be made in the frequency of this athlete's training? If so, what kind?

Problem 2
A pole-vaulter is tested and found to have good lower body strength but poor upper body strength after an 8-week training cycle during which he exercised the upper and lower body 2 days/week each, on alternate days. Each workout took slightly over 1 hour. Now the athlete has only 1 day/week (Friday) on which he has more than 1 consecutive hour to spend on supervised strength training. The athlete is mildly hypertensive and seeks no additional body weight; he is 6 ft tall and weighs 82 kg. Design a program to best meet his needs.

References

1. Berger, R. (1972, August). Strength improvement. *Strength & Health*, pp. 44-45, 70-71.
2. Fleck, S.J., and W.J. Kraemer. *Designing Resistance Training Programs*. Champaign, IL: Human Kinetics. 1987.
3. Garhammer, J. *Sports Illustrated Strength Training*. New York: Harper & Row. 1986.
4. Hoffman, J.R., W.J. Kraemer, A.C. Fry, M. Deschenes, and M. Kemp. The effects of self-selection for frequency of training in a winter conditioning program for football. *J. Appl. Sport Sci. Res.* 4(3):76-82. 1990.
5. Hunter, G. Changes in body composition, body build and performance associated with different weight training frequencies in males and females. *NSCA Journal* 7(1):26-28. 1985.
6. Lombardi, V. *Beginning Weight Training*. Dubuque, IA: Brown. 1989.
7. Pauletto, B. Rest and Recuperation. *NSCA Journal* 8(3):52-53. 1986.
8. Spassov, A. (1989, June). *Bulgarian training methods*. Paper presented at the symposium of the National Strength and Conditioning Association, Denver, CO.
9. Stone, M., and H. O'Bryant. *Weight Training*. Minneapolis: Burgess International. 1987.
10. Tesch, P., and L. Larson. Muscle hypertrophy in body builders. *Eur. J. Appl. Physiol.* 49:301-306. 1982.
11. Weiss, L. The obtuse nature of muscular strength: The contribution of rest to its development and expression. *J. Appl. Sport Sci. Res.* 5(4):219-227. 1991.
12. Westcott, W. *Strength Fitness*. Boston: Allyn & Bacon. 1982.

CHAPTER 30

PERIODIZATION: CONCEPTS AND APPLICATIONS

Dan Wathen

A system of **periodization** has been established to prevent overtraining and optimize peak performance through training. Periodization organizes training into cycles of training objectives, tasks, and content. Historically, periodization was adapted in the 1960s by Russian physiologist Leo P. Matveyev and Romanian sport scientist Tudor Bompa from Canadian endocrinologist Hans Selye's General Adaptation Syndrome (GAS) theory (2,5,6). American exercise scientists Stone and O'Bryant further modified Matveyev's work, adding distinct phases to the preparatory period (2,6).

ADAPTATION TO STRESS

Selye's GAS theory describes an individual's ability to adapt to stress. This theory proposes three distinct phases when the body is faced with a training stimulus. The first phase is termed the *shock* or *alarm* phase (6). During this phase, lasting 1 to 2 weeks, there may be soreness, stiffness, and a temporary drop in performance. In the second phase, *resistance*, the body adapts to the stimulus, or, as described by Stone and O'Bryant (6), "The athlete adapts by making various biochemical, structural, mechanical and likely physiological adjustments that lead to increased performance." This phase of adaptation is sometimes termed *supercompensation*. In the third phase (maladaptation), staleness, overtraining, overwork, or exhaustion may occur when there is no variety in the stimulus or when the total stress

from the work load and extraneous stress are too great and a decrease in performance occurs. It is this phase one wishes to avoid. By manipulating the basic principles proposed by Matveyev and Bompa, the strength and conditioning professional is able to "reduce the potential for overtraining and bring strength to . . . peak levels" (6). Periodization is a system that helps structure this manipulation.

PERIODIZATION CYCLES

The overall training period is termed a **macrocycle**, which usually refers to the entire training year, but can also refer to a period of many months to 4 years, as with the Olympics. Within the macrocycle, two or more **mesocycles** occur, which consist of many weeks to months, depending on the goals of the athlete and the number of competitions contained within the period. Each mesocycle comprises a number of **microcycles**, which are generally periods of 1 week (7 days) of training.

Periods of a Mesocycle

A mesocycle comprises distinct periods: a preparatory period, a competition period, and transitional periods within and between the other two periods (see Table 22.1, p. 404). The duration of each period is dictated by the goals of the cycle and the amount of time between competitions.

Following a season of competition and before the next season's preparatory phase, there is a transition period, which begins with a phase of active rest lasting 1 to 4 weeks. During this period there is little formal training, with recreational activities being the norm, to allow the athlete to recover from the stresses of the competition period and help prepare him or her for a new training period. For example, after a basketball season, team members may engage in light, low-volume, nonspecific weight training and in such recreational activities as volleyball, racquet sports, and swimming in a leisurely manner.

The preparatory period comes next. Preparation usually takes place when there are no important competitions (i.e., the off-season), so the major emphasis is conditioning, with sport-specific skill practices and game strategy sessions limited. Conditioning activities are begun at relatively low intensity and high volume: long, slow distance running or swimming; low-intensity plyometrics; and high-repetition weight training done with light to moderate resistances. These activities progress in weekly microcycles that gradually add intensity while lowering volume.

Stone and O'Bryant (6) divide the preparatory period into three phases that differ in the intensity and volume of training.

- The *hypertrophy phase* (Phase I) has the largest volume (3-5 sets* of 8-12 repetitions) and the lowest intensity (50%-75% of 1RM).
- The *strength phase* (Phase II) has moderate volume (3-5 sets* of 5-6 repetitions) and intensity (80%-88% of 1RM).
- The *power phase* (Phase III) has low volume (3-5 sets* of 2-4 repetitions) and high intensity (90%-95% of 1RM).

*Does not include warm-up sets.

Between the preparatory and competition periods, another transition period may be undertaken. The period often includes slightly more intense training and is shorter than the transition period at the end of the season, between the competition and preparatory periods.

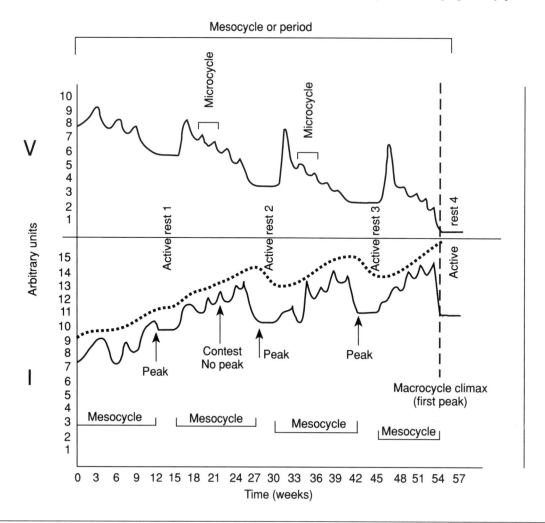

Figure 30.1 Training cycles of a weightlifter training for nationals. V = volume, I = intensity, ▬ = emphasis on sport technique.

The competition period is the late preseason and the season itself for many sports. It begins with a shift to very high intensity work with lower volume. Practice in skill technique and game strategy increase dramatically, as conditioning work decreases proportionally in duration. The goal in this period is for the athlete to reach the highest level of fitness and performance for the most important competitions (see Figure 27.2, p. 449).

The results of competition should substantiate that the athlete had a higher level of fitness than previously. The intensities of the next mesocycle can then be increased to bring about a still higher level of fitness and performance (Figures 30.1 and 30.2). The length of each phase is dictated by its goals. For example, in Figures 30.3 and 30.4, the various cycles for a tennis player and the interaction of strength conditioning and skill acquisition goals are outlined (2).

Manipulating Training Variables

Many trainers and athletes find the whole notion of periodization confusing and frustrating. In practical terms, the strength and conditioning professional needs to know how to manipulate intensity and volume for the seasonal demands of a particular sport and athlete. The professional should realize the need for regular variation in training. This breaks up the monotony and staleness that can occur when the body has adapted to the imposed demands and then encounters no further overload stimulus. We will use specific cases to elucidate the types of manipulations available.

Most scholastic, intercollegiate, and professional sports have an annual schedule that consists of off-season, preseason, and in-season periods and phases (see Table 22.1, p. 404). In the examples given here, the period between the last contest and 6 weeks prior to the first contest of the next season is considered the off season, which would contain a transition period and part of the preparatory period. The preseason begins 6 to 8 weeks prior to the first contest. The competitive period contains all the contests scheduled for that year. The competitive period would be a mesocycle if it is over 3 weeks in length. The off season could be divided

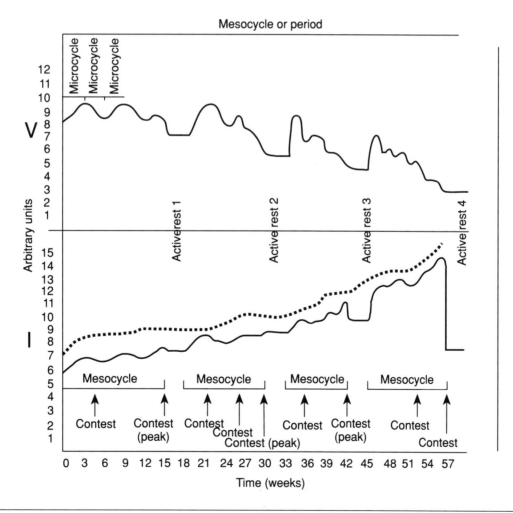

Figure 30.2   Training cycles of a shot-putter training for the Olympics. See Figure 30.1 for key.

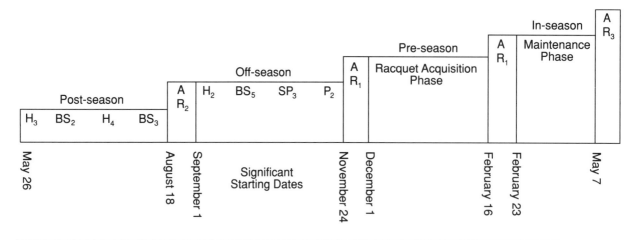

Figure 30.3   The training year: Tennis. AR = active recovery; BS = basic strength; H = hypertrophy; P = peaking; SP = strength and power. The subscript beside the letter indicates the number of weeks spent in that phase.
Adapted from Chargina et al. (1987).

Hypertrophy phase
Load: 70% of the estimated 1RM
Reps: 10
Sets: 3-4
Rest: 2-3 min between sets
Training sessions/week: 3 (MWF)
Exercises:
   Power clean
   Trunk rotation (using pulley systems)
   Hip sled
   Twisting and weighted crunches
   Bench press
   Rowing
   Shoulder press
   Biceps curls
   Wrist curls

Basic strength
Load: 86%
Reps: 5
Sets 3-5
Rest: 2-4 min
Training sessions/week: 3 (MWF)
Exercises: same as hypertrophy phase

Strength and power
Load: 92%
Reps: 3
Sets: 3-5 plus 1 warmdown set of 10 reps
Rest: 3-4 min
Training sessions/week: 3 (MWF)
Exercises: same as hypertrophy phase

Peaking power
Load: 93-100%
Reps: 1-2
Sets: 2-3
Rest: 4-7
Training sessions/week: 2 (MF)
Exercises:
   Power clean
   Bench press
   Hip sled

Figure 30.4   Phases of the off-season cycle.
Adapted from Chargina et al. (1987).

into two or more mesocycles if it is a long period of time (8 to 16 weeks).

For example, if the sport has 6 months between major competitions, two to four mesocycles, lasting from 8 to 16 weeks each, could be engaged. Many sports have long in-season periods that necessitate multiple mesocycles arranged around the most important contests. Some authors feel that the goal of in-season training should be maintenance of condition developed in the off season and preseason (2,4,6). This is exemplified by the in-season (competitive) period seen in Figures 30.3, 30.4, and 30.5.

It is difficult to maintain peak levels of fitness for more than a few weeks (1). Thus, a long competitive period (4-16 weeks) presents some unique challenges in terms of designing a training program. One solution is to treat the competitive period as a mesocycle and develop a training schedule that peaks the athlete for the most critical contests, which are usually at the end of the regular season. This is not to imply that the athlete will not be in good condition for the other events, but that the shifts in volume and intensity will reflect greater intensity and less volume for the most critical events.

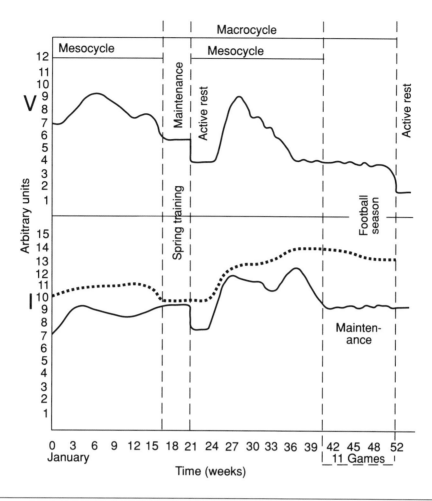

Figure 30.5 Macrocycle for a team sport. See Figure 30.1 for key.

The following is an example of a 4-week mesocycle during the competitive period:

Week 1
1 set* of 10 repetitions at 75% of 1RM

Week 3
1 set* of 3 repetitions at 92.5% of 1RM

Week 2
1 set* of 5 repetitions at 85% of 1RM

Week 4
1 set* of 1 repetition at 102% to 105% of 1RM

*Does not include warm-up sets.

This example could be further modified according to the type of athlete. Endurance athletes might increase their RM each week. A higher RM may also be used with many single-joint exercises, such as calf raises and abdominal flexion movements. Then, a 1-week transition period could be used, with fewer training sessions and moderate to light intensities and volumes. In this fashion, strength gains are not only maintained but improved upon during the competitive period.

In any event, one should not feel bound by periodization, but should feel free to manipulate the variables to suit the needs and goals of each situation.

Example of a Macrocycle

We will look at the 1-year macrocycle of a 17-year-old female high school volleyball player. The preseason for this athlete begins August 1. Her first contest takes place on September 15, and she will have 2 or 3 contests each week thereafter until November 1; tournaments could last until December 1, depending on how the team progresses through various levels of championships. This leaves a long off-season, from December 1 to August 1. This is typical of many team sports. We will assume that our athlete has not engaged in any formal training prior to this macrocycle. The schedule for the athlete's macrocycle follows.

First Preparatory Mesocycle (Off-Season)

Transitional Period (Dec. 1-31)

The transitional period comprises active rest, with no formal or structured workouts. Recreational games and fitness activities include swimming, jogging, circuit weight training (at low volume and low intensity), basketball, racquetball, and informal volleyball.

Preparatory Period (Jan. 1–Apr. 29; 17 weeks)

The following is the basic training schedule for each week during the preparatory period. The activities conducted during this period are described next.

Monday: strength training (heavy load)

Tuesday: endurance or other training (running, skill drills)

Wednesday: strength training (moderate to light load)

Thursday: endurance or other training (running, skill drills)

Friday: strength training (moderate to light load)

Early Hypertrophy/Endurance Phase (Jan. 1–Feb. 11; 6 weeks)

Flexibility training: Part of warm-up and cool-down for all workouts.

Strength training: 3 days/week, 1 to 1.5 hr/workout. The athlete does three to five sets based on 8RM to 12RM on heavy days and 75% to 90% of the heavy-day load on other days; volume is 8 to 12 repetitions. Each week, she adds 5 percentage points to the percentage of RM on the heavy day. Exercises are nonspecific movements, such as leg presses, dumbbell deadlifts, bench presses, calf raises, knee curls, leg raises, lateral raises, and biceps curls.

Endurance training: 2 days/week, 20 to 30 min/workout. Endurance training should be geared to maintenance of desirable levels of body fat rather than building a high level of endurance, which is not required and may be counterproductive relative to strength and power gains. Training can include 6-player volleyball and traditional aerobic activities, such as cycling, swimming, rowing, and running.

Unloading Week (Feb. 12-18)

An unloading week is included here to prepare the body for the shift to the next phase. Both volume and load are reduced significantly.

Strength Phase (Feb. 19–Mar. 18; 4 weeks)

Flexibility training: Part of warm-up and cool-down for all workouts.

Strength training: 3 days/week, 1 to 1.5 hr/workout. The athlete does three to five sets based on 5RM on heavy days and 80% to 95% of the heavy-day load on other days; volume, at five to six repetitions, is reduced from the previous phase. Each week, she adds 5-10 percentage points to the percentage of RM on the heavy day. Exercises are nonspecific and specific movements, such as push presses, calf raises, knee curls, leg raises, lateral raises, squats, and clean pulls.

Other training: 2 days/week, 20 to 30 min/workout. Activities include some skill drills, short-interval (≤ 50-m) sprints, and low- to moderate-intensity plyometric drills for the upper and lower extremities.

Unloading Week (Mar. 19-25)

Volume and load are reduced to prepare the athlete for the power phase.

Power Phase (Mar. 26–Apr. 15; 3 weeks)

Flexibility training: Part of warm-up and cool-down for all workouts.

Strength training: 3 days/week, 1 to 1.5 hr/workout. The athlete does three to five sets based on 2RM to 4RM on heavy days and 70% to 90% of 2RM to 4RM on other days; volume, at two to four repetitions, is reduced from the previous phase. Additional warm-up sets may be added as needed. Exercises are nonspecific and specific movements, such as calf raises, knee curls, sit-ups, lateral raises, pullovers, front squats, snatch pulls, and push jerks.

Other training: 2 days/week, 20 to 30 min/workout. Activities include sport-specific agility drills and high-intensity plyometric drills.

Unloading Week (Apr. 16-22)

An unloading week allows the athlete complete recuperation from the previous weeks of very intense training.

Competition Week (Apr. 23-29)

A new maximal effort is achieved during this week. Because this is the first mesocycle of the off season, the new maximum may be from 5% to 10% above the previous maximal effort. As the athlete gets into increasingly better condition, the percent of increase between the last RM test and the current test maximally may drop to 5% or below.

The strength training schedule for the entire preparatory period is delineated as follows.

Early Strength Phase (Weeks 1-6)

Week 1 (Jan. 1-7)		*Intensity*
Mon.	3-5 sets of 8-12 reps with 75% of 10RM	H
Wed.	Same sets and reps as Mon. with 90% of Mon. load	L-M
Fri.	Same as Wed.	M-L

Week 2 (Jan. 8-14)		
Mon.	3-5 sets of 8-12 reps with 80% of 10RM	H
Wed.	3-5 sets of 8-12 reps with 85% of Mon. load	L
Fri.	3-5 sets of 8-12 reps with 90% of Mon. load	M

Week 3 (Jan. 15-21)		
Mon.	3-5 sets of 8-12 reps with 85% of 10RM	H
Wed.	3-5 sets of 8-12 reps with 85% of Mon. load	L
Fri.	3-5 sets of 8-12 reps with 90% of Mon. load	M

Week 4 (Jan. 22-28)		
Mon.	3-5 sets of 8-12 reps with 90% of 10RM	H
Wed.	3-5 sets of 8-12 reps with 85% of Mon. load	L
Fri.	3-5 sets of 8-12 reps with 90% of Mon. load	M

Week 5 (Jan. 29–Feb.4)		
Mon.	3-5 sets of 8-12 reps with 95% of 10RM	H
Wed.	3-5 sets of 8-12 reps with 80% of Mon. load	L
Fri.	3-5 sets of 8-12 reps with 90% of Mon. load	M

Week 6 (Feb. 5-11)		
Mon.	3-5 sets of 8-12 reps with 105% of 10RM	H
Wed.	3-5 sets of 8-12 reps with 80% of Mon. load	L
Fri.	3-5 sets of 8-12 reps with 90% of Mon. load	M

Unloading Week

Week 7 (Feb. 12-18)

Mon.	1-3 sets of 5-6 reps with 85% of 10RM	H
Wed.	1-3 sets of 5-6 reps with 85% of Mon. load	L
Fri.	1-3 sets of 5-6 reps with 95% of Mon. load	M

Strength Phase (Weeks 8-11)

Week 8 (Feb. 19-25)

Mon.	3-5 sets of 5-6 reps with 85% of 5RM	H
Wed.	3-5 sets of 5-6 reps with 85% of Mon. load	L
Fri.	3-5 sets of 5-6 reps with 95% of Mon. load	M

Week 9 (Feb. 26–Mar. 4)

Mon.	3-5 sets of 5-6 reps with 90% of 5RM	H
Wed.	3-5 sets of 5-6 reps with 85% of Mon. load	L
Fri.	3-5 sets of 5-6 reps with 95% of Mon. load	M

Week 10 (Mar. 5-11)

Mon.	3-5 sets of 5-6 reps with 95% of 5RM	H
Wed.	3-5 sets of 5-6 reps with 85% of Mon. load	L
Fri.	3-5 sets of 5-6 reps with 90% of Mon. load	M

Week 11 (Mar. 12-18)

Mon.	3-5 sets of 5-6 reps with 105% of 5RM	H
Wed.	3-5 sets of 5-6 reps with 80% of Mon. load	L
Fri.	3-5 sets of 5-6 reps with 90% of Mon. load	M

Unloading Week

Week 12 (Mar. 19-25)

Mon.	1-3 sets of 2-4 reps with 85% of 5RM	H
Wed.	1-3 sets of 2-4 reps with 85% of Mon. load	L
Fri.	1-3 sets of 2-4 reps with 90% of Mon. load	M

Power Phase (Weeks 13-15)

Week 13 (Mar. 26–Apr. 1)

Mon.	3-5 sets of 2RM-4RM	H
Wed.	3-5 sets of 2-4 reps with 75% of 2RM-4RM	L
Fri.	3-5 sets of 2-4 reps with 85% of 2RM-4RM	M

Week 14 (Apr. 2-8)

Mon.	3-5 sets of 2RM-4RM	H
Wed.	3-5 sets of 2-4 reps with 85% of 2RM-4RM	L
Fri.	3-5 sets of 2-4 reps with 90% of 2RM-4RM	M

Week 15 (Apr. 9-15)

Mon.	3-5 sets of 2RM-3RM	H
Wed.	3-5 sets of 2-4 reps with 70% of 2RM-3RM	L
Fri.	3-5 sets of 2-4 reps with 85% of 2RM-3RM	M

Unloading Week

Week 16 (Apr. 16-22)

Mon.	1-3 sets of 2-4 reps with 85% of 2RM-3RM	H
Wed.	1-3 sets of 2-4 reps with 75% of 2RM-3RM	L
Fri.	1-3 sets of 2-4 reps with 80% of 2RM-3RM	M

Competition Week

Week 17 (Apr. 23-29)

Mon.	1-2 sets of 1 rep with 1RM	H
Wed.	1-2 sets of 1 rep with 70% of 1RM	L
Fri.	1-2 sets of 1 rep with 90% of 1RM	M

> **Intensity Level**
> L= low, M = moderate, H = high

Transitional Phase (Apr. 30–May 13; 2 weeks)

A transitional phase at this point is similar to the earlier transitional period prior to the preparatory period, except that some formal volleyball drills could be included.

Second Preparatory Mesocycle (Off-Season)

During the previous mesocycle the athlete worked with RMs other than 1RM because of a lack of training background. Having established a 1RM, she can now work with a percentage of 1RM.

The second preparatory period steps up the general intensity in all areas. It is shorter than the previous mesocycle. More sport-specific activities are included, and plyometric drills are more intense and include jumping activities. Endurance activities comprise interval/sprints with change of direction (agility) moves. Volleyball skill activities may be inserted 2 days/week after the moderate- and low-intensity weight sessions.

The following is the basic training schedule for each week during this mesocycle.

Monday: strength training (heavy load for clean pulls and push jerks; moderate load for squats)

Tuesday: plyometrics, interval sprints, agility drills

Wednesday: strength training (light load), volleyball drills

Thursday: plyometrics, interval sprints, agility drills

Friday: strength training (moderate load for clean pulls and push jerks; heavy load for squats), volleyball drills

Preparatory Period (May 14–Jul. 15; 9 weeks)

Flexibility training: part of warm-up and cool-down with each training session.

Strength training: 3 days/week; 1 to 1.5 hr/workload. Exercises are more activity specific than before, with the inclusion of back squats, cleans, pulls, push jerks, lunges, rotator cuff exercises, pullovers, calf raises, standing leg curls, and decline sit-ups. During this phase, the multiple-joint activities (squats, clean pulls, push jerks) are alternated as seen in the weekly schedule just noted. Single-joint exercises typically done on machines, such as calf raises and knee curls, are often not subject to all periodization principles because the mechanical advantage that the machine gives often allows a moderate to high number of repetitions once the first repetition has been achieved. Volume and load are manipulated so that a moderate to high number of repetitions and sets are done in general accord with the period of training. For example, during the hypertrophy phase, the repetitions for single-joint exercises should be higher than in the strength and power phases, and the intensity a little lower.

Endurance training: 2 days/week for 20 min/workout. Anaerobic interval sprints and agility drills.

Plyometrics: 2 days/week prior to interval sprint training; 15 to 20 min/workout. Done at low intensity and moderate to high volume (number of foot touches = 200-300). Hops and bounds only; no jumps (2).

The weekly schedules for strength training volume and load are as follows. The athlete uses this schedule in conjunction with the previously given weekly outline. Thus, for example, Monday is a "heavy day" for clean pulls and push jerks and a "moderate day" for squats. All loads are based on the athlete's most recent 1RM figure.

Hypertrophy Phase (Weeks 1-2)

Week 1 (May 14-20)

Heavy day	3-5 sets of 8-12 reps with 70% of 1RM
Moderate day	3-5 sets of 8-12 reps with 60% of 1RM
Light day	3-5 sets of 8-12 reps with 50% of 1RM

Week 2 (May 21-27)

Heavy day	3-5 sets of 8-12 reps with 75% of 1RM
Moderate day	3-5 sets of 8-12 reps with 70% of 1RM
Light day	3-5 sets of 8-12 reps with 60% of 1RM

Strength Phase (Weeks 3-4)

Week 3 (May 28–Jun. 3)

Heavy day	3-5 sets of 5-6 reps with 85% of 1RM
Moderate day	3-5 sets of 5-6 reps with 80% of 1RM
Light day	3-5 sets of 5-6 reps with 70% of 1RM

Week 4 (Jun. 4-10)

Heavy day	3-5 sets of 5-6 reps with 85% of 1RM
Moderate day	3-5 sets of 5-6 reps with 80% of 1RM
Light day	3-5 sets of 5-6 reps with 70% of 1RM

Unloading Week

Week 5 (Jun. 11-17)

Heavy day	1-3 sets of 2-4 reps with 80% of 1RM
Moderate day	1-3 sets of 2-4 reps with 70% of 1RM
Light day	1-3 sets of 2-4 reps with 60% of 1RM

Power Phase (Weeks 6-9)

Week 6 (Jun. 18-24)

Heavy day	3-5 sets of 2-4 reps with 90% of 1RM
Moderate day	3-5 sets of 2-4 reps with 80% of 1RM
Light day	3-5 sets of 2-4 reps with 70% of 1RM

Week 7 (Jun. 25–Jul. 1)

Heavy day	3-5 sets of 2-4 reps with 92.5% of 1RM
Moderate day	3-5 sets of 2-4 reps with 80% of 1RM
Light day	3-5 sets of 2-4 reps with 70% of 1RM

Week 8 (Jul. 2-8)

Heavy day	3-5 sets of 2-4 reps with 95% of 1RM
Moderate day	3-5 sets of 2-4 reps with 85% of 1RM
Light day	3-5 sets of 2-4 reps with 75% of 1RM

Week 9 (Jul. 9-15)

Heavy day	1-2 sets of 1 rep with 105%-110% of 1RM
Moderate day	1-2 sets of 1 rep with 100% of 1RM
Light day	1-2 sets of 1 rep with 70% of 1RM

Third Preparatory Mesocycle (Preseason)

After a 2 week transition period, it should be around the first week in August. The preseason now begins. This mesocycle will see a very abrupt drop in volume of strength training with a maintenance of load. Volleyball drills and practices dramatically increase. Endurance and plyometrics sessions are reduced to once or twice weekly, and weight training sessions are modified and reduced to twice weekly. Exercise selection is as sport-specific as possible. Multiple-joint activities, such as front squats, snatches, and push presses, are augmented by such single-joint activities as calf raises, pullovers, and a variety of abdominal exercises. This mesocycle will last roughly 6 weeks, from August 1 to September 15. The weekly schedule is as follows.

Monday: Heavy weight work followed by light volleyball practice

Tuesday: Volleyball practice followed by high-intensity endurance activities, such as agility, sprint, and shuffle intervals for 20 min

Wednesday: Volleyball practice

Thursday: Volleyball practice followed by moderate weight work

Friday: Plyometric drills for 15 min followed by light volleyball practice

The specific weekly schedules for strength training volume and load are as follows.

Phase I

Week 1 (Aug. 1-7)

Mon.	1-3 sets of 8-10 reps with 70% of 1RM
Thurs.	1-3 sets of 8-10 reps with 75% of 1RM

Phase II

Week 2 (Aug. 8-15)

Mon.	1-3 sets of 5-6 reps with 80% of 1RM
Thurs.	1-3 sets of 5-6 reps with 70% of 1RM

Week 3 (Aug. 16-23)

Mon.	1-3 sets of 5-6 reps with 85% of 1RM
Thurs.	1-3 sets of 5-6 reps with 80% of 1RM

Phase III

Week 4 (Aug. 24-31)

Mon.	1-3 sets of 2-4 reps with 90% of 1RM
Thurs.	1-3 sets of 2-4 reps with 80% of 1RM

Week 5 (Sept. 1-8)

Mon.	1-3 sets of 2-4 reps with 92.5% of 1RM
Thurs.	1-3 sets of 2-4 reps with 80% of 1RM

Week 6 (Sept. 9-16)

Mon.	1-3 sets of 1 rep with 105% of 1RM
Thurs.	1-3 sets of 1 rep with 100% of 1RM

Competition Mesocycle (In-Season)

At this point, the athlete is ready to begin the competition period of training. The volume of conditioning activities remain very low, with intensity varying from moderate to very high. Plyometrics activities are alternated with weight training and are conducted once or twice weekly, depending on the number of contests. Resistance training may be limited to 30 min once or twice weekly, with sport-specific multiple-joint activities that cover as many muscle groups as possible. For example, a squatting movement may be performed on one day and a pulling/pushing movement such as clean pulls and push presses/jerks on the other day. Single-joint exercises, such as calf raises and lateral raises, could be done in circuit training fashion to conserve time. Fifteen to 20 min of various short sprint intervals could be performed once or twice weekly during practice on days when no lifting is done. Two to 3 days should be given between lifting, plyometrics, and interval sessions, depending on the contest schedule. Much like the previous mesocycle, 90% to 95% of the athlete's time is spent on skill and strategy development, the remainder on conditioning. The in-season period spans 7 to 10 weeks. The athlete is in good condition from the previous mesocycles, so she should not only maintain that condition but peak again for the tournament period, which could last for 3 weeks.

The lifting schedule is as follows during this mesocycle. The number of sets do not include warm-up sets. The athlete's 1RM is determined from the results of the previous mesocycle.

Week 1 (Sept. 17-24)

1 set of 10 reps with 75% of 1RM

Week 2 (Sept. 25–Oct. 2)

1 set of 5-6 reps with 80% of 1RM

Week 3 (Oct. 3-10)

1 set of 5-6 reps with 85% of 1RM

Week 4 (Oct. 11-18)

1 set of 2-4 reps with 90% of 1RM

Week 5 (Oct. 19-26)

1 set of 2-4 reps with 92.5% of 1RM

Week 6 (Oct. 27–Nov. 3)

1 set of 2-4 reps with 95% of 1RM

Week 7 (Nov. 4-11)

1 set of 1-3 reps with 102.5% of 1RM

If the team continues in the tournament, begin with the Week 2 workout; progress to Weeks 3 and 4 if the team makes it to the finals. Should the game schedule not allow for more than one lift during a week, do both multiple-joint exercises in that workout, skipping the single-joint circuit. Two examples of specific weekly schedules follow.

Week A (two matches)

Mon.	weight work and practice
Tues.	match
Wed.	practice and interval sprints
Thurs.	match
Fri.	plyometrics and practice

Week B (three matches)

Mon.	match
Tues.	match
Wed.	weight work and practice
Thurs.	match
Fri.	practice and interval sprints

REVIEWING THE EXAMPLE

For a program such as the previous model to function optimally, the skill and strategy coach and the strength and conditioning professional must plan the program together and share goals and strategies. Without the cooperation of all involved parties, optimal performance cannot be fully achieved.

This is one model of the implementation of periodization principles of cyclic variation of volume and intensity in training. Other athletes and events will require subtle to radical variations from the example. This is where the training art melds with the science of adaptation. Readers who wish more examples of periodization models may consult references 1-4 and 6.

CONCLUSION

Periodization is based on Selye's General Adaptation Syndrome. Training is organized into cycles for the purpose of bringing the athlete to peak condition for the most important competitions. The year's training, or macrocycle, is divided into one or more mesocycles, which contain preparatory, competition, and transition periods. Each period has one or more weekly microcycles that are often divided into heavy, moderate, and light training days. The mesocycles begin with high-volume and low-intensity training and progress to low-volume and high-intensity training just prior to the competition period. Transition periods of active rest follow each competition period and may be interspersed in long preparatory periods. The nature of the sporting season dictates the length and number of mesocycles during the training year.

Key Terms

macrocycle	459	microcycle	459	periodization	459
mesocycle	459				

Study Questions

1. Periodization was first developed by

   a. Stone
   b. Selye
   c. Matveyev
   d. O'Bryant

2. The macrocycle is generally

   a. one year of training
   b. part of a year of training
   c. a week of training
   d. a day's training

3. Volume of training during the hypertrophy phase of the preparatory period is
   a. moderate
   b. low
   c. low to moderate
   d. high

4. During a short competitive period (1-3 weeks), the goal of training should be
   a. active rest
   b. maintenance of fitness
   c. development of strength
   d. development of endurance

Applying Knowledge of Periodization

Problem 1

The wrestling team has a 22-match (12-week) season that precedes the conference tournament. What type of volume and intensity of training should be undertaken during the competition period that contains the 22 matches?

Problem 2

How do you keep the stress of training from becoming so great that it causes maladaptation or overtraining?

References

1. Bompa, T. *Theory and Methodology of Training*. Dubuque, IA: Kendall/Hunt. 1983.
2. Chargina, A., M. Stone, J. Piedmonte, H. O'Bryant, W.J. Kraemer, V. Gambetta, H. Newton, G. Palmeri, and D. Pfoff. Periodization roundtable. *NSCA Journal* 8(5):12-23. 1986. 8(6):17-25; 9(1):16-27. 1987.
3. Matveyev, L. *Fundamentals of Sport Training*. Moscow: Progress. 1981.
4. Pauletto, B. Let's talk training: Periodization-peaking. *NSCA Journal* 8(4):30, 31. 1986.
5. Pedemonte, J. Historical perspectives on periodization, Part 2. *NSCA Journal* 8(4):26-29. 1986.
6. Stone, M., and H. O'Bryant. *Weight Training: A Scientific Approach*. Minneapolis: Burgess International. 1987.

PART V

ORGANIZATION AND ADMINISTRATION OF THE STRENGTH TRAINING AND CONDITIONING FACILITY

We would like to thank the following individuals who were members of the NSCA's Standards for Weightroom Safety Panel, and who contributed to the ideas and guidelines presented in chapters 31 through 34: Mike Burke, CSCS; Mike Carter; Boyd Epley, CSCS; Rick Huegli, CSCS; Bill Kroll, CSCS; Ray Moran, CSCS; Gary Polson, CSCS; Ron Thomson, CSCS; and Paul White, CSCS.

We acknowledge that chapters 31 through 34 contain several ideas from Gary Polson's *Institutional Weight Room Design Manual*. Stillwater, OK: Strength Tech. 1989.

CHAPTER 31

FACILITY LAYOUT AND SCHEDULING

Stephanie L. Armitage-Johnson

The lack of time, facility space, equipment, and qualified supervisory staff are major concerns for a facility coordinator. It is a challenge to effectively utilize the space and time and to do so in a safe manner. As the facility coordinator you are responsible for not only knowing how to organize athletes for strength training and conditioning activities, but also for knowing how to arrange equipment safely in order to meet the challenge.

In some cases you might be responsible for developing a facility from almost nothing. Planning the facility takes many hours of creating and reviewing floor plans and deciding what equipment will be needed, how space may be best utilized, what surfaces are needed in various areas, and other factors. For development from scratch, it is worthwhile to contact professionals in other programs who have built a facility and to compile information on specific needs. A committee of people who represent various areas of expertise may be organized to help in the planning of the facility. Such a committee may consist of an administrator, contractor, lawyer, student-athlete, sport coach, instructors who would use the facility, various experts in the field of sport conditioning, and any other people who could give valuable input on design.

In most cases, however, you will "inherit" an existing facility. Therefore, this discussion is limited to existing facilities and how you might improve and reorganize them to best suit the needs of the **philosophy** (the ideals and values shaping the program), **goals** (the desired outcome), and **objectives** (the individual steps toward a goal) of a program.

ASSESSING NEEDS

After defining the program goals and objectives (see chapter 32), the facility coordinator should assess existing equipment and the needs of the various sport groups that plan to use the facility. As the coordinator, you will need to answer these questions:

- What are the specific training goals of each group?
- What types of training does each require (e.g., circuits, machines, free weights, platform lifts, plyometrics)?
- What are the seasonal priorities of each group?
- What are the training ages (training experience) of the athletes in the groups?
- When will weight training fit into each group's schedule?
- What repairs, adaptations, and modifications must be made to meet the athletes' needs?
- How should the equipment be placed to best utilize the space in a safe and efficient manner?

ARRANGING EQUIPMENT

Find out who will be using the facility and list existing equipment. Draw a floor plan to visualize the present and potential locations of equipment; to plan for safety and the most efficient use of space, exits, and entrances; to identify areas of frequent travel; to develop **facility flow** (pathways in the facility); and to plan supervisor station locations for maximum supervision of the whole facility, especially areas of increased risk (such as the platform area). Safety should always be a priority (1).

Station all high-risk activities, including platform lifts, squats, overhead presses, bench and incline presses, and exercises that require spotters, away from windows, mirrors, exits, and entrances to avoid breakage of glass, distraction, or collision with the bar or lifter. Place the equipment for these activities in areas that are readily supervised to ensure safety and the execution of proper technique.

Supervision is effective only if all areas of the facility can be observed at any given time (3). Therefore, place supervisor stations in locations with full visibility to all areas of the facility, to allow quick access to athletes in need of spotters or immediate assistance.

Arrange the tallest machines or pieces of equipment along the walls, with the shorter, smaller pieces in the middle to improve visibility (as well as appearance) and maximize use of space. Place weight racks with enough distance away from bar ends and spotter areas for ease of movement without obstruction. Tall pieces of equipment, such as squat racks, may need to be bolted to the walls or floors for increased stability.

The following are guidelines suggested by a panel of safety experts at the National Strength and Conditioning Association (NSCA) for safety and efficient use of equipment:

- All weight machines and apparatus must be spaced at least 2 ft (61 cm) from one another, and preferably 3 ft (91 cm) apart.
- Platform areas should have sufficient overhead space (at least 12 ft [3.7 m]), which should be free of such low-hanging items as beams, pipes, lighting, and signs.
- The proper spacing of Olympic bars is 3 ft (91 cm) between ends (12 ft [3.7 m] × 8 ft [2.4 m] = 1 platform lifting area).

Maintain a clear pathway 3-ft (91-cm) wide in the facility at all times, as stipulated by federal, state, and local laws. Machines and equipment must not be allowed to block or obstruct this flow. Place equipment at least 6 in. (15 cm) from mirrors and mirrors 20 in. (51 cm) above the floor. Place free-weight equipment well away from exits and entrances to avoid obstruction and give participants ample room for passage and guarantee safety to the pedestrian and lifter. Organize equipment into "priority sections," such as free-weight areas, machine areas, power training areas, aerobic areas, and so on. This allows the supervisor to identify and focus on the higher risk areas and keep equipment orderly in the facility.

You may wish to make several blank copies of the floor plan and draw in possible designs to suit the needs of the participants and conform with program goals. The floor plans shown in Figures 31.1, 31.2, and 31.3 are examples of efficient use of space in high school, club, and university settings. These examples show reasonable traffic flow without obstruction, high-risk areas located away from traffic and obstruction, lack of "dead space," and equipment placement for safety and ease of supervision of the whole facility.

ORGANIZING GROUPS OF ATHLETES ACCORDING TO FACILITY

When organizing groups of athletes, you should consider the size of the facility and assess the needs of each group in terms of the following:

- Sport-specific training needs (e.g., strength, endurance, circuits, and power)
- Seasonal priority (i.e., when sports occur, such as football in the fall and baseball in the spring)
- Group size and equipment availability (e.g., a football team with 150 members may not be able to efficiently and safely use a facility without being split into groups; other sports groups may have to be scheduled at times other than that of football groups to ensure sufficient use of the equipment)
- The athlete-staff ratio (1:10 to 1:30, depending upon the training group)
- The minimum space requirement per lifter is 30 ft² (2.8 m²) and the maximum is 60 ft² (5.6 m²) (2)

Schedule facility usage so that different groups of athletes train in the facility at more or less constant "density" throughout the day; avoid large, congested groups, which increase the potential for injury and inefficient use of equipment. If the facility is designed for high school athletes, groups may be organized through physical education classes that offer beginning, intermediate, and advanced strength and conditioning to the students. Teams may organize facility usage time before or after practice according to seasonal priority. See Figure 31.4 for a sample training schedule for teams using the strength facility.

CONCLUSION

Designing the strength and conditioning facility for safety and for effective use of equipment, time, and space can be a challenging task. In most cases, a facility coordinator "inherits" an existing facility and therefore must assess needed modifications to suit its users.

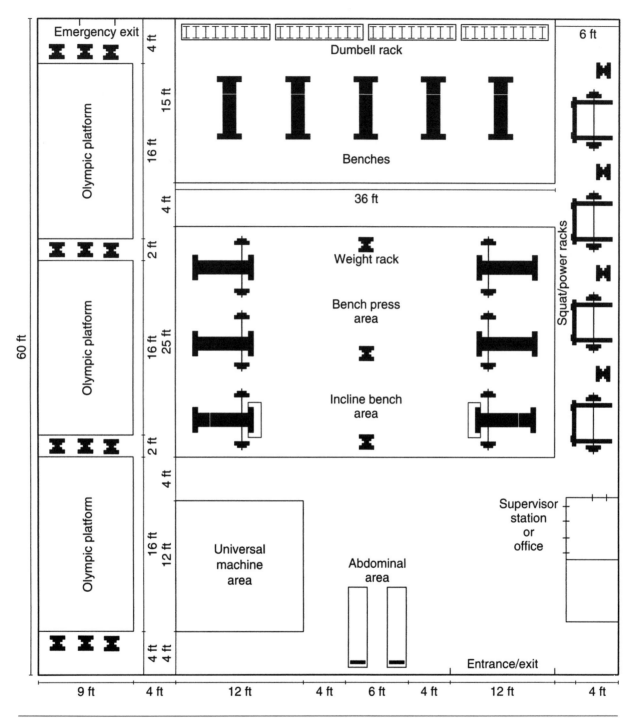

Figure 31.1 Floor plan of a high school training facility.

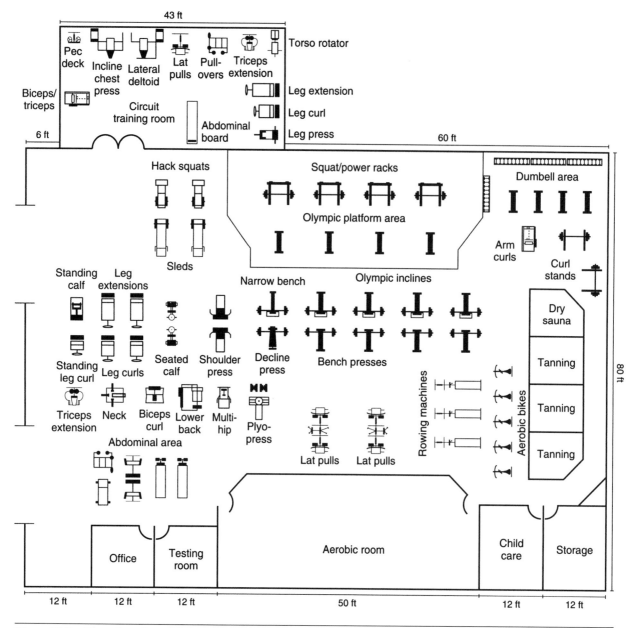

Figure 31.2 Floor plan of an athletic club's training facility.

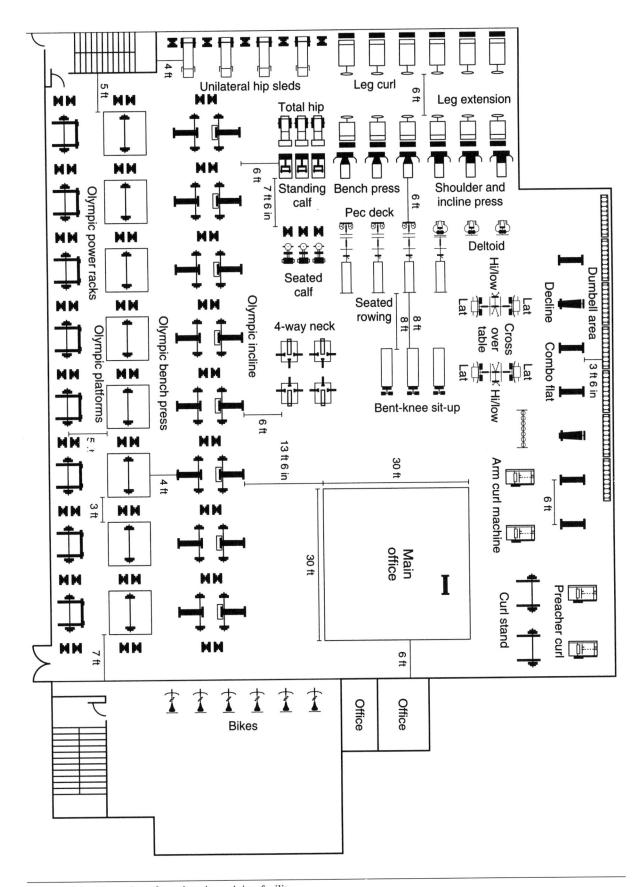

Figure 31.3 Floor plan of a university training facility.

	Mon.	Tues.	Wed.	Thurs.	Fri.	Sat.
7-8	Crew	Crew	Crew	Crew	Crew	
8-9	Gymnastics		Gymnastics		Gymnastics	
9-10	Swimming		Swimming		Swimming	
10-11						
11-12						
12-1						
1-2	Track/ cross-country	Volleyball	Track/ cross-country	Volleyball	Track/ cross-country	
2-3	Golf/soccer		Golf/soccer		Golf/soccer	
3-4	Track	Basketball	Track	Basketball	Track	
4-5	Football offense	Football defense	Football offense	Football defense	Football offense	Football defense
5-6						
6-7	Softball/ baseball/ tennis		Softball/ baseball/ tennis		Softball/ baseball/ tennis	

Figure 31.4 Schedule of team usage of a strength and conditioning facility during the fall semester (September-December). Some teams are scheduled in the morning hours to avoid extremely large numbers of athletes in the facility simultaneously. A large block of time is open from midmorning to early afternoon to let athletes with class or other conflicts train; such athletes may also use a Tuesday/Thursday/Saturday schedule, using the 9 a.m. to 1 p.m. time slot. A large team like football may split into two or more groups (such as offense and defense). This allows smaller numbers to train, avoiding congestion and making equipment more available.

Changes may include placement or arrangement of equipment for safety and efficient use. Floor plans are useful in designing safe pathways in the facility. Taller equipment should be placed near the walls and shorter equipment toward the center of the room to increase visibility, maximize useable space, and improve appearance. When organizing athlete groups, the facility coordinator must assess the specific training needs of each sport group, determine seasonal priorities, and evaluate equipment availability relative to group size.

Key Terms

facility flow	475	objective	475	philosophy	475
goal	475				

Study Questions

1. When designing or reorganizing a facility, the use of a floor plan is valuable for determining
   a. location of equipment
   b. most useful placement of a supervisor station
   c. facility flow or pathway
   d. all of the above

2. When making up a schedule for use of the facility by groups of athletes, the facility coordinator should assess

   a. sport-specific training needs
   b. sport seasonal priority
   c. group size and availability
   d. all of the above

3. Taller equipment should be placed along the walls of the strength and conditioning facility because

   a. taller equipment may tip over
   b. observation of the whole facility is enhanced
   c. all such equipment must be bolted to the walls
   d. none of the above

4. High risk activities include

   a. leg presses
   b. dumbbell lifts (excluding over-the-face and overhead lifts)
   c. overhead lifts
   d. lunges in place

Applying Knowledge
of Facility Layout and Scheduling

Problem 1
Jim was just beginning his first year as the assistant track coach and strength coach for a small private college. When he wasn't out on the field coaching the jumpers and hurdlers, he was in the weight room coaching athletes of various sports. With only two lifting platforms and four squat racks, training sessions proved to be quite hectic as well as pretty "scary," according to Jim. It seemed that the morning hours and early afternoon hours were the low activity times of the day. At 3 p.m., athletes and other students filled the room beyond capacity. This made it very difficult to do one-on-one instruction and to make sure individuals completed their programs without skipping exercises. What should Jim do to properly address his concerns?

Problem 2
Look at the floor plan on p. 482 and make any needed changes to improve the flow, safety, and efficient use of the facility and its equipment.

References

1. Adams, S., M. Adrian, and M. Bayless. *Catastrophic Injuries in Sports: Avoidance Strategies*. Salinas, CA: Coyote Press. 1984.
2. Kroll, W. Structural and functional considerations in designing the facility, Part I. *NSCA Journal* 13(1):51-58. 1991.
3. Nygaard, G., and T. Boone. *Coaches Guide to Sport Law*. Champaign, IL: Human Kinetics. 1985.

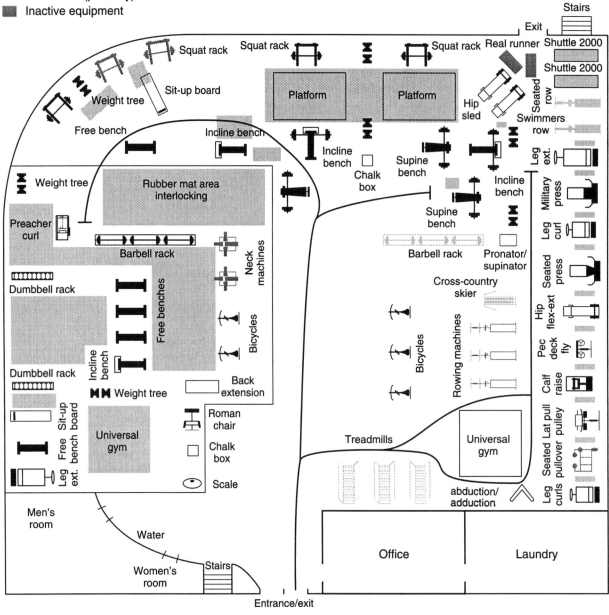

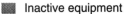

Problem floor plan of a facility and equipment.

CHAPTER 32

DAY-TO-DAY OPERATIONS: DEVELOPING POLICIES AND PROCEDURES

Stephanie L. Armitage-Johnson

Liability is now a concern common to all people responsible for sport and movement activities. Liability concerns heighten the need for quality instruction and supervision of participants in a program and for continual inspection and maintenance of the facility and its equipment. The National Strength and Conditioning Association (NSCA) has established policy and procedure guidelines to assist the strength and conditioning professional in assuring participants, family members, educators, and administrators that a safe facility free from hazards is being maintained. The guidelines in this chapter are based on those developed by the NSCA.

Policies and procedures concern both athletes (and other users) and staff members. *Policies* are essentially a facility's rules and regulations; they reflect the goals and objectives of the program. *Procedures* describe the approach to how policies are met. Before detailing specific policies and procedures, we need to look at program goals and objectives, because these are the basis on which policies and procedures are determined.

PROGRAM GOALS

Program goals are the desired end products of a strength and conditioning program. The following is a sample goal statement that a facility coordinator may use:

The major goal of a strength and conditioning program is to provide to competitive athletes the means by which they may train consistently, sensibly, and systematically over designated periods of time, in a safe, clean, and professional environment in order to help prevent injury and improve athletic performance.

PROGRAM OBJECTIVES

Program objectives are individual means of attaining program goals. To state program goals without listing ways in which these goals might be attained may result in athletes never achieving them. Program objectives should encompass all areas of the program to ensure that goals are attained. The following is a sample list of program objectives that lead to the previously stated goal:

1. To design and administer strength, stretching, aerobic, and plyometric and other anaerobic training programs that reduce the likelihood of athletic injuries and improve athletic performance

2. To design resistance training programs that maximize physical performance by using various strength training methods and modes

(a) To select appropriate exercises for athletes that produce training outcomes specific to each athlete's needs

(b) To apply the principles of exercise sequence to ensure the desired training outcomes

(c) To prescribe appropriate training volumes, rest periods, frequencies, and load resistances based on the athlete's health status, strength and conditioning levels, sport, and goals of training

3. To design a strength and conditioning program that uses the principles of periodization to meet the specific needs of a sport

4. To prescribe exercises that develop and maintain muscular balance between antagonistic muscle groups in order to decrease susceptibility to injury and enhance performance

5. To instruct athletes in how to execute resistance training exercises safely and correctly and thus obtain the desired results

6. To develop individual programs to account for biomechanical and physiological differences among individual athletes, taking into account their age, gender, training status, physical limitations, and past injuries

7. To recognize acute and chronic physiological responses and adaptations to training and their implications to the design of sport-specific training programs

8. To utilize information on body composition to prescribe training programs that bring about the desired results in body composition, hypertrophy, strength, muscular endurance, and cardiovascular endurance

9. To educate athletes on the importance of good nutrition and its role in health and performance

10. To educate athletes on the abuse and effects of performance-enhancing substances, on relevant school policy and legal legislation, and on viable alternatives

Based upon these statements, your first tasks as a facility coordinator are to establish policies in written form and to set up meetings to familiarize both participants and staff with written goals, objectives, and procedures.

FACILITY POLICIES

Strength and conditioning facility policies, or rules, are important to providing the participants with guidelines for conduct and behavior, keeping order, and maintaining the program on course toward the goal of providing a safe, clean, and professional training environment.

The following is a checklist of facility rules and policies for athletes and other users. These should be posted in the training area where they can be easily seen.

Checklist of Facility Rules and Policies

☐ Operating hours

☐ Policy on recognized users and/or membership (recognized users may include athletes, students, guests, staff, faculty, alumni, family members, visiting teams, and fitness program clientele)

☐ Emergency procedures (see chapter 34)

☐ Staff members and area responsibilities (brief comment on whom to go to if a problem arises)

☐ Specific rules on use of the facility

✓ No one is allowed in the training facility without a qualified supervisor present.

✓ Prior to participation, you must get a medical check-up and receive a doctor's approval in writing.

✓ Prior to participation, you must undergo an orientation on common risks involved in strength training, on the proper execution of various exercises, and on the possible consequences if proper technique is not employed.

✓ Prior to participation, you must undergo an orientation on equipment and its proper use.

✓ Do not use equipment unless you are knowledgeable about how to properly use it.

✓ Observe weight room etiquette and demonstrate courtesy toward others in the room at all times.

✓ No horseplay; loud, offensive language; or temper tantrums are permitted.

✓ Wear proper training attire, particularly shirts and athletic shoes, at all times. No jeans are allowed.

✓ Show respect for equipment and facilities at all times. Do not drop or throw weights.

✓ You may be expelled from the facility immediately if you misuse any equipment or facilities. If you fail to leave when asked, you may be expelled from a team and assisted out by security personnel.

✓ Utilize spotters and locks when necessary (e.g., for overhead lifts, squats, bench presses, and platform lifts).

✓ Keep equipment off the floor and return it to its proper rack when lifting is completed.

✓ Keep the facility flow path clear; remove any obstructions.

✓ Check out weight training equipment from a supervisor and return it when finished.

✓ The on-duty supervisors have the authority over all room conduct and use of equipment, including the sound system.

✓ Immediately report any facility-related injury or facility/equipment irregularity to the supervisors on duty.

✓ Use the minimum space requirement per lifter of 30 ft^2 (2.8 m^2) and take up no more than 60 ft^2 (5.6 m^2).

✓ Tobacco, food, chewing gum, glass bottles, and cans are not allowed in the training facility; plastic water bottles are acceptable.

✓ Alcohol, drugs, and banned substances are not allowed in the training facility.

✓ Weight equipment is not allowed in the mat area.

✓ Supervisors are not responsible for users' personal belongings or lost or stolen items.

✓ Keep feet off of the walls.

✓ Minimize chalk and powder on the floor.

✓ Do not spit in the facility.

✓ Never attempt to ''save'' Olympic-style lifts (i.e., power snatches and power cleans).

✓ Use belts when attempting extremely heavy lifts where the bar is placed on the back (e.g., squats).

✓ All guests and visitors must report to the facility coordinator for signing of liability forms and approval for use of the facility.

✓ Follow the posted rules and policies when using the saunas, showers, whirlpools, and other rehabilitation and treatment equipment.

To ensure that athletes adhere to the facility rules, the facility coordinator might want to have each athlete sign an agreement, such as the ''Weight Room Policies'' form on page 486.

MEDICAL SERVICES

Chapter 34 discusses medical services, basic life support, and first aid in some detail. Medical services are briefly introduced here as part of the day-to-day operations of the strength and conditioning facility.

Medical services at high school, university, and health club facilities may vary greatly. Staff members at all settings should have current first aid and cardiopulmonary resuscitation (CPR) certifications. If an athlete sustains a catastrophic injury (one that threatens life or the long-term quality of life) in which immediate CPR or first aid is required, staff members near the injured person should follow American Red Cross guidelines for CPR and first aid. Medical personnel and/or medical trainers should then be notified; medical personnel may call upon emergency hospital aid directly if necessary. If medical services are needed for a non-

catastrophic injury (one that warrants care but is not threatening to life or the long-term quality of life), the emergency may be handled in the training facility by the staff and then referred to athletic trainers.

A first aid box should be stocked and located in a visible site in the training facility and the staff informed of its location and contents.

SCHEDULING AND PROGRAMMING

The scheduling and programming of athletes or groups in the training facility is an important part of time management and efficient facility use. In chapter 31 we covered how to schedule groups of athletes according to facility size, equipment available, seasonal priority, and group size.

EQUIPMENT OPERATION AND MAINTENANCE

Equipment is expensive and usually not easy to replace; maintenance of the equipment is important for protecting the investment of the institution. As the facility coordinator, you are responsible for instructing staff members on the operation and maintenance of equipment. Staff members may be assigned the responsibility for maintaining certain pieces of equipment and for instructing individuals and groups about equipment usage, during orientation and periodically throughout the year when needed. Equipment maintenance is discussed in detail in chapter 33.

JOB TITLES AND RESPONSIBILITIES

One of your responsibilities as coordinator of the day-to-day operations of a facility is to clearly define the job descriptions of those under your management. The title and responsibilities of the traditional strength coach, for example, are changing as the strength and conditioning field grows and becomes more recognized. Because specific responsibilities will vary according to the institution, only general descriptions will be given in this chapter (see pp. 488-491 for job descriptions for various positions).

In the school setting, according to NSCA guidelines, the *strength and conditioning coordinator* (also commonly referred to as the *head strength coach*) is both a coach and administrator who is a *Certified Strength and Conditioning Specialist* (CSCS). This person organizes the strength and conditioning programs and the

Weight Room Policies

1. Only intercollegiate athletes are permitted to use the Weight Room.
2. You must sign in each time you use the facility.
3. You must have a workout program, follow it, and record workout content on your own.
4. If you have an injury that in any way inhibits a portion of a workout, you must first see a trainer and receive a written slip explaining the injury, which movements are to be avoided, and which ones may be substituted.
5. Lifters are required to use collars once there is more than one plate on the end of the bar.
6. Lifters are required to use spotters on every set after the initial warm-up set.
7. Move weights from the racks to the bar only. Never set them on the floor or lean them against equipment.
8. Strip all bars immediately after use. Return dumbbells to the rack in the proper order.
9. Keep bars and weights off the vinyl at all times to prevent tearing.
10. Food, drink, gum, tobacco, and toothpicks are not permitted.
11. Walkmans are allowed on the exercise bikes and stairmasters only.
12. Spitting in or defacing the facility is not tolerated and will result in immediate expulsion.
13. Horseplay will not be tolerated.
14. The staff offices and telephones are off limits to athletes, unless permission to use them is given.
15. The strength and conditioning staff is not responsible for holding personal items.
16. Follow all instructions given by the coaches.
17. Failure to follow any of the policies could result in loss of Weight Room privileges.

I, _____ , have read all the Weight Room policies and hereby agree to follow them. I also acknowledge that failure to comply with these policies may result in loss of Weight Room privileges.

Adapted by permission from *Huskies History Questionnaire* by the University of Washington Athletic Department (1991).

coaches assigned to individual sports. The coordinator is responsible for the overall program, facility, equipment, and staff, and for such administrative tasks as preparing a budget, purchasing equipment, preparing proposals, and dealing with the administration.

A *strength coach* or an assistant to the strength and conditioning coordinator, as defined by the NSCA, is responsible for many of the same duties as the coordinator, but he or she may not be a CSCS and may be responsible for one team and not the whole program. This person may be a full-time or part-time staff member responsible for the strength and conditioning programs of several teams, with additional cleaning, maintenance, and supervisory tasks.

The training facility *supervisor* is usually a part-time student assistant responsible for observing the participants to ensure safe and effective use of equipment. The supervisor is also responsible for assisting the strength coaches and coordinator when necessary and for assigned cleaning and maintenance tasks. *Volunteer assistants* may be utilized as well; they perform a variety of tasks to assist the coordinator, while gaining valuable experience in the field.

In the club setting, the equivalent of the coordinator may have the title *fitness manager* or *fitness director*. The staff members under the direction of the fitness manager may be called *fitness specialists* or *personal trainers* and may be responsible for many of the same tasks as assistant strength and conditioning coordinators and supervisors.

The facility coordinator is responsible for the proper instruction and education of supervisors and assistants on the written policies and procedures directed to them. The coordinator should make sure each staff member understands the coordinator's program goals and objectives, coordinate each staff member's schedule and responsibilities, and communicate requirements concerning the professional conduct of each staff member.

The following checklist may be used as a guide in developing and communicating expectations to staff members.

Checklist for Staff Requirements

☐ Demonstrated knowledge of the coordinator's program goals and objectives

☐ Demonstrated willingness to learn and instruct proper exercise and spotting techniques

☐ Fulfillment of continuing education requirements, which may include CPR and first-aid; participation in clinics and conferences to stay current in the field of strength and conditioning

☐ Demonstrated knowledge of emergency procedures

☐ Professional etiquette consistent with the requirements of the coordinator, including the following points:

✓ Display of positive attitude toward all recognized users of the facility

✓ Display of willingness to readily assist participants in spotting, demonstration, instruction of techniques, and explanation of exercise usefulness

✓ Display of willingness to effectively and properly motivate individuals to achieve maximum potential in all areas of performance without increased potential for injury

✓ Promotion of a healthy body and mind to participants by presenting the advantages of strength and conditioning for improved self-image, health, and improved performance without the need for performance-enhancing substances

✓ Promotion of strength and conditioning techniques and a hard-work ethic for the improvement of performance

✓ If approached by a participant concerning performance-enhancing substances, education of the participant on the facts and legal implications (and following specific guidelines given by the coordinator)

✓ Demonstration of willingness to cooperate with other staff members in all aspects of facility operations, including cleaning, inspecting, and maintaining facilities and equipment

✓ Demonstration of diplomacy and good judgment when dealing with participants by interacting with members of both sexes without bias or prejudice

✓ Avoidance of flirtation or intimate relationships with student athletes

✓ Avoidance of conversations that may be classified as gossip or slander

✓ Display of a high level of attentiveness concerning proper instruction and supervision at all times while on duty

✓ Maintenance of confidentiality when dealing with the coordinator, staff, and individual participants

✓ Display of prudent judgment, common sense, and foresight when making decisions or inspecting and maintaining the facility and equipment

✓ Demonstration of an understanding and willingness to monitor assigned training programs daily, make observations, and perform any other requirement dealing with monitoring and record keeping

✓ Display of willingness to attend required meetings held by the facility coordinator

✓ Demonstration of willingness to perform specific and general supervision as well as other performance tasks requested by the facility coordinator

Sample job descriptions for six types of university and club positions are provided on pages 488 to 491. These may be useful for developing and defining positions. The reader may also want to consult the *ACSM Guidelines for the Health and Fitness Industry* (4th ed. published by Lea & Febiger, Philadelphia, 1991).

CONCLUSION

Program goals give the program direction and purpose; objectives help keep the program on task by providing steps toward these goals. Based on goals and objectives, rules and policies are developed to guide participant conduct and ensure safety. People in the field of strength and conditioning have numerous responsibilities, outlined in the various lists in the chapter.

Responsibilities of the Coordinator of a Strength and Conditioning Facility (University and Health Club Setting)

1. Instructing athletes in the safe and correct execution of flexibility, plyometrics, and speed development exercises in order to obtain the desired result
2. Providing instruction in safe and effective spotting procedures to ensure the maximum effect of the exercise and the safety of the athlete
3. Establishing policies and procedures for athletes in the form of written staff procedures, to facilitate the day-to-day operation of the facility
4. Administering basic life support and other first-aid procedures to facility users in need of immediate care
5. Possessing equipment maintenance skills to provide a safe training environment
6. Knowing proper procedures in designing strength and conditioning facilities to most effectively utilize the space and time allotted and reduce the potential for injury
7. Selecting, organizing, and administering testing procedures in a manner that ensures the collection of valid and reliable data
8. Evaluating test data to determine special needs, appropriate training procedures, and motivational strategies
9. Understanding human muscle physiology in order to appropriately design exercise programs
10. Understanding human bioenergetics and metabolism so that training programs are designed specific to the activity
11. Possessing factual knowledge of neuroendocrine responses to physical activity so that appropriate training programs are designed to obtain the desired results
12. Applying knowledge of neurological adaptations to training so that safe and effective programs can be designed
13. Understanding cardiovascular anatomy and physiology at rest and in response to various forms of exercise so that appropriate and effective exercise programs can be designed
14. Understanding bone, muscle, and connective tissue adaptation; possessing the ability to apply this knowledge in program design so that the potential for injury is reduced and the probability of enhanced performance increased
15. Understanding muscle and skeletal anatomy; applying the principles of the biomechanics of human movement in order to select appropriate exercises and promote their safe, effective, and proper execution
16. Possessing knowledge of performance-enhancing substances; recognizing symptoms of their use and providing persuasive evidence to athletes on effects, risks, and appropriate alternatives
17. Communicating effective approaches in implementing sport psychology techniques to enhance training and performance

18. Recognizing nutritional factors (including vitamins and minerals) that affect health and performance; providing appropriate nutritional counseling
19. Recognizing symptoms and behaviors associated with eating disorders; being able to utilize physical performance evaluations and observations
20. Generating income and budgeting available funds for maintenance and improvement of the facility
21. Effectively and properly motivating athletes to achieve maximum potential in the activity of their choice
22. Defining job responsibilities and managing subordinates
23. Working and communicating with other coaches in the athletic department
24. Developing and monitoring the facility's safety inspection and maintenance programs
25. Selecting new equipment and developing bid specifications for equipment
26. Traveling with sports teams and providing remote-site strength training and flexibility programs, including pregame stretching
27. Closing facilities temporarily if unsafe conditions warrant this
28. Properly installing new equipment according to a manufacturer's installation instructions, with staff assistance
29. Maintaining a strength library for professional improvement and the training of others

Responsibilities of an Assistant Strength and Conditioning Coordinator (University Setting)

1. Developing and monitoring strength and conditioning programs for assigned varsity athletic teams
2. Assisting in fitness testing, computation of results, and evaluation of individual athletes
3. Organizing team and supervisor orientation and follow-up meetings, in-service training meetings for supervisors, and nutrition and weight management meetings
4. Analyzing the nutritional habits of athletes to determine the steps necessary for modifying and providing a balanced diet (may include data entry into computer system)
5. Teaching proper lifting technique and assisting in spotting heavy lifts when necessary
6. Assisting in the general maintenance and cleaning of the facility and its equipment
7. Anticipating potential risks of injury, taking measures to remove them, and, in the event of an injury, having the ability to implement emergency medical procedures
8. Assisting the facility coordinator with all tasks for which he or she is responsible and with the general operation of the facility in the coordinator's absence
9. Effectively and properly motivating athletes to achieve maximum potential in all areas of performance
10. Working and communicating with other coaches in the athletic department
11. Assisting with equipment check-out
12. Performing other duties as assigned by the facility coordinator

Responsibilities of Volunteer Assistants, Student Assistants, and Supervisors (University Setting)

1. Supervising the facility during assigned times
2. Enforcing facility policies and rules

3. Maintaining and cleaning the facility and its equipment
4. Anticipating potential risks of injury and taking measures to remove them and alert participants to them
5. Assisting in spotting heavy lifts when necessary and teaching proper lifting technique
6. Monitoring equipment check-out
7. Assisting in testing of athletes
8. Attending all required meetings
9. Performing duties assigned by the coordinator or assistant coordinator
10. Effectively and properly motivating athletes to achieve their maximum potential in all areas of performance
11. Performing other duties as assigned by the staff

Responsibilities of a Fitness Program Director (Health Club Setting)

1. Managing the development, implementation, and evaluation of all fitness programs
2. Managing the development of procedures and training manuals for all programs
3. Managing the maintenance and cleaning of the facility and equipment
4. Preparing and monitoring the operating plan and budget for the fitness center
5. Preparing and presenting reports to company management concerning the operations of the fitness center
6. Developing promotional literature
7. Coordinating special fitness center events and activities
8. Developing and managing program schedules on a quarterly basis, providing creative and interesting programs and activities for employees
9. Managing and supervising the staff of the fitness center
10. Scheduling and conducting weekly staff meetings
11. Monitoring and evaluating staff performance
12. Coordinating the flow of information between fitness center staff and company management
13. Keeping abreast of trends and issues in the health and fitness industry to integrate state-of-the-art techniques and equipment into the operations of the facility
14. Identifying special topics of research, taking part in data collection, and submitting publications of scientific studies
15. Representing the company at conferences and health and wellness clinics and events

---

Responsibilities of a Fitness Specialist (Health Club Setting)

1. Conducting fitness assessments and health risk profiles for new members and when otherwise requested
2. Evaluating profiles and assessments and conducting private consultations with members to develop individualized exercise prescriptions
3. Conducting individualized instruction sessions, teaching and demonstrating exercise technique, and informing members of the risks and benefits of exercises
4. Developing and instructing group exercise classes
5. Ensuring that the facility and its equipment are safe, clean, and in proper working order

6. Helping compile fitness data on members
7. Assisting the director in the development of promotional literature and conducting special events for the fitness center
8. Keeping abreast of trends and issues in the health and fitness industry

---

Responsibilities of a Facility Attendant (Health Club Setting)

1. Cleaning and maintenance, including laundering and folding towels and cleaning the locker rooms, grooming areas, whirlpool, and pool area
2. Assisting the staff member responsible for inventory and ordering of toiletries and cleaning supplies
3. Learning to perform duties such as security, lights, and pool and jacuzzi maintenance
4. Assisting the director in other areas, as requested

Study Questions

1. Which of the following are the major goals of a strength and conditioning program?

   a. improving performance and lowering the potential for injury
   b. providing a safe and orderly environment
   c. producing winning teams and developing an individual's potential
   d. improving participation and attracting recruits

2. Effective organization and efficient administration of a strength and conditioning program require of the coordinator skill in

   a. supervision
   b. cooperation
   c. observation
   d. instruction

3. Without _____ , the program goal(s) may not be achieved.

   a. objectives
   b. competition
   c. performance
   d. new equipment

4. Strength and conditioning facility _____ are important for offering to participants guidelines on equipment and facility use and personal conduct.

   a. goals and objectives
   b. rules and policies
   c. cleaning and maintenance
   d. organization and administration

Applying Knowledge of Day-to-Day Operations

Problem 1

Coach Hart was optimistic about this new school year. It was her third year of trying to organize a competitive softball team in a very competitive league, and the team had, she felt, finally shown a maturity that winning teams display. The area of strength and conditioning was a valuable part of the team's development, and Coach Hart was looking forward to discussing the team program with the new assistant in the training facility. The students were 2 weeks into classes. Several players came to complain about the new weight training program (run by the new assistant), saying, "We do a lot of the same exercises, and it takes us 2 hours to get it all done." Looking at one of the player's training programs, Coach Hart was under the impression that the new assistant had designed somewhat of a bodybuilding program, with 20 exercises/workout, 4 days/week. "This is too much," she thought as she headed toward the weight room.

How might the facility coordinator have avoided this problem? What should Coach Hart do to solve the problem?

Problem 2

Thirty thousand dollars worth of new equipment was purchased last year. Looking over the training facility in the club, Terry thought it looked reasonably good for a high-volume facility. As the fitness manager, Terry was responsible for overseeing the cleaning and maintenance of the facility and equipment and had instructed his staff to clean up during their shifts. Several suggestions and comments were written in the suggestion box concerning the condition of the floors and walls of the weight room. "Is there anything we can do about the holes and peeling wallpaper next to the squat rack?" one said. "I am tired of tripping on the curled ends of the rubber mat in the dumbbell area!" wrote one member. "The slits and wear spots in the carpet by the bench and incline racks are showing through to cement now—hint, hint!" said another frustrated member.

What should Terry do to solve these concerns?

CHAPTER 33

EQUIPMENT MAINTENANCE

Stephanie L. Armitage-Johnson

A safe training environment is the result of proper instruction and supervision, reasonable facility design, appropriate rules and policies, and cleaning and maintenance of a strength and conditioning facility and its equipment. The facility coordinator is responsible for the orchestration of these elements to provide for the safety of athletes.

Maintenance and cleaning may be seen as means of extending the life span of a facility and its equipment and enhancing the safety of users. Supervisors and assistants may be called upon to clean and maintain equipment. The facility coordinator is also responsible for the purchase of new equipment. Staff members should become familiar with the function, proper use, maintenance, and cleaning of new equipment and be aware of **product liability**.

Product liability refers to the responsibilities a product manufacturer has concerning the quality of their product. If the product is defective, the manufacturer is sometimes liable for certain claims. The facility coordinator should thoroughly inspect new equipment for any defects of production, and should also be aware of any recalls or warning announcements concerning older equipment. If equipment breaks due to a manufacturer error, the coordinator should contact the manufacturer to have the equipment repaired or replaced.

LITIGATION ISSUES

Coaches Guide to Sport Law by G. Nygaard and T. Boone (published by Human Kinetics, Champaign, IL, 1985) was written for sport instructors and physical educators because more lawsuits are directed toward coaches' actions and inaction in sport and physical education than ever before. Every movement activity entails risk of injury. Coaches and instructors must be aware of the **inherent risks** involved in the exercises performed and in the use of equipment by athletes in the training facility. (Inherent risks are those that exist under normal circumstances in a safe environment, when the participant in an activity appreciates the risks of the activity following explanation by qualified personnel.) If the facility and equipment are not maintained and pose a threat of injury to participants, the coordinator may be held liable (legally responsible) for a negligent situation. If a piece of equipment breaks down, signs warning participants to keep off until repairs are made should be placed on the equipment. If equipment is modified in any way or if parts not designed for a particular piece of equipment are used, documentation of such changes must be filed in the **documentation file**. (Kept in the coordinator's desk, this file documents all safety procedures, emergencies, accidents and injuries, modifications to the facility and its equipment, and rationales for specific methods of teaching and specific exercises.)

MAINTENANCE PROCEDURES

Maintaining a facility involves making sure equipment is functional and useful to the goals of the program. The facility coordinator should frequently assess the facility's overall design; the condition of walls, ceilings, and floors (wear, tears, holes, etc.); and accessibility and safe placement of equipment.

Cleaning is usually handled by the custodial staff, but strength and conditioning staff should also be aware of proper procedure. Frequent cleaning and maintenance of equipment ensures safe training, protects investments, and maintains the facility's appearance. Equipment that is constantly used (or abused) and not consistently cleaned or maintained is unsafe, may present health hazards, may be frequently out of order, and must be replaced frequently. This process consumes funds from already limited budgets that may be used more appropriately elsewhere. Therefore, the professional should take proper care to clean and maintain equipment on a regular basis.

Assessing Surfaces

Maintenance and cleaning of the training facility and its equipment begins by assessing what types of surfaces exist in the facility and what maintenance difficulties could arise relative to each of them. The following lists may assist the coordinator in organizing the basic cleaning and maintenance of the facility.

Flooring. Flooring can be composed of such materials as wood, tile, rubber, interlocking mats, and carpet. The custodial staff and the assistant strength and conditioning staff need to maintain floors to the following standards:

- Wooden flooring on platforms must be kept free of splinters, holes, protruding nails, uneven boards, and screws. The boards should run in the direction of the bar so that the lifter does not catch his or her foot against the grain of the wood when widening the stance; this is the safest flooring for Olympic-style lifts.
- Tile flooring and antistatic floor should be treated with antifungal, antibacterial agents in the aerobic machine area. Tile should also be resistant to slipping, resistant to moisture accumulation, and free from chalk accumulation.
- Resilient rubber flooring in the free-weight and machine areas should be similar to aerobic flooring. It must be kept free of large gaps between pieces, cuts, and worn spots.
- Interlocking mats must be secure and arranged so as not to pull apart or become deformed (with protruding tabs). The stretching area must be kept free of accumulated dust. Mats or carpets should be nonabsorbent and contain antifungal and antibacterial agents.
- Carpet must be free of tears. High-use areas should be protected with throw mats.
- All areas must be swept and vacuumed or mopped on a regular basis.
- Flooring must be kept glued and fastened down properly.

- Fixed equipment must be attached securely to the floor.

Walls. Wall surfaces include mirrors and windows, exits, storage areas, and shelves. The custodial staff and the assistant strength and conditioning staff need to maintain wall surfaces to the following standards:

- Walls in high activity areas must be kept free of protruding apparatus (e.g., extended bars and lighting fixtures).
- Mirrors, shelves, and other fixtures must be fixed securely to the walls.
- Mirrors and windows must be cleaned regularly (at least twice weekly; more often in high-activity areas, such as around drinking fountains and in doorways).
- Mirrors, if present in any area, must be attached to the wall at least 50 cm off the floor.
- Replace cracked or distorted mirrors.

Environmental Factors

Environmental factors that should be considered in helping make the facility safe and effective include noise control, temperature, ventilation, humidity, lighting, electrical cords and outlets, and posted signs. Music can be a form of motivation for many, but it can also pose a problem if the stereo system is not properly managed. Volume should be low enough to allow for clear communication between spotters or instructors and lifters at all times. The stereo system should be controlled by the facility coordinator and qualified supervisors only.

Air temperature should be kept constant at 22° to 26° C to offer a reasonable training environment. If the room is too cold, athletes may become chilled after they finish warming up; if too hot, participants may become overheated or lose motivation to continue. Proper ventilation is important to maintaining air quality and keeping humidity to a minimum (relative humidity <60%). The ventilation system should provide at least 8 to 10 air exchanges/hr and optimally 12 to 15 air exchanges. The result should be no detectable strong odors in the room and equipment free of slickness or rust due to high humidity.

Proper lighting of the facility is important for safety and motivation. A facility is well lighted if it is free of dark areas and all equipment and areas can be observed from one end of the facility to the other. Bulbs, tubes, and other lighting apparatus should be checked and changed on a regular basis; optimum lighting is 75 to 100 footcandles. Exit signs should also be well lighted and all exits well marked. All extension cords should be large enough for the electrical load and routed, secured, and grounded. Because some aerobic equipment requires 220 V, both 110 V and 220 V outlets are needed.

All safety, regulation, and policy signs should be posted in clear view, in two or three central places within the facility; more postings may be needed in a large facility.

PROCEDURES FOR MAINTAINING EQUIPMENT

In a large training facility, the facility coordinator may organize staff members for cleaning and maintenance according to specialty area. This method is useful even in smaller facilities with limited staff. Common specialty areas are noted as follows.

• *Aerobic/anaerobic fitness area:* rowing machines, bikes, sprint machines, stair machines, skiing and climbing machines. In this area, surfaces that come into contact with human skin should be cleaned and disinfected daily. This not only protects participants from unsanitary conditions, but also extends the usefulness and maintains the appearance of equipment surfaces. The moving parts of the equipment should be properly lubricated and cleaned when needed so that they are not unnecessarily stressed. Connective bolts and screws need to be checked for tightness or wear and replaced if needed. Straps and belts should be secure and replaced if necessary. Measurement devices such as rpm meters should be properly maintained (this is usually done by the manufacturer but the life span of the equipment can be extended by wiping off sweat and dirt regularly). Equipment parts such as seats and benches should be easily adjustable.

• *Machines area:* isokinetic, variable resistance, single-station, multistation machines.

• *Rehabilitation and special-population machine area:* The cleaning and maintenance of both the machines and rehabilitation areas are similar to those processes in the aerobic/anaerobic fitness area. Bench and machine surfaces that come into contact with skin should be cleaned and disinfected daily to provide a clean surface. Padded and upholstered areas should be free of cracks and tears. Moving parts should be cleaned and lubricated (guide rods on selectorized machines cleaned and lubricated two to three times/week). These areas should be free of loose bolts, screws, cables, chains, and protruding or worn parts that need replacing or removal. Pins that were designed for the machines and belts should be kept in stock; chains and cables should be adjusted for proper alignment and smooth function. Machines should be spaced so that they are easily accessed, with a minimum of 2 ft (61 cm) on all sides, preferably 3 ft (91 cm).

• *Body weight resistance apparatus area:* sit-up board, pulleys, hyperextension benches, plyometric boxes, medicine balls, climbing ropes, pegboard climb, jump ropes. This area should have secured apparatus with well-padded flooring. If mats are used they should be disinfected daily and free of cracks and tears. The flooring below plyometric boxes and jumping equipment should be padded to protect the jumper from impact with a hard surface. The tops and bottoms of boxes should have nonslip surfaces for safe use.

• *Stretching area:* mats, stretching sticks, medicine balls, elastic cords, wall ladders. Mats in stretching areas should be cleaned and disinfected daily and be free of cracks and tears. Areas between mats should be swept or vacuumed regularly to avoid dust and dirt buildup. The area should be free of benches, dumbbells, and other equipment that may clutter the area and tear mat surfaces. Medicine balls and stretching sticks should be stored after use, and elastic cords should be secured to a base, checked for wear, and replaced when necessary.

• *Free-weight area:* bench presses, incline presses, squat racks, dumbbells, weight racks. Equipment should be spaced (see chapter 31) to allow easy access to separate areas. All equipment, including safety equipment (belts, locks, safety bars) should be returned after use to avoid pathway obstruction. Benches, weight racks, and standards may be bolted to the floor or walls. In the squat area, the flooring should be of a nonslip surface and cleaned regularly. Equipment such as curl bars and dumbbells should be checked frequently for loose hex nuts. Nonfunctional or broken equipment should be posted with ''out of order'' signs or, if a long delay in repairs is expected, removed from the area or locked out of service. All protective padding and upholstery should be free of cracks and tears and cleaned and disinfected daily.

• *Lifting platform area:* Olympic bars, standards, bumper plates, racks, locks, chalk bins. The cleaning and maintenance of the lifting platform includes ensuring that all equipment is returned after use to prevent obstruction of the area and hazardous lifting conditions. Olympic bars should be properly lubricated and tightened to maintain the rotating bar ends. If standards are used in the area, the base of each should be secure and each standard stored out of the way when not in use. Bent Olympic bars should be replaced and the knurling kept free of debris and chalk buildup by cleaning and brushing occasionally. All locks should be functioning, and wrist straps, knee wraps, and belts should be stored properly. The platform should be inspected for gaps, cuts, slits, and splinters (depending on the type of surface) and properly swept or mopped to remove chalk. The lifting area should be free of benches, boxes, and other clutter to give the lifter sufficient room.

CLEANING SUPPLIES

Cleaning supplies should be kept in a locked cabinet located near the office or supervisor station. Supplies should be inventoried and restocked on a regular basis (once or twice each month). These items should be kept in stock:

- Disinfectant (germicide)
- Window and mirror cleaner
- Lubrication sprays
- Cleaning sprays
- Spray bottles (about four)
- Paper towels
- Cloth towels
- Sponges
- Broom and dust pan
- Small vacuum cleaner
- Vacuum cleaner bags
- Whisk broom
- Mop and bucket
- Shower caps (for bicycle meter equipment)
- Gum and stain remover (for carpet and upholstery)

MAINTENANCE SUPPLIES

Maintenance supplies should be kept in a tool box located in a locked cabinet. The tool box should contain these items:

- File
- Hammer
- Pliers (standard and needle-nose)
- Screwdrivers (Phillips and standard)
- Allen wrenches
- Crescent wrench
- Rubber mallet
- Carpet knife
- Cable splicer parts and appropriate tools
- Chain splicer parts and appropriate tools
- Heavy-duty stapler
- Nuts, bolts, washers, nails, and screws in various sizes
- Heavy-duty glue
- Transparent tape
- Masking tape
- Duct tape
- Drill and drill bit set
- Lubricant spray
- Socket set
- Vise grip

The safety checklist on pages 498 to 500 provides an easy format in which to evaluate the maintenance and cleaning status of a facility.

CONCLUSION

Cleaning and maintenance may be seen as a means of extending the life span of a facility and its equipment and enhancing the safety of users. Supervisors and assistants may be called upon for cleaning and maintenance. Supervisors should be made aware of the function and care of new equipment as well as the product liability of all equipment. Organizing the facility and equipment into specialty areas may be helpful for keeping track of regular cleaning and maintenance.

If the facility and its equipment are not properly cleaned and maintained, accidents, injuries, and illness may occur, any of which may be considered a result of negligence if proper precautions have not been taken.

Cleaning and maintenance supplies should be readily available and restocked when necessary.

Key Terms

documentation file   493   inherent risk   493   product liability   493

Study Questions

1. Frequent cleaning and maintenance of the facility and equipment provide for

   a. safe participation
   b. protection of investments
   c. maintaining the appearance of the facility
   d. all of the above

2. The equipment in the facility should be

    a. functional and useful to the goals of the program

    b. fun to use

    c. easy to maintain and trouble free

    d. attractive and match the decor of the facility

3. Product liability refers to

    a. a manufacturer's responsibility for producing a defective product

    b. professional misuse of equipment

    c. participant misuse of equipment

    d. high risk equipment

Applying Knowledge of Equipment Maintenance

Problem 1

"It is so frustrating," thought Jan as she left the club. "It always seems to be so dirty, and it's falling apart. Where do all of my membership dues go? Certainly not for cleaning and upkeep." That morning as Jan walked into the club, she had noticed finger marks all over the glass door of the entrance. The locker room floor had lint and hair all over it, and the weight room had dust balls clinging to the bases of the machines. The bicycles and stair machines had sweat drips that had collected dirt. Jan sought out a spray bottle of disinfectant to cover any surface her hand might touch. She stepped up to a stair machine, sprayed and wiped the handlebars, and began her workout. Two minutes later the right foot pedal suddenly dropped. The machine had malfunctioned and the tension had been lost. Jan didn't feel like trying another machine. She went to the manager to complain, but he wasn't there. As she left his office she noticed that her back and right knee hurt. What should the owner of the club do?

Problem 2

A facility has the following problems:

    a. worn carpet or tile at dumbbell area

    b. curled ends of interlocking mat or throw mat

    c. holes in wall near squat rack

    d. cracked mirror at a lifting platform area

    e. dustballs under machines and equipment and between mats in the stretching area

For each item, explain the changes you would make in the equipment and how you would organize staff to maintain the area.

NSCA Safety Checklist for Maintenance and Cleaning of a Strength and Conditioning Facility and Its Equipment

I. Facility

   A. Flooring

      _____ Wooden flooring on platform free of splinters, holes, protruding nails, and screws
      _____ Tile flooring resistant to slipping; no moisture or chalk accumulation
      _____ Rubber flooring free of cuts, slits, and large gaps between pieces
      _____ Interlocking mats secure and arranged so as not to pull apart or become deformed (no protruding tabs)
      _____ Carpet free of tears; wear areas protected by throw mats
      _____ Area swept and vacuumed or mopped on a regular basis
      _____ Flooring glued and fastened down properly
      _____ Fixed equipment attached securely to floor

   B. Walls (including mirrors and windows, exits, storage areas, and shelves)

      _____ Walls in high-activity areas free of protruding apparatus
      _____ Mirrors and shelves securely fixed to walls
      _____ Mirrors and windows cleaned regularly (twice weekly)
      _____ Mirrors (if present in platform areas) minimum of 50 cm off the floor
      _____ Mirrors not cracked or distorted

   C. Environmental factors (noise control, temperature, ventilation, humidity, lighting, electrical cords and outlets, and posted signs)

      _____ Volume of stereo system set low enough to allow clear communication between the spotter and lifter at all times
      _____ Stereo system controlled by the facility coordinator and qualified supervisors
      _____ Air temperature kept constant at 22° to 26° C
      _____ Ventilation systems working properly (minimum of 8-10 air exchanges/hr and optimally 12-15 air exchanges/hr); no detectable strong odors in the room
      _____ Equipment not slick due to high humidity
      _____ Facility well lighted and free of dark areas; bulbs changed on regular basis
      _____ Exit sign is well lighted
      _____ Extension cords are routed, secured, and grounded and large enough for electrical load
      _____ All safety, regulation, and policy signs posted in clear view (two or three central places within facility; more postings in large facilities)

II. Equipment

   A. Aerobic/anaerobic fitness area (rowing machines, bikes, sprint machines, stair machines, skiing and climbing machines)

      _____ Easy access to each work station (minimum of 2 ft [61 cm] between machines; 3 ft [91 cm] optimal)
      _____ Bolts and screws tight
      _____ Functioning parts easily adjustable
      _____ Parts and surfaces properly lubricated and cleaned
      _____ Foot and body straps secure and nonripping
      _____ Measurement devices for tension, time, rpms, etc., properly functioning
      _____ Surfaces that contact human skin cleaned and disinfected daily

B. Machines area (isokinetic, variable resistance, single-station, multistation machines)

_____ Easy access to each work station (minimum of 2 ft [61 cm] between machines; 3 ft [91 cm] optimal)
_____ Area free of loose bolts, screws, cables, and chains
_____ Proper pins used
_____ Securing straps functional
_____ Parts and surfaces properly lubricated and cleaned (guide rods on selectorized machines cleared and lubricated two or three times/week)
_____ Protective padding free of cracks and tears
_____ Surfaces that contact human skin cleaned and disinfected daily
_____ All parts smoothly functioning and lubricated regularly
_____ No protruding screws or parts that need tightening or removal
_____ Belts, chains, and cables aligned with machine parts
_____ No worn parts (frayed cable, loose chains, worn bolts, cracked joint screws, etc.)

C. Rehabilitation and special-population machine area

_____ Easy access to each work station (minimum of 2 ft [61 cm] between machines; 3 ft [91 cm] optimal)
_____ Parts and surfaces properly lubricated and cleaned
_____ Area free of loose bolts, screws, cables, and chains
_____ Proper use of attachments, pins, and other apparatus
_____ Surfaces that contact human skin cleaned and disinfected daily
_____ Securing straps functional
_____ Protective padding free of cracks and tears
_____ All parts smoothly functioning
_____ No protruding screws or parts that need tightening or removal
_____ No worn parts

D. Body weight resistance apparatus area (sit-up board, dips, pulleys, hyperextension benches, plyometric boxes, medicine balls, climbing ropes, pegboard climb, jump ropes)

_____ Apparatus properly lubricated
_____ Surfaces that contact human skin cleaned and disinfected daily
_____ Protective padding free of cracks and tears
_____ Securing straps and apparatus functional
_____ Climbing apparatus secured with well-padded floor area
_____ Properly padded floor area below plyometric boxes
_____ Nonslip material on the top surface and bottom or base of plyometric boxes
_____ Apparatus for holding feet for sit-ups, hyperextension, etc., secure

E. Stretching area (mats, stretching sticks, medicine balls, elastic cords, wall ladders)

_____ Mat area free of weight benches and equipment
_____ Mats free of tears
_____ No large gaps between stretching mats
_____ Area swept and disinfected daily
_____ Stretching sticks and medicine balls properly stored after use
_____ Elastic cords secured to base with safety knot and checked for wear

F. Free-weight area (bench presses, incline presses, squat racks, dumbbells, weight racks)

_____ Proper spacing of racks and weight standards to allow access to all areas
_____ All equipment returned after use to avoid obstruction of pathway
_____ Safety equipment (belts, collars, safety bars) used and returned
_____ Protective padding free of cracks and tears
_____ Surfaces that contact human skin cleaned and disinfected daily
_____ Securing bolts and apparatus parts (collars, curl bars) tightly fastened
_____ Nonslip mats on squat rack floor area
_____ Olympic bars turn properly and are properly lubricated and tightened
_____ Benches, weight racks, standards, etc., secured to the floor or wall
_____ Nonfunctional or broken equipment removed from area or locked out of service

G. Lifting platform area (Olympic bars, standards, bumper plates, racks, locks, chalk bins)

_____ Olympic bars properly spaced (3 feet [91 cm] between ends; lifting area is 12 × 8 ft [3.7 × 2.4 m])

_____ All equipment returned after use to avoid obstruction of lifting area

_____ Base on all lifting standards secured

_____ Olympic bar rotates properly and is properly lubricated and tightened

_____ Bent Olympic bars replaced; knurling clear of debris

_____ Collars functioning

_____ Sufficient chalk available to lifters

_____ Wrist straps, belts, and knee wraps available, functioning, and stored properly

_____ Benches, chairs, boxes kept at a distance from lifting area

_____ No gaps, cuts, slits, splinters in mat

_____ Area properly swept and mopped to remove splinters, chalk, etc.

_____ Ceiling space sufficient for overhead lifts (12 ft [3.7 m] minimum) and free of low-hanging apparatus (beams, pipes, lighting, signs, etc.)

III. Cleaning supplies

_____ Disinfectant (germicide)

_____ Window and mirror cleaner

_____ Lubrication sprays

_____ Cleaning sprays

_____ Spray bottles (about four)

_____ Paper towels

_____ Cloth towels

_____ Sponges

_____ Broom and dust pan

_____ Small vacuum cleaner

_____ Vacuum cleaner bags

_____ Whisk broom

_____ Mop and bucket

_____ Shower caps (for bicycle meter equipment)

_____ Gum and stain remover (for carpet and upholstery)

_____ Items in locked cabinet near supervisor's station, inventoried, replenished once or twice monthly

IV. Maintenance supplies: Tool box contents and other items

_____ File

_____ Hammer

_____ Pliers (standard, needle-nose)

_____ Screwdrivers (Phillips and standard)

_____ Allen wrench

_____ Crescent wrench

_____ Rubber mallet

_____ Carpet knife

_____ Cable splicer parts and appropriate tools

_____ Chain splicer parts and appropriate tools

_____ Heavy-duty stapler

_____ Nuts, bolts, washers, nails, and screws in various sizes

_____ Heavy-duty glue

_____ Transparent tape

_____ Masking tape

_____ Duct tape

_____ Drill and drill bit set

_____ Lubricant spray

_____ Socket set

_____ Vise grip

_____ Items in locked cabinet

CHAPTER 34

PREPARING FOR EMERGENCIES

Stephanie L. Armitage-Johnson

The possibility of injury and litigation exist in any facility in which people are present. Today there seems to be a societal preoccupation with litigation, with plaintiffs searching for the "deepest pocket" from which to win compensation for personal injury as a result of what the courts judge as negligence. It is therefore vitally important for professionals who manage facilities to realize the potential for litigation and to establish a comprehensive safety program that will help to avoid it.

We describe such a program here; however, readers should refer to American Red Cross materials for specific protocols. Discussed in this chapter are important elements of a comprehensive safety program, including risk awareness, preparticipation procedures, facility preparedness, and staff preparedness.

RISK AWARENESS

Athletes must be made aware of the most common injuries associated with a given activity (contusions, scrapes, strains, broken bones, and joint injuries) and possible catastrophic injuries (injuries that result in death, paraplegia, quadriplegia, or blindness).

When sport teams report to the training facility during the first week or two of the new school year, the strength coach or assistant strength coach should explain facility rules and policies. Additionally, instructors should demonstrate and explain specific exercises and explain the risks associated with them. Athletes should be made aware of injuries that may occur as a result of equipment

misuse or inappropriate conduct. To educate athletes on potential risks and to guard against litigation, the facility coordinator might want to require athletes to sign an assumption of risk form. An example of an assumption of risk form for the university level is shown on page 506.

The actual content of the initial meeting with teams may be summarized as follows.

- Introduce supervisory staff.
- Hand out "Assumption of Risk" form (see p. 506), to be signed (by parent or guardian if necessary) and returned.
- Explain rationale for strength and conditioning training and weight room purpose.
- Explain weight room rules, policies, and etiquette.
- Walk through the weight room. Review specific exercises and provide instruction on techniques. Include a discussion of possible consequences if proper technique is not followed, injuries common to each exercise, and means of avoiding injuries. (Documentation by the professional of all orientations and instruction sessions is necessary.)
- Discuss abuse of performance-enhancing substances, narcotics, diet drugs, and other drugs (may be handled by sports medicine personnel).
- If available, notify athletes of nutrition, drug abuse, and weight gain/loss counseling sessions.

Instructors, assistant strength coaches, and facility coordinators are all responsible for ensuring that participants understand and appreciate the risks of injury. The facility coordinator is responsible for making sure that these staff members appreciate the risks associated with the exercises they are demonstrating, as well as these other risks:

- The risk of illness or infection from treating someone in an emergency or from unsanitary conditions due to improper cleaning of equipment
- The risk of injury due to improper maintenance of the facility or its equipment
- The risk of legal action against instructors and supervisors as a result of their own negligence or lack of foresight
- The risk of injury as a result of poor conduct by an athlete

The facility coordinator should ensure that staff members are aware of the necessity of foresight and common sense during instruction and supervision. Foresight is the act of ''seeing ahead,'' or anticipating potential emergencies or injuries. By thinking ahead, instructors and supervisors may help participants avoid mishaps or injuries. Foresight should be used during instruction, by warning participants of potential risks, and also during overall supervision of the facility. When a potential problem with a piece of equipment or area of the facility is noted, the staff member observing it should alert the facility coordinator and make efforts to eliminate or prevent the problem.

PREPARTICIPATION PROCEDURES

The facility coordinator should consider requiring athletes to undergo physicals and obtain medical approval prior to participation. In high school and college settings a preparticipation physical is required of all athletes. Individuals considered ''health risks'' *must* undergo a physical and receive a physician's approval prior to participation. All physicals and medical approvals should be copied, dated, signed, and filed by either the fitness coordinator (if in a club setting) or by the school nurse or training room personnel.

The ''PAR-Q and You'' questionnaire on page 507 can be used to screen athletes beginning low-intensity exercise. The facility coordinator can use such a questionnaire to see which athletes should be referred for additional medical screening. The ''Risk Factor Questionnaire'' on page 508 can be used in the same way. The facility coordinator might want to use a health and fitness history questionnaire such as the one on pages 509 to 511 to learn about the athlete's health habits, medical history, and fitness goals. The ''Health History Questionnaire'' on pages 512 to 514 might be used by physicians to evaluate athletes' participation risks.

FACILITY PREPAREDNESS

For convenience, facility preparedness may be divided into three areas: (a) overall facility preparedness, (b) maintenance of athletes' files, and (c) first-aid equipment. Each is covered in the following checklists.

Checklist for Overall Facility Preparedness

☐ The following phone numbers should be posted prominently in key areas throughout the facility (if the facility does not have a telephone, a map showing the location of the nearest phone should be included in this posting):
- ✓ Training room
- ✓ Athletic trainers' offices
- ✓ Hospital emergency room
- ✓ Emergency doctors/nurses
- ✓ Police department/campus security
- ✓ Fire department

☐ The room capacity and an evacuation plan must be posted.

☐ Signs delineating policies, regulations, and safety specifications should be posted in high-visibility areas throughout the facility.

☐ An emergency plan includes staff preparedness: emergency medical training, what staff should learn, who conducts sessions, and when training sessions should take place. This plan also includes the people to be contacted if an emergency occurs.

☐ A fire extinguisher must be present and easy to access.

Checklist for Maintenance of Athletes' Files

☐ Emergency cards for individual athletes should be kept on file either in the weight room office or with the athletic trainer (wherever more appropriate); duplicate cards may be kept on file with the school health officials. Emergency cards should include the following information:
- ✓ Athlete's home phone number
- ✓ Phone numbers of family members
- ✓ Whom to contact when parents are unavailable
- ✓ Name and number of athlete's physician
- ✓ Special instructions and considerations

Checklist for First-Aid Equipment

☐ A first-aid box should be kept in the supervisor's station. It should be clearly visible to staff and athletes.

☐ The first-aid box should be restocked regularly and contain the following items:

- ✓ 1 box of 1-in. adhesive bandages
- ✓ 1 box of 2-in. adhesive bandages
- ✓ 1 box of 4-in. adhesive bandages
- ✓ 2 rolls of gauze
- ✓ 1 roll of 2-in. tape
- ✓ 1 roll of 1/2-in. tape
- ✓ 1 box of butterfly adhesive bandages
- ✓ 1 triangle bandage
- ✓ 5 pairs of rubber gloves
- ✓ 10 tongue depressors
- ✓ 1 box of smelling salts (ammonia capsules)
- ✓ 1 can of disinfectant spray
- ✓ 1 box of alcohol wipes
- ✓ 1 tube of neosporin disinfectant salve
- ✓ 2 ace bandages
- ✓ 1 pair of scissors
- ✓ 1 box of safety pins (clips)
- ✓ 1 wrist splint
- ✓ 1 finger splint
- ✓ 10 "instant cool" bags

STAFF PREPAREDNESS

To prepare staff members for their responsibilities in emergencies, the facility coordinator should hold meetings at the beginning of the year and periodically throughout the year to communicate concerns, create a dialogue between coordinator and staff, and introduce and review first-aid and cardiopulmonary resuscitation (CPR) training (taught by American Red Cross–certified personnel). All instructors and supervisors must demonstrate the ability to administer basic life support as well as appropriate first-aid procedures to athletes in need of immediate care. Of course, preventing the occurrence of an injury is preferred to having to deal with an injury, but all instructors and supervisors must be qualified to act should an emergency take place.

All emergencies, injuries, and preventive discussions with individuals (e.g., warning them that a specific action is dangerous) should be documented using a form such as the "Documentation Form" on page 515. This form can also be used to document equipment modifications or maintenance issues as explained in chapter 33.

The following is a checklist for emergency procedures for facilities and their personnel.

Checklist for Staff Preparedness

☐ All supervisors and instructors must hold up-to-date American Red Cross certification cards in first aid and CPR prior to the beginning of the school year.

Certifications must be renewed on a regular basis. Certificates must be kept on file.

☐ During the first week of class or at the beginning of a new year, a meeting should be held with all assistants and full-time supervisory personnel. The meeting should include the following agenda.

- ✓ Review of rudimentary first-aid procedures (review a first-aid certification course offered by local fire departments or hospitals) covering common training facility injuries and their prevention
- ✓ CPR review
- ✓ Location of emergency medical personnel
- ✓ Location of phone; emergency phone numbers (nurse, training room, hospital)
- ✓ Location of first-aid box and ice machines
- ✓ Understanding the policy that, prior to participation, all participants or athletes must fill out a health-risk questionnaire. If health risk is high, the participant or athlete must have approval to participate in the program, as well as a list of limitations, if they exist, signed and dated by a physician
- ✓ Discussion of *foresight*, *liability*, *negligence*, and other legal terms
- ✓ Discussion of coach liability insurance programs
- ✓ Reminder not to attempt to motivate athletes or individuals beyond physical limitations
- ✓ Review of documentation of all injuries, incidents, and consultations (including date, time, occurrence, and names of witnesses)
- ✓ Encouragement of membership in professional organizations
- ✓ Discussion of foresight reports and evasive action reports, with rationales
- ✓ Reminder of the need to have contents of injury reports verified by physicians, with attached statements from witnesses and the injured person
- ✓ Discussion of rules and policies, including rationale and checklists for cleaning and maintenance
- ✓ Reminder that staff supervisors are identified by wearing a standard shirt provided by the department
- ✓ Discussion of the head coach's philosophy of instruction and program
- ✓ Discussion of body composition guidelines and nutritional consultation
- ✓ Showing and discussing technique videotapes on strength training and conditioning
- ✓ Reminder that confidential documentation is required of all athlete consultations on use of performance-enhancing substances
- ✓ Review of the need for documentation of all meetings

CONCLUSION

Any strength and conditioning facility risks the possibility of participant injury and litigation. Because there seems to be a societal preoccupation with litigation, it is very important for the facility coordinator to establish a comprehensive safety program for the facility that he or she manages.

The safety program comprises staff and participant awareness; understanding and appreciation of common and catastrophic injury risks associated with specific activities within the facility; staff foresight concerning potential injury situations; preparticipation activities, such as medical examinations and orientation of athletes to the facility and equipment; preparing the facility for emergencies by posting emergency numbers, filing emergency cards on individuals, supplying a first-aid box and posting it in a visible and accessible place; and preparing staff for emergencies by requiring updated first-aid and CPR training and certification.

Study Questions

1. A catastrophic injury is any injury that

   a. endangers two or more people
   b. causes multiple contusions and abrasions
   c. results in death, paraplegia, quadriplegia, or blindness
   d. is easily treated by the facility staff, allowing the victim to go home

2. Prior to participation, each athlete should

   a. have written permission from his or her parent or guardian
   b. have medical approval for participation
   c. have a written training program
   d. take a written test demonstrating the appreciation and understanding of the risks of the exercises

3. At the beginning of the school year, athletes should be given an orientation of the facility and equipment. This orientation should include

   a. facility rules and policies
   b. demonstration of equipment use and risks of misuse
   c. demonstration of exercises in the program
   d. all of the above

4. Prior to participation, it is important that athletes _____ the risks associated with various exercises.

   a. feel and describe
   b. see and experience
   c. understand and appreciate
   d. study and memorize

Applying Knowledge of Preparing for Emergencies

Problem 1

Joe, a student supervisor, was working the early shift in the student weight room, and he had a lot of studying to do before his first class of the day at 10:00 a.m. There were about 10 people in the room, mostly students like himself, trying to get a start on the day and perhaps a little tired from finals week preparation. Suddenly a student rushed up to Joe, saying, "Come quick. A guy at the dumbbell rack just cut off his finger!" Joe grabbed a clean towel and ran to the injured lifter. "He cut his finger off trying to replace the dumbbell to the rack," said one of the students who observed the accident. Joe wasn't sure what to do, but common sense told him to put pressure on the hand. He looked for the first-aid box but wasn't sure which cabinet it was in; they were all locked, anyway. There was blood everywhere and the victim was going into shock. "Here's his finger," said one of the students, picking it up.

What are the important steps that Joe should follow? What procedural changes would you make based on what Joe did or did not do?

Problem 2

Janet had enjoyed teaching the adult fitness class at a local high school 2 years ago. When the recreation director asked if she would teach the class again, she agreed immediately. Even though she had not led the class recently, she felt that she had not forgotten anything important. It was a great way to make extra money for the school sports clubs, meet people, and involve adults of all ages in fitness. Tonight was the first night of the new session. People began arriving, and before long Janet turned on the music and started the class on a warm-up. Many in her group were over 50 and seemed to be going strong. After about 15 min, Janet noticed one man in the back corner stop and grasp his arm. The woman next to him stopped to see if he was all right. Janet asked one of the women to stop the stereo and went to the corner of the room to see what was going on. The man had fallen unconscious and was no longer breathing. Janet asked if anyone knew CPR.

What would be the precautions in organizing a class such as this? State any additional safety measures that may be necessary.

Shared Responsibility for Sport Safety

Assumption of Risk

The responsibility for sport safety must be shared by administrators, coaches, physicians, trainers, and student-athletes. I, the undersigned, am aware and appreciate that there are risks of injury involved in my participation in intercollegiate athletics at [school name]. I and the school understand that my signature below in no way relieves the school of its responsibilities for my welfare. Signing this statement is intended to make me aware of my responsibilities in preventing potential injuries or harm, reporting actual injuries, and complying with the treatment plan of my health care providers and indicates that I understand and appreciate the risks involved with my participation. I understand that this includes the risk of brain and spinal cord injury that may result in paralysis, other permanent injury, or possibly death.

Female athletes with menstrual irregularities may experience a devastating effect on bone density that results in osteoporosis (decrease in bone density). I understand and appreciate the increased risk of stress fractures due to the loss of bone density that results from menstrual irregularities and know that I should seek prompt medical attention if this condition develops or exists, ensuring appropriate preventive measures.

I acknowledge that the above statements of Awareness of Risk were read to me and that I understand them.

_____   _____

Student-athlete's signature   Date

Adapted by permission from *Shared Responsibility Form for Sport Safety: Assumption of Risk* by the University of Washington Athletic Department (1993).

PAR - Q & YOU

(A Questionnaire for People Aged 15 to 69)

Regular physical activity is fun and healthy, and increasingly more people are starting to become more active every day. Being more active is very safe for most people. However, some people should check with their doctor before they start becoming much more physically active.

If you are planning to become much more physically active than you are now, start by answering the seven questions in the box below. If you are between the ages of 15 and 69, the PAR-Q will tell you if you should check with your doctor before you start. If you are over 69 years of age, and you are not used to being very active, check with your doctor.

Common sense is your best guide when you answer these questions. Please read the questions carefully and answer each one honestly: check YES or NO.

YES	NO		
☐	☐	1.	Has your doctor ever said that you have a heart condition <u>and</u> that you should only do physical activity recommended by a doctor?
☐	☐	2.	Do you feel pain in your chest when you do physical activity?
☐	☐	3.	In the past month, have you had chest pain when you were not doing physical activity?
☐	☐	4.	Do you lose your balance because of dizziness or do you ever lose consciousness?
☐	☐	5.	Do you have a bone or joint problem that could be made worse by a change in your physical activity?
☐	☐	6.	Is your doctor currently prescribing drugs (for example, water pills) for your blood pressure or heart condition?
☐	☐	7.	Do you know of <u>any other reason</u> why you should not do physical activity?

If you answered

YES to one or more questions

Talk with your doctor by phone or in person BEFORE you start becoming much more physically active or BEFORE you have a fitness appraisal. Tell your doctor about the PAR-Q and which questions you answered YES.

- You may be able to do any activity you want — as long as you start slowly and build up gradually. Or, you may need to restrict your activities to those which are safe for you. Talk with your doctor about the kinds of activities you wish to participate in and follow his/her advice.
- Find out which community programs are safe and helpful for you.

NO to all questions

If you answered NO honestly to <u>all</u> PAR-Q questions, you can be reasonably sure that you can:

- start becoming much more physically active — begin slowly and build up gradually. This is the safest and easiest way to go.
- take part in a fitness appraisal — this is an excellent way to determine your basic fitness so that you can plan the best way for you to live actively.

DELAY BECOMING MUCH MORE ACTIVE:

- if you are not feeling well because of a temporary illness such as a cold or a fever — wait until you feel better; or
- if you are or may be pregnant — talk to your doctor before you start becoming more active.

Please note: If your health changes so that you then answer YES to any of the above questions, tell your fitness or health professional. Ask whether you should change your physical activity plan.

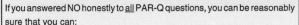

<u>Informed Use of the PAR-Q</u>: The Canadian Society for Exercise Physiology, Health Canada, and their agents assume no liability for persons who undertake physical activity, and if in doubt after completing this questionnaire, consult your doctor prior to physical activity.

Risk Factor Questionnaire

Name _____

Address _____

Phone (home) (_____) _____ (work) (_____) _____

Age _____ Birth date _____ Occupation _____

Physician's name _____

Physician's address _____ Physician's phone (_____) _____

Yes	No	
☐	☐	1. Have you ever had, or has your doctor ever diagnosed you as having, heart trouble or coronary disease?
☐	☐	2. Do you have a family history of heart problems or coronary disease?
☐	☐	3. Do you have a history of high blood pressure (above 140/90)?
☐	☐	4. Have you recently had surgery or experienced bone, muscle, tendon, or ligament problems (especially in your knees or back)?
☐	☐	5. Do you have diabetes?
☐	☐	6. Do you smoke cigarettes?
☐	☐	7. Are you overweight?
☐	☐	8. Is your diet heavy in fatty foods and red meat?
☐	☐	9. Do you ever have pains in your heart/chest?
☐	☐	10. Do you ever feel faint or have dizzy spells?
☐	☐	11. Has your doctor ever said you have high cholesterol?
☐	☐	12. Are you over 65 and sedentary?
		13. Resting EKG: _____
		14. Total cholesterol/HDL ratio: _____

Adapted from Peterson and Bryant (1992).

Health and Fitness History

Name _____ Date _____

1. Are you presently involved in a regular exercise program? If yes, please list activity, duration, frequency, and intensity:

2. Do you now smoke or have you ever smoked? ☐ Yes ☐ No

    (a) If you previously smoked, how long did you smoke, how often, and when did you quit?

    (b) If you currently smoke, how much?

3. Do you use alcohol? ☐ Yes ☐ No

    (a) If yes, how much per day? _____

    (b) How much per week? _____

4. Do you drink coffee or colas that contain caffeine? ☐ Yes ☐ No

    (a) If yes, how much per day? _____

5. Are you now or have you ever been on a diet? ☐ Yes ☐ No

    (a) If yes, please explain.

6. Do you consider yourself overweight or underweight? (If yes, please circle which.)

7. How many meals do you usually eat each day? _____

8. Do you usually eat breakfast? ☐ Yes ☐ No

9. How many eggs do you eat per week? _____

10. How many times each week do you usually eat the following?

    Beef _____ Pork _____ Fowl _____ Fish _____

    Desserts _____ Fried foods _____ Fast foods _____

11. Do you regularly use any of the following? (Please circle.)

    Butter   Sugar   Sweeteners   Salt   Whole milk

12. How active do you consider yourself? (Please circle.)

    Sedentary   Lightly active   Moderately active   Highly active

13. How would you describe your nutrition habits? (Please circle.)

    Good   Fair   Poor

14. How would you characterize your life? (Please circle.)

    Highly stressful   Moderately stressful   Low in stress

15. Please describe your knowledge of exercise and fitness. (Please circle.)

    Good   Fair   Poor

16. Please describe your knowledge of nutrition. (Please circle.)

    Good   Fair   Poor

(continued)

Health and Fitness History *(continued)*

Medical History and Present Medical Condition

1. Check any conditions or diseases you now have or have had in the past.

   ☐ Heart attack; coronary bypass or other cardiac surgery   ☐ Cold hands or feet

   ☐ Diabetes   ☐ Unusual shortness of breath

   ☐ Stroke   ☐ Light-headedness or fainting

   ☐ Peripheral vascular disease   ☐ Epilepsy or seizures

   ☐ Phlebitis or emboli   ☐ Anemia

   ☐ Rheumatic fever   ☐ Asthma

   ☐ High blood pressure   ☐ Emphysema

   ☐ Low blood pressure   ☐ Bronchitis

   ☐ Chest discomfort   ☐ Pneumonia

   ☐ Extra, skipped, or rapid heart beats or palpitations   ☐ A chronic recurrent cough

   ☐ Heart murmur   ☐ Increased anxiety or depression

   ☐ Ankle swelling   ☐ Emotional disorders

   ☐ Trouble sleeping   ☐ Fatigue or lack of energy

   ☐ Migraine or recurrent headaches   ☐ Ulcers

   ☐ Swollen, stiff, or painful joints   ☐ Stomach or intestinal problems

   ☐ Foot problems   ☐ Hernia

   ☐ Back problems   ☐ Limited range of motion in joints

   ☐ Shoulder problems   ☐ Arthritis

   ☐ Neck problems   ☐ Bursitis

   ☐ Broken bones

   If you checked any of these, please explain here.

2. Please list any prescribed medications you are now taking.

3. Please list any over-the-counter medications or dietary supplements you are now taking.

4. Please list any illness, hospitalization, or surgical procedure within the past 2 years.

5. Please list any drug allergies.

6. Please list date of last physical examination and results.

Fitness Goals

Please check specific goals and list dates for achieving them.

- ☐ Improve strength
- ☐ Improve flexibility
- ☐ Improve cardiovascular fitness
- ☐ Improve muscle tone and shape
- ☐ Improve diet/eating habits
- ☐ Lose weight
- ☐ Gain weight/muscle

- ☐ Reduce stress
- ☐ Increase energy
- ☐ Stop smoking/drinking
- ☐ Injury prevention
- ☐ Rehabilitate injury
- ☐ Additional goals (list):

Adapted from Peterson and Bryant (1992).

Health History Questionnaire

Name _____ Date _____

Answer all questions; write N/A if something does not apply to you.

Family history:	Age	Health	Age at death	Cause
Mother	_____	_____	_____	_____
Father	_____	_____	_____	_____
Siblings	_____	_____	_____	_____
	_____	_____	_____	_____
	_____	_____	_____	_____
	_____	_____	_____	_____

Has any blood relative ever had any of the following? (Check the appropriate lines.)

Sudden death before the age of 50	_____	High blood pressure	_____
Cancer	_____	Diabetes	_____
Tuberculosis	_____	Stroke	_____
Heart disease	_____	Epilepsy	_____
Blood diseases (sickle cell anemia, leukemia)	_____		

Have you had, or do you currently have, any of the following?

High blood pressure	_____	Frequent skin infection	_____
Frequent headaches	_____	Skin disorders	_____
Migraine headaches	_____	Heat exhaustion	_____
Concussion/fainting/unconsciousness	_____	Heat stroke	_____
Chronic sore throat	_____	Kidney/bladder infection	_____
Mononucleosis	_____	Thyroid disease	_____
HIV infection	_____	Seizures disorder	_____
Heart problem	_____	Hepatitis	_____
Heart disease	_____	Tuberculosis	_____
Rheumatic fever	_____	Bruise or bleed easily	_____
Scarlet fever	_____	Hemorrhoids	_____
Ulcer	_____	Hernia	_____
Nervous stomach	_____	Sickle cell anemia	_____
Appendicitis	_____	Diabetes	_____
Congenital abnormality	_____	Pneumonia	_____
Loss of a paired organ	_____	Cancer, tumor, growth, cyst	_____
Frequent diarrhea	_____	Arthritis	_____
		Other: _____	

Have you ever had or do you currently have any of the following?

Neck

Pinched nerve _____

Burners/stingers _____

Fractures _____

Sprain/strain _____

Disc problems _____

Unexplained pain _____

Surgery _____

Other: _____

Hand, wrist, fingers

Fracture _____

Sprain/strain _____

Surgery _____

Other: _____

Spine/back

Fracture _____

Muscle spasm _____

Ruptured/herniated disc _____

Stiffness _____

Pain with lifting _____

Congenital deformity _____

Spondylogenic problems _____

S-I joint pain _____

Surgery _____

Other: _____

Pelvis/hip

Fracture _____

Subluxation/dislocation _____

Contusion/hip pointer _____

Groin strain _____

Tendinitis _____

Surgery _____

Other: _____

Shoulder/clavicle

Fracture _____

Subluxation/dislocation _____

Separation _____

Tendinitis _____

Other: _____

Arm

Fracture _____

Calcium deposits _____

Ruptured muscle _____

Other: _____

Elbow

Fracture _____

Subluxation/dislocation _____

Sprain/strain _____

Tendinitis _____

Surgery _____

Other: _____

Thigh

Quadriceps strain _____

Hamstring strain _____

Fracture _____

Surgery _____

Ruptured muscle _____

Calcium deposits _____

Tendinitis _____

Other: _____

Knee, lower legs, ankles, feet, toes

Fracture _____

Ligament damage _____

Cartilage damage/removal _____

Subluxation/dislocation _____

Patella-femoral problems _____

Do you wear orthotics? _____

Tendinitis _____

Surgery _____

Strain/sprain _____

Shin splints _____

Compartment syndrome _____

Other: _____

(continued)

Health History Questionnaire *(continued)*

Are there any other comments you would like to give concerning your health?

_____

_____

_____

I do hereby state that I have, to the best of my knowledge and belief, given a correct and accurate medical history report.

_____   _____
Athlete's signature   Date

Documentation Form

Date _____ Location _____

Subject _____ Persons or company involved _____

Comments:

Signed _____ Date _____

This form may be used to document incidents involving discussions with individual athletes, as well as such actions as changing program protocols or modifying the facility or its equipment.

CHAPTER 35

REHABILITATION CONCERNS

Dan Wathen

The role of the strength and conditioning professional has expanded in recent years. The growing need for rehabilitation beyond the clinical setting has found the strength and conditioning professional in a unique position to provide for conditioning maintenance during healing and the early stages of clinical rehabilitation. Once the athlete progresses to the point where normal conditioning activities such as multijoint free weight exercises and locomotor drills (various types of running and plyometric activities) can be safely initiated, the strength and conditioning specialist can supervise these activities under the guidance of the physician, athletic trainer, or therapist in charge of the athlete's rehabilitation. Where and at what level the strength and conditioning professional becomes involved in an athlete's rehabilitation will vary in accordance with the professional's relationship with the medical specialist. Hopefully, the information collected by the strength and conditioning specialist on the physical status of the athlete prior to injury can be utilized to better assess the athlete's readiness to return to activity. This chapter will examine some of the problems and solutions the strength and conditioning professional may encounter in this area of rehabilitation.

COMMUNICATION

Effective communication is paramount in maintaining safe and effective conditioning during the rehabilitation process. The strength and conditioning professional must have an open and regular dialogue with the health care professional (usually a physician, athletic trainer, or physical therapist) in charge of rehabilitation. (Occasionally, a strength and conditioning professional with the proper background and qualifications may be placed in charge of the rehabilitation.) Ineffective communication means lost time during the conditioning process. Problems can be minimized or eliminated if all parties in the rehabilitative process communicate freely with each other and understand the goals and objectives of each member of the rehabilitation team.

Strategy

The strength and conditioning professional in charge of a facility should discuss the latest advances in the theory and practice of conditioning activities with the person in charge of medical care at the facility. This discussion should take place before implementing a general program or an individual athlete's rehabilitation protocol, since many medical professionals are unfamiliar with modern conditioning techniques and rationale. Be prepared to support yourself with hard data; disagreements will no doubt arise on occasion. The strength and conditioning professional also needs to communicate the rehabilitation plan clearly to the athlete being rehabilitated. This requires good interpersonal skills.

The final decisions on a program for an injured athlete must be left with the medical professional in charge of the case, for legal reasons (7). Do not deviate from the established program without first receiving approval from the medical professional in charge of the athlete.

516

Types of Communication

There are five communication skills in which the strength and conditioning professional must become proficient in order to effectively communicate with the medical community:

1. *Reading skills* are necessary for understanding the directives of the medical personnel in charge of an athlete's rehabilitation and for keeping abreast of the literature.

2. *Writing skills* are needed to convey ideas that cannot be conveyed orally owing to time or logistical constraints. Written documentation is also needed if subsequent legal action should arise. Exercise programs, test results, and conditioning recommendations need to be stated in an orderly, readable format for medical personnel, coaches, and athletes. Do not be verbose; medical professionals are inundated with reading material and greatly appreciate concise reporting.

3. *Body language* cannot be overlooked as a communication skill. Your facial expressions, eye movements, and carriage may convey a message different from what you happen to be saying at the time. Make eye contact when giving or receiving directions.

4. *Listening* is an almost lost communication art but one that is critical to success in dealing with medical staff. Many misunderstandings are directly linked to not listening to oral commands. Facial expression can be a strong indication of your listening skill. As points are being made by the speaker, facial expressions allow the speaker to gauge your reactions. Lack of eye contact and an overly relaxed posture may communicate disinterest, which can jeopardize future communications.

5. *Oral skills* are perhaps the most important communication skills. When time is of the essence, oral communication is generally most expedient. Areas of confusion are often cleared up with the proper questions to the appropriate medical personnel.

When seeking approval from medical personnel, a nondogmatic approach will result in the most favorable outcome. A statement such as, "In light of recent biomechanical and clinical evidence [state the evidence], it seems best to use safety bar squats or power squats for postoperative ACL patients" will likely give a better response than, "I'm going to get the athlete on a squatting program right away." Never place anyone on the defensive unnecessarily if their approval or support is sought. By maintaining a friendly dialogue and at the same time supplying enough hard evidence to make the request undeniable, effective change in program policy can be made.

Medical Terminology

Effective communication requires understanding medical terms used often in describing certain physical conditions or rehabilitative exercises. Familiarity with anatomical and kinesiological terms to describe body position and joint ranges of motion (ROM) can be critical in following medical guidelines. Terms such as *prone, supine, flexion, extension, abduction, adduction, pronation, supination, external rotation, internal rotation, lateral, isokinetic, isometric, agility,* and *flexibility* should be part of the strength and conditioning professional's working vocabulary. However, some terms that do not come up in the training of healthy populations are helpful to know in working with injured athletes. These terms are listed here with a brief definition (1,3,8).

ACL—abbreviation for *anterior cruciate ligament*

Active-assisted exercise—an exercise in which the patient is helped through a ROM through which they are unable to move by themselves

Active exercise—an exercise in which the movement is done entirely by the patient

Brachial plexus—a large nerve tree that begins in the lower cervical and upper thoracic vertebrae and branches off at the axilla and runs to the fingers in each extremity

Closed-chain exercise—any exercise in which the exercising body segment is attached to a fixed surface, such as the floor, at the distal end, requiring the entire limb to bear the resistance—for example, push-ups for the arm or squats for the legs

Cross transfer—a neurological phenomenon in which training the contralateral limb provides strength increases to an immobilized limb; also called *cross education*

DAPRE—abbreviation for *daily adjustable progressive resistance exercise*, a program often used in rehabilitation (discussed in more detail later in this chapter)

LCL—abbreviation for *lateral collateral ligament*

Limited ROM exercise—an exercise in which the ROM is limited to a certain range owing to injury or the biomechanics of an injury; also called *short-arc ROM exercise*

MCL—abbreviation for *medial collateral ligament*

Non–weight bearing exercise—an exercise in which the body's weight is not borne by the lower extremities

Open-chain exercise—an exercise in which the end of the exercising body segment is not fixed to a surface such as the floor, wall, or foot plate and the segmental distal end is freely movable—for example, knee extensions or neck flexion using a machine

Passive exercise—an exercise in which the patient is taken through a ROM by another person or a machine

PCL—abbreviation for *posterior cruciate ligament*

Proprioceptive exercise—an exercise in which balance is a factor due to proprioceptive activity—for example, balance board, beam, and standing free-weight exercises

Reconditioning—the restoration of preinjury or pre-deconditioning levels of fitness through a program of prescriptive therapeutic exercise; interchangeable with *rehabilitation*

Rotator cuff—a group of four muscles (supraspinatus, subscapularis, teres minor, and infraspinatus) that function to give the shoulder stability and allow for internal and external rotation; they originate on the scapula and insert on the humerus

EQUIPMENT USED IN REHABILITATION PROGRAMS

Items typically found in weight rooms that can serve a dual purpose for both rehabilitation and general training include knee extension/flexion units, hip abduction/adduction units, hip flexion/extension units, leg press units, safety squat bars, wall pulley units, dumbbells, surgical tubing, flex bands, therabands, neck flexion/extension units, balance boards, calf-raise units, back extension benches, weight vests, and ankle weights. When purchasing exercise machines, choose some units that allow for comparatively inexpensive accommodating or semiaccommodating resistance provided by a braking or hydraulic system. These devices help facilitate the early stages of rehabilitation and can often be substituted for the more expensive isokinetic devices used in some rehabilitation settings. Some such devices have gauges that are beneficial in motivating the patient and allowing for some quantification of improvement.

Upper body devices that do not require a hand grip to perform the movement can be useful in rehabilitation (Figure 35.1); these are invaluable when an athlete has a broken hand or wrist that is immobilized. A number of companies make resistance training units with ROM-limiting devices (Figure 35.2). These are needed for exercising a patient in pain-free, biomechanically safe ROMs following injury or surgery. Commonly seen on knee extension/flexion units, such devices can also be useful when strength in specific ROMs needs to be developed in an isolated manner similar to functional isometric training.

Some facilities may be equipped with sophisticated equipment capable of isokinetic testing and rehabilitation and sometimes of eccentric as well as concentric

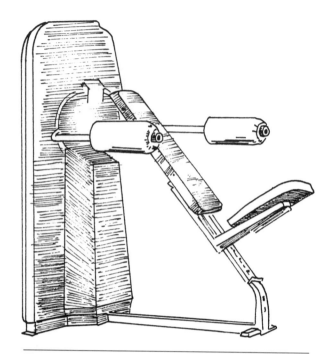

Figure 35.1 Upper body device without hand grips.

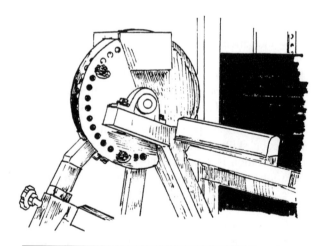

Figure 35.2 Range of motion–limiting device.

resistance. Although rehabilitation can generally be conducted with the ordinary equipment found in most weight training facilities, the more expensive testing devices are helpful in quantifying joint imbalances bilaterally and unilaterally. Much of the rehabilitation equipment used in clinical settings is not designed to biomechanically equate the forces that many body parts encounter in sporting activities; rather, it is used to isolate single-joint action and may only provide concentric resistance capability, even though most sporting activity involves multiple-joint movements and utilizes all types of muscle actions.

Equipment for Different Stages of Rehabilitation

Light or accommodating resistance—manual resistance, isokinetic devices, ankle weights, surgical tubes and flex bands, light dumbbells, and rubber balls and grippers—is commonly employed to provide resistance for the affected body parts during the early phases of rehabilitation. Pools, exercise bicycles, rowers, and arm-cranking devices are invaluable in the maintenance of cardiovascular endurance when running is contraindicated (8). Resistance machines can be used when the sense of balance has been affected by an injury and free-weight apparatus cannot be used. For example, when an ankle sprain contraindicates weight bearing, a leg press device can be employed to provide hip and knee extension exercise for the noninvolved extremity, as well as possibly the involved extremity, with less than body weight in a pain-free ROM.

In many cases the strength and conditioning professional has contact with athletes toward the end of the rehabilitation process to return them to the general conditioning activities in which they were involved prior to injury. This final step requires the professional to reintroduce many activities, such as free-weight training, agility, and power (plyometric) activities. A recent trend is to introduce closed-chain kinetic activities earlier in the rehabilitation process; reports indicate excellent results (2,3,8). Activities such as squatting, step-ups, lunging, deadlifting, and other pulling movements from a standing position create forces that are similar to actual sport activity and allow athletes to achieve better function in a biomechanically more specific and safer mode of exercise (2,3,8). As athletes progress in these activities, they can begin walking, running, plyometric drills, and other functional activities at an earlier stage of the recovery process (2,3). Athletes should not be considered fully rehabilitated until they are performing at or near previous levels of strength, power, agility, endurance, and flexibility in a variety of activities.

As a final note, the strength and conditioning professional must keep records of athletes' performance in the aforementioned areas.

Rehabilitating Specific Sites

The following list indicates the type of equipment that can be used in the rehabilitation of specific parts of the body.

Neck—manual resistance, four-way neck units, free weights for shrugging

Shoulder—dumbbells, surgical tubes and flex bands, lateral raise units, rotator cuff units, manual resistance, various isokinetic units

Low back—back extension machine, free weights, back extension (hypertension) bench

Thigh, knee, and hip—manual resistance, safety squat bars and units, knee extension/flexion units with ROM limiters, hip abduction/adduction units, hip flexion/extension units, calf raise units, various isokinetic units, free weights (barbells), balance/wobble boards, ankle weights, rotation boards, leg press units

Ankle and lower leg—calf raise units, surgical tubes and flex bands, wobble/balance boards, ankle weights, manual resistance, various isokinetic devices, rotation boards

Hand, wrist, and elbow—dumbbells, manual resistance, surgical tubes and flex bands, grippers, various isokinetic devices, rubber balls

Endurance training devices—stationary bicycle, rowing machine, arm-cranking devices, shallow and deep water pools

REHABILITATION PROGRAMS

Rehabilitation programs are varied but generally based on the work of DeLorme in the 1940s and 1950s. Known as Progressive Resistance Exercise (PRE), DeLorme's regime was based on 10RM (repetition maximum) weights (2). Rehabilitation sessions consisted of warm-up sets of 10 repetitions at 50% and 75% of 10RM, with one to seven sets of maximal repetitions at the 10RM load. If more than 10 repetitions were achievable with the 10RM load, the load was adjusted upward at the next session. This regime has been modified over the years but still remains one of the most commonly utilized protocols.

A protocol that has been used with great success is the Daily Adjustable Progressive Resistance Exercise (DAPRE) system introduced by Dr. Ken Knight (5,6). The DAPRE system is based on 5RM to 7RM and is designed to take into account daily variations in individual strength levels. It is a four-set program with the first two sets being progressive warm-ups similar to the DeLorme method. The third set is done at the 5RM to 7RM with maximal repetitions, which determines the weight level for the fourth set of maximal repetitions;

this in turn determines the weight for the third set of the next session (Tables 35.1 and 35.2). The workout can be modified to accommodate isometric exercise by substituting seconds of contraction for repetitions (6).

Many conditions call for joint motion to be restricted due to pain or inflammation. Maximal isometric exercise to the patient's tolerance can be utilized in these cases to maintain and improve strength. It is rare for a condition to warrant complete rest for a prolonged period of time. When limbs and joints have to be immobilized, other body parts, especially contralateral limbs, should be regularly treated with strength and flexibility exercises.

Cardiovascular conditioning is conducted with exercise bicycles for upper body immobilizations and with arm-cranking devices for lower body immobilizations. In many cases, rowing can be substituted for arm cranking, and either deep- or shallow-water pool work is excellent when indicated and available. Every effort should be made to maintain overall condition during the recovery phase of an injury because loss of conditioning is more acute in competitive athletes than in untrained individuals.

CONCLUSION

In order to maintain safe and effective conditioning during the rehabilitative process, effective communication with medical personnel is essential. Familiarity with pertinent medical terms and rehabilitative procedures will enable the strength and conditioning professional to interact successfully with medical personnel. In order to assist in the rehabilitative process, a facility should have equipment that can be used for both conditioning and rehabilitation. The more sensitive the conditioning professional is to the needs of the athlete in the rehabilitative process, the better communication will be with the medical staff. Positive interaction will allow the conditioning professional a more prominent role in rehabilitation beyond fitness maintenance.

Table 35.1 The DAPRE Technique

Set	Weight	Number of repetitions
1	One half of working weight	10
2	Three quarters of working weight	6
3	Full working weight	Maximum[a]
4	Adjusted working weight[a]	Maximum[b]

[a]The number of repetitions performed during the third set is used to determine the adjusted working weight for the fourth set according to the guidelines in Table 35.2.

[b]The number of repetitions performed during the fourth set is used to determine the working weight for the third set of the next session according to the guidelines in Table 35.2.

Table 35.2 Guidelines for Adjustment of Working Weight in the DAPRE Technique

Number of repetitions performed during the third set	Adjusted working weight for the fourth set
0-2	Decrease 5-10 lb
3-4	Decrease 0-5 lb
5-6	Keep the same
7-10	Increase 5-10 lb
≥ 11	Increase 10-15 lb

Number of repetitions performed during the fourth set	Adjusted working weight for the third set of the following week
0-2	Decrease 5-10 lb
3-4	Keep the same
5-6	Increase 5-10 lb
7-10	Increase 5-15 lb
≥ 11	Increase 10-20 lb

Study Questions

1. Which of the following methods of communication is most effective from a legal standpoint in supporting your actions?
   a. written
   b. oral
   c. reading
   d. body language

2. Which of the following types of equipment should be equipped with ROM limitation devices?

a. shoulder flexion equipment
b. safety squat bar
c. flex bands
d. rowing units

3. Which of the following is not a closed-chain exercise?

a. leg curl machine
b. deadlift with dumbbells
c. dumbbell bench press
d. barbell front raise

Applying Knowledge
of Rehabilitation Concerns

Problem 1

You are directed to allow an athlete recovering from major reconstructive knee surgery to perform knee extension exercise using 30° to 60° of flexion with a DAPRE protocol. What frequencies of exercises and types of equipment would be called for?

Problem 2

A runner has a fractured ankle and has been placed in a fiberglass walking cast for 6 weeks. Which multiple-joint lower body strength and cardiovascular exercise modes would be most appropriate?

References

1. Arnheim, D. *Modern Principles of Athletic Training.* St. Louis: Mosby. 1986.

2. Blair, D., and R. Willis. Rapid rehabilitation following anterior cruciate ligament reconstruction. *Athletic Training* 26(1):32-43. 1991.

3. Case, J., DePalma, B., and R. Zelco. Knee rehabilitation following anterior cruciate ligament repair/reconstruction an update. *Athletic Training* 26(1):22-31. 1991.

4. Gieck, J. Psychological considerations of rehabilitation. In: *Rehabilitation Techniques in Sports Medicine*, W. Prentice, ed. St. Louis: Times Mirror/Mosby. 1990. pp. 1-12.

5. Knight, K. Knee rehabilitation by the daily adjustable progressive resistive exercise technique. *Am. J. Sports Med.* 7:336-337. 1979.

6. Knight, K. Rehabilitating chondromalacia patellae, *Physician Sports Medicine* 7:147-148. 1979.

7. Wathen, D., Communication: Athletic trainer/conditioning coach relations—communication is the key. *NSCA Journal* 6(5):32-33. 1984.

8. Wathen, D. Exercise prescription notes #4: Athletic rehabilitation: The role of the C.S.C.S. *NSCA Journal* 11(2):29-34. 1989.

ANSWERS TO STUDY QUESTIONS

CHAPTER 1
1. c, 2. b, 3. e,
4. b, 5. a, 6. c

CHAPTER 2
1. b, 2. a, 3. a,
4. d

CHAPTER 3
1. c, 2. c, 3. d,
4. c, 5. a, 6. c,
7. b

CHAPTER 4
1. a, 2. a, 3. a,
4. c, 5. a, 6. d,
7. a, 8. a, 9. a

CHAPTER 5
1. d, 2. b, 3. a,
4. c, 5. a, 6. d,
7. b, 8. a

CHAPTER 6
1. a, 2. b, 3. d,
4. a

CHAPTER 7
1. c, 2. a, 3. c,
4. d, 5. b, 6. d,
7. d

CHAPTER 8
1. b, 2. b, 3. d,
4. a, 5. c, 6. c,
7. c, 8. a, 9. c,
10. b

CHAPTER 9
1. c, 2. d, 3. a,
4. c, 5. c, d
6. d

CHAPTER 10
1. d, 2. b, 3. b,
4. c, 5. a, 6. c,
7. b, 8. a, 9. b,
10. d

CHAPTER 11
1. d, 2. c, 3. b,
4. a, 5. c, 6. c,
7. d, 8. d, 9. a,
10. a, c, d

CHAPTER 12
1. d, 2. d, 3. d,
4. d, 5. b, 6. d

CHAPTER 13
all a

CHAPTER 14
all c

CHAPTER 15
1. d, 2. b, 3. c,
4. a

CHAPTER 16
1. a, 2. c, 3. d,
4. b

CHAPTER 17
1. b, 2. d, 3. a,
4. d, 5. b, 6. c

CHAPTER 18
all a

CHAPTER 19
1. a, 2. c, 3. a,
4. c

CHAPTER 20
1. a, 2. a, 3. c,
4. c, 5. a, 6. c

CHAPTER 21
1. d, 2. b, 3. b,
4. b

CHAPTER 22
1. b, 2. d, 3. a

CHAPTER 23
all a

CHAPTER 24
1. a, 2. a, 3. a,
4. c

CHAPTER 25
all a

CHAPTER 26
1. a, 2. a, 3. a,
4. d

CHAPTER 27
1. d, 2. a, 3. c,
4. c

CHAPTER 28
1. a, 2. b, 3. c,
4. d -

CHAPTER 29
1. b, 2. a, 3. c,
4. d

CHAPTER 30
1. c, 2. a, 3. d,
4. b

CHAPTER 31
1. d, 2. d, 3. b,
4. c

CHAPTER 32
1. a, 2. a, 3. a,
4. b

CHAPTER 33
1. d, 2. a, 3. a

CHAPTER 34
1. c, 2. b, 3. d,
4. c

CHAPTER 35
all a

SUGGESTED SOLUTIONS FOR APPLIED KNOWLEDGE QUESTIONS

CHAPTER 2

Problem 1
Select three exercises for training that focus on whole-body power output and emphasize the importance of the intensity, not volume, of training.

Problem 2
Explain that the hypertrophic response to resistance training occurs gradually, so that neural factors are mainly responsible for increased strength during the first month of training.

CHAPTER 3

Problem 1
Improved strength-to-mass ratio is essential for propelling the body upward. This can be accomplished by both reducing overall body mass and increasing strength in muscles involved in jumping. The high-volume, high-repetition, short-rest features of a bodybuilding program should be replaced by a low- to medium-repetition, high-resistance exercise program with ample interset rest periods. Exercises such as the squat, power clean, and front dumbbell raise, which parallel high jump movements, should be central to the training program. Plyometric exercises can be incorporated when the athlete is physically ready for them.

Problem 2
There is a considerable amount of lateral body acceleration in tennis, propelled by frontal plane hip abduction and adduction. Because it is quite difficult to exercise these movements using free weights, the purchase of weight stack machines designed to exercise these movements should be recommended.

Problem 3
Increased squatting ability with the bands is a direct mechanical effect. There is no evidence of increased muscular force or an improved training effect using them, and they pose risks of detrimental side effects, including skin damage and chondromalacia patellae. Thus, advise the athlete against the use of such bands.

CHAPTER 4

Problem 1
Goals:

1. Improve physique
2. Increase bone mineral density

Methods:

1. Choose an exercise to cover each of the major muscle groups.
2. To increase bone marrow density in the axial skeleton, choose exercises that direct weight bearing forces through the axial skeleton. Core exercises are the exercises of choice so include at least one core exercise for the upper and lower body.
3. Order the exercises so the core exercises are performed first when the individual can put the most effort into the exercises.
4. Example: Upper body core exercise: Bench press. Lower body core exercise: Squat. Other exercises: Pulldown, shoulder press, biceps curl, leg curl, abdominal crunch.
5. Choose the appropriate intensity and volume of exercise.

   - Core exercises—Use a standard periodization scheme that alternates a hypertrophy phase with a basic strength phase. For example: hypertrophy phase of 8 to 12RM, 3 to 4 sets, and 1 to 2 min rest between sets; basic strength phase of 5 to 8RM, 3 to 5 sets, and 2 to 5 min rest between sets.
   - Body part exercises—8 to 12 repetitions, 3 to 4 sets, 1 to 2 min rest between sets.

Problem 2
Responses to a muscular strength program: Increases in cross-sectional area of Type II fibers (especially Type IIb), which promotes increases in lean muscle mass. The outcome is an increase in the muscle's force output and contraction velocity.

Responses to a hypertrophy program: Possible increases in fiber number and increases in collagen and other noncontractile connective tissue. Type I fibers are somewhat larger in hypertrophied muscle from bodybuilding-type training than from strength training. The outcome is an increase in total power output that can be extended over a greater time period.

Responses to a muscular endurance program as promoted by aerobic exercise: Decreases in initial size of Type II fibers and an influential alteration in Type IIb fibers toward the functional characteristics of Type IIa fibers. Type IIa fibers, in conjunction with the capabilities of Type I fibers, contribute to an increase in the endurance capacity of the overall muscle.

CHAPTER 5

Problem 1

It is possible that Runner A has an LT and OBLA at a higher percentage of maximal oxygen uptake than Runner B; consequently, Runner A is able to run at a higher percentage of maximal oxygen uptake and thus likely at a faster pace than Runner B without the accumulation of lactic acid. Lactic acid accumulation would likely inhibit performance during a 5,000-m race by interfering with muscle excitation-contraction coupling. An interval training program with appropriate exercise and rest intervals will likely improve Runner B's performance by pushing LT and OBLA to the right, allowing the runner to run at a faster pace (higher percentage of maximal oxygen uptake) than before.

Problem 2

No, adding aerobic training will likely not improve his weightlifting performance and is in direct conflict with the principle of metabolic specificity of training. Combined anaerobic and aerobic training can reduce muscle girth, maximum strength, speed, and anaerobic power–related performance. Therefore, aerobic exercise should not be included in the training of a competitive weightlifter.

Problem 3

No, his current training program is not appropriate to the metabolic demands of collegiate wrestling. Wrestling, like many other sports, relies on a series of high-intensity exercise periods interspersed with rest periods of various durations. It is very unlikely that jogging 3 miles stimulates the proper energy system for the development of optimal wrestling performance. The wrestler's conditioning should include more high-intensity training with exercise-rest ratios that approximate those commonly experienced during a wrestling match. These may include a series of sprint activities (30-90 s in duration) with 5 to 30 s rest between bouts. However, depending on wrestling style, technique, and

competition, the appropriate exercise and rest intervals may vary considerably.

CHAPTER 6

Problem 1

Anabolic hormones—testosterone, growth hormone, insulinlike growth factors, and insulin
Catabolic hormones—cortisol and progesterone

The characteristics of a program that will elevate the anabolic hormones include higher volume exercise protocol (multiple sets), a 10RM resistance, exercises that recruit a large percentage of the body's muscle mass, and rest periods of 1 to 2 min. Little is known about insulin's response to resistance exercise. Few data have shown that insulin decreases in response to resistance exercise unless dietary intakes of carbohydrate and protein are taken prior to and during the recovery period. One study has shown that increases in insulinlike growth factors have been observed with resistance exercise but increases appear to be more related to chronic changes with training rather than acute increases with exercise, which may be small. In addition, increases in insulinlike growth factors may happen in the muscle cells themselves due to autocrine mechanisms.

Designing a program that will elevate testosterone but will probably not elevate growth hormone is related to the fact that testosterone may influence nervous system function. Therefore, a heavier protocol (5RM) with longer rest periods (3 min) again using a large amount of muscle mass and multiple sets may increase testosterone without a concomitant increase in growth hormone. The reason appears to be related to the reduction of signal cues (e.g., increase in hydrogen ions) to the brain that signals growth hormone release. From a program standpoint this is related to the length of the rest period (3 min results in less lactic acid formation than 1-2 min) and the duration of the set (10RM longer than the 5RM) performed.

The exercise protocols that elevate these various hormones could be performed at various times during a training program. For example, the short-rest program could be used in the "hypertrophy phase" of a periodized program. The short-rest program could also be used within a week's training program where two days may be used for strength/power and one or two days dedicated to hypertrophy type programs and increasing local muscular endurance. Thus, the use of very specific styles of workouts will be dependent upon the theoretical framework of the training cycle for the year. One protocol design (short-rest) focuses on muscle tissue growth, local muscular endurance, and toleration of acidic conditions in the body, while the other protocol design (longer rest, heavier resistances) focuses on strength and power development. These protocols can be used in sequence or within the same week. Typically they are not used together.

CHAPTER 7

Problem 1

Football players whose positions require a significant amount of running during this activity, such as offensive and defensive backfielders as well as offensive ends, should place greater emphasis on increasing maximal oxygen uptake, particularly during the off-season training program. Although it is potentially of less importance for some positions, all players should be somewhat concerned about their aerobic capacity (maximal oxygen uptake). Development of aerobic capacity is important because it provides a basis for anaerobic development, allows faster recovery between plays, and helps prevent injuries due to fatigue late in the game. The attainment of an athlete's greatest potential for maximal oxygen uptake should be primarily focused on that period of time preceding the football season as aerobic training programs are more difficult to schedule during in-season practice periods. As for cross-country skiing, it has been found that one of the main factors in performance of this activity is the oxygen supply to the working muscles. This supply is directly dependent upon the efficiency of the cardiovascular system. An endurance sport activity such as cross-country skiing must be associated with a greatly increased maximal oxygen uptake (aerobic capacity). Again, particularly during the off-season and preseason periods, exercise training should be of the type that emphasizes the development of aerobic capacity.

Problem 2

The Fick equation, made up of the parameters heart rate, stroke volume, and arteriovenous oxygen difference, can be impacted by both endurance as well as resistance training. Prolonged endurance exercise training will result in significant increases in both stroke volume and arteriovenous oxygen difference at maximal exercise while heart rate may be unaffected or slightly decreased with such training. The degree to which resistance training will impact these parameters will be the result of the contribution of aerobic versus anaerobic training and to the extent that increased muscle mass can be developed. The greater the endurance portion of resistance training, the more likely the impact on maximal oxygen uptake resulting from potential increases in stroke volume and arteriovenous oxygen difference. If a significant increase in muscle tissue is the result of resistance training, this may also impact the degree of

maximal oxygen uptake particularly as expressed in liters of oxygen per minute.

CHAPTER 8

Problem 1

Strength training is usually characterized by high intensity (85% to 100% of an individual's 1RM) and low volumes (3-5 sets of 1-6 repetitions). Strength gains can be made by both neural and muscle tissue adaptations. It has been suggested that neural adaptations occur within the first few weeks of training and are most responsive to high intensity and low volume training programs. For untrained individuals, at least four weeks of training are necessary to see an increase in muscle size, which would contribute to additional strength gains.

Training for power follows a similar regimen to a strength training program, with an emphasis on the speed or velocity of the particular exercise movement. To increase power output, you must either increase the amount of work you do in a given period of time by increasing force production or decrease the amount of time in which you do a given amount of work by increasing the velocity of that particular movement (Power = Work/Time). Power training programs usually consist of 3 to 5 sets of 2 to 6 repetitions with intensities of either 85% to 95% of an individual's 1RM or 8RM or less. The concentric phase of the movement must be accelerated as quickly as possible.

To maximize muscular endurance, a training program should consist of high volumes, low intensities, and short rest periods. Both the number of repetitions and the number of sets should be high compared to a strength training program. The number of repetitions should be greater than 12, and intensity should usually be 12RM or greater. A typical repetition range would be from 15 to 25, but repetitions above this range are still effective for muscular endurance. The number of sets should be approximately 3 to 5. The purpose of endurance training is to prepare a muscle for resistance to fatigue, therefore increasing the amount of time that a particular muscle can produce adequate force for a given task.

Strength training (very low volume)	Power training (low volume)	Endurance training (high volume)
1-6 repetitions	2-6 repetitions	15-25 repetitions
1-3 sets	1-3 sets	1-2 sets
(untrained)	(untrained)	(untrained)
3-5 sets (trained)	3-5 sets (trained)	2-3 sets (trained)

Multijoint exercises for power development (e.g., squats, pulls, cleans, bench press). Strength and endurance can be utilized for both isolated-joint and multijoint exercises.

Trained and untrained states are defined by physiological adaptations to a training program. As an individual begins a training program, adjustments must be made within this program to ensure that the desired training effects continue. New and different types of stimuli are necessary as the time of past training exposure increases. Within the three training programs listed above, the stimuli for trained individuals is altered by increasing the number of sets per muscle or muscle group, thus increasing the total volume for each muscle or muscle group.

Some physiological reasons for increased volumes of training for trained individuals include

- increases in muscle fiber size
- increases in enzyme activity within the muscle (i.e., creatine kinase, myokinase, phosphofructokinase), and
- increases in ATP, creatine phosphate, and glycogen stores.

For these adaptations to continue it is necessary to provide new and more demanding stressors to the muscle fibers. Therefore, trained individuals require a more intense stimulus as opposed to untrained individuals.

Problem 2

- Wrestling has the highest lactic acid response to competition
- The ranking of wrestling, soccer, and basketball according to their glycolytic component is as follows:

  1. Wrestling
  2. Basketball
  3. Soccer

- Soccer has the highest aerobic component of these three sports
- The ranking of wrestling, soccer, and basketball according to their aerobic component is as follows:

  1. Soccer
  2. Basketball
  3. Wrestling

Basketball—Basketball has a relatively low aerobic component because most of the action within the game occurs in spurts. An intense sprint during a breakaway or a jump for shooting or rebounding would require an immediate energy source. This energy source would be supplied by stored ATP and regenerated ATP via creatine phosphate stores. These two components as a whole form the phosphagen system. The phosphagen system is the main supplier of energy for strenuous activity lasting less than 30 s. Energy for high intensity activity from 30 to 180 s is supplied primarily from anaerobic glycolysis. A good portion of the energy necessary during basketball would be supplied by the phosphagen system followed closely by anaerobic glycolysis. Aerobic metabolism would also begin to play a significant role at this point, tying in all three of the energy pathways.

Wrestling—Wrestling has an even lower aerobic component than basketball. All of the maneuvers involved with this sport would be very demanding of both the phosphagen system and anaerobic glycolysis. Explosive movements such as takedowns and throws would exclusively use the ATP and creatine phosphate stores by means of the phosphagen system. Anaerobic glycolysis again, as in basketball, would be necessary to supply energy for periods of maximum exertion lasting longer than 30 s. Aerobic metabolism would only be significantly important if these periods of exertion were unusually long.

Soccer—Soccer is very unique in comparison to wrestling and basketball due to the fact that it is very demanding of all three of the energy supplying pathways. During movements such as kicks and short-burst sprints, the phosphagen system is extensively used. For longer periods of sprinting, anaerobic glycolysis is necessary to provide the necessary ATP. Aerobic metabolism is a much more important factor in soccer due to the large playing field. Each player must cover a large area, which requires a considerable amount of low intensity jogging or running. It may be necessary to sustain this activity for relatively long periods of time. Aerobic metabolism would be absolutely necessary to supply this type of energy requirement. There is almost an equal contribution of the phosphagen system, anaerobic glycolysis, and aerobic metabolism in the sport of soccer.

With wrestling, basketball, and soccer, as well as other sports, there is a continuum among the three energy supplying systems. In any activity there is not just one source of energy at any given time. One pathway or another may be the main supplier of energy at that time, but that does not mean that the other systems are not active. These descriptions are in terms of the main contributor of energy for a specific period of time.

Resistance Training Program

Wrestling—The two primary energy pathways used in wrestling are the phosphagen system and anaerobic glycolysis. It would then be necessary to provide a stimulus through resistance training that would cause performance enhancing adaptations within these energy pathways to occur. A power training routine would be used to mimic the demands on the phosphagen system during wrestling competition. Synchronously, a routine using 3 to 5 sets of 8 to 10 repetitions and 1 min rest periods between sets would be used to mimic the high lactic acid responses seen during wrestling competition, thus causing the desired performance enhancing adaptations. To cover the crossover area of these two routines, one day would consist of a strength training routine. One week would consist of three workouts. Each workout would cover all body parts used in wrestling competition. The first workout would consist of 3 sets per body part of 8 to 10 repetitions with 1 min or less of rest between sets. On the second workout, again 3 sets per body part would be completed, although each set would consist of 4 to 6 repetitions. The workout poundages should be of adequate weight to ensure that the suggested repetition range is a repetition maximum. The last workout for that week would be a power workout of 3 sets per body part of 2 to 3 repetitions. The subsequent week would again begin with the higher volume workout. It is important that the body learns to tolerate the extreme stress on the acid-base mechanisms of the body. Thus, short rest programs are important to gain such initial toleration.

Basketball—The main energy pathway used in basketball is the phosphagen system. A resistance program would involve primarily power training due to the explosive nature of the skills involved in this sport. Higher repetitions would be employed on alternating days to account for the use of anaerobic glycolysis for energy at times during competition. One week would consist of three workouts, the first workout would be 3 sets for all relevant body parts of 8 to 12 repetitions with 1 min rest periods, the second workout would be 3 sets per body part of 4 to 6 repetitions, and the last workout would be 3 sets per body part of 2 to 3 explosive repetitions.

Soccer—It is known that soccer involves all three energy pathways. It would then be necessary to mimic all three metabolic demands with resistance training. One week would consist of three workouts. The first workout would be a muscle endurance workout. It would entail 3 sets per relevant body part of 15 to 25 repetitions per set. Rest periods would be kept to a minimum. The second workout would be 3 sets per body part of 8 to 12 repetitions with 1 min rest periods to provide stimuli for anaerobic glycolysis. The third workout would be 3 sets of 2 to 3 explosive repetitions. Weights should be heavy enough that suggested repetition ranges are repetition maximums.

Problem 3

Overtraining syndrome is identified by some as decrements in sports performance due to an overtraining stimulus. This may result from inadequate rest or recovery time between training. It may also be caused by high intensity or excessive volumes of training. There is some speculation that overtraining syndrome is more likely to occur in athletes participating in anaerobic sports as compared to aerobic sports. Sympathetic and parasympathetic syndrome are the two types of overtraining syndromes. Sympathetic syndrome seems to precede parasympathetic syndrome and is more commonly found in speed and power athletes.

There are many physiological variables used as markers for overtraining and there are unique differences for aerobic and anaerobic overtraining.

- Resting heart rates in aerobic overtraining may increase, decrease, or stay the same. In anaerobic training there is an increase in resting heart rate.
- Body weight may decrease in aerobic overtraining, but does not change in anaerobic overtraining.
- Total testosterone levels decrease in aerobic overtraining. In anaerobic training these levels are unchanged at rest.
- Luteinizing hormone levels at rest increase with anaerobic overtraining, but are unchanged at rest in aerobic overtraining.

	Month					
	1	2	3	4	5	6
Aerobic overtraining						
Muscle glycogen	—	—	—	—	D	D
Exercise induced max heart rate	—	—	—	—	—	D
Lactate concentrations	—	—	—	—	D	D
Anaerobic overtraining						
Resting heart rate	—	—	—	—	I	I
Motor coordination	—	—	—	—	D	D
Force production	—	—	—	—	—	D

D = decrease, I = increase.

Recovery could be affected by many variables such as psychological stress of competition, shortened rest periods between training, and inadequate nutrition. Aerobic overtraining may be identified prior to the 6-month point in the above situation by decreases in maximal oxygen uptake, altered blood pressure, increased muscle soreness, altered cortisol concentrations, and decreased sympathetic tone. Anaerobic overtraining prior to the 6-month point might be identified by increased resting heart rate and blood pressure, decreased muscle glycogen, and decreased motor coordination. An important point to consider when comparing aerobic and anaerobic overtraining syndrome is that many physiological variable changes between the two are similar.

Responses to overtraining among athletes can be very different. The amount of prior training experience and the genetic potential of that athlete can dramatically affect that individual's response to overtraining. Predictors of overtraining should be used as general guidelines, but episodes of overtraining syndrome should be considered on an individual basis.

CHAPTER 9

Problem 1

Check for weightlifting shoes with sufficient heel height, or have the athlete stand on a weight plate or chock. Is the athlete inflexible in the hips or the ankles? Add appropriate stretches before and after squatting. Continue to have the athlete squat regularly, the depth determined by the ability to keep the feet flat on the floor, and encourage the athlete to keep the chest up and back tight. Over a period of weeks and months, form and strength in the movement should improve. Remember that the best squatters have short legs relative to their torsos and that not everyone has the proportions to be a champion at every exercise.

Problem 2

Although these adolescents are in the same grade and probably about the same age, there are clues that the first boy is an early maturer: mesomorphic, showing secondary sex characteristics, and near adult stature. He is probably ready for a demanding strength training program. The second boy seems to be a late maturer, not yet finished with height and weight development (compared with his parents) and not yet exhibiting secondary sex characteristics. Explain to the boys and the parents that the boys can train together and perform the same kinds of exercises, but that their program goals will be different because they are at different stages of growth. That means the sets and reps and weight amounts will be different. For now, the goal of the second boy's program won't be to maximize strength, but rather to increase overall fitness and exposure to a variety of motor skills. Both boys can practice agility skills like the shuttle run or tumbling. If you feel that it is appropriate, tell them to ask their doctor about the Tanner Scale. Reassure everyone that these differences in physical maturity are normal, show the boys how to track height and body weight and keep a training log, and tell the first boy that in 2 or 3 years his friend will be taller and heavier and maybe able to challenge him in strength.

Problem 3

Tell her that because of her fine training background (specialized movement phase reached during the sensitive period of adolescence and stabilizing, locomotor, and manipulative movements all well developed by gymnastics), her youth, and her recent active lifestyle, you will create a demanding workout. You will make program adjustments based on progress in strength and power and the appearance of overtraining symptoms. Training frequency will increase from 3 days/week to 4 or more. Her goal is no longer to maintain general fitness, but to develop the strength and then the power required by a thrower, so the intensity of weight will increase and workouts will be longer. You plan to switch her to multijoint, free-weight exercises such as squatting, pressing, snatching, cleaning, and jerking because these are more specific to the demands of javelin than machines and permit more variety in her program. She will notice rapid initial increases in strength, and she will probably experience some muscle hypertrophy and perhaps some related increases in body weight over the coming months, but body fat will likely not increase. Emphasize to her that she needs to eat well to gain more muscle mass and strength than in gymnastics. Point out that the body image of the top level throwers she saw in the Olympics is much more developed than that of top-level gymnasts.

Problem 4

With a physician's permission, take this man for a visit to a local weight room, preferably one with a variety of equipment and a clientele of a variety of ages. Seeing other people with similar goals and participating in a group setting could help the depression. Finding an older weight room buddy who has had a degree of success would be ideal. Demonstrate a selection of machine and free-weight exercises and see what attracts him and what exercises he can perform properly that are as similar as possible to the demands of his yard work. Explain that strength can be improved at any age and that since part of regaining lost strength is regaining lost muscle mass, he need not give away the clothes just yet. Tell him that his progress and recovery time may be slower than that of the youngsters in the room, but that with a regular schedule of 3 days/week of training, or even 2 days/week, he'll notice definite improvement after 4 or 5 months, and in a year he should feel a lot more confident about his yard work. Show him how to keep a training log to track his responses.

CHAPTER 10

Problem 1

Given that you have five 1-hour sessions to teach your athletes about sport psychology, you decide there is ample time to teach the team both a few theoretical points and then provide them with several practical skills. You stress to your athletes that the basis of a strong mental training program is sound physical and nutritional preparation. This includes strict adherence to both strength and conditioning work and skill work during practice. Without maximal preparation, you stress, the athlete is leaving more to chance.

You define mental training as "the ability of the athlete to mentally manage her physical resources, thereby managing the stress of competition and maintaining concentration and focus in order to take one moment at a time.'' You believe that the athlete should first understand what sport psychology, thus mental training, can do and then how to use it to maintain mental and physical consistency.

Session 1—First, you decide to teach them basic sport psychology theory. During this session you teach them to understand the relationship between arousal, anxiety, attention, and performance. You discuss the arousal-performance relationship explained by inverted-U theory. You explain performance decrements are more likely to occur when you become overaroused. You describe the box of attentional capacity and the arousal–attention–performance relationship of cue utilization. You stress the importance of understanding the relationship between arousal, anxiety, attention, and performance. Some arousal is needed for optimal performance. An overabundance of arousal in the form of anxiety or worry will cause performance decrements. Overarousal in any form has the potential to negatively effect the athlete's ability to attend to the appropriate cues.

Session 2—You teach hands-on relaxation techniques to reduce stress and improve concentration. These include diaphragmatic breathing for relaxation and progressive muscular relaxation to learn to release muscular tension.

Session 3—You begin to introduce the team to mental imagery techniques to improve concentration and focus.

Session 4—You further develop the mental routine to teach the athletes to take one moment at a time.

Session 5—You assist your athletes in designing a mental game plan. This includes goal setting, motivation, and learning from failure in order to improve.

Problem 2

The ability to relax is entirely under your control. First, it is important to understand how stress can negatively affect your ability to perform. You want to play as well as possible, but cannot worry so much that you paralyze yourself. When you are tense, your muscles are not as well coordinated, and you hamper your ability to concentrate. If you concentrate on controlling your breathing, your mind will remove worry and tension and replace them with a higher degree of focus. Then you will be able to attend to the important cues related to the game. Anytime you get tense and short of breath, remember to control your breathing. The first step in relaxing is to control your breathing. Diaphragmatic, or belly, breathing focuses thought on breathing. Relax your entire body, particularly your neck and shoulders.

Next, relax your abdominal muscles so that they protrude as if you have a large abdomen. You need to breathe from the stomach as opposed to the chest. Each breath is initiated with the abdominal muscles. This is the first of six stages in breaking down your breathing in order to relax. The process of inhalation occurs over three steps. First, with the initiation of the breath, the lower abdominal area expands, then the mid-chest region, and finally, the upper chest region. At the end of the inhalation phase there is a slight pause in breath (not a breath hold) followed by a slow and controlled exhalation. At the end of the exhalation there is another slight pause as you prepare to inhale again. The entire sequence is listed here:

1. Initiate your inhalation by relaxing your abdominal muscles while filling the lower portion of your lungs with air.
2. Expand the mid-chest region.
3. Fill the upper chest and shoulders.
4. To complete the process of inhalation, a momentary pause in breathing should occur. Don't hold your breath but instead experience a slight pause.
5. Relax your entire body while you slowly and passively exhale.
6. At the end of your exhalation, take another brief pause in breathing.
7. Repeat steps 1 to 6.

Problem 3

Basic goal-setting concepts can be applied to strength and conditioning, both to motivate an athlete and to decrease the chances of overtraining and injuries occurring. The first step in helping these athletes is to learn what their goals are and if their goals are congruent with proper training principles. It is important to find out what each athlete is willing to do and what he expects from the effort. Because chronic injuries are occurring, it would be wise to educate these athletes to the signs of overtraining. In addition, educate them to fully understand the concepts of periodized training and the importance of proper warm-up. If they don't maintain your prescribed program, they will continue to be injured and be of little use to the team. The basic design of a periodized program sets the daily lifting goals for the athlete according to his or her given training cycle. The design of the periodized program exemplifies the building blocks of goal attainment, namely, process-oriented or performance-related goals. The long-term outcome goal may be to gain a certain amount of muscle weight or max a given weight; however, of utmost importance is what the athlete has to do on a given day. If you attain your daily goals by staying within the guidelines of your training program, the design of and adherence to the program will help you increase the likelihood of attaining your long-term goals. Not adhering to the program decreases the chance of success. Judge your success by attainment of your daily goal, which the strength and conditioning specialist has set for you. Be patient and trust the periodization principles.

Problem 4

You stress to the athlete that she has been extremely successful in attaining all her training goals over the last 6 months. Emphasize where she started and how far she has come in such a short period of time. Reiterate to her the keys to successful performance: maximal physical preparation and sound nutritional practices. Further emphasize that during the last 6 months she focused on controlling every aspect of her life in order to attain her goals of qualifying for the world championships and also competing at her best. Remind her that during that time she never worried about things that she had no control over, such as other opponents. Instead she focused only on what she could control. Be sure to help her realize that she has attained her goals: With that she will increase her perceived success. That will have the effect of reducing her frustration, thus enabling her to stay focused without burning out. To complete her task she needs only to focus on what she does best, and that is her preparation for each event. Finally, stress that she take one moment at a time, just as she did in training. Taking one moment at a time during her training resulted in her qualifying for the world championships. Taking each moment at a time during competition will result in her performing at her best.

CHAPTER 11

Problem 1

None of these extreme points of view are accurate; steroids almost certainly help some types of athletic performance *and* they do carry health risks, risks that are increased by the doses and methods in which athletes use them. The strength and conditioning specialist should be honest with his/her athletes and give accurate information. Any discussion should also include emphasis on sportsmanship and development of personal strengths without pharmacological crutches. If anabolic steroid use was permitted, athletes hoping to compete in sports where steroids give a significant edge would be compelled to use the drugs. Instead of relying on exercise techniques and proper training, athletes would become dependent on drug regimens and hormonal manipulation pushing beyond understood limits and normal effects; ''sport'' would be an abomination.

Problem 2

The athlete should be counseled to not waste his money on this ''witches' brew'' or jeopardize the athletic performance he has worked so hard to perfect. He could be given some examples of how bogus these products and their claims of performance enhancement are. For example, he could be told how misconceptions about boron arose from a study of menopausal women that did not conclude that athletes would benefit from supplementation. Another example could be the logical equivalence of the claims for eating smilax and eating butter, with the main difference being that we don't know what health risks might be associated with smilax. This is the time to review with the athlete their training program and set them back on course with advice about sensible sports nutrition.

Problem 3

Indications of steroid use by an athlete should trigger some direct discussion between the athlete and coach or strength and conditioning specialist; ignoring suspicions of steroid use amounts to tacit approval and can indicate to athletes that win-at-all-costs is your leadership view. The athlete should be told that you suspect he may be using anabolic steroids. You should review for him what your position on steroid use is and what the penalties for him and the team are if he is caught. If he chooses to tell you that he is using steroids, you must decide whether or not to suspend him from competition. This decision will depend on your school's policy; however, in this example, the athlete is likely to test positive even if he stops injecting steroids immediately. If he wants to stop but needs help, you should consider getting him counseling support.

CHAPTER 12

Problem 1

One solution is to try a modified carbohydrate loading regimen with a slow 6-day taper of training before the race. Another solution is to have this runner ingest about 150 g of carbohydrate about 5 to 10 min before the race and drink a 10% carbohydrate solution every 15 to 20 min during the race. Not taking in carbohydrates during a marathon will almost certainly lead to a decrease in blood glucose.

Problem 2

Extensive weight training can markedly reduce muscle glycogen. Her diet suggests that she may not be ingesting enough carbohydrates and likely too much fat. A change in diet so that fat intake is reduced to about 30% and carbohydrate is increased to about 55% may be advantageous in enhancing recovery. Also, ingesting a carbohydrate drink during exercise *may* reduce fatigue. Ingesting carbohydrates immediately after exercise can help replenish glycogen and speed recovery.

Problem 3

This is a difficult problem. There are two possible solutions. First, the percentages of carbohydrate, protein, and fat can remain the same, and she can simply ingest more total calories, including more carbohydrate drinks. However, this may not be an easy solution because the amount of food that has to be ingested may cause some discomfort. This may be alleviated by eating more meals each day, with less food at each meal. The second solution is to add some fat back into the diet until stable body mass and body composition values are achieved.

CHAPTER 13

Problem 1

Because training has not yet started, it may be advisable to wait and see if the training for basketball will cause a significant weight reduction without dietary intervention. An important consideration here is the playing ability of the athlete as well as his health. Caloric restriction at the initiation of fall basketball practice may produce maladaptations, resulting in a change in vitamin and mineral status, loss of glycogen, marked loss of lean body mass, and other overtraining symptoms. However, if the strength and conditioning professional and physician feel that a player is too heavy to begin practice, a lighter training schedule with some caloric restriction may be advisable (see chapter 14). Additionally, body composition measures should be performed to assess lean body mass and percent body fat. It is possible that this athlete will be able to play at this body mass, provided that he possesses a reasonable body composition.

Problem 2

Detraining can produce marked changes in body mass and body composition. Body composition should be assessed on a regular basis during the 6-week detraining period. However, some training can usually be continued during an injury period. For example, if the injury is in the lower body, then upper body training may be continued, and vice versa. A modified training program can help maintain body composition (as well as performance). Additionally, modifications in diet may be of some benefit. For example, if body composition measures show an increase in fat mass, then a reduction in fat calories in the diet may be in order.

CHAPTER 14

Problem 1

Approach the athlete and discuss his performance problems and eating habits. Emotional problems may be contributing to his poor performance. It is also possible that he is eating extra calories in the evening after his normal meals. If extra calories are being consumed, a simple recommendation not to eat at night may help resolve the problem. If performance continues to fall, counseling is advisable.

Problem 2

This is a very difficult situation. If you suspect that anorexia is a problem with this athlete, some consultation with a clinician is in order. It is possible that in the early stages of anorexia, endurance performance can be enhanced. However, amenorrhea predisposes the athlete to bone loss and increased connective tissue injury. Modification in her training program (if any) should be worked out with the team physician.

CHAPTER 15

Problem 1

There are six areas of preparatory information that are pertinent for choosing the most appropriate tests: *Age related factors*—consider the range of physical and mental maturity for your team, i.e., the age range may be 14 to 19 years. *Sex-related factors*—if both the men's and women's teams are to be tested, separate norms for evaluation would be appropriate. *Experience related factors*—what is the training age of your athletes? *Environmental factors*—heat, humidity, altitude, terrain, etc. *Positions within the sport*—tests should match the physical requirements of the sport position whenever feasible. *Unbiased test*—the tests should be appropriate for the training methods used by the athletes, i.e., if training is on machines, testing should be conducted with these machines.

Problem 2

It is important for physical conditioning and sport-specific tests to have a high degree of validity to ensure the tests are measuring the constructs they are supposed to measure. They should also have a high degree of reliability to promote repeatability of test scores to ensure posttest scores are the result of physical fitness program adaptations and not other confounding factors. A high degree of objectivity is necessary to ensure a low level of discrepancy due to the way multiple scorers perceive and record the data. When selecting the most valid and reliable tests, the following 10 criteria are appropriate:

1. It should measure important abilities (be relevant)
2. It should involve game like situations
3. It should encourage good form

4. It should involve one performer only
5. It should be interesting and meaningful
6. It should be of suitable difficulty
7. It should differentiate between levels of ability
8. It should provide accurate scoring
9. It should provide a sufficient number of trials
10. It should be judged by statistical evidence

CHAPTER 16

Problem 1

This four-test battery should be conducted in the following order:

1. *Edgren Side Step*—tests requiring high-skill movements should be administered before tests that are likely to produce muscle fatigue. Allow one warm-up run and record the best of two trial runs. One minute rest between trial runs is appropriate. Allow 3 to 5 min rest before beginning the 40-yard dash.
2. *40-yard dash*—this is also a running test but is more strenuous than the Edgren Side Step and may produce minor fatigue; therefore, it should be conducted second. Two submaximal warm-up runs are recommended. Record two test trials and average times to the nearest 0.1 s for the criterion score. Allow 5 min rest before the 1RM squat test.
3. *1RM squat*—allow several submaximal warm-up lifts (i.e., 3 to 5) and record the best of three maximal attempts. A 3 to 5 min rest interval between trial lifts is appropriate. Allow 5 to 10 min rest before beginning the line drill test.
4. *The line drill test* is a fatiguing anaerobic capacity test and should be conducted last in the testing battery.

Problem 2

The steps to follow when preparing test administrators would be to have them review written protocols and participate in a *mock* testing session (i.e., supervisors test each other) and talk through administrative decisions regarding positioning of equipment and supervisors, flow of traffic, etc. Strict adherence to the testing protocol, including rest periods, is essential. It is advisable to read prepared test directions to the athletes to enhance reliability. The experienced supervisor should conduct the Edgren Side Step and 40-yard dash tests since they require skilled use of a stopwatch. The novice tester can judge the squat along with the experienced tester. The novice tester can conduct the line drill test. Athletes to be tested should be informed concerning the nature of the tests well in advance of test day so they

can prepare physically and psychologically. A short pretest practice session often promotes test reliability.

CHAPTER 17

Problem 1

The appropriate tests for female, high school-aged soccer players are as follows:

Aerobic power: 2-mile run
Anaerobic power: Line drill test or 300-yard shuttle run
Speed: 40-yard dash
Agility: T-test or Edgren Side Step
Lower body strength: Back squat or leg press
Flexibility: Sit and reach test

Problem 2

Football, lacrosse, basketball, rugby, and soccer.

CHAPTER 18

Problem 1

Evaluation based solely on difference scores has two major limitations that preclude their exclusive use. First, athletes who begin the training period at a higher fitness level and therefore pretest well will not improve as much as untrained athletes who perform poorly at the beginning of the training period. Second, athletes may deliberately perform poorly on a pretraining test with the intent of achieving an inflated improvement score on the posttraining test. A more sound method of representing the data would be to reference test scores with a percentile rank table of norms.

Problem 2

To be able to compare physical test scores with differing units of measurement the first step would be to transform all scores to standard or *z* scores. These scores are then converted to T scores, which are a form of standard score where the mean is 50 and the standard deviation is 10.

CHAPTER 19

Problem 1

Low back—use the Semi-Leg Straddle to stretch the low back only because the knees are flexed and the legs are relaxed so the hamstrings are not a limiting factor and therefore the range of motion in the low back is increased. Or use the Spinal Twist stretch for the low back (and external obliques). This stretch also contains a rotational element for the low back.

Quadriceps—use the Side Quadriceps stretch, which will stretch primarily the quadriceps and will not place any rotational stress on the knee joint (as with the hurdlers stretch). Or use the Kneeling Quadriceps stretch, which will also slightly stretch the hip flexors.

Low back and quadriceps—to stretch both of these areas use the Sitting Toe Touch.

Problem 2

To increase the intensity of the stretch, move the knee backward and slightly elevate the knee. Do not create excessive stress in the knee by pulling the foot too close to the buttocks. Slowly move from the easy stretch to the developmental stretch by moving the knee back and slightly up. The slow movement will inhibit the stimulation of the muscle spindles and therefore allow the quadriceps to relax and range of motion will increase.

CHAPTER 20

Problem 1

Running speeds of approximately 60 to 75 percent of maximum should be used to develop correct running form. The development of correct running form is a motor learning process that requires a speed slow enough that errors may be identified and corrected. However, the speed must also be fast enough to allow for normal high-speed running mechanics to be efficient but also correctable.

Problem 2

Stride frequency is increased by assisted (overspeed) training, leg turnover drills, and improved running mechanics. Assisted running methods include downhill running and towing (using mechanical or surgical tubing). These drills increase the rate at which the feet contact the ground. Leg turnover drills include running and stationary high-knees and rear heel kicks and stationary running drills. These drills will help increase the rate at which a leg moves through one cycle. Correct running technique will allow for more efficient movement.

Problem 3

The most important program considerations before beginning a plyometric program are the sport (position or event), training phase of the year, sport specific directional movements, footwear, surface, equipment, and facilities. Athlete considerations include physical maturity level, adequate strength base, adequate sprint base, coachability, fitness level, and previous or current injuries. Failure to address these key program and athlete considerations may lead to overtraining and possible injury.

CHAPTER 21

Problem 1

- A minimum of two spotters are needed, preferably three
- If two spotters, one should be on each end of the bar during the exercise
- If three spotters, one should be on each end of the bar and one should be behind the lifter
- All spotters should follow the bar and lifter throughout the exercise phases, being careful to not interrupt the movement of the bar and lifter
- The spotters should be prepared to assist the lifter when necessary

Problem 2

- The grip width is similar in the power clean, hang clean, and power (high) pull, but the snatch grip is much wider
- The bar begins on the floor in the power clean and snatch
- The bar begins at the thighs in the hang clean and power (high) pull
- The position of the feet in all four exercises is similar
- The action (movement) phases of the four exercises begin differently due to the variations in the beginning positions, but once the bar is moving the second pull is similar in the four exercises
- The catch in the power clean and hang clean is similar (the bar is racked at the shoulders)
- There is no catch phase of the power (high) pull
- The catch phase of the snatch is with bar supported by the arms overhead

CHAPTER 22

Problem 1

The athlete needs to concentrate on strength-building exercises, with emphasis on the lower extremities, as his scores indicate weakness in the area.

Problem 2

All but isokinetic resistance training could be made available. The equipment or means to get the equipment for other types of training are available.

CHAPTER 23

Problem 1

Lunges, back extensions, chest presses, bent-arm pullovers, neck harness, knee curls, calf raises on leg press, upright rows, and lateral raises.

Problem 2

Set up a conference with the throwing coach, medical personnel, yourself, and the athlete to discuss the situation. Have a copy of a nationally recognized throwers' lifting exercise protocol for the athlete.

CHAPTER 24

Problem 1

Supine flys, leg curls, abdominal curls, and external shoulder rotations.

Problem 2

The athlete needs to spend more time and place more emphasis on functional activities, such as regular weight training, and running activities.

CHAPTER 25

Problem 1

Clean pulls, push presses, squats, calf raises, pullovers, supine flys, knee curls, lat raises, and torso rotations.

Problem 2

Dips, back extensions, calf raises, lat pulldowns, knee extensions, torso rotations, straight-arm pullovers, leg curls, abdominal curls; or any order that alternates muscle groups in preferably an upper body–lower body sequence.

CHAPTER 26

Problem 1

Load assignments would be between 50% and 110% of 10RM. Lower percentages would be used during the early part of the phase and higher percentages assigned toward the end of the phase.

Problem 2

An intensity of 50% to 60% of this RM, or 37.5 to 45 lb.

CHAPTER 27

Problem 1

She should gradually decrease the volume by the number of repetitions per set.

Problem 2

Given the athlete's training background and lack of muscle hypertrophy, along with his excellent power

level, the preparatory period should have a long hypertrophy phase, with high volume, and relatively brief strength and power phases.

CHAPTER 28

Problem 1

Approximately 12 min/station should be sufficient to allow for each player to complete a set of exercise and have about 3 min recovery time while their partners are completing their sets, on an alternating basis.

CHAPTER 29

Problem 1

The athlete's schedule should be curtailed to a week or more of low-intensity recreational activities of a voluntary, unsupervised nature. No structured training of any type should be done during this time. As baseball season approaches, an in-season program of training 1 or 2 days/week can be instituted on days of light or no baseball practice or games.

Problem 2

With fewer blocks of over 1 consecutive hour for training, the athlete will have to engage in more frequent sessions of lesser duration. Because the upper body needs more attention, the athlete could devote three sessions of less than 1 hr to upper body training and maintain his leg strength with one or two sessions/week.

CHAPTER 30

Problem 1

Volume should be kept low and intensity kept above 80% of 1RM (1RM-8RM range) with an occasional unloading week prior to critical matches, in which the intensity can drop below 80% of 1RM

Problem 2

Stress is controlled by the weekly variations in training so that days of low to moderate intensity surround days of high intensity. The progression of low to high intensity along with high to low volume allows for proper adaptation to training stress. Periods of active rest further enhance both mental and physical recovery from the stress of competition and intense training.

CHAPTER 31

Problem 1

Jim's main task is to find out when he can organize the teams into a weight training schedule based on the facility's size and equipment limitations. The order of exercises may vary according to the number of people on the teams and types of exercises required. If the intended order of exercises is to complete all platform lifts first, but there are only two platforms for a 15-member team, the order would have to be changed. For example, 2 people could share a platform and then perform the incline bench while their teammates squat and then do cleans. Although performing quick lifts, like cleans, after a slow/strength lift, like squats, may not be ideal, it is often necessary to make this type of change to accommodate groups in a smaller or limited-equipment facility.

Team members may find it impossible to train during the morning because of classes, but it may be possible to organize groups of 4 to 6 athletes to come and train during weight training classes in the mornings. This way, Jim could give the athletes one-on-one instruction and specific supervision. It also appears that Jim needs help in general supervision. A supervisor should be on duty whenever the facility is open. Jim may need to develop a proposal to the school's administration stating his concerns in light of national guidelines on supervision and safety.

Problem 2

The figure on p. 536 shows a redesigned floor plan. The following safety concerns were considered in the new layout:

1. Platform area
   - Space between platforms
   - Space behind platforms
   - Space to the sides of platforms
   - Space in front of platforms (away from high activity areas involving pathways and equipment)
   - Positioning—beneath speakers
   - Interlocking mat strips on platform

2. Placement of supine benches
   - In front of platforms
   - Too close to other equipment and room pathways (exposure of bar ends)

3. Placement of incline benches
   - In front of platforms
   - Too close to other equipment and room pathways (exposure of bar ends)

4. Placement of squat racks
   - Behind platforms (poor footing)
   - Around the corner of the room (exposure of bar ends)
   - No safety mechanisms on wall squat racks

5. Pull-up bar apparatus
   - Open hooks for attachment to straight bars (easily detached)

6. Shuttle 2000 machines
   - Detached and bent foot platforms
   - Broken handles and strap devices
   - Eroding cords and connective devices

7. Hip sled
   - Narrow foot platform
   - Slick material on foot platform

CHAPTER 32

Problem 1

The strength coach and Coach Hart, the women's softball coach, should have had a conversation prior to the beginning of the team's involvement in the facility. This would have communicated Coach Hart's goals to the strength coach. It sounds as if the assistant strength coach has a bodybuilding background and may not have checked with the head strength coach before administering the program he had written. There is no real harm done. Coach Hart just needs to meet with the assistant strength coach and communicate her ideas abut what needs to be accomplished and what she expects. The head strength coach needs to oversee the outcome of what is designed by his or her assistant.

Problem 2

The facility's equipment may be clean and new, but the facility itself needs repair and maintenance as well. The staff was doing the cleaning, as Terry had asked, but because it was a high-volume club, a good deal of wear on the facility itself was taking place. Terry should organize a cleaning and maintenance schedule that would take care of basic cosmetic or surface maintenance and create a sanitary environment for participants. Money should be budgeted for maintenance, and basic repairs (peeling paint on the wall, worn carpet, curled ends on rubber mats) taken care of.

CHAPTER 33

Problem 1

The owner of the club should find out why the facility and equipment hasn't been maintained and cleaned.

Problem 2

a. Place a throw mat here until funds can be budgeted for a carpet section or full-carpet replacement or the purchase of an interlocking mat for the dumbbell area to place over the existing worn carpet. Ask the staff to make sure that athletes replace

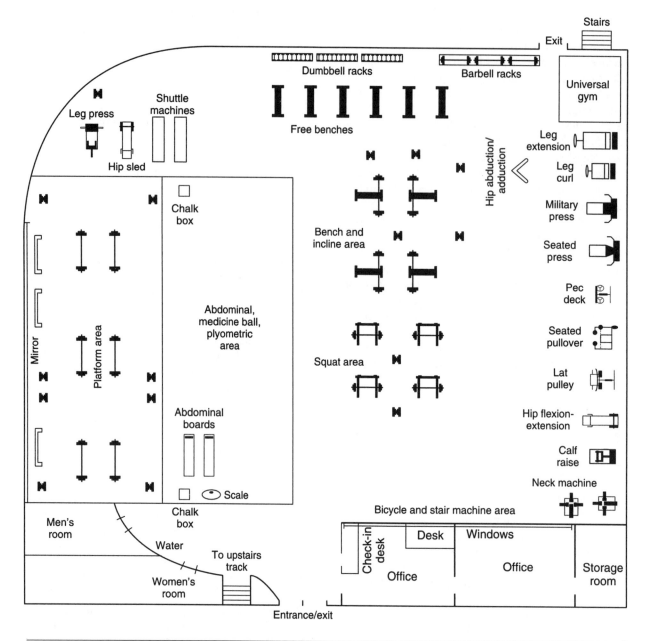

Solution to the problem floor plan of a facility and equipment.

dumbbells after use and that they do not drop equipment on the floor at the completion of a set.

b. Turn over or replace mat.

c. Cover with plywood and carpet. Instruct staff to make sure athletes do not lean equipment or weight plates against the wall.

d. The mirror should be removed immediately. When the budget allows, the mirror should be replaced and the new one placed 50 cm (20 in.) off the floor surface. Platforms should be placed 1 m (39 in.) from the wall and mirrors.

e. Organize the staff by specialty area to clean under and around equipment and in mat areas. Provide dust brooms and vacuum cleaners for cleaning where the janitorial staff do not.

CHAPTER 34

Problem 1

Joe should not have been studying; he should have been circulating in the facility as the general supervisor. It sounds like he didn't really know the procedures for handling an emergency—he should have been trained in first aid. He should also have known where the first-aid box was and have had a key to that cabinet. Joe should handle the finger in as sanitary a manner as possible, placing it in ice. Joe needs to first direct a bystander to call an emergency number (e.g., 911) and then treat the victim for shock and care for the injury according to the guidelines established by the American Red Cross.

Problem 2

Janet, as the instructor of the fitness class, should have been trained in first aid and CPR. She should have run a comprehensive fitness and health risk profile based on questionnaires and reviewed them before the class to check for high-risk participants. Those that scored as health risks should have been required to get prior medical approval. If Janet had been trained in CPR she would have approached the victim and followed the standard CPR guidelines of the American Red Cross.

CHAPTER 35

Problem 1

Daily workouts using a knee extension or leg press unit with a ROM limiting device would be appropriate.

Problem 2

For strength, the leg press would be appropriate for endurance, rowing or cycling.

INDEX

DATE DUE

FE24 '97			
MR20 '97			
MR03 '97			
AP09 97			
FE16 98			
866 0			
09			

Demco, Inc. 38-293